Handbook of Geriatric Psychiatry

Preface

The editors have taken an eclectic orientation to the theory and practice of geriatric psychiatry. This book brings together a number of contributors who are considered to be highly respected physicians. They are predominantly psychiatrists, biomedical and behavioral scientists. The contributors were selected because the editors believe that, in addition to their special area of clinical and scientific competence, they are particularly aware of the skills and knowledge that are needed by many health professionals charged with the care of the elderly. This eclectic and broad orientation is pragmatic in that there is and will continue to be an under supply of psychiatrists to deal with the elderly in the community, in the hospitals, and in various institutions. For example, a statistician[1] estimated that as of 1975 there were approximately 1,200,000 residents in nursing and personal care homes in the United States. Data supplied by the National Institute of Mental Health indicate that over half of this group has a diagnosable mental disorder of the aged. If each of these patients were to receive each week a minimum of one hour of service from a psychiatrist, and if one assumes that the psychiatrist will work 1,500 hours per year, it would require 40,000 psychiatrists to do nothing but serve the needs of this elderly population in nursing and personal care homes. Assuming by 1980 there will be 30,000 to 31,000 psychiatrists in practice in the United States, there will continue to be a serious deficit in the number of psychiatrists available to meet the mental health needs of our institutional population of older adults, much less the community based elders. It will continue to be necessary that other physicians and members of the health professions help to meet the needs of these individuals.

The content and organization of the material presented in this handbook is, according to the editors, consistent with its objectives. It is believed that information from the basic sciences must be incorporated into a comprehensive approach to patient care. With this in mind, the editors have devoted the first ten chapters of this book to the biological and psychosocial basis of geriatric psychiatry. The common disorder of depression in late life provides an excellent example, as one must understand the neurophysiological changes in the brain, the organic and physiological body changes, which take place with aging, the changes in perception, cognition and orientation, and the relationship of the older person to his or her social environment, in order to treat effectively the patient with a depression.

The second section of this book is devoted to the diagnosis and treatment of psychiatric disorders in late life. A significant change is occurring in American psychiatry with the evolution and gradual implementation of the third edition of the *Diagnostic and Statistical Manual*. Changes have been made and will be made in DSM–III, as DSM–III has the rather specific objectives of establishing operational and predictive validity to the nomenclature as well as developing a multiaxial approach to diagnosis. Therefore the nomenclature in this *Handbook* may not completely reflect the final version of the *Diagnostic and Statistical Manual*. Operational criteria diagnosis means that the categories of mental disorders are defined by the criterion. Such a nomenclature is of great importance in research settings in that it greatly increases reliability (repetition without distortion). The inability to agree upon the diagnosis has been a particular problem for researchers and clinicians alike who work with the elderly.[2] Prediction of outcome is dependent, at least in part, upon the operational validity of diagnostic criteria. At present, many of the categories in DSM-III have insufficient evidence of their predictive validity in the sense of providing useful information for treatment assignment or outcome, but the operational definitions of the disorders should allow accurate studies of outcome not formerly possible. The multiaxial approach is to insure that other data, besides the categorization of psychiatric disorder, are included in the diagnosis. These data include nonmental disorders, the severity of psychosocial stresses which are thought to have contributed to the development or exacerbation of the current episode of mental disorders,

and the level of adaptive functioning.[3] The change to operational criteria and the multiaxial approach will present problems to clinicians who are accustomed to more traditional forms of psychiatric diagnosis. It is hoped and believed that this new nomenclature will benefit communication between clinicians and investigators. It will facilitate the development of collaborative research and should prove to be very useful in testing in various locations treatment procedures and their effectiveness.

The third section of this book considers future directions in geriatric psychiatry. The chapter on "The Continuum of Care" represents a medical sociologist's approach to conceptualizing geriatric psychiatry in the context of total patient care of the older adult. Future clinicians will of necessity be involved in numerous decisions which are relevant to evaluating changes in health care systems. The practice of psychiatry will move closer to the mainstream of medicine. Therefore the geriatric psychiatrist must have a working knowledge of health services in the total delivery of care. In the last chapter the editors have presented some thoughts about the future directions of research and the practice of geriatric psychiatry.

The body of knowledge available to a geriatric psychiatrist and other clinicians involved in the care of the elderly patients has grown rapidly over the past two decades. The editors have attempted to be comprehensive while limiting information to a manageable level. Consequently the content only includes that knowledge which is believed pertinent and essential to the practice of geriatric psychiatry. This book is not primarily disease oriented but represents an attempt to place our current knowledge about certain disease processes in the context of normal life development and aging.

Styles of learning for various individuals are frequently different but equally effective. Some learners prefer to have a firm grasp of the "clinical picture" prior to acquiring basic science information, as such learners feel they better appreciate the

Isadore Rossman, Ph.D., M.D.
Medical Director, Home Care & Extended Services Department,
    Montefiore Hospital
Associate Professor Medicine and Community Medicine,
    Albert Einstein College of Medicine
New York, New York

T. Samorajski, Ph.D.
Head, Gerontology Research Section, Texas Research Institute of Mental
    Sciences
Faculty of the University of Texas Graduate School of Biomedical
    Sciences
Adjunct Professor of Biology, Texas Women's University
Texas Research Institute of Mental Sciences
Houston, Texas

Ilene C. Siegler, Ph.D.
Assistant Professor of Medical Psychology, Department of Psychiatry
Duke University Medical Center
Durham, North Carolina

James Spikes, M.D.
Assistant Clinical Professor of Psychiatry, Albert Einstein College
    of Medicine
Acting Director, Division of Liaison Psychiatry
Montefiore Hospital and Medical Center
New York, New York

Michael C. Storrie, M.D.
Clinical Investigator, American Lake Veterans Administration Hospital
Instructor, Department of Psychiatry and Behavioral Sciences,
    University of Washington
Seattle, Washington

Roy V. Varner, M.D.
Chief, Geriatric Services, Texas Research Institute of Mental Sciences
Assistant Clinical Professor of Psychiatry, University of Texas Medical
    School and Baylor College of Medicine
Houston, Texas

Adrian Verwoerdt, M.D.
Professor of Psychiatry, Department of Psychiatry
Duke University Medical Center
Durham, North Carolina

John Ingram Walker, M.D.
Assistant Professor of Psychiatry, Department of Psychiatry
Duke University Medical Center
Staff Psychiatrist, Veterans Administration Hospital
Durham, North Carolina

H. Shan Wang, M.B.
Professor of Psychiatry, Department of Psychiatry
Duke University Medical Center
Durham, North Carolina

Jack Weinberg, M.D.
Director, Illinois Mental Health Institutes
Professor of Psychiatry, Rush Medical College
Professor of Psychiatry, Abraham Lincoln School of Medicine
Rush-Presbyterian-St. Luke's Medical Center
University of Illinois at the Medical Center
Chicago, Illinois

Alan D. Whanger, M.D., D.T.M. & H. (London)
Associate Professor of Psychiatry, Department of Psychiatry
Director, OARS Geriatric Evaluation and Treatment Clinic
Duke University Medical Center
Durham, North Carolina

William W. K. Zung, M.D.
Professor of Psychiatry, Department of Psychiatry
Duke University Medical Center
Durham, North Carolina

Contributors

Dan G. Blazer, M.D., M.P.H.
Assistant Professor of Psychiatry, Department of Psychiatry
Associate Director for Programs, Center for the Study of Aging
  and Human Development
Duke University Medical Center
Durham, North Carolina

H. Keith H. Brodie, M.D.
Professor and Chairman, Department of Psychiatry
Chief, Psychiatry Service
Duke University Medical Center
Durham, North Carolina

Harold Brody, Ph.D., M.D.
Professor and Chairman, Department of Anatomical Sciences
State University of New York at Buffalo
Buffalo, New York

Ewald W. Busse, M.D., Sc.D.
Associate Provost and Dean, Medical and Allied Health Education
J. P. Gibbons Professor of Psychiatry, Department of Psychiatry
Duke University Medical Center
Durham, North Carolina

Carl Eisdorfer, Ph.D., M.D.
Professor and Chairman, Department of Psychiatry and Behavioral
  Sciences
University of Washington
Seattle, Washington

Charles M. Gaitz, M.D.
Head, Clinical Services Division and Department of Applied Research,
  Texas Research Institute of Mental Sciences
Clinical Professor of Psychiatry, Baylor College of Medicine
Houston, Texas

James T. Hartford, M.D.
Research Associate, Gerontology Research Section
Texas Research Institute of Mental Sciences
Houston, Texas

Lawrence W. Lazarus, M.D.
Director of Geriatric Services, Illinois State Psychiatric Institute
Assistant Professor of Psychiatry, Rush Medical College
Chicago, Illinois

George L. Maddox, Ph.D.
Director, Center for the Study of Aging and Human Development
Professor of Sociology and Medical Sociology, Department
  of Psychiatry
Duke University Medical Center
Durham, North Carolina

Gail Marsh, Ph.D.
Associate Professor, Medical Psychology, Department of Psychiatry
Associate Director for Research, Center for the Study of Aging and
  Human Development
Duke University Medical Center
Durham, North Carolina

Walter D. Obrist, Ph.D.
Research Professor of Neurosurgery and Neurology, Division
  of Neurosurgery
University of Pennsylvania
Philadelphia, Pennsylvania

Erdman Palmore, Ph.D.
Professor of Medical Sociology, Department of Psychiatry
Duke University Medical Center
Durham, North Carolina

Eric Pfeiffer, M.D.
Professor of Psychiatry, Department of Psychiatry, University of South
  Florida College of Medicine
Chief, Psychiatry Service, James A. Haley Veterans Administration
  Hospital
Tampa, Florida

Murray Raskind, M.D.
Assistant Professor, Department of Psychiatry and Behavioral Sciences,
  University of Washington
Director, Geriatric Research, Education and Clinical Center
American Lake Veterans Administration Hospital
Seattle, Washington

Handbook of Geriatric Psychiatry

EDITED BY
Ewald W. Busse, M.D.
Dan G. Blazer, M.D.
Duke University Medical Center

 VAN NOSTRAND REINHOLD COMPANY
NEW YORK   CINCINNATI   ATLANTA   DALLAS   SAN FRANCISCO
LONDON   TORONTO   MELBOURNE

Van Nostrand Reinhold Company Regional Offices:
New York   Cincinnati   Atlanta   Dallas   San Francisco

Van Nostrand Reinhold Company International Offices:
London   Toronto   Melbourne

Library of Congress Catalog Card Number: 79–18955
ISBN: 0–442–20896–0

Manufactured in the United States of America

Published by Van Nostrand Reinhold Company
135 West 50th Street, New York. N.Y. 10020

Published simultaneously in Canada by Van Nostrand Reinhold Ltd.
15   14   13   12   11   10   9   8   7   6   5   4   3   2   1

Library of Congress Cataloging in Publication Data

Main entry under title:

Handbook of geriatric psychiatry.

   Includes bibliographical references and index.
   1. Geriatric psychiatry.   2. Aging.   I. Busse,
Ewald W. II. Blazer, Dan G. [DNLM: 1. Aging-Hand-
books.   2. Mental disorders—In old age-Handbooks.
3. Mental processes—In old age—Handbooks. WT150
H235]
RC451.4.A5H36   618.9′76′89   79–18955
ISBN 0–442–20896–0

relevance of the basic science to the clinical or applied area and hence the total information is better integrated. There are other learners who prefer to use the building block approach; that is, they learn first the basic sciences and then the applied or clinical areas. To accommodate these various types of learning it is possible that some readers will want to read Section 2 before Section 1. Others will do the reverse, and undoubtedly, a certain number will want to move back and forth from one section to another; to make this possible the index has been given special attention. It is hoped that this book is organized in such a manner that flexibility can be achieved without disruption to the learning styles of the readers.

The editors wish to acknowledge the continued help, encouragement and patience of Mr. Ashak M. Rawji, senior editor at Van Nostrand, during the entirety of this project. Our deepest appreciation is also extended to our secretaries, Mrs. Ann Rimmer and Mrs. Thelma Jernigan for the long hours spent in typing, editing and organizing the manuscript.

REFERENCES

1. Gurel, L. (Memo). Psychiatric Manpower Estimates, February 1976, American Psychiatric Association.
2. Freeman, F. A. *Theory and Practice of Psychological Testing.* New York: Holt, Rinehart and Winston, p. 89, 1962.
3. Spitzer, R. L., Sheely, M. and Endicott, J. DSM-III: Guiding Principles. Presented at the 4th C. M. Hincks Memorial Lectures, Symposium on Psychiatric Diagnosis, University of Toronto, November 18, 1976.

Ewald W. Busse, M.D.
Dan Blazer, M.D.

Contents

Handbook of Geriatric Psychiatry

Part I
The Biological and Psychosocial Basis of Geriatric Psychiatry

Chapter 1
The Theories and Processes of Aging

Ewald W. Busse, M. D.
Duke University Medical Center

Dan Blazer, M. D.
Duke University Medical Center

THE ELDERLY IN THE WORLD POPULATION

In the United States population, those 65 years and over account for approximately 10.9% of the population. By 1980, it is predicted that it will increase to at least 11%. In the total population of the world, currently about 8% are 65 years of age and older. This percentage will also gradually increase achieving about 9% in the year 2000.

Based upon data supplied by the United Nations, it is found that there is considerable difference in various parts of the world when one looks at those 60 years of age and over.[1] One must be aware that population reports in the developed nations are usually based at age 65 years as the beginning of late life rather than age 60 years as used by the United Nations' report. As of 1970, in Africa only 4.7% of the total

Preparation of this chapter was supported in part by Research Career Development Award #1 K01 MH 00115-01A1 (Dr. Blazer).

Preparation of this chapter was supported in part by Grant #5 P01 AG00364 from the National Institute on Aging (Dr. Busse).

population were 60 years of age and over. In South America it was 5.8%, in North America, 13.8%, and in Europe, 16.7%. Clearly, the so-called developed nations had a much greater number of people 60 years and older. It is estimated that in the year 2000 all of these percentages in the developed as well as the less developed countries will continue to increase. The actual number of elderly people is more important than the percentage. As of 1970, there were 304 million 60 plus years persons in the world. By the year 2000 this will increase to 581 million persons. A further complication is that those 80 years and older will better than double, reaching 58 million by the year 2000.

In 1970 the expectation of life at birth for the population of the world was 53 years. This undoubtedly has increased, but considerable differences persist in some regions of the world. The following countries in South America exceed a life expectancy of 60 years at birth: Uruguay, Venezuela, Argentina, Brazil, Guyana, and Surinam. This calculation is combining the life expectancy of both sexes. As of 1970, Uruguay apparently had the best life expectancy. Males were 65.15 and females, 71.56. The lowest life expectancy is reported to be in Ecuador where males live 51.04 and females, 53.67.[2] It should be noted that these reports are subject to some question as they are not necessarily based upon the same years in reporting, but merely show up in the 1970 report derived from the United Nations. One of the nations with the lowest life expectancy reported in the *Demographic Yearbook* is Afghanistan, where the life expectancy for both sexes is 37.5. Even this figure excludes infants dying within the first 24 hours of birth. Consequently, the life expectancy is probably less as the majority of nations include infants that die within the first 24 hours of birth.

AGING DEFINED

What is aging? Is it normal? Is it a disease? Can it be prevented or altered? *Normal* is a word with several meanings. Normal when used in systemic studies of a population is a standard for comparison of deviations, the standard being based on a set of observations that can be measured and the average or the median determined. Often a normal individual is one who is considered to be relatively free of disease and disability and whose life expectancy is not reduced by the presence of serious pathology. Usually a normal individual is one who has the capacity, and has demonstrated the ability, to meet his basic human needs and to solve the usual problems of living in a manner acceptable to himself and to society. Hence an individual who successfully copes with disability can be considered a normal individual. From a biochemical viewpoint normality is usually based upon a standard derived from medical statistics. But in the behavioral sciences normality may be successful adaptation to deficiencies and losses.

The term *aging* can also have several meanings. As a biological term it is used to identify inherent biological changes that take place over time and end with death.

Some investigators prefer to define biological changes that take place over time and end with death. Some investigators prefer to define biological aging as a progressive loss of functional capacity after an organism has reached maturity, while others insist that aging processes can be identified with the onset of differentiation. Of course there are some who contend that any attempt to separate aging processes and to identify them is not useful or possible. The terms *growth* and *development* usually represent biological processes which are the opposite of aging.

For operational purposes declines in functioning can be separated into primary aging (senescence) and secondary aging (senility). *Primary aging* is a biological process whose first cause is apparently rooted in heredity. The inborn first cause of age changes produces inevitable detrimental changes that are time-related but are etiologically relatively independent of stress, trauma, or acquired disease. *Secondary aging* refers to defects and disabilities whose first cause comes from hostile factors in the environment, particularly trauma and disease.

All of the aging processes are not recognizable in all people, and those that are present do not progress at the same rate. This operational definition of primary aging clearly has limitations. For example, it does not adequately distinguish between the so-called "normal" aging processes and the diagnostic entities related to inborn errors of metabolism. Of course the ultimate question is: Can biomedical science through research provide the diagnostic skills and the techniques for prevention and intervention that will control both the primary and the secondary aging processes?

BIOLOGICAL AGING

There are numerous theories of aging. A few are ancient, and many more of recent origin. Some of the theories are fascinating, but esoteric, while a number are relevant to an understanding of the information included in this handbook. Consequently only those theories believed to be important to geropsychiatry will be reviewed. Theories that attempt to explain the phenomenon of aging are based upon certain assumptions and definitions; for example, primary and secondary aging.

The bodies of humans and higher animals all consist of three biological components— two are cellular and one is noncellular. Within the living body there are cells capable of reproducing themselves throughout the life span. Skin cells and white blood cells are examples of such cells that have the capacity to reproduce. There are other cells that cannot reproduce and when lost cannot be replaced. Such cells are the neurons of the brain and of the nervous system, the noncellular component being the material that occupies the space between cells. Obviously there would be considerable gain if it could be demonstrated that a single process of aging occurred in the three components of the body. Unfortunately this is not the case, as the aging theories and processes that have been developed do not have uniform application. Consequently many of the theories are limited, others are overlapping, some simple and some complex.

Exhaustion and Watch Spring Theories

The *exhaustion theory of aging* was put forth many years ago. This explanation of aging rests on the assumption that a living organism contains a fixed store of energy diffusely or strategically located, and that as time passes the energy is depleted and because it cannot be restored, the organism dies. A similar theory is the *watch spring theory*. Although these two simplistic theories have essentially disappeared, certain of their basic assumptions continue, and they as theories have been replaced by more sophisticated approaches consistent with our current scientifc knowledge.

The Hypothalamus — The Location of the Aging Clock?

Over the past 20 years the expanding knowledge of neurohumoral physiology has resulted in the replacement of the pituitary

gland by the hypothalamus as the major controller of many body processes.[3] The hypothalamus has numerous roles including the regulation of the pituitary gland. This major function was demonstrated by Andrew V. Schally[4] and Roger Guillemen[5] who for their work shared a Nobel Prize in 1977 Schally initially identified a substance, corticotropin-releasing factor (CRF), that produced an increase in the release of ACTH from anterior pituitary tissue. Subsequently at least nine other hypothalamic hormones or factors have been identified that control the release of pituitary hormones including thyrotropin-releasing hormone (TSH), growth hormone (GH-RIH) release-inhibiting hormone, and growth hormone releasing factor (GH-RF).

It is certain that the cells within the hypothalamus have their own internal controls, but their actions are clearly responsive via a feedback mechanism to other changes within the body to changes stimulated by the environment. The hypothalamus accomplishes its task by neuroendocrines (hormones) and neurotransmitters. Sometimes it appears that there is a very fine line between these two classes of biological substances.

As is well known, cell loss is a common feature of aging. The disappearance of a few cells in the hypothalamus may have far-reaching consequences. The number of dying cells may be overshadowed by the death of cells of critical importance. The death of such critical cells may be genetically determined or may be the result of acquired disease or trauma. There is no doubt that much more information is required regarding the role of the hypothalamus in the regulation of homeostasis, with particular emphasis upon its loss of ability to coordinate the various physiological processes and to be responsive to stress, as frequently observed in late life.

Deliberate Biological Programming

Another biological explanation for aging that is receiving considerable attention and seems to have considerable validity, is the theory of *deliberate biological programming*. This theory holds that within a normal cell are stored the memory and capability of terminating the life of the cell. Obviously this means that all normal human diploid cells will die. It is held that either the memory or the capability of carrying out the order to die has been destroyed in mixoploid or cancer cells. It appears that only the mixoploid cell is immortal while the diploid cell is doomed to eventual death. However, 40 years ago this was not the situation. Based on the assumption or hope that immortality exists in the lower and simpler forms of life, it was reported that cultured fibroblasts from chicken embryo heart tissue could be held in a state of continuous proliferation for many years. This finding—if it could be proven to be true—would demonstrate that biological aging is not the result of intrinsic failure within the individual cell, but was the result of disorganization of the entire organism. This work was originally reported by Carrell and Ebeling in 1921. Subsequently it was demonstrated that these respected investigators had made an error in their methodology that resulted in improper conclusions. The apparently immortal cell culture was fed with a crude extract taken from chick embryos. This extract actually contained a very few but significant number of new viable cells. Hence the introduction of the new cells permitted the culture to survive. It was found that if the extract was carefully prepared removing all new cells, the cell colony would die.

The mystery of why, how, and when a colony of normal cells capable of dividing eventually dies was partially solved by Hayflick and Moorhead who in 1961 reported that normal human fibroblasts when cultured underwent a finite number of population doublings and then died.[6] Further information was forthcoming a few years later when Hayflick and coworkers reported that human fibroblast cultures derived from embryo donors as a group underwent significantly more population doublings, that is, 40–60 doublings, than those derived from an adult group. In this group,

doublings were between 10–30. Other experiments demonstrated that cells could be removed from the culture, stored in subzero temperatures for as long as 20 years, and when removed and returned to a culture medium, they would begin to divide. Furthermore, the stored cells seemed to contain an inherent mechanism for remembering at what doubling level they were stored in the cold. This obvious memory ability is strong evidence in support of the deliberate biological programming theory.

Hayflick contends that this *in vitro* demonstration can be repeated *in vivo* by marking cells and injecting them into a host animal from which they can be withdrawn later and then reinjected into new host animals. A similar limit to the number of possible doublings can be demonstrated. There is another interesting aspect to these studies as they provide an opportunity to determine if there is an inherent biological difference in the cells of males and females. Again Hayflick and coworkers have reported that the number of doublings is not different in male or female cells.

There are those who doubt the validity of Hayflick's conclusions. Holliday and coworkers[7] believe that when a cell divides, some of the daughter cells are "committed to senescence," while the other cells would under proper circumstances be capable of continuous reduplication. One of the obvious problems would be to provide a proper circumstance, and undoubtedly the commitment theory of cellular aging will get additional attention. Furthermore, Holliday and his coworkers expressed the belief that the error theory which is also reviewed in this chapter may be compatible with the commitment theory, as the aging of fibroblasts is accompanied by alterations or defects in genes, chromosomes, DNA replication, and repair.

The error theory and mutation theory have some similarities. The error theory of cellular aging mentioned above proposes that production errors are made that are not necessarily based upon mutations but result in the transmission of faulty messages and the ultimate production of defective enzymes. If the number of defective or inactive enzymes proceed to a point at which synthesis within the cell is sufficiently defective that life cannot be sustained, the cell dies. Eventually a sufficient number of cells die or malfunction to the point that death of the organism is inevitable. The error theory seems to be more applicable to nondividing cells, such as the neurons of the brain and the muscle cells of the heart.

Chromosomal aberrations can be demonstrated in aging animal and human cells.[8] Therefore the mutation theory is linked with these chromosomal changes and is similar to the error theory in that defects then result within the cellular metabolism and eventually death ensues. Exposure to ionizing radiation increases the number of chromosomal aberrations, and exposure to ionizing radiation reduces the life span of a living organism. Numerous attempts have been made to study the changes brought about by radiation for any possible similarity to the aging process. Longevity in an aging animal is inversely proportional to the rate at which mutations develop in the animal. This is a spontaneous or unexplained appearance of mutations. However, it appears that the changes that accompany aging, and mutations that are brought about by radiation are not the same. When one compares the number of chromosomal aberrations produced by radiation to the life-shortening effect that would be expected proportional to the number of aberrations, there is not nearly the amount of life-shortening that would be expected. Aging produces fewer chromosomal aberrations, yet in proportion produces more life-shortening. The reparative life processes of these aberrations also appear to be different. There is no satisfactory explanation for these observed discrepancies.

The Accumulation of Waste

The accumulation of deleterious material is a relatively simple theory of aging that continues to hold the interest of some biomedi-

cal scientists, particularly neuropathologists who have yet to explain the origin and significance of the accumulation of certain pigments such as lipofuscin within neurons and other cells. There are other late-appearing accumulations with brain cells that are unexplained such as the hirano bodies.

Hirano bodies are fusiform or spheroidal eosinophilic bodies that are commonly observed in the hippocampi of the elderly and are especially numerous in patients with various dementias or degenerative diseases.[9]

Lipofuscin is one of the pigments that accumulates in certain cells with the passage of time. There is no direct evidence in the support of harmful effects of the pigment, but it is held that the age association wear and tear within the cells underline pigment formation, and could still be detrimental to the cells. The accumulation of lipofuscin is limited to those cells which are incapable of dividing. Nandy has demonstrated that if tumor cells which are capable of dividing are prevented from further division by the use of chemicals, the neuroblastoma cells show aging changes including the accumulation of lipofuscin just as do normal neurons. The evidence that is available as to the origin of lipofuscin implicates lysosomes, mitochondria, and other organelles. The major culprit in the deposition of lipofuscin appears to be the lysosomes.[10]

The Immune System and Aging

In recent years information regarding the immune system has rapidly expanded. Consequently psychiatrists and other physicians who completed medical school some years ago often do not have sufficient knowledge to understand this complex system and its relations to the brain, aging, and the somatoform disorders.

The immune system as a primary defense mechanism of the body is essential for the preservation of life. The immune system is extremely complex and is widely dispersed throughout the tissues of the body. When a foreign substance is introduced into the body, the immune system can respond in two ways. The first is the humoral immune response which is characterized by the production of antibody molecules which specifically bind the introduced substance. The second is the cellular immune response. Cells are mobilized which can specifically react with and destroy the invader. The immunological theory of normal aging advocated by Walford[11] and Burnet[12] holds that with the passage of time, alterations transpire within the immune system. Surveillance is impaired and there is a decline in the protective mechanism. Furthermore, the system may be distorted so that it functions in a self-destructive, that is autoaggressive, manner.

Cells that cannot divide, for example, neurons and cardiac muscle cells, may be particularly vulnerable to alteration in the immune system. Such nondividing cells are gradually lost in the latter part of the life span, and it may be that this loss is the result of the inability of the immune system to protect these nonreplaceable cells, or they may be lost as the result of autoaggressive processes. In old mice the loss of cortical neurons characteristic of aging has been associated with a specific brain reactive antibody.[13]

The protective mechanisms of the immune system reach a peak during adolescence and then decline in conjunction with the involution of the thymus. With the passage of years the body demonstrates an increased susceptibility to infection, and, in general, effective immunization cannot be induced in late life.

Walford and Burnet hold somewhat different points of views of the immune system and aging. Burnet considers the thymus gland the clock of aging, as its removal produces immunodeficiencies not unlike those associated with aging. Walford is concerned with autoimmune responses, but according to Kent[14] a critical issue is what comes first—immunodeficiency or autoimmunity. In contrast, there is evidence that prolonged survival in humans accompanied by preservation of efficient mental and physical ac-

tivities may be associated with an intact immune system.

The Cellular Immune Response. The cells of the immune system are derived from stem cells located in the bone marrow. From the stem cells one line becomes promonocytes, then monocytes, and finally macrophages. A second line is lymphocytes that pass through the thymus gland and are there altered to become T cells. The third line is the B cells.

When bacteria invade the body, monocytes are activated into more aggressive macrophages. T cells are also stimulated to actively resist the invader, to signal for the production of more T cells, and also to send messages to the B cells. B cells also proliferate and become plasma cells that produce and release antibodies. Hence T cells are responsible for cellular immunity, while B cells are important to humoral immunity.

In peripheral blood, about 34% of the circulating lymphocytes are B-type cells and 66% are T-type. T cells have a variety of functions that are not thoroughly understood. T cells are more effective against fungi, acid-fast bacilli, and viruses. Some T cells seem to cooperate or help with B cells in synthesizing antibodies, while other T cells suppress antibody synthesis, and still others seem to be directly involved in cellular responses. One category of suppressor T cells prevents autoantibody formation; hence autoimmunity diseases may increase with age because of a decline in suppressor T cells.[15] The B cell system handles a variety of organisms including pneumococci, streptococci, and meningococci.

There are changes in T and B cells with age. T cells proliferate more slowly and their numbers decline. Antibody production indicative of B cell activity also declines with age.

The Humoral Immune Response. A cross-sequential longitudinal study of immunoglobulin serum levels at the Center for the Study of Aging and Human Development at Duke University found that in elderly subjects early death is likely in those who have relatively low levels of IgG and high levels of IgM. However, in many old people both IgG and IgA increased with age. The immunoglobulin IgA is concentrated in the fluids of the respiratory and gastrointestinal system, and here acts as a first line defense against invading organisms. IgM, although in some respects similar to IgG, is a much larger molecular structure than IgG, and is therefore likely to remain in the blood stream. Serum IgG is a major defense against virus, bacteria, and fungi wherever they may be found in the body. IgM has a cleaning-up-of-debris function and appears to direct its effort to fighting disease in blood vessels. Why high IgM contributes to increased risk to life is not established.

There are two other major classes of antibodies (immunoglobulins): IgE and IgD. IgD is found in very low concentrations in humans. Its role is speculative. IgE is involved in the release of molecules like histamines associated with symptoms of allergies. Both the cellular and humoral responses require additional scientific attention.[16]

The major categories of immunoglobulins are divided into subclasses: for example, there are at least four subclasses of IgG and two subclasses of IgA and IgM. IgM has the largest molecular weight. Generally IgM is the first antibody formed in response to a new antigen.

The basic structure of immunoglobulins consists of four polypeptide chains joined by disulfide bonds. Each contains two identical chains—two light and two heavy. The heavy chains determine class specificity.

Emphysema is becoming an increasingly serious disease in the United States. It is generally associated with chronic lung infections and heavy smoking. An individual with an impaired immune system is even more vulnerable to the possibility of emphysema.

Amyloidosis is a condition that affects many people. *Amyloid B* is found in senile plaques. It is believed to be caused by a malfunctioning immune system and affects the connective tissue of nearly every part of the brain, as well as throughout the body. It is said to act like rust in a complicated machine, reducing the effectiveness of the body cells.

Performance and Immunity. Attempts have been made to determine the relationship between serum immunoglobulins and intellectual performance. Cohen and Eisdorfer[17] found no significant relationship between immunoglobulin level and the WAIS subtest scores in 23 women with a mean age of 73.2 years who reported that they were in good health. However, in 14 elderly men, age 74.2 years, Cohen and Eisdorfer report significant correlations between performance, both vocabulary and digit symbol, and heightened serum IgG and IgA.

Cohen and Eisdorfer found that among the men IgG was negatively correlated to both vocabulary and digit performance, and IgA was negatively correlated with vocabulary. The authors agree that these findings are difficult to explain, and the sex differences are particularly annoying. It is evident that much work needs to be done to understand the relationship of the central nervous system to the immune responses.

The progressive failure and perversion of the immune system with advancing age are thought to contribute to a number of diseases in late life, including the increasing incidence of cancer, maturity-onset diabetes, emphysema, and amyloidosis.

Maturity-onset diabetes occurs in a severe form in about 13% of people over the age of 75 and in a mild form in almost half of the population over 65. This, too, is considered to be an autoimmune phenomenon, and it is assumed that it is an autoimmune reaction to insulin and to the cells that produce it.

Genetics and Aging

Molecular Genetics. It is anticipated that the rapidly expanding area of molecular genetics will do much towards establishing or repudiating certain theories of aging. Molecular genetics is concerned with the unraveling of genetic code and understanding its ambiguities and subtleties as well as its evolution. Molecular genetics is concerned with the translation of information stored in the code as DNA into protein, the synthesis and chemistry of protein, the synthesis of DNA and RNA, and the nature and cause of mutations, the biochemistry of enzyme regulation, and DNA repair.

Chromosome Loss in Senile Dementia. Until 1970 when the so-called banding technique was developed to identify chromosomes, it was difficult to distinguish sex chromosomes from autosomal chromosomes. Banding has made it possible to show that the most frequent missing chromosome in cultured female leucocytes is an X chromosome. There is also evidence that suggests that the Y chromosome is frequently lost in male cells in late life.

In 1968 Nielsen examined a group of females with senile dementia and compared them to normal females of the same age. He found that the highest levels of hypodiploidy, that is, a loss of chromosomes, were observed in the demented group.[18,19] This type of work with considerable elaborations has been carried on by Jarvik and associates. Jarvik[8] has clearly demonstrated that women with a diagnosis of chronic organic brain syndrome excluding those showing clinical evidence of multiple infarct dementia show a high frequency of hypodiploidy when compared to normals.

Genetics and the Environment. Genetics and the environment influence health, behavior, and length of life.

The term *environment* is inclusive of the physical and social milieu. The social milieu is the result of reciprocal interactions between humans as individuals and groups. The physical environment includes human interaction with the inanimate and nonhuman organisms.

As to human genetics, it is the study of the existence of transmitted "inborn" characteristics, particularly those qualities that distinguish humans from nonhumans and those qualities that characterize human individuals, families, and groups.

Behavioral geneticists generally agree that normal behaviors tend to be polygenically determined representing the concerted action of many genes interacting with the environment resulting in the physiological processes expressing the normal behavior. In contrast, abnormal behaviors may be caused by a single abnormal gene that interferes with any one of an extensive number of essential normal steps. The expression of the abnormality stemming from the gene can be environmentally influenced, but the range of the expression is probably narrower than the normal behaviors.

To study the interaction of genetic and environmental determinants is complicated by processes of development and aging. In infancy not all of the genetically controlled physiological processes have been released, and the environment of the infant is restricted. The stimuli responses of the infant are relatively simple as compared to those of the adult. The older the human, the more diversified biologically he becomes, life experiences accumulate, environmental influences expand, social values and expectations become more complex. Animal experimentation has presented clear evidence that genetic differences that result in variations in behavior can be influenced by the environment and the age of the animal.

Hereditary and genetic determinants are roughly synonymous, but the term "familial" is used to identify disorders which cluster in families but are not yet proved to be genetically determined. Alcohol preference studies indicate that different strains of mice will vary their consumptions of alcohol at different ages. This occurs despite the fact that the environment is held constant.

All humans have recognized that there are certain individuals who seem to age prematurely or rapidly. Often such observed aging changes are considered to be inherited but sometimes are held to be acquired either through disease or trauma or through stress within the social environment. Unfortunately, the explanation is not that simple, as genes may turn off and on at different ages. Furthermore, this turning on or off may be the result of internal stimuli, an external stimulus, or a combination of stimuli. Also, the physiological processes that intervene between the turning on or off of a gene and the behavioral manifestations of this change may be altered by age. As to the social environment, chronological age to a large measure determines social expectations, and the behavioral manifestation can be very much influenced by social attitudes and opportunities.

Genes which are likely to be the first cause of age changes are inherited, but the behavioral manifestation is not. Furthermore, a single gene may influence several types of behavior (pleiotropic effect), or, as has been demonstrated in numerous animal experiences, one behavior can be the result of several genes (polygenic effect).

The heritability of many age changes can be estimated by constructing a ratio between the amount of variance attributable to the genotype and the amount attributable to environment. It is likely that all genotypically determined behavior is modified to some degree by the environment, but inherent biological behavioral manifestations cannot be forever abolished by environmental influences.

Genetic Determinants of Longevity. The significant difference in the life span of the female and the male in developed nations raises the question of the importance of genetic differences as opposed to, or combined with, a favorable environment for the female.

At the turn of the century, there were slightly more older men than women—90 women to 100 men. By 1940, the situation had reversed itself, and thereafter the preponderance of older women grew rapidly. This imbalance has important social and medical implications. Most older men are married, while most older women are widowed or single, that is, divorced or never married. The sex imbalance is enhanced by the practice of men to marry younger females, thus expanding the pool of older unmarried women. The recognition of the preponderance of women in our society in part motivates the women's liberation movement and has a profound impact on the type and amount of health care that is needed.

For all races that constitute the population of the United States of America, after the age of 55 there are 128 women for every 100 men. Between the ages of 65 and 74, there are 130 women to every 100 men; and for those after the age of 75, there are 171 women to every 100 men. Again, assuming this trend continues, in 2000 for all over 65 years of age the ratio will be 154:100. After the age of 75 years, there will be 191 females to 100 males.

Contrary to the reasonable expectation of the equality in males and females at birth, among the whites in the United States the ratio is approximately 106 newborn boys to 100 girls. Among the Unites States blacks the sex ratio is less biased in favor of males. There are 102.6 black males for every 100 black females born. In greater contrast is the ratio found in Korea where it appears that there are 113 males to 100 females at birth. It is reported that in black populations of several islands in the West Indies there are fewer males than females at birth.

Numerous environmentalist influences have been investigated to determine their influence upon sex ratio at birth. In England and Wales it has been reported that upper socioeconomic groups are likely to have a higher ratio of males to females than the lower socioeconomic groups. In fact, this applied to the upper and middle classes, while skilled workers had more male offspring than unskilled workers. During World War II many European countries observed the fact that the ratio of males was higher than during times of peace. This not only occurred in the warring countries but also in the neutral European countries. It is possible that this is due to the fact that the births occurred in younger parents as opposed to older parents. The order of birth does influence the sex ratio as the ratio of males is highest for first births. As to age of parents, it is possible that the age of the father is more important than the age of the mother.

As to the difference in death rates in adulthood, recent data indicate that 40% of the excess male mortality is due to arteriosclerotic heart disease. An additional one-third is due to the male having a higher rate of suicide, fatal motor accidents and other accidents, cirrhosis of the liver, carcinoma of the lung, and emphysema. It is claimed that these conditions account for 75% of the causes of the excess male mortality. It is clear that cultural behavioral patterns which are more prevalent among men than women contribute to arteriosclerotic heart disease, as well as habits of excess smoking and drinking and a risk-taking behavior found so often in men as compared to women.

Sex-controlled Traits. For the relatively uninformed individual it is easy to assume that traits including longevity which appear more frequently or predominantly in one sex as opposed to the other are the result of the presence or the absence of the male Y-chromosome. The primary etiology of these sex-related traits may not be in the sex chromosome at all but rather in an autosomal gene, and the difference in its frequency of expression is really the result of what is called sex-controlled or sex-modified traits. A good example of a sex-controlled trait is gout. This condition is based on an excess of uric acid in the blood. Its genetic basis has been described as that of a dominant autosomal gene and its penetrance, that is, the percentage of cases that manifest the disease, is estimated as more than 80% in males but less than 12% in females.

Furthermore, there are some traits that are sex *limited*, that is, the manifestations only appear in one sex. Most sex-limited genes are autosomal. But even this limitation should not be confused with sex-linked. *Sex-linked* is the term that means that the inheritance determined by a gene is located in a sex chromosome.

As to sex chromosome and longevity, it has been suggested that the greater constitutional weakness of males may be due to their having only one X-chromosome. This possibility is related to the redundant message theory of Medvedev.[19a]

Current knowledge regarding the female X-chromosomes is much greater than that of the Y-male chromosome. At least 150 detrimental traits are X-linked. X-linked traits include color blindness, brown teeth, Duchenne type of muscular dystrophy, and hemophilia. Some traits have been considered Y-linked, but only one has been proven, and this is hairy ear rims. This single Y-linked trait can hardly be considered detrimental. Although women are more likely to develop Alzheimer's disease or senile dementia, these difficulties are probably sex-modified and are not sex-linked disorders. The defects are probably in the autosomal genes, and the principle of "genetic heterogeneity" may be in operation. This holds that the pheno-type similarity, that is, the clinical manifestations of the disease, is produced by genotypically different conditions.

The Y-chromosome which appears exclusively in males is smaller than the paired X-chromosomes in the female. Furthermore, in normal human males the Y-chromosomes may be of significantly different lengths. Again, using modern staining techniques, it has been found that the size difference may actually result from different amounts of chromosomal substance. Obviously the Y-chromosome does not contain genetic material necessary for the normal development or the well-being of a human as it is absent in the female. Its only function is to provide the male characteristic of the human. It is noteworthy to recognize that some racial groups differ from others in the average length of the Y-chromosome. The Y-chromosome in Japanese males has a mean length greater than that found in Jews, American blacks, Asian Indians, and Caucasians. The Caucasian is likely to have the shortest Y-chromosome.

To briefly summarize the current situation

regarding the genetic determinants of primary aging, there is no known gene responsible for the extension of the life span, but there are genes that cause defects resulting in the shortening of life.

Hypothermia, L-dopa, and Prolongation of Life

Temperature is one of the most potent and widely studied variables in the control of the life span in poikilothermic animals. A tiny aquatic poikilothermic animal—the rodifer—in 1968[20] was found to respond to an environmental temperature reduction by a substantial increase of life span. A similar prolongation of life could result from the reduction of food intake. However, Barrows and Strehler reported that a reduced diet resulted in a gain in life span when applied to younger animals, while the reduction in temperature was effective in animals who had reached full maturity and had ceased to lay eggs. The extension of such studies to homeothermic animals including man requires an ability to adjust and control thermostatic mechanisms in a large cohort over an extended period of time. At the present time there is no clearly demonstrated pharmacological agent that will reduce temperature in man that would favorably influence the life span.

However there are some intriguing leads. Cotzias and his coworkers[21] showed that rats fed large amounts of L-dopa in their diet exhibited a 73% increase in life span and a concomitant prolongation of vitality when compared to nontreated controls. The question of course was, how does L-dopa favorably influence the life span of these laboratory animals? Janoff and Rosenberg have presented evidence that L-dopa and other agents such as reserpine reduce the core body temperatures of mice and rats.[22] It is postulated therefore that this is the underlying reason for the extension of life. However, it is interesting to note that the feeding of large amounts of L-dopa is reflected in an enormous increase of that substance in the brain. There is no observation regarding the neuromuscular activity of the animals and their behavior.

PROGERIA

There are several syndromes that are linked with premature aging. The victims of these disorders do, to a limited extent, provide an opportunity to study accelerated bodily changes that resemble those attributable to aging. The appearance of these individuals is indeed striking as the initial impression is that the person is a very old man or woman. Although all of these syndromes are quite rare, two have received the most attention. These are the Hutchinson-Gilford syndrome[23,24] (see illustrations) Figs. 1-1, 1-2, 1-3, 1-4 and Werner's syndrome. The Hutchinson-Gilford syndrome is characterized by dwarfism, physical immaturity, and pseudosenility. These individuals have a peculiar form of hypermetabolism and generally die during their mid-teens of coronary heart disease. Progeria affects both sexes and has also been described in Caucasians, blacks, and Asians. It is believed to be an inherited defect based upon an autosomal recessive trait. The affected individuals look like very old, wizened, small distorted humans. This is because their heads are comparatively large, while the face is small, and the ears and nose are small. Scalp, hair, eyebrows, and eyelashes are lost.

In 1904, Otto Werner described in his doctoral dissertation for graduation from the Ophthalmological Clinic in Kiel an unusual disorder under the title "Cataract in Connection with Scleroderma."[25] Werner reported the condition in siblings, two brothers and two sisters, between the ages of 36 and 40 years of age. Parents, grandparents, and one sister were healthy.

Werner's syndrome is a later onset type of progeria. As the disease develops, the individual looks 20 to 30 years older than their actual years, and their life span is shortened. As the disease usually appears before growth is completed, they frequently will have thin limbs and are of smaller stature and not as

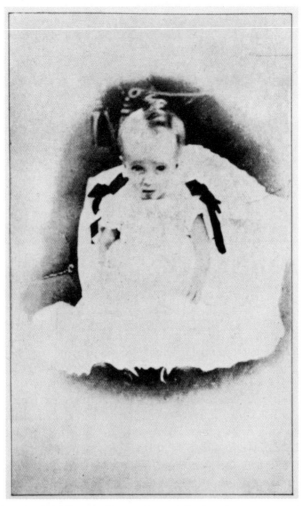

Fig. 1-1. Progeria. Case I.—Age 1½ years. From a photograph taken about one year after the disorder was first noticed. He looks thin and wizened, and much of the hair has gone. The head seems large. This and the downcast appearance of the face suggest hydrocephalus. But the former was probably only relative, the result of wasting of the face, while the hanging down of the head was due to weakness of the neck-muscles.

well developed as would be expected. Their appearance is striking in that the face develops a tightly drawn pinched expression. There is a pseudoexophthalmos, a beak nose, protubcrant tccth, and a recessive chin. Cataracts develop early and in addition to hypogonadism they are likely to have diabetes. Not infrequently they develop cancer which contributes to their shortened life expectancy. The connective tissue cells and fibroblasts of these patients have been studied. For instance, Hayflick mentions that the fibroblast cells derived from such individuals and cultured *in vitro* undergo significantly fewer doublings than their age-matched controls.[26] At this time no neuro-anatomical description of the brain of patients with progeria could be found. According to a recent review approximately 25% have mild neurological defects such as loss of distal deep tendon reflexes, but no systematic psychological or EEG studies have been reported. It is highly likely, however, that psychological problems are common.[27]

Since 1904, at least 150 patients have been reported with similar clinical findings and have been labeled "Werner's syndrome." A recent publication reviews this disease and reports 15 patients with progeria—12 males

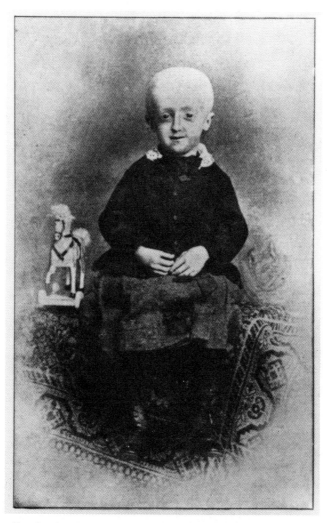

Fig. 1-2. Progeria. Case I.—Age 7 years. He is bald, the eyes are prominent, and the knuckles rather conspicuous. The lobule of the left ear is present, but is evidently wasting. The photograph has been much "touched up" by the photographer.

and 3 females—ranging from 17 to 59 years of age. All 15 patients showed the following signs and symptoms: short stature and light body weight, slender extremities with a stocky trunk, beak-shaped nose, high-pitched and weak voice or hoarseness, juvenile bilateral cataracts, flat feet and hyperreflexia of the patellar and Achilles tendons. Thirteen of the 15 patients had parents who were consanguineously married, although the article does not indicate any further information regarding their consanguineous relationship. It was noted, however, that a consanguineous marriage is common in Japan. They were able to collect a total of 100 cases in Japan and found that the sex ratio was one to one. They do note that the patients were so similar in their facial characteristics that they could be easily mistaken for identical twins. In an attempt to determine the genetic causation, they found no chromosomal abnormalities.

As to the immunological data, only in one patient did they find any differences in the titers of IgG, IgA, IgM, and IgE. The only deviation occurred in one patient who had an elevated IgE. They also note that the ratio of the T-cell subpopulation has been reported to decrease with age; that is, it declines in a normal aging group. However,

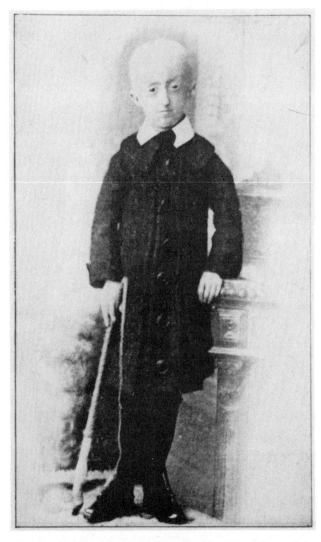

Fig. 1-3. Progeria. Case I.—Age 12 years. He looks much older. The outlines of the nasal cartilages can be seen. There is a distinct fold curving down from the nose, but the finer markings of the face, head, and hands have been obliterated by the photographer.

utilizing the method of Nakai, they found there was a decrease in the T-cell subpopulation. Goto *et al.* do not report the age of death of any of the subjects studied.[28]

Progeria is a rare human phenomena and although a progerialike familiar syndrome has been reported in rabbits,[29] these disorders have not contributed important information pertinent to primary aging.

PSYCHO-SOCIAL AGING

Personality Theory in Old Age

There is no personality theory which is more than minimally satisfactory when applied to the entire life span. Freudian theory which dominated psychiatric thinking for the 20 years immediately following World War II emphasized infancy, childhood, and adolescence, considered adulthood, but virtually ignored old age. For many psychiatrists interested in the latter part of the life span, Erikson's "The Eight Stages of Man" provides a useful basis for thought, investigation, and application.[30]

The eight stages in the life cycle as delineated by Erikson are represented by a choice or crisis for the expanding ego. As one moves from the identity versus confusion problem of adolescence into young

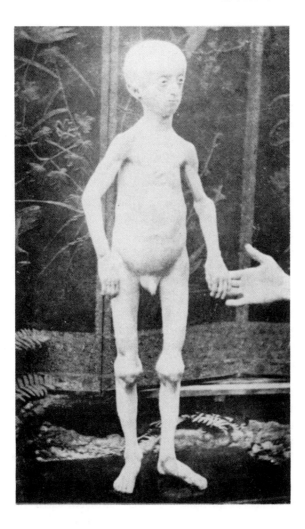

Fig. 1-4. Progeria. Case I.—Age 17. The beaked nose showing outlines of cartilages, thin lips, ill-developed lower jaw and clavicles, wasted ear lobules, and scanty white hair are all shown: also the extreme leanness, poor muscular development, the large knuckles of the hands, the absence of sexual hair, and backward sexual development. A normal adult hand is introduced to show the proportions.

adulthood, the focus shifts to intimacy versus isolation, that is, the ability to merge oneself with the self of another. Adulthood, the next stage, is concerned with generativity versus self-absorption (investment in the product of one's own creation and identification with the future), and in late adulthood the crisis of ego integrity (the view that one's life has been the product of one's own making that it could not be different and that it had been a meaningful life), versus disgust and despair.

To demonstrate that there are frequent if not consistent personality changes in old people that come about as the result of ag-

ing, it would be necessary to demonstrate that there exists an orderly sequential pattern of changes of personality traits that alter behavior in old age. So far this is not the case, as repeated cross-sectional studies often show variable results although certain investigators or research teams are more consistent in their findings. The failure to demonstrate consistent personality changes accompanying aging is in part accounted for by the use of research instruments which are of unknown reliability or validity, particularly when applied to older persons. At this time, it appears that aging *per se* does not independently alter personality. Rather, the passing of time, the biological status of the individual, and the time, degree, and the time of the event in the life cycle all influence personality and behavior.

In recent years the psychoanalytic method as a therapeutic approach has been severely criticized.[31] However, as a method of investigation the psychoanalytic method is ideal for observing a relationship between biological and social factors and their effect upon the individual. The psychoanalytic method has the capability of making important contributions to the study of personality structure and function in late life.

The psychosocial approach to the study of personality has traditionally focused on so-called personality traits. That psychophysiological disposition underlies traits is accepted, but the measure of the trait is how the individual responds in a social or interpersonal situation. This approach permits the utilization of standardized tests.

Psychoanalysis and psychodynamics add another dimension, as such studies are concerned with the events within the individual, the feelings within the individual, and the cause and consequences of anxiety, guilt, hostility, depression, etc. Although the distinction is not sharp in these two approaches to the study of personality, both have particular value for the study of personality in old age.

Personality and developmental theories of aging are to a remarkable degree complicated by the fact that as humans pass through their life experiences they become increasingly different rather than similar. Infants at 6 months of age are more similar than children at age 12. This divergence continues throughout the life span as a response to a large array of possible learning and living experiences. It is possible that this divergence phenomenon reverses in extreme old age, as very old people show considerable similarity in certain characteristics, but this may result from the fact that they are a biologically elite group and that very old people are usually treated by society in a relatively uniform manner, that is, protected and respected.

Personality traits are theoretically the result of various combinations of endogenous and exogenous factors. In late middle life the menopause in women is the most commonly recognized physiological alteration associated with personality change and the appearance of various psychiatric disorders. A wide variety of biological age changes has been identified, but their often subtle impact upon personality and psychic well-being has been given relatively little attention.[32] This lack of attention in part is attributed to the fact that these age changes and the onset of chronic diseases and disabilities do not interfere with the capacity to work until relatively late in life. They do, however, have considerable influence in many other spheres of living, including sexual behavior and recreational or leisure time activities. Included in the significant biological alterations associated with aging are presbycusis, presbyopia, declines in muscle mass and strength and reaction times, significant changes within the endocrine and nervous systems (neuronal loss), decline of gustatory sensation, loss of teeth, and numerous other system, organ, and cellular changes.[33]

Bernice L. Neugarten and associates[34] published a study of personality in middle and late life. Eight empirical approaches were utilized, each focusing upon a personality theory. A study of Erikson's theory of ego development concluded that Erickson's model of personality in assessing adult personality was relatively successful, as it was concluded "the hypothesized interdependence of ego dimensions and their proposed hierarchical order has some validity." It appears, however, that adulthood is more homogeneous then the theory would indicate. This study included a model of personality based upon psychoanalytic and ego concepts. This study found that personalities maintained their characteristics in middle and late life, and personality changes or disintegration were not related to age *per se* but to losses, particularly those involving health and social support systems. Neugarten does believe there are sex differences in certain personality traits in late life. Men are more affiliative, that is, they ally themselves with groups of men in male group identity. Males are more nurturant, as their patterns of response are more affected by the supplies from their environment, yet they are more responsive in their stimuli; for example, in their eating and drinking patterns. In contrast, women become more individualistic, in effect, egocentric, and more aggressive.

Increasing cautiousness or conservatism is often associated with advancing age. A number of reports deal with this subject, but perhaps the most enlightening is that of Botwinick.[35] Botwinick utilized groups of young adult volunteers as well as older subjects and paid attention to the influence of education and socioeconomic factors. He utilized a questionnaire of 24 life situations, 12 of which had been previously employed by other investigators. He considered not only the age of the participants but also the age of the central character in the life situation or life problem that was presented. In responding, the subjects had a choice of two alternatives. One alternative was rewarding but risky, and the other alternative was less rewarding but safer. The overall results were that elderly subjects were more cautious in their decisions than younger subjects, and neither sex nor education was related to the cautiousness. Moreover Botwinick found that both young and old adults were less cautious when solving problems of the aged than they were when solving problems of younger adults. It appears that cautiousness does increase with advancing age, but the degree of the cautiousness is influenced by the type of problem and by when it is placed in the life span.

A recent study by Okun, Siegler, and George[36] suggests that cautiousness is not strictly an age effect but is a "multidimensional construct." These reported differences can be attributed to the cohort influence.

Psychological Theories

According to Birren and Renner[37] there is no pressure on the field of psychology to produce a unifying theory or to explain how behavior is organized over time. They view the psychology of aging as predominantly a problem and data-oriented area of research. Baltes and Willis[38] reach a number of conclusions including "all existing theories (of psychological aging and development) are of the prototheoretical kind and are incomplete."

The psychological theories that have appeared are often the extension of personality and developmental theories into middle and late life. Personality theories usually consider the innate human needs and forces that motivate thought and behavior and the modification of these biologically based energies by the experiences of living in a physical and social environment.

Schaie[39] has recently advanced what he calls "a stage theory of adult cognitive development." His tentative scheme involves four possible cognitive stages. These sequential stages are denoted as acquisitive (one-childhood and two-adolescence), achieving (young adulthood), responsible and executive (middle age), and reintegrative (old age). During middle life he postulates two overlapping cognitive patterns—a "responsible" component and "executive" abilities—neither can be judged by common psychometric testing. He suggests that during the life span there is a transition from "what should I know" through "how should I use what I know" to "why should I know" phase of life. Schaie believes that numerous new strategies and techniques will have to be developed in order to fully test a stage theory that alterations in the theory will emerge.

Kalish and Knudtson[40] recommend the extension of the *concept (theory) of attachment* common in infant and child psychology to a lifetime conceptual scheme for understanding relationships and involvements of older people. They further state that the *concept (theory) of disengagement* is not functional and that it should be eliminated. Attachment is a relationship established and maintained by "social bonds" and is distinguished from social contact. Elderly people lose significant early objects of attachment. New attachments are often much weaker and frequently not mutual and therefore vulnerable. Kalish and Knudtson argue that an appreciation and understanding of attachments will provide a better approach to explaining the psychological changes in elderly people. Relevant to the attachment concept is the finding by Lowenthal and Haven[41] that more than any other single factor having a confident appeared to discriminate between elderly persons who were institutionalized and those who could remain in the community.

Social Theories

The term *social* in its broadest usage and as applied to human beings "refers to any behavior or attitude that is influenced by past or present experience of the behavior of other people (direct or indirect), or that is oriented (consciously or unconsciously)" toward other people. Normally the term is morally neutral.[42]

Social scientists are usually concerned with the social role or place (status) of the aged in society. Aging to a social scientist may refer not only to a decline in social usefulness but also to an alteration of status. Social theories relevant to the aging and elderly are affected by the structure of society and social change. One such theory holds that the status of the aged is high in static societies and tends to decline with rapid social change. According to another theory, the status of the aged is high in societies where there are few elderly, and the value and status of the aged decline as they become more numerous. A third theory holds that the status and prestige of the aged are high in those societies in which older people, in spite of physical infirmity, are able to continue to perform useful and socially valued functions. This last theory has a particularly pessimistic quality when applied to Western society, because early retirement and rapid social change are making it difficult for the elderly person to be involved in socially valued functions although attempts are being made to improve the situation.

Two social theories are frequently discussed by behavioral scientists: One is *the disengagement theory* targeted by Kalish; the second is *the activity theory*. The disengagement theory maintains that high satisfaction in old age is usually present in those individuals who accept the inevitability of reduction in social and personal interactions. The activity theory holds that the maintenance of activity is important to most individuals as a basis for obtaining and maintaining satisfaction, self-esteem, and health.

A third psychosocial theory of aging is referred to as *the continuity theory*. This theory is often offered as an alternative to both the disengagement and the activity theory. Generally it is held that those whose lifestyles are altered the least will exhibit the highest life satisfactions. To attain long life and happiness, continuity is preferred over discontinuity. As in all of the behavioral theories of aging, there are some obvious strengths and weaknesses; for example, the social scientists who believe that an orderly career is a great predictor of success in work. It would appear that this would be consistent with the continuity theory. However, there is a limitation in the fact that if an individual's life is too controlled and consistent, it could become a very dull and nonstimulating experience. If one looks at a socioeconomic data, it certainly does appear that economic security for many people provides a continuity which in turn permits them to avoid the dull boring lifestyle while maintaining control of deviations from their usual patterns of living.

PREJUDICE AND THE MINORITY STATUS OF THE ELDERLY

The vast majority, if not all, of the men and women who work in the field of geriatrics believe that elderly Americans constitute a deprived minority group. The elderly differ from many other minority groups in the way in which they have come by their status. They were neither born into it, nor did they achieve it through any action on their part. Rather, they have had their minority status thrust upon them as a result of the accumulation of a certain number of birthdays. Whether lifelong discrimination or recently acquired discrimination is harder to bear is a question that is unresolved, but it is important to those individuals who are concerned with the impact of discrimination upon social and economic well-being as well as health. Regardless of the answer to this particular question, it does appear to geriatricians and to an expanding number of the leaders of our society that elderly people are deprived of human rights and opportunities.[43]

The advocates of the elderly contend that they have a positive attitude and that this positive attitude must be adopted by our society. If a change is to be made from a negative attitude to a positive one, it is important to examine the causes of such a negative attitude. One must understand the first cause as well as the mechanisims which perpetuate an unfair and unreasonable approach.

Gerontophobia

It is important to understand the nature of prejudice.[44] In primitive societies, social and health problems are often complicated by the existence of folklore, myths, and superstitions. In so-called civilized or developed societies, unexpressed and unrecognized individual prejudices and group biases can be equally troublesome. The complications arising from prejudices and biases are often difficult to recognize since they are sufficiently distinct that they cannot be recognized as myths or superstitions. Nevertheless, they do have serious impact upon thought and behavior and can result in misinterpretation of facts, inappropriate reactions to events or ideas, or a lack of interest and neglect.

The psychiatrist and behavioral scientist recognize that the abode of prejudice is largely in the unconscious mind. The conscious recognition that a prejudice exists, resulting in illogical behavior, is usually transient. Prejudices can be acquired throughout the life span, but the facilities that make possible these developments require the continuation of in-childhood modes of thinking and responses to stimuli. Because the mechanisms of prejudice are rooted in childhood, they are also likely to carry the intense emotional patterns of childhood, so that anxiety, despair, anger, as well as laughter and happiness, can be exaggerated. When adults are confronted with prejudice and explanations are required, responses are couched in adultlike terms, while the origin and the intense feelings accompanying the prejudice resist reality and logic. To dispel the negativity generated by prejudice, the individual must first recognize that the excessive feelings that accompany their attitude or behavior are indeed unreasonable, and they must be willing to unlearn the faulty learning by actual personal experience replacing prejudice with a rational approach.

Many professionals including physicians and psychiatrists are reluctant to become involved with elderly persons. Far too often this reluctance is the result of prejudice. Hence many members of the health and welfare profession have difficulty relating effectively to elderly persons. If one assumes that this is a prejudice that is acquired in some phases of life rather than in early childhood, one will turn attention to events that transpire during the years of education. At some point during the educational years, a person observes that age can be associated with physical and mental decline. Children will observe in their grandparents the loss of physical strength and stamina, a decline in mental vigor, and the loss of the attractiveness of the body. Of particular importance to the bodily changes is the loss of smoothness of contour and asymetrical body changes. Added to this are many other unattractive changes, including the loss of hair, changes in skin pigmentation, wrinkles, and the dullness of the eyes. The developing person sees the undesirable changes accompanying age and unconsciously moves from disliking the aging process to disliking those who have become aged.

The health professional has an added problem. When deterioration of a patient is obvious despite medical and social intervention, the observers are reminded of their own vulnerability and inevitable death. Members of the health disciplines are frequently frustrated because elderly patients often have multiple chronic physical and psychological complaints that moreover are often exaggerated by the patient's life circumstances; for example, social isolation and economic limitations. The physician is made to feel that he or she has little to offer. The symptoms cannot be completely relieved, and a cure is impossible. Furthermore, the health professional has neither the skill nor the prerogative to alter the socioeconomic conditions. These circumstances have resulted in what has become known as gerontophobia.

Economic Status

Although the older persons in our society remain a deprived minority, changes have been made to improve their lot. The automatic increases in income derived from Social Security have played a role in the improved economic status. Palmore sees the current situation as follows. Poverty continues to be more prevalent among the elderly than other sections of society, if judged by poverty levels of income. However, there are several factors which offset the decline in money income among the aged. For example, there are reductions in property tax, a double personal exemption on income tax, and tax-exempt income such as Social Security benefits, etc. In addition, there are substantial transfer payments to the aged such as Medicare benefits and housing subsidies which do not show up as income. Palmore concludes that the aged actually receive more of the nation's personal income, that is, 14%, than their proportion in the population, which is 10–11%. Palmore does not agree with the widespread belief that "most aged are poor."[45] This improvement in economic status is further reflected in a change between 1969 when 27.3% were below the poverty level, to 1975 when 14% were below the poverty level.[46]

Employment

Since 1900, there has been a steady decline in persons who continue to work after reaching age 65. In the year 1900, two of three males 65+ were employed; in 1950, less than one in two, and in 1975, one in five. Assuming that the new laws regarding retirement have no widespread impact, it is predicted that in 1990, one in six will be employed after the age of 65.

As to employment between the ages of 65 and 69, 4% are employed full time, and 14%, part-time. Between the ages of 70 and 79, 3% are employed full time, and 8% are employed part-time. After the age of 80, only 1% is employed full time and 3% are employed part-time.[47]

The policy of Social Security in permitting additional income has gradually changed over the years, but it appears to be designed to keep the older worker out of the labor force and to assure that only a minimal additional income will be generated. In 1970, the Social Security provisions requiring an earning on retirement test was somewhat liberalized and resulted in the fact that for every two dollars earned in excess over $4,000 for those up to the age of 65, one dollar could be lost from Social Security.

Mandatory Versus Flexible Retirement

In the fall of 1978 the United States Congress amended the Age Discrimination in Employment Act of 1967. Congress made it unlawful to forcibly retire most nonmilitary federal workers at any age and most other public or private workers under the age of 70. Exceptions include air-traffic controllers, fire fighters, some law-enforcement personnel, executives who are entitled to an immediate and nonforfeitable retirement benefit of $27,000 a year or more, and employees of companies with fewer than 20 workers. The effective dates for these changes are September 30, 1978, for federal workers; January 1, 1979, for workers in the private sector and state and local government workers; January 1, 1980, for workers under union contracts that were in effect on September 1, 1977; and July 1, 1982, for tenure college and university professors.[48] It is believed highly likely that the amendment will again be altered prior to the effective dates of the requirements. There have been numerous previous attempts to reduce or eliminate mandatory retirement, but the attempts have been frustrated by the harsh reality of economic limitations and the pressure of the labor market. However, the passage of the bill was undoubtedly influenced by the threat to the Social Security system and the belief that maintaining people in the labor force would reduce the drain on Social Security as well as the drive to insure human rights regardless of sex, race, religion, handicap, and age. In the event that the law remains essentially unaltered, the critical issue will be the availability of valid indicators of functional status to determine the work or retirement status of an individual. It is likely that performance evaluations will become much more critical and will be applied to younger workers as well as to older workers,[49] and there will be attempts to drive out the marginal employee through pay cuts, demotions, transfers, denial of bonuses, or other disagreeable assignments. It is possible companies will offer older workers various inducements to retire early; for example, a somewhat larger pension, special insurance, medical benefits, and other positive features.

THE CENTENARIANS

In the United States as determined by the census of 1970, there were 106,000 Americans 100 years of age or older. This is approximately one-half of 1% of the population 65 years of age and older. For many years the news media has reported the existence of three pockets of people widely distributed in the world who reportedly live very long lives frequently exceeding 100 years of age. One group lives in Vilcabamba, a small mountain village in Ecuador. The two other pockets are in widely separated regions of Asia, the Hunzukuts of the Karakoram Range in Kashmir and the Abkhazians of the Republic of Georgia, U.S.S.R. Particular attention has been given to the Los Viejos (the very old), the residents of Vilcabamba, because of the skillful writing of Grace Halsell.[50]

Over the past decade a number of individuals have visited the two pockets in Ecuador and Georgia, U.S.S.R. In February 1978, the National Institute on Aging brought together a number of the scientists who have visited Vilcabamba. Two investigators, Dr. Richard Mazess and Dr. Sylvia H. Forman[51] of the University of Massachusetts visited the village in 1974, 1976 and 1978. Utilizing a careful reconstruction of family genealogy and comparison to the records of civil agencies, they concluded that the ages of the elderly in Vilcabamba were greatly exaggerated. The age exaggeration began at about age 70 and amounted to as much as 20 to 40 years. Furthermore, the increase in the percentage of elderly people was not due to longevity, but was due to the outflux of younger people. Those remaining, however, did seem to be healthy, and shared some unusual characteristics including the fact that they were not overweight, they had lower blood pressure than expected and hypertension was rare, their blood cholesterol levels were slightly lower than average, and their heart rates were lower than expected especially after exertion. According to their calculations, the oldest person in the community was 96 years of age. Scientists now generally agree that the claim of the high number of centenarians in the Andes and the Soviet Caucasus is a hoax. As to the evidence refuting the claim of the Russians, this is clearly presented by the distinguished Russian geneticist, Zhores Medvedev, who cites a large series of reasons why the claims are false.[52] Medvedev cites the lack of birth records, the rapid increase in the number claiming to be centenarians, the greater number of men as compared with women, the discrepancies of life expectancies of other members of the same group, and the proved falsification by at least one deserter or draft dodger and so on.

Apparently the Hunzukuts because of their remoteness have received little attention. According to one account supposedly based on visits by Art Linkletter and Lowell Thomas, Hunza is a 2000-year-old country that has remained virtually isolated from the rest of the world. It is claimed that this civilization originated in 330 B.C. when an army division of Alexander the Great of Macedonia broke away, took Persian wives, and purposely lost themselves in the vastness of the Himalayas. These individuals supposedly live from 120 to 140 years of age, and men father children at 100 years and older. Hunza women of 80 "look like American women of 40." Their longevity is attributed to a number of factors including exercise, diet, periods of relaxation, and moderation in many things including the consumption of wine.[53]

Based on the results of scientific inquiry of the Los Viejos and the Abkhazians, it is a reasonable assumption that the tale of Hunza longevity is also essentially a distortion of fact. It appears that the hope for a lengthened life span will continue to result in wish fulfilling reports.

PSEUDOSCIENCE IN GERIATRICS AND PSYCHIATRY

Zhores Medvedev, a distinguished Russian scientist who has made many contributions to biological aging including the redundant theory of aging, is discussed elsewhere in this chapter. He has published two books that are important and are relevant to geriatric psychiatry. Medvedev was the author of the historical account of pseudoscience. This account, *The Rise and Fall of T. D. Lysenko,* first appeared in the science underground of Russia in 1961 and was finally published in the United States in 1969. The second book, *A Question of Madness*, coauthored with his brother Roy was published in 1971 in London and in the United States in 1972. This book is a vivid account of the problems of utilizing psychiatry for political purposes. For those

who are unaware, Medvedev is now living in London. His first book vividly recounts how Lysenko between 1937 and 1964 utilized a false doctrine and fabricated scientific data to achieve fame and power. The book illustrates how a pseudoscientific doctrine can achieve great acceptance by political leaders who in order to remain in power must have explanations for failure and promises of great improvement consistent with their political orientation. There is little doubt that the value system and the methods of problem-solving which are characteristic of the skillful and dedicated scientist are remarkably different and often incompatible with the goals and the methods utilized by politicians.

Of further interest to the geriatric psychiatrist is the account by Medvedev of a technique of rejuvenation advocated by a disciple of Lysenko, a woman by the name of O. B. Lepeshinskaya. In approximately 1949, she began to advocate the use of soda baths. Bags of soda were added to bath water to prolong life and restore vigor. This practice was warmly supported by Lysenko. This approach quickly moved to the drinking of soda water and finally to the introduction of soda into the body by enema. Apparently the latter two techniques were used as substitutes for those who were unable to take frequent soda baths. Lepeshinskaya also claimed that she could make living matter from nonliving material. Geriatrics is vulnerable to the pseudoscientist.

The Prolongation of Youth

Attempts to prolong youth or to restore sexual vigor and physical vitality have existed for many centuries and are found today. Many such attempts of rejuvenation carry a distinct risk. In fact, Greek mythology teaches that the risk is greater than the gain. The goddess Aurora (also called Eos) with great effort persuaded Zeus to grant her husband Tithonus immortality. Regretfully, she neglected to mention that she also wanted him to remain eternally young. As the years passed, Tithonus became more and more disabled, praying frequently for death.

In one account Tithonus escaped his misery by turning into a cicada. The male of this insect produces a shrill sound similar to the voice of a demented person. Ancient Greek tales do contain one success story. The sorceress Medea claimed to hold the key that unlocked the door to eternal youth. She mixed a ram's blood, a snake's skin, an owl's flesh, roots, herbs, grass, and other ingredients and then proceeded to fill the veins of King Aeson. The king promptly leaped from his sick bed, bursting with energy and youthful vitality. But how long this lasted is unclear. A similar injection ended in a catastrophe.

Pope Innocent VIII (1432-1492) was appropriately named as he requested his physicians to transfuse the blood of young men into his veins. Obviously the blood type was incompatible, for he died almost immediately.

During the nineteenth century there were two famous rejuvenists. Serge Voronoff (1866-1951), a Russian physician in Paris, continued in his efforts to restore youth. He claimed great success by grafting testicles of a monkey into an aging male. Elie Metchnikoff (1845-1916), another Russian, had a different approach to the prolongation of life. He advocated the removal of the large intestine and the ingestion of large amounts of yogurt. Advertising seen on television today suggests that long-lived Cossacks achieve this status by consuming large amounts of yogurt.

During the past 30 years at least two rejuvenating techniques have been given considerable publicity. The first was developed by Paul Neihans of Geneva, Switzerland. He injected living cells derived from a lamb embryo into his clients. Considerable success was claimed, and the technique continues to be utilized. But there is no doubt that the introduction of a foreign protein into a human body can result in disaster.

Gerovital H3

Gerovital H3 has been an exceedingly controversial compound that has received attention for over 30 years. It is claimed by its advocates to have a variety and remarkable curative and restorative power for disabilities and diseases affecting the elderly. The most active advocate of Gerovital H3 is Professor Anna Aslan of the Geriatric Institute of Bucharest, Romania. Although procaine hydrochloride has been utilized in Europe as a general tonic for over 50 years, it was not until 1945 when Professor Aslan began to utilize and proclaim its value that this particular drug began to receive considerable attention. Many of her claims are probably exaggerated, and this may mask its potential usefulness. She reports beneficial results in a wide variety of conditions including depression, degenerative arthritis, hypertension, angina pectoris, reversal of graying of the hair, and improvement in texture and appearance of the skin. Originally Aslan utilized a commercially available 2% solution of procaine hydrochloride. In 1955, she dropped the treatment with commercially available procaine and started to make and treat with Gerovital H3. Gerovital H3 is a solution of 2% hydrochloride with benzoic acid added as a preservative and potassium metabisulfite as an antioxidant. The solution is buffered at pH 3.3 in order to ensure maximum (shelf) stability.[54] Each 5cc ampule contains 100 milligrams of procaine hydrochloride. Assuming that it does have some pharmaceutical effect, the question is, how is this accomplished? One explanation is that it is an effective inhibitor of monoamine oxidase. Another explanation involves the presence of benzoic acid which positively influences the availability of the needed substances to a cell. An alternative is that presence of benzoic acid enhances the action of the metabolic products which include paraaminobenzoic acid and at least one other substance which is believed to have favorable effects upon the organism.[55]

A review of 285 articles and books addressing themselves to the subject of procaine hydrochloride was recently reported.[56] This review concluded that except for the possible antidepressant effect there is no convincing evidence that procaine or Gerovital H3 has any value in the treatment of disease of older patients. Inasmuch as its sole capability may be a mild antidepressant effect, it is possible that the improvements that are reported may be the relief of complaints referrable to the depressive condition.

REFERENCES

1. Beattie, W. M. Aging—a framework of characteristics and consideration for cooperative efforts between the developing and developed regions of the world. *The Graying of Nations,* Appendix 3, 155–167. U. S. Printing Office, 99–586, November 10, 1977.
2. Life Tables, Expectation of Life, *Demographic Yearbook,* United Nations, p. 718, 1970.
3. Samorajski, T. "Central neurotransmitter substances and aging: A review." *J. Am. Geriatrics Soc.* 25: 337–348 (1977).
4. Schally, A. W. Aspects of hypothalamic regulation of the pituitary gland. *Science* 202: 18–18. (1978).
5. Guillemin, R. Peptides in the brain: The new endocrinology of the neuron. *Science* 202: 390–401 (1978).
6. Hayflick, L. and Moorhead, P. A. The serial cultimation of duman diploid cells. *Exp. Cell Research* 25: 585–621 (1961).
7. Holliday, R., Hutschtscha, L. I., Tarrant, G. M., and Kirkwood, T. B. L. Testing the commitment theory of cellular aging. *Science* 190: 136–137 (1977).
8. Jarvik, Lissy F. The aging central nervous system: Clinical aspects. In H. Brody, D. Harmon, and J. M. Ordy (eds.) *Aging.* New York: Raven Press, vol. 1., 1975.
9. Ogatha J., Budzilovich, G. N., and Crarioto, H. A study of rodlike structures (hirano bodies) in 240 normal and pathological brains. *Acta Neuropath* 21: 40–60 (1972).
10. Nandy, Kalidas. Morphological changes in the aging brain. In K. Nandy (ed.) *Senile Dementia, A Biomedical Approach.* Amsterdam: Elsevier North-Holland Biomedical Press, pp. 19–29, 1978.
11. Walford, Roy. *The Immunological Theory of Aging.* Copenhagen: Munksgaard, 1969.
12. Burnet, F. M. An immunological approach to aging. *Lancet* 2: 358 (1970).
13. Nandy, K., Fritz, R. B., and Threatt, J. Specificity of brain-reactive antibodies in serum of old mice. *J. Gerontol.* 30: 269–274 (1975).
14. Kent, S. Can normal aging be explained by the immunologic theory? *Geriatrics* 32: 112–138 (1977).
15. Mackay, I. R., Whittingham, S. F., and Mathews, J. D. The immunoepidemiology of aging. In T. Makinodan and E. Yunis (eds.) *Immunology and Aging.* New York and London: Plenum Medical Book Company, pp. 35–49, 1977.
16. *Immunology—Its Role in Disease and Health,*
17. Cohen, D. and Eisdorfer, C. Behavioral-immunologic relationships in older men and women. *Experimental Aging Research* 3: 225–229 (1977).
18. Schneider, Edward L. *The Genetics of Aging.* New York and London: Plenum Press, 1978.
19. Nielsen, J., Jensen, L., Lindhardt, H., Stroltrup, L., and Sondergaard, A. Chromosomes in senile dementia. *Br. J. Psychol.,* 114–303 (1968).
19a. Medvedev, Z. Possible role of repeated nucleotide sequences in DNA in the Evolution of life spans of differentiated cells. *Nature* 237: 453–454, 1972.
20. Barrows, C. H. and Strehler, B. L. Program biological obsolescence. *Johns Hopkins Med. J.* 19: 18 (1968).
21. Cotzias, G. C., Miller, S. T., Nicholson, A. R., Maston, W. H., and Tang, L. D. Prolongation of the life span in mice adapted to large amounts of L-dopa. *Proc. Natl. Acad. Sci.* USA pp. 2466–2469, 1974.
22. Janoff, A. S. and Rosenberg, B. Chemically evoked hypothermia in the mouse: Towards a method for investigating thermodynamic parameters of aging and death in mammals. *Mech. Aging and Dev.* 3: 335–349 (1978).
23. Hutchinson, J. Case of congenital absence of hair and mammary glands with atrophic condition of the skin and its appendages. *Lancet* 1: 473–477 (1886).
24. Hastings, G. Progeria: A form of senilism. *The Practitioner* 73: 188–217 (1904).
25. Werner, O. Über Katarakt im Verbindung mit Sklerdermie. Kiel, 1904. (Thesis)
26. Hayflick, L. Cellular basis for biological aging. In C. E. Finch and L. Hayflick (eds.) *Handbook of Biology of Aging.* New York: Van Nostrand Reinhold, pp. 159–186, 1977.
27. Omenn, G. S. Behavior Genetics. In J. Birren and W. Schaie (eds.) *Handbook of the Psychology of Aging.* New York: Van Nostrand Reinhold, pp. 209–211, 1977.
28. Goto, M., Horiuchi, Y., Tanimoto, K., Ishii, T. and Nakashima, H. Werner's syndrome: Analysis of 15 cases with a review of the Japanese literature. *J. Am. Geriatrics Soc.* 26: 341–347 (1978).
29. Pearce L. and Brown, W. H. Hereditary premature senescence in the rabbit. *J. Exp. Med.* 111: 485–516 (1960).
30. Erikson, E. H. Identity and the life cycle. *Psychological Issues.* New York: International Universities Press, p. 120, 1959.
31. Gross, Martin L. *The Psychological Society.* New York: Random House, 1978.
32. Busse, E. W. Physiological changes and disease (functional consequences of aging). In A. N. Exton-Smith and J. G. Evans (eds) *Care of the Elderly.* London: Academic Press, pp. 33–41, 1977.

DHEW Publication No. (NIH) 77–940, National Institute of Allergy and Infectious Diseases, Bethesda, Maryland (1977).

33. Busse, E. W. How mind, body and environment influence nutrition in the elderly. *Postgrad. Med.,* **63:** 118–125 (1978).

34. Neugarten, Bernice L. (ed). Personality in Middle and Late Life. New York: Atherton Press, 1964, 225 pages.

35. Butwinick, J. Cautiousness with advanced age. *J. Gerontol.* **21:** 347–353 (1966).

36. Okun, M. A., Siegler, I. C. and George, L. K. Cautiousness and verbal learning. J. Gerontol. **33:** 94–97 (1978).

37. Birren, J. E. and Renner, V. J. Research on the psychiatry of aging. In J. E. Birren and K. W. Schaie (eds.). *Handbook of the Psychology of Aging.* New York: Van Nostrand Reinhold, pp. 3–38, 1977.

38. Baltes, P. A. and Willis, S. L. Toward psychological theories of aging and development In J. E. Birren and K. W. Schaie (eds.). *Handbook of the Psychology of Aging.* New York: Van Nostrand Reinhold, pp. 128–150, 1977.

39. Schaie, K. W. Toward a state theory of adult cognitive development. *Journal of Aging and Human Dev.* **8:** 129–138 (1977–78).

40. Kalish, R. A. and Knudtson, F. W. Attachment versus disengagement: A life-span conceptualization. *Human Development* **19:** 171–181 (1976).

41. Lowenthal, M. F. and Haven, C. Interaction and adaptation: Intimacy as a critical variable. In B. L. Neugarten (ed.). *Middle Age and Aging.* Chicago: University of Chicago Press, pp. 390–400, 1968.

42. Gould, J. and Kolb, W. L. *Dictionary of the Social Sciences.* New York: Free Press of Glencoe, p. 643, 1964.

43. Busse, E. W. Prejudice and gerontology. *Gerontologist* **8:** 66 (1968).

44. Busse, E. W. The aged: A deprived minority. *N. C. J. Ment. Health* **4:** 307 (1970).

45. Palmore, Erdman. Personal communication—The socioeconomic status of the aged. Fall, 1978.

46. Statistical Notes. *National Clearing House on Aging.* No. 2 (1978).

47. *Fact Book on Aging.* National Council on the Aging. Inc. February (1978).

48. What the new retirement law says. *Changing Times* 15–16. (1978).

49. Busse, E. W. and Kreps, J. M. Criteria for retirement: A reexamination. *Gerontologist* **4:** 115–120 (1964).

50. Halsell, Grace. *Los Viejos—Secrets of Long Life from the Sacred Valley.* Emmaus: Rodale Press, 1976.

51. Mazess, Richard. Did Methuselah lie about his age? National Institute on Aging (NIH) Conference on the Longerous Population of Vilcabamba, Ecuador (Fogarty International Center) February 1978.

52. Medvedev, Z. A. Caucasus and Altay longevity: A biological or social problem? *Gerontologist* **15:** 196 (1975).

53. *The Bio Calendar Health System.* American Health Institute, Canton, Ohio, 1978.

54. *Gerovital H3 Injectable,* prepared for the FDA by Rom-Amer Pharmaceuticals, Ltd., April 1973.

55. Busse, E. W. Longevity and rejuvenators. In *Mental Illness in Later Life,* E. W. Busse and E. Pfeiffer (eds). Washington D. C.: American Psychiatric Association, p. 168, 1973.

56. Ostfeld, A., Smith, C. M. and Stotsky, B. A. The systemic use of procaine in the treatment of the elderly: A review. *J. Am. Geriatrics Soc.* **25:** 1–19 (1977).

Figs. 1-1, 2, 3, 4—Illustrations and explanations reproduced from the 1904 publication of Hastings Gilford, F.R.C.S. (Eng.) in *The Practitioner.*

Chapter 2
Neuroanatomy and Neuropathology of Aging

Harold Brody, Ph.D., M. D.

State University of New York at Buffalo

INTRODUCTION

At the time of the 1971 White House Conference on Aging, it was estimated that of the 20 million persons in the United States past the age of 65 years, approximately four million had suffered moderate to severe psychiatric impairment secondary to either cerebral arteriosclerosis, senile dementia, functional psychoses, alcoholism or various other medical conditions. Of this four million, 20% were not legally competent to manage their personal and business affairs.

It appears obvious from this information, that paramount among organ systems affected to a large degree in the older individual, the central nervous system is particularly susceptible to change which may alter to a perceptible degree, the ability of an individual to function satisfactorily in the general environment. Unfortunately, the level of our knowledge and understanding of the mechanisms involved in central nervous system function and dysfunction is not equivalent to the degree of clinical involvement of this system in the aging. Only comparatively recently has the research literature on the aging central nervous system shown growth, and hopefully the basic anatomical and pathological mechanisms involved will be understood sufficiently to provide some morphological knowledge upon which functional concepts may be developed. The gross and microscopic changes which appear during normal and abnormal aging of the nervous system will be reviewed in this chapter and some specific disease entities which commonly affect the aging person will also be examined.

MACROSCOPIC AND MICROSCOPIC CHANGES WITH NORMAL AND ABNORMAL AGING

Brain Weight

Among the gross changes which have been described in the aging brain are thickening, increasing opacity and an adherency of the leptomeninges to the underlying cerebral cortex. This is accompanied by a decrease in the weight of the brain and a questionable change in the size of the ventricles. [1,2] However, it should be emphasized that studies described in the literature have failed to set specific criteria for the weighing of the brain, failed to provide information on the exact caudal extent of the brain removed for weight determination, or to indicate the weight of the cadaver from which the brain specimen was taken. One does not know whether the lower brain stem has been severed from the spinal cord at the level of the pyramidal decussation, or above or below this point. This will undoubtedly provide some error in calculation. It is also generally accepted that brain size is directly related to body size and weight. Since body size and weight of the average 25-year-old male dying today is greater than that of the average 75-year-old male, one would expect the weight of the brain to be greater in the younger person. Without information regarding body size, data forthcoming would bias the investigator to relating brain weight with increasing age. It is therefore necessary that studies regarding this aspect of brain aging be performed with better information provided. At any rate the importance of brain weight loss in the total picture of central nervous system aging remains a moot point at this time. Boyd[3] described an increase in weight in the male from 493 grams at 3 months of age to 1,374 grams between 14 and 20 years after which there was a loss of approximately 90 grams up to the 80-year-old specimens. While the weight of the female brain was less (in keeping with a generally smaller stature) the decrease was relatively similar to that of the male. Broca[4] found the same decrease in brain weight, although he reported the maximum weight to occur between 25 and 35 years of age but Pearl,[5] after examining more than 3100 brain specimens, observed a linear regression in brain weight after 20 years of age amounting to a 7% decrease by 80 years.

Confirmation of brain weight loss with age in man has been provided by other studies[6,7,8] while no change in wet brain weight was found between 10–12 month old and 28–30 month old C57B1/63 male mice which were at a stable, maximum value of skeletal size and body weight.[9]

Neurofibrillary Tangles

In 1907, Alzheimer[10] had described an alteration in neurons of the cerebral cortex consisting of a thickening and twisting of the neurofibrillary network within the cytoplasm. In silver stained preparations, they take two forms. The triangular type was an earlier form of a coarse twisting band extending from the apical dendrite along the cell membrane to the base of the neuron. It is more commonly seen in the frontal and temporal cortex. The second type of change found in the pyramidal cells of the hippocampus was composed of a finer network of fibrils which fill the cell as a collection of fibers curved parallel to each other resulting in the appearance of a spool. These neurofibrillary tangles may appear in the normal aging brain but are a feature of Alzheimer's disease.

One cannot discuss the neurofibrillary tangle without citing the work of Wiśniewski, Terry and their coworkers. In a series of contributions to the electron microscopic structure of the neurofibrillary tangle[11,12,13] they have identified a new class of fibrillary material not present in normal cells. These fibers were composed of paired helical filaments which in narrowed regions of the filament had an increased density band about 100°A wide. In wide areas of the paired helical filaments which measured up to 350°A there were frequent spaces up to 50°A wide between two 100°A bands. The bands in twisting, sometimes lie close together and have a variable periodicity, with constructions occurring at an average of 650°A. The paired helical filaments are found especially in the cerebral cortex, mesencephalon, and rostral rhombencephalon[14] and occur in Alzheimer's disease, Guam Parkinsonian dementia, Dementia "Psychistics," Down's Syndrome, postencephalitic Parkinsonism, subacute sclerosing pan encephalitis and Pick's disease.[12,14] In animals, they may be found in the aged rhesus monkey, although the dimensions of the filaments differ from those described above.[14] Of particular interest is the correlation between the quantity of paired helical filaments and the degree of mental deterioration.[2,15]

Senile (Neuritic) Plaques

Another characteristic neuropathological structure is the senile or neuritic plaque. It is especially common in Alzheimer's disease, but is only occasionally seen in the frontal cortex and the hippocampus of the normal aged brain. Tomlinson and Henderson[16] compared the presence of senile plaques in 28 nondemented and 50 demented elderly subjects by counting the number of plaques per low power field in frontal, temporal, parietal and occipital cortex of both hemispheres. They reported that plaques were present in small numbers in 15% of subjects in the fifth decade. This percentage increased to more than 50% by the seventh decade and 75% by the ninth decade. However, in the intellectually well-preserved individual, the number was quite small. Less than 10 plaques were found per field in 90% of normal elderly subjects and another 70% of such individuals had less than 5 plaques per field. However, in the demented older subjects, 50% had more than 13 plaques per field. The mean plaque count between the normal (3.3 per field) and demented (14.7 per field) was significantly different. From this information, the authors have concluded that there is a direct relationship between numbers of plaques and degree of dementia and that in the person with intact intellect, one should expect to find few plaques.

The presence of argyrophilic plaques was first noted by Blocq and Marinesco[17] in the brain of an epileptic subject and named "senile plaques" by Simckowicz[18] in 1910. With silver impregnation preparations, it was noted that the plaque (range 10–150 μm in diameter) is composed of silver staining granular or filamentous particles surrounding a central amyloid material. Around the periphery there may be astrocytes and mi-

croglial cells. Plaques appear only in gray matter suggesting that the central amorphous material may have been formed from a degenerated neuron or its processes and the periphery of the plaque is a tissue reaction to the degeneration within its center. In electron microscopic studies,[19,20] the plaque has been substantiated to consist of the elements earlier identified in light microscopic studies: degenerative neuronal elements, reactive glial cells and amyloid. This constitutes the classical senile or neuritic plaque while those which are chiefly composed of the central core are called amyloid, compact or burned out plaques. The neuronal processes within the plaque are to the largest extent, presynaptic terminals containing synaptic vesicles in varying number, possibly related to the degree of degeneration and marked by an intact plasma membrane. It has been suggested that there exists the possibility of future functional recovery of these terminals because of the continued presence of these specialized membranous structures.[13]

Lipofuscin

One of the few changes in central nervous system morphology which is consistently reported, continually occurring and involves the majority of neurons to some degree in the aged brain is the deposition of lipofuscin, known in earlier literature as "aging" pigment or "wear and tear" pigment. Light microscopic examination of unstained preparations demonstrates a yellow-brown intracellular granular material which increases with age in dividing and nondividing cells including liver, spleen, adrenal gland, seminal vesicles, corpus luteum, prostate, interstitial cells of the testes and neurons. The age-correlated relationship has been well demonstrated by numerous investigators, among whom only several are cited.[21,22,23,24,25,26]

The composition of lipofuscin pigment is not revealed by any single histochemical method, indicating a heterogeneity in its structure. It has been demonstrated to contain lipid, carbohydrate and protein, to have an affinity for lipid stains as well as methyl-green, periodic acid Schiff and nile blue, and it is probable that there may be more than one type of lipofuscin pigment, or that the pigment itself may be undergoing an aging change within the cell resulting in a structure receptive to different staining preparations and providing a different colored autofluorescence.[27,28] Mention at this point should be made of the difficulty of drawing a sharp distinction between lipofuscin and another lipopigment, ceroid, which may represent different degrees in the autoxidative polymerization of unsaturated fatty acids.[29]

There is general agreement at this time that lipofuscin originates from lysosomes.[30,31] Ultrastructurally, lipofuscin bodies are revealed as electron-dense, osmiophilic particles bound by a single membrane with polymorphic internal structures which vary from fine particles to coarse dense granular material,[32] and it has been suggested[33] on the basis of its ultrastructural composition that neuronal lipofuscin may be classified into four types, I granular; II homogeneous; III lamellated; IV compound (consisting of combinations of I, II and III).

Quantitative examination of lipofuscin deposition within its normal neuronal environment requires examination by light microscopy and on the basis of the amount and distribution pattern it is possible to divide cells containing lipofuscin granules into several types,[23] the number depending upon the specific area of the nervous system examined: I, cells without pigment; II, cells whose pigment granules are scattered throughout the cytoplasm (Fig. 2-1); III, cells whose pigment granules are clumped and concentrated in one pole (Fig. 2-2), and IV, cells in which the pigment occupies the entire cytoplasmic region, pushing the nucleus into an eccentric position and commonly found in the inferior olive. Neurons in human cerebral cortex characteristically show pigment deposition of the first three types (Fig. 2-3) and it should be emphasized that at least in four separate cortical regions

there is a relatively low percentage of group III cells. This is in contrast with the nucleus of the inferior olive where, after the fourth decade, in a series of randomly selected brains of several age categories, more than 90% of cells may be included within group IV (see Table 2-1).

The functional significance of pigment accumulation in nerve cells is as unclear today as it was when lipofuscin was first described.[34,35] It forms early in life in both animals and man and in some areas accumulates to a large degree during adulthood. It may be a reasonable deduction to assume that the pigment granules in occupying the cytoplasm of a neuron must interfere with cell metabolic processes. In fact, if this concept is carried to a natural conclusion, one might expect that an alteration in cell metabolism (if this indeed results) eventually could cause the loss of the nerve cell. However, it must be emphasized that in the inferior olive, while there are a preponderance of group IV cells, there is no decrease in cell number over the life span,[36,37] indicating that whatever the lipofuscin may or may not do, it does not have any impact on the life of the cell. A question remains as to the possible interference by lipofuscin accumulation with the activity level of a group of cells. Clarification of this issue depends upon a complete quantitative survey of the distribution of the pigment throughout the nervous system,[38] correlated with functional changes during a lifetime, as well as single unit electrical and microchemical studies which may provide direct experimental evidence concerning the functional consequences at the cellular level.[39]

Neural Vascular Relationships

In the human the arterial supply of the brain is obtained completely by way of the internal carotid and the vertebral arteries. Branches of these arteries form the major vessels located on the base of the brain which supply the entire aspect of the hemispheres, brain stem and the cerebellum. Smaller branches of these vessels pass into

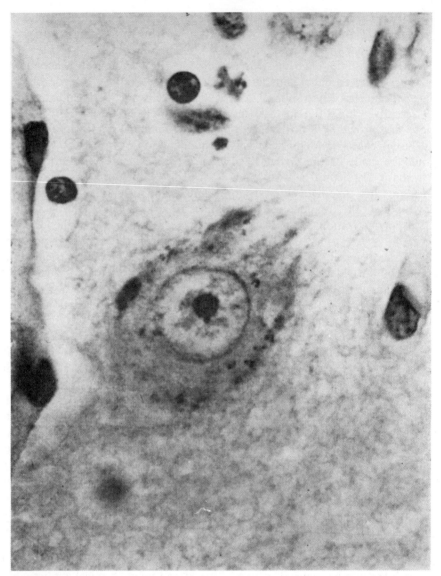

Fig. 1.   Photomicrograph of a Group 2 cell from layer III of the precentral gyrus of human cerebral cortex indicating pigment granules scattered in the cytoplasm. PAS preparation with hematoxylin counterstain. Oil immersion. (From Brody, *J. Geront.* **15**, 1960)

the brain substance where they functionally become end arteries providing a system which at that level is poorly adapted to establish an effective collateral circulation. While the larger cerebral and meningeal arteries are similar structurally to equally sized vessels in other areas of the body, those arteries less than 100μm in diameter display a thin total vessel wall although the internal elastic membrane is thicker than in other vessels. The media is composed of collagenous connective tissue with rare muscle cells and is relatively thicker than the intima or adventitial layers. The adventitia may be variable, ranging from a few collagenous fibrous strands, to a thickness equaling the media of that vessel.

The density of the capillary network is proportional to the concentration of neurons, being rather slight in white matter but more dense in gray matter, related to the metabolic needs of the tissue being supplied.

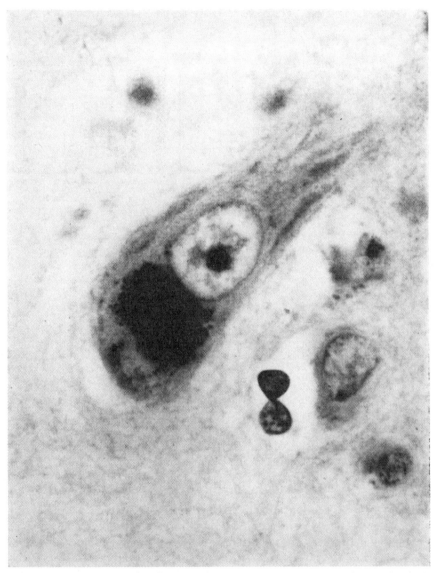

Fig. 2.   Photomicrograph of a Group 3 cell from layer III of the precentral gyrus of human cerebral cortex indicating congregation of pigment granules in the cytoplasm. PAS preparation with hematoxylin counterstain. Oil immersion. (From Brody, *J. Geront.* **15,** 1960)

Even within specific neuronal regions, because of a localized higher level of activity, the capillary network may be variable.

It is apparent from an examination of the literature, that there is a paucity of information available on changes with age of the cerebral vasculature and microcirculation. Fang has observed the microscopic changes occurring in blood vessels of subjects 55 years and older, citing the following findings:[40] coiling or looping of perforating blood vessels which extends through the thickness of the cerebral cortex into the underlying white matter; the intracerebral microvasculature develops knoblike structures and enlargement along the course of draining cerebral venules; areas of decreased local vascularity especially in the deeper layers of the cerebral cortex. The relationship between these changes and neuronal viability is impossible to assess at this time due to a lack of experimental evidence, but

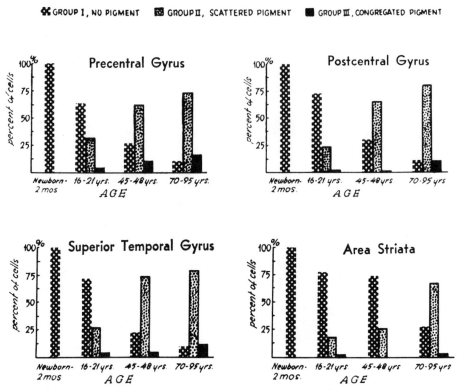

 GROUP I, NO PIGMENT   GROUP II, SCATTERED PIGMENT   GROUP III, CONGREGATED PIGMENT

Fig. 3.   The relationship according to age of the distribution of pigment within cells of layer III in the human cerebral cortex. (From Brody, *J. Geront.* **15,** 1960)

it is obvious that this topic is a concern for the understanding of the role of the circulation and the aging neuron.

Mention needs to be made of the blood-brain barrier and its possible role in aging in the nervous system. There is evidence that certain circulating substances are unable to pass from the cerebral vascular system into the central nervous system. The site of this barrier is considered to be at the level of the blood-vessel endothelium,[41] where tight junctions may play a role in transport mechanisms between nerve tissue and the blood vessel. When a breakdown in the blood brain barrier occurs, as in brain trauma, infections, tumors, etc., protein molecules may diffuse into the nervous system.[42] While it has been suggested that there is a breakdown in the blood-brain barrier with advancing age,[43,44] resulting in nervous system changes, experimental evidence is lacking in the human. A recent study by Rapoport *et al.*[45] while verifying an earlier demonstration by Bondareff and Narotsky[46]

of a reduction of the extracellular space in the brains of older animals, does not support experimentally the hypothesis of a breakdown of the blood-brain barrier with age. Unless there is a species difference, Rapoport having used the Fisher 344 male rat while Nandy's subjects were C57BL/6 female mice, it appears obvious that further work is needed to clarify this issue.

Cell Changes in Relation to Time

Jacobson has suggested that the number of neurons that reach maturity is the result of a balance between cell proliferation and cell death during neurogenesis.[47] He wonders as to how and why the remarkable constancy in neuronal number is controlled or achieved. Must there be a specific number of neurons present to perform a specific function? While one should expect that optimum activity relates to maximum number of related cells, could the individual suffer a 10% or even a 50% loss in cells without functional

Table 2-1.   Lipofuscin in the chief nucleus of the human
inferior olive.

AGE	CELL NUMBER	AGE	CELL NUMBER
Prenatal	100	32 years	0
	0		3
	0		13
	0		84
Newborn	100	44 years	0
	0		1
	0		7
	0		92
3 months	65	56 years	0
	35		0
	0		5
	0		95
9 years	6	65 years	0
	19		0
	75		2
	0		98
12 years	0	85 years	0
	9		0
	91		0
	0		100
19 years	0		
	7		
	81		
	12		

effect, or could a 10% loss result in impairment of activity? Are certain areas of the nervous system more or less susceptible to cell change than other regions, because they may prove to be capable of maintaing function without the maximum number of cells? Are some of the manifestations of neurological disease due to cell loss, or morphologic changes in neurons, or to an altered activity in remaining cells as a compensation for the loss of neighbor cells? When nerve cells are lost due to neurological disease, trauma, drugs or toxins or as a consequence of the normal aging process, we may assume that the axonic terminals of those cells upon other cells will be vacated. Are the remaining neurons capable of continuing proliferation (plasticity) so that these vacated synaptic sites may be reoccupied? What might be the functional effect of such reorganization occurring after the nervous system is well constituted?

The neurons of the human nervous system are postmitotic, indicating that they are not capable of division postnatally. This is probably fortunate since it is difficult to imagine how a later developing cell would be capable of fitting itself into the existent circuitry. Having the total and largest number of nerve cells at birth within a comparatively small brain, emphasizes the fact that as further enlargement of the brain occurs with an increase in processes, blood vessels, myelin, etc., the nerve cells will be spread farther apart and the original number of cells will now be situated in a larger, heavier structure. This deserves emphasis since it indicates that a cell population determined in specimens before 20 years of age may be compared in structures which lend themselves to total cell counts, e.g. a brain stem nucleus, and are not useful in structures where total cell counts are not possible and unit areas must be considered, e.g. cerebral cortex. After the brain reaches maximum weight, cell counts of unit areas of cerebral cortex will have validity.

The topic of nerve cell loss has been controversial, primarily due to a confusion among investigators who have failed to appreciate that there may be species differences as well as regional differences in areas of the brain examined.[48] It should be evident that a comparison can not be made anatomically, physiologically or in response to stress between disparate areas of the central nervous system.[24,49,50] Since the brain is not a unit structure, (the time sequence of development of the neurons even within a single region may be variable) it is probable that cell activity varies and that cell loss in turn, may not be equal.

Cerebral Cortex

Examination of the cerebral cortex requires a careful sampling of the material in order to compare cortical regions in as like a manner as possible.[51,52] Several studies have now demonstrated a decrease in the nerve cells of the cerebral cortex in man[16,51,53,54,55,56,57] and in Rhesus monkey.[58] This decrease has been significant in the superior temporal gyrus, precentral gyrus, superior frontal gyrus and the visual cortex (area striata) and was not significant in the postcentral gyrus or the inferior temporal gyrus. Generally, although some dissimilarities exist in cell number, there was a clustering by decades and a linear decrease with advancing age. The most remarkable loss occurred in the external and internal granule layers, layers 2 and 4 where Golgi Type II short axoned cells are to be found. These are local circuit neurons that form central integrating circuits and are characteristic of the associational cells of the human cerebral cortex.

In addition to these reports of cell decrease in cerebral cortex, two separate studies in rat and man have demonstrated aging changes in the dendrites of cortical cells. In the rat[59] a loss of dendritic spines from pyramidal cells of layer 5 of the visual cortex has been described, while in the human,[60] a ''progressive multi-stepped process'' is noted in the neocortex involving the small pyramidal cells of layers 2 and 3 and a lesser number of cells in layer 4 stellate and layer 5 large pyramidal cells. This results in a loss of the basilar dendrites and a decrease in the number of horizontal and oblique branches of the apical dendrite so that the neuron appears to be returning to a denuded structure of early formation. As noted by the Scheibels, the interruption of intracortical circuits may influence the undulating or inhibitory components of cortical activity and may additionally result in a loss of whatever stored programs may be located within the dendritic processes.

Therefore, two concomitants of aging of cortical neurons are cell loss which may be specific to a greater degree in certain regions, occurring in a linear fashion throughout the adult life of the individual, and a decrease and loss of dendritic processes and spines. Taken together this may result in the interruption of intracortical circuitry, so vital in the functioning of the mammalian brain.

Several recent reports have appeared analyzing the hippocampus and its relation to aging. These have demonstrated a loss of pyramidal cells and an unusual hypertrophy of astroglia in rats which have exhibited impaired memory retention.[61,62] Repetitive stimulation of hippocampal slices from these animals showed a marked deficit in frequency and post-tetanic potentiation considered to be related to synaptic depression.[63] The description of an increase in subsynaptic plate perforations occurring in the synapse in occipital cortex layer 3 cells of the rat postnatally[64] is of interest in this regard and deserves examination in the older animal.

Other Central Nervous System Structures

In the cerebellum, a very careful study of Purkinje cell populations[65] has demonstrated that although there may be a wide individual variation among subjects, there is a tendency for these cells to decrease in number during adult life. A final decrease of 25% was however not appreciable until the sixth decade of life. This is a confirmation of earlier work by several investigators in human[66,67,68,69,70] and in rat[71] although at variance with other studies in human[72] and in guinea pig.[73]

To emphasize central nervous system differences in response to age, the usual picture in the brain stem indicates a stability in cell populations as examined by several workers. No change has been noted in cell number in the nucleus of the facial nerve,[36,37] the trochlear[76] or the abducens nuclei.[77] However, recent studies of these separate areas in the human brain indicate cell decreases occurring in the substantia nigra,[78] the locus coeruleus[79] and the putamen.[80] The decrease in cell number in the locus coeruleus is approximately 40% by the ninth decade, with the significant change beginning during the seventh decade. Changes in the catecholamine neurotransmitter system may be of consequence in relation to this cellular change and since the locus coeruleus projects widely within the central nervous system, this change may be related directly to alteration of activity in the older individual. Bugiani et al.[80] note in relation to changes in the putamen, that the neuronal decrease affects both large and small cells so that while the numbers of both cell types decrease, the ratio remains the same as at an earlier age, in effect permitting a balance within the system.

It appears obvious from this review that a quantitative approach to the study of the central nervous system may provide valuable information for an understanding of the effect of increasing age upon the cellular unit, the neuron. This must be joined by continuing studies of changes in axonal and dendritic processes and when possible supported by associated physiological and functional investigation.

Slow Virus Diseases

About 20 years ago, a progressive degenerative disease of the central nervous system was noted in a native tribe in New Guinea which practiced cannibalism. This disease, kuru[81,82,83,84] was particularly evident in women, and in male and female children who ate the brains of their victims, while it was generally not seen in men who rarely ate visceral organs. Kuru, whose major effects involve the cerebellum, has been characterized as one of a group of slow virus diseases, which have as their features:[85] (1) an incubation period lasting from months to years; (2) a progressive illness usually resulting in death; (3) pathological findings limited to the central nervous system, and (4) a limited number of susceptible hosts.

The slow virus diseases include scrapie, which may infect sheep and goats and which has been experimentally transmitted to goats, mice, rats, hamsters, gerbils and monkeys, and the human slow virus diseases which include kuru and Creutzfeldt-Jakob disease. While the principal site of involvement may vary in these three conditions, medulla in scrapie, cerebellum in kuru and cerebral and cerebellar cortex in Creutzfeldt-Jakob disease, microscopic changes include:[86] (1) vacuolation in neuronal cell bodies, dendrites and axons resulting in a spongy appearance (status spongiosis); (2) chromatolysis, degeneration and loss of nerve cells; (3) extensive astroglial hypertrophy, hyperplasia, and fibrillary gliosis with a spongy vacuolation within glial cells as seen with the electron microscope (4) development of amyloid-containing, double refractive birefringent plaques resembling the neuritic plaques of Alzheimer's disease.

Creutzfeldt-Jakob disease, an example of a subacute spongiform encephalopathy generally occurs in late middle age, in all temporate climates and worldwide, and has been transmitted through direct tissue contact between individuals (corneal transplant). It is marked by behavioral, memory and reasoning changes. and visual difficulties. Hallucinations may occur early in the disease and there is rapid progression of the process. Myoclonus, hyperesthesia, ataxia and dysarthria occur. The EEG pattern also changes from diffuse slowing to high voltage synchronous sharp waves, and coma continues to death in one year or less from the onset of the disease.

It appears obvious that this group of disorders, which may have a long incubation period and may mimic senile dementia in either the clinical course or specific pathological (histological) features, is of great importance and interest to investigators in senile dementia. This is illustrated by the question proposed by Katzman et al.,[87] as to whether viral infections may cause the neurofibrillary tangle found in Alzheimer's disease.

DEGENERATIVE DISEASES

The anatomical and pathological changes in the central nervous system which have been described earlier could be expected to be reflected in alteration of function. While this specificity might simplify our thinking about the relationship between structure and function, no such relationship has been demonstrated. The role of lipofuscin or the effect of senile neuritic plaques or neurofibrillary tangles upon a specific activity are not known and we only assume that these conditions are pathological because they may appear in the malfunctioning brain. The question as to whether there is a relationship between dementia and specific degeneration has not been answered although there is evidence that the brain of the more seriously impaired will demonstrate a constancy in the presence of degenerative changes. The diseases which are considered to be degenerative in classification are noted as developing in middle or later life after a long period of normal functioning, and deterioration is continuous and progressive. We may include in this group, Alzheimer's disease, Pick's disease, Huntington's Chorea and Parkinson's disease. Major features of the first two conditions are progressive dementia with other obvious findings, while the third is an example of progressive dementia with other neurological signs. Parkinson's disease is typified by progressive abnormalities in posture and movement. It should be noted that other disease entities exist as examples of progressive neurological syndromes but only these four will be described in this review. These reviews will be brief and the reader is encouraged to refer to standard textbooks in neurology and neuropathology for further information.

Alzheimer's Disease

It has been estimated[88] based on prevalence studies from Scandinavia[89] that severe dementia occurs in 4.4% of those older than 65 years while mild to moderate dementia occurs in 11–12%. Projected onto the fact that by 1980, it is estimated that 12% of the population in the United States will be 65 years or older, this prevalence data suggests "that there are approximately one million severely demented persons and another three million mildly to moderately demented persons in this country today." Katzman[90] has indicated that survival of severely demented persons is one-third to one-half that of age-matched controls and a projected 100,000 annual mortality would place senile dementia as the fourth or fifth leading cause of death in the United States.

Because it has been noted that the same pathological changes occur in the brains of those below 65 years of age with Alzheimer's disease as are found in patients over 65 with clinically defined senile dementia, it has been recommended that the disease may be distinguishable only on the basis of age and because this separation is not logical, should be spoken of as "Alzheimer's disease" in the younger aged group and "senile dementia of the Alzheimer type" in the older group. Some of the clinical features which may be noted in Alzheimer's disease are loss of memory, difficulty in speaking and writing (presumably related to memory deficit), loss of conceptualization and arithmetic ability, and forgetfulnes in common activities such as finding one's home, performing relatively stereotyped acts (dressing, eating, washing) and relating to others. Frequently altered personality and paranoia may result in serious problems with family relationships, particularly if the family does not have an appreciation of the basic problem and its ramifications. In its final stages, the process may cause deterioration of the overall health of the patient and death occurs usually due to an aspiration pneumonia.

The brain will show widespread atrophy with a loss of several hundred grams in weight. This atrophy is characteristically symmetrical, although the frontal and temporal lobes may be more involved. The two major microscopic changes are the presence of senile or neuritic plaques throughout the cerebral cortex, and oftentimes in the basal ganglia, and neurofibrillary tangles which were originally described by Alzheimer.[10] The neurofibrillary tangles occur especially in pyramidal cells of the third and fifth layers and are numerous in Sector H_1 and the subiculum of the hippocampus. These latter areas also undergo neuronal loss although this occurs in all cortical regions to a slightly lesser degree.

While lipofuscin accumulation is often cited as being present in neurons in Alzheimer's disease, it probably should not be included as a feature since it is a normal concomitant of aging, appearing to some considerable degree in brain stem and cortical neurons.[23] However, granulovascular degeneration as seen in Alzheimer's disease affects the neuron and is demonstrated by cells containing small cytoplasmic vacuoles, each with a small, argentophilic 1μm granule which also stains with hematoxylin. This occurs to the greatest extent in hippocampal neurons of the subiculum and H_1 and H_2 sectors.

Pick's Disease

This is a rare disease usually occurring during the seventh decade with a slightly greater percentage of occurrence in women. The duration of the disease is generally between one and ten years and based on the studies of Sjögren *et al.,*[91] Pick's disease is probably transmitted by a dominant gene.

Pick's disease is marked by extreme shrinkage of localized cortical areas in contrast to the diffuse involvement of Alzheimer's. Typically the gross changes of shrinkage in frontal and temporal lobes may be sufficient to provide a diagnosis. The shrinkage may cause a narrowing of the cortex so that the term "knife edge" has been used to describe the appearance of the gyri in affected lobes of the brain. The process of atrophy may involve the underlying white matter and the basal ganglia, especially the caudate nucleus. Histologically, there is a large decrease in neurons in the affected cortex and an astrocytic hyperplasia and gliosis which may occur in response to the neuronal loss or as a primary change in the involved cortex.

While cells may atrophy or lose their Nissl structure, some cells may undergo swelling and become rounded, with displacement of the nucleus to an eccentric position, and may demonstrate a diffuse argentophilic material within the cytoplasm or a well defined homogeneous argentophilic inclusion (Pick cells). While there may be evidence of granulovacuolar degeneration, senile plaques and neurofibrillary tangles are present infrequently.

Clinically, there is a gradual increase in confusion and loss of concentration with increasing disorientation, depression and apathy. Language disorders usually occur with dysphagia and dyslexia and finally mutism. The disease runs a course of from one to ten years, and affects women slightly more than men.

Huntington's Chorea

This condition has been of great interest since its accurate and precise description by Huntington[92] who recognized the fact that the process was one of autosomal dominant inheritance marked by choreoathetosis and dementia. This extrapyramidal degenerative disease usually begins between 25 and 45 years of age in individuals of either sex who usually have not demonstrated any abnormality in activity or behavior before the first indication of the disease. In this regard, the disease is particularly insidious as it is impossible beforehand to know whether the children of a Huntington patient have the disease. It is therefore difficult for a genetic counselor to advise young adults with a familial history of Huntington's disease on the advisability of having children of their own. From the time of the first manifestation of the disease, the duration for the process is about 15 years, progressing without remission to death. Typically, the Huntington patient is first fidgety or nervous, and over some years this progesses to jerking and choreiform movements, accompanied by memory loss, irritability and paranoia. Finally, the patient is rarely still, moving constantly. Behavior may be altered to a state of psychosis.

Major findings in this disease involve the superior part of the caudate nucleus and the posterior two-thirds of the putamen as well as marked atrophy of the cortex of the frontal lobe. Due to the atrophy in the head of the caudate nucleus, the configuration of the anterior horns of the lateral ventricle will be changed and its flattening, with resultant enlargement of the ventricle, may be seen in the pneumoencephalogram or by computerized tomography.

Microscopically, there is a severe neuronal loss of small cells in the caudate nucleus and putamen. There is also a large degree of astroglial proliferation and gliosis.

It is of particular interest that in Huntington's chorea dopamine and homovanillic acid levels are generally normal, indicating a higher amount of dopamine for each surviving neuron in caudate nucleus or putamen. When L-dopa is administered to such a patient, the condition is aggravated possibly as a response to dopamine overload.

Parkinson's Disease

This degenerative disease of the extrapyramidal system is included among a larger classification of basal ganglia diseases. The basal ganglia are a complex consisting of the caudate nucleus and putamen (striatum), globus palladus, claustrum, amygdaloid nucleus, subthalamic nucleus, red nucleus and the substantia nigra. These structures primarily located in the more rostral regions of the brain are characterized by anatomical pathways which are short (in contrast to the long pyramidal pathway from cerebral cortex to lower motor neurons in cranial nerve nuclei and the spinal cord), interconnecting basal ganglia structures with cerebral cortex and with each other by a series of loops and playing an important role in the modification of posture for cortically induced movements. Notwithstanding the considerable clinical importance of basal ganglia disease, and the surgical experiences with laboratory animals and human patients, little is known functionally about the mode of action and the function of the specific nuclei included in this system. This is very likely due to the anatomical, physiological, and as has been demonstrated more recently, the biochemical[93] interrelationships of the basal ganglia nuclei, so that no one nucleus is capable of action without influencing other components of the system. As an example, dopamine is contained within the nerve endings in the striatum and the cell bodies of the substantia nigra. The nigrostriatal pathway is the means of transfer of dopamine to the striatum, and depletion of the cells of the substantia nigra or its stimulation will decrease or increase respectively the amount of dopamine found in the striatum. Since the major pathology in Parkinson's disease is the loss of pigmented cells of the zona compacta of the substantia nigra (cells particularly rich in dopamine), with subsequent decrease of dopamine in the striatum, one therapeutic approach has been to replace the level of dopamine in the striatum by administration of a pharmacological agent, in this case L-dopa (a precursor of dopamine), which is capable of passing the blood brain barrier to be converted to dopamine and utilized by the striatum. Certainly this has been one of the major therapeutic advances for the alleviation of the symptoms of a dreaded disease.

Parkinson's disease has a worldwide distribution, may involve the sexes equally, has its onset in middle age with a peak level during the sixth decade and its cause is unknown. This degenerative disease should be considered to be idiopathic although other types of Parkinsonism which may present some clinical signs of the disease (the rigidity, tremor, akinesia) have been described as: (1) drug toxicity; (2) arteriosclerotic; (3) postencephalitic; (4) traumatic. While arteriosclerosis of vessels of the brain has been implicated as a causative agent of Parkinson's, no evidence exists to warrant this assumption. One would hope that this will not continue to be referred to in this context, just as it has become apparent with time that age changes in the brain are not related to impairment of circulation.

In addition to the loss of melanin containing cells of the substantia nigra which can be observed with the naked eye, another constant finding is the presence of inclusions (Lewy bodies)[94] within remaining pigmented cells. These round structures have a protein central core containing alpha amino acids and ultrastructurally have been shown to be composed of loosely packed filaments surrounding a core of granular material and tightly packed filaments.

Metabolic and Nutritional Conditions

It is fitting that some attention be given to a consideration of neurological disease in the aged person as a reflection of nutritional deficiency. The diet of the older individual may be lacking in nutritional value either in quality or quantity, or may be composed of large amounts of one food type while deficient in others. Poor dentition and altered physiological activity within the gastrointestinal tract may also result in deficient intake and absorption of certain foods. An additional but separate problem relates to the poor economic status of many elderly which makes the purchase of essential foods difficult. Among the essential nutrients are

vitamins and particularly for the disease entity to be discussed, there is a need for sufficient amounts of thiamine. Alcoholism is an increasing problem for this segment of the population, and in addition to the decrease in the intake of necessary foods, the alcohol supplies additional carbohydrates which may encourage a thiamine deficiency. In less usual circumstances, thiamine deficiency may result from the administration of parenteral fluids (glucose) without adequate thiamine additives in a seriously ill medical or surgical patient.

Wernicke-Korsakoff Syndrome. Wernicke's disease appears suddenly, is marked by paralysis of ocular movements, ataxia and mental confusion and results from a deficiency of thiamine. Wernicke described the pathology[95] in the brains of three patients to be consistently in the periventricular gray matter of the third ventricle, aqueduct of Sylvius and fourth ventricle. Grossly visible petechial hemorrhages occur in the mammillary bodies and microscopically there is a secondary degeneration of neurons, astrocytic proliferation and an increased cellularity in lesioned areas due to capillary proliferation.

Korsakoff's psychosis is usually associated with Wernicke's disease in the patient who is nutritionally deficient and alcoholic and may be considered as the "psychic manifestation of Wernicke's disease."[96] This is an amnesic psychosis with impaired retentive memory for old and new events in an otherwise alert and responsive individual. The pathological findings are similar to those of Wernicke's disease with the additional involvement of the dorsomedial thalamic nucleus in a patient with Korsakoff's psychosis. Fortunately, aggressive and immediate treatment with thiamine may halt or reverse those lesions in Wernicke's disease which have not caused permanent structural changes and may also prevent the later development of a psychosis. However, once the amnesic psychosis occurs, recovery may not be complete, regardless of the amount of thiamine administered, indicating the probability of permanent structural damage in Korsakoff's psychosis.

CONDITIONS SECONDARY TO CEREBRAL VASCULAR ABNORMALITIES

Multi-infarct Dementia

It had been traditionally assumed that senile dementia was due to cerebral arteriosclerosis. However, more recently the term of multi-infarct dementia was introduced[97] to indicate that cerebral infarction is responsible for approximately a third of dementias while the majority are of the Alzheimer type unrelated to cerebral arteriosclerosis. The process of narrowing of cerebral vessels does not contribute to dementia unless actual closure or emboli result in small or large infarctions. Measurement of cerebral blood flow[98,99] is of diagnostic value as there is a significantly greater reduction in cerebral blood flow in patients with multi-infarct dementia when compared with patients with dementia of a primary degenerative type (Alzheimer's disease) as well as an inverse relationship between the degree of dementia and cerebral blood flow in the multi-infarct dementia group.

Acceptance of the difference between these two processes may prove beneficial in the approach taken by the physician in dealing with these problems.

Lacunar State

This term originally introduced by Pierre Marie was used to define small areas of ischemic infarction resulting from occlusion of the small penetrating branches of cerebral arteries. Removal of the infarcted area leaves small cavities or lacunae which may be from 2–15 mm in diameter and tend to be located in the striatum, thalamus, pons and white matter of the cerebrum and cerebellum.[100,101,102] The lacunar state is often seen in association with hypertension and atherosclerosis. The neurological picture depends upon the size of the lacunae and the area involved and oftentimes, a small lesion may not cause any symptoms.

REFERENCES

1. Tomlinson, B. E., Blessed, G. and Roth, M. Observations on the brains of non-demented people. *J. Neurol. Sci.* **7**: 331–356 (1968).
2. Tomlinson, B. E., Blessed, G. and Roth, M. Observations on the brains of demented old people. *J. Neurol. Sci.* **11**: 205–242 (1970).
3. Boyd, R. The average weights of human body and brain. Philosophical Transactions. In Schafer and Thane (eds.) *Quain's Anatomy* (reference) p. 219. London: Longmans and Green, 1895.
4. Broca, P. Anatomie comparée des circonvolutions cérébrales le grand lobe limbique et al scissure limbique dans la série des mammifères. *Rev. Antropol.* **1**: 384–498 (1878).
5. Pearl, R. *The Biology of Death.* Philadelphia: J. B. Lippincott, 1922.
6. Appel, F. W. and Appel, E. M. Intracranial variation in the weight of the human brain. *Human Biol.* **14**: 48–68 (1942).
7. Appel, F. W. and Appel, E. M. Intracranial variation in the weight of human brain. *Human Biol.* **14**: 235–250 (1942).
8. Pakkenberg, H. and Voigt, J. Brain weight of the Danes. *Acta Anat.* **56**: 297–307 (1964).
9. Finch, C. E. Catecholamine metabolism on the brains of aging male mice. *Brain Res.* **52**: 261–276 (1973).
10. Alzheimer, A. Über eine eigenartige Erkrankung der Hirnrinde. *Zbl. Nervenh. Psychiatr* **18**: 177–179 (1907).
11. Wiśniewski, H. M., Narang, H. K. and Terry, R. D. Neurofibrillary tangles of paired helical filaments. *J. Neurol. Sci.* **27**: 173–181 (1976).
12. Wiśniewski, H. M., Terry, R. D. and Hirano, A. Neurofibrillary pathology. *J. Neuropathol. Exp. Neurol.* **29**: 163–176 (1970).
13. Wiśniewski, H. M. and Terry, R. D. Neuropathology of the aging brain. In R. D. Terry and S. Gershon (eds.) *Neurobiology of Aging.* New York: Raven Press, 1976.
14. Iqbal, K., Wiśniewski, H. M., Grundke-Iqbal, I. and Terry, R. D. Neurofibrillary Pathology: An Update In K. Nandy and I. Sherwin (eds.) *The Aging Brain and Senile Dementia.* New York: Plenum Press, 1977.
15. Wiśniewski, H. M., Narang, H. K., Corsellis, J. A. N. and Terry, R. D. Ultrastructural studies of the neuropil and neurofibrillary tangles in Alzheimer's disease and post-traumatic dementia. *J. Neuropathol. Exper. Neurol.* **35**: 367 (1976).
16. Tomlinson, B. E. and Henderson, G. Some quantitative cerebral findings in normal and demented old people. In R. D. Terry and S. Gershon (eds.)

Neurobiology of Aging. New York: Raven Press pp. 183–209, 1976.

17. Blocq, P. and Marinesco, G. Sur les lésions et la pathologie de l'epilepsie dite essentiale. *Semin. Med. Pans,* **12:** 445–446 (1892).

18. Simchowicz, T. Histoligische Studien über die Senildemenz. *Hist. histopath. Arb.* **4:** 267 (1910).

19. Wiśniewski, H. M., Johnson, A. B., Raine, C. S., Kay, W. J. and Terry, R. D. Senile plaques and cerebral amyloidosis in aged dogs. A histochemical and ultrastructural study. *Lab. Invest.* **23:** 287–296 (1976).

20. Wiśniewski, H. M., Ghetti, B. and Terry, R. D. Neuritic (senile) plaques and filamentous changes in aged Rhesus monkeys. *J. Neuropathol. Exp. Neurol.* **32:** 566–584 (1973).

21. Jayne, E. P. Cytochemical studies of age pigments in the human heart. *J. Gerontol.* **5:** 319–325 (1950).

22. Strehler, B. L., Mark, D. D., Mildvan, A. S. and Gee, M. S. Rate and magnitude of age pigment accumulation in the human myocardium. *J. Gerontol.* **14:** 430–439 (1959).

23. Brody, H. The deposition of aging pigment in the human cerebral cortex. *J. Gerontol.* **15:** 258–261.

24. Dayan, A. D. Comparative neuropathology of aging. Studies on the brains of 47 species of vertebrates. *Brain* **94:** 31–42 (1971).

25. Brizzee, K. R., Ordy, J. M. and Kaack, B. Early appearance and regional differences in intraneuronal and extraneuronal lipofuscin accumulation with age in the non-human primate (*Macaca mulatta*). *J. Gerontol.* **29:** 366–381 (1974).

26. Miquel, J., Tappel, A. L., Dillard, C. J., Herman, M. M. and Bensch, K. G. Fluorescent products and lysosomal components in aging *Drosophila melanogaster. J. Gerontol.* **29:** 622–637 (1974).

27. Braack, H. Über das Neurolipofuscin in der unteren olive und dem Nucleus dentatus cerebelle in Gehirn des Menschen. *Z. Zellforsch* **121:** 573–592 (1971).

28. Nandy, K. Properties of neuronal lipofuscin pigment in mice. *Acta Neuropathol.* **19:** 25–32 (1971).

29. Nishioka, N., Takahata, N. and Iizuka, R. Histochemical studies on the lipopigments in the nerve cells. A comparison with lipofuscin and ceroid pigment. *Acta Neuropathol.* **11:** 174–181 (1968).

30. Pallis, C. A., Duckett, S. and Pearse, A. G. E. Diffuse lipofuscinosis of the central nervous system. *Neurol.* **17:** 381–394 (1967).

31. Brünk, U. and Ericsson, J. L. E. Electron microscopical studies on the rat brain neurons. Localization of acid phosphotase and mode of formation of lipofuscin bodies. *J. Ultrastruct. Res.* **38:** 1–15 (1972).

32. Porta, E. A. and Hartroft, W. S. Lipid pigments in relation to aging and dietary factors (lipo-

fuscin). In M. Wolman (ed.) *Pigments in Pathology.* New York: Academic Press, 1969.

33. Miyigashi, T., Takashata, M. and Iijuka, R. Electronmicroscopic studies on the lipopigments in the cerebral cortex nerve cells of senile and vitamin E-deficient rats. *Acta Neuropathol.* **9:** 7–17 (1971).

34. Hannover, A. *Videnskapsselsk Naturvidensk.* Math. Afh. Copenhagen, 10, 1842.

35. Borst, M. *Pathologishe Histologie.* Leipzig, **210:** Vogel, 1922.

36. Moatamed, F. Cell frequencies in human inferior olivary complex. *J. Comp. Neurol.* **128:** 109–116 (1966).

37. Monagle, R. D. and Brody, H. The effects of age upon the main nucleus of the inferior olive in the human. *J. Comp. Neurol.* **155:** 61–66 (1974).

38. Reichel, W., Hollander, J., Clark, J. H. and Strehler, B. L. Lipofuscin pigment accumulation as a function of age and distribution in rodent brain. *J. Gerontol.* **23:** 71–78 (1968).

39. Brody, H., and Vijayashankar, N. Anatomical changes in the nervous system In C. E. Finch and L. Hayflick (eds.) *Handbook of the Biology of Aging.* New York: Van Nostrand Reinhold, 1977.

40. Fang, H. Observations on aging characteristics of cerebral blood vessels, macroscopic and microscopic features. In R. D. Terry and S. Gershon (eds.) *Neurobiology of Aging.* New York: Raven Press, 1976.

41. Reese, T. S. and Kainovsky, M. J. Fine structural localization of a blood-brain barrier to exogenous peroxidase. *J. Cell Biol.* **34:** 207–217 (1967).

42. Bakay, L. Alteration of the brain barrier system in pathological states. In A. Lajtha (ed.) *Handbook of Neurochemistry,* Vol. 7: *Pathological Chemistry of the Nervous System.* New York: Plenum Press, 1972.

43. Nandy, K. Neuronal degeneration in aging and after experimental injury. *Exp. Gerontol.* **7:** 303–311 (1972).

44. Nandy, K. Significance of brain-reactive antibodies in serum of aged mice. *J. Gerontol.* **30:** 412–416 (1975).

45. Rapoport, S. I., Ohno, K. and Petigrew, K. D. Blood-brain barrier permeability in senescent rats. *J. Gerontol.* (In Press) (1979-March).

46. Bondareff, W. and Narotzky, R. Age changes in the neuronal microenvironment. *Science,* **176:** 1135–1136 (1972).

47. Jacobson, Marcus. *Developmental Neurobiology,* 2nd edition. New York: Plenum Press, 1978.

48. Konigsmark, B. W. and Murphy, E. A. Volume of ventral cochlear nucleus in man: Its relationship to neuronal population and age. *J. Neuropathol. Exp. Neurol,* **31:** 304–316 (1972).

49. Ordy, J. M. and Schjeide, O. A. Neurobiological aspects of maturation and aging. In D. H. Ford (ed.) *Progress in Brain Research.* Vol. 40. Amsterdam: Elsevier, 1973.

50. Wright, E. A. and Spink, J. M. A study of the loss of nerve cells in the central nervous system in relation to age. *Gerontologia* **3**: 277–287 (1959).

51. Brody, H. Organization of cerebral cortex III. A study of aging in the human cerebral cortex. *J. Comp. Neurol.* **102**: 511–556 (1955).

52. Brody, H. Aging of the vertebrate brain. In M. Rockstein and M. L. Sussman (eds.) *Development and Aging in the Nervous System* New York: Academic Press, pp. 121–133, 1973.

53. Brody, H. Structural changes in the aging nervous system. In H. T. Blumentahl, (ed.) *Interdisciplinary Topics in Gerontology,* Vol. 7, New York/Based: Karger pp. 9–21, 1970.

54. Hanley, T. "Neuronal Fallout" in aging brain: A critical review of the quantitative data. *Age and Ageing* **3**: 133–151 (1974).

55. Colon, E. J. The elderly brain. A quantitative analysis of cerebral cortex in two cases. *Psychiat. Neurol. Neurochir.* **75**: 261–270 (1972).

56. Shefer, V. F. Absolute number of neurons and thickness of cerebral cortex during aging, senile and vascular dementia and Pick's and Alzheimer's Disease. *Neurosci. Beh, Physiol.* **6**: 319–324 (1973).

57. Henderson, G., Tomlinson, B. E. and Weightman, D. Cell counts in the human cerebral cortex using a traditional and an automatic method. *J. Neurol. Sci.,* **25**: 129–144 (1975).

58. Brizzee, K. R. Gross morphometric analyses and quantitative histology of the aging brain. In J. M. Ordy and K. R. Brizzee (eds.) *Neurobiology of Aging.* New York: Plenum Press, 1975.

59. Feldman, M. L. and Dowd, C. Loss of dendritic spines in aging cerebral cortex. *Anat. Embryol.* **148**: 279–301 (1975).

60. Scheibel, M. E. and Scheibel, A. B. Structural changes in the aging brain. In H. Brody, D. Harman, and J. M. Ordy (eds.) *Clinical, Morphologic and Neurochemical Aspects in the Aging Central Nervous System.* New York: Raven Press, 1975.

61. Landfield, P. W., Rose, G., Sandles, L., Wohlstadter, T. C. and Lynch, G. Patterns of astroglial hypertroply and neuronal degeneration in the hippocampus of aged, memory-deficient rats. *J. Gerontol.* **32**: 3–12 (1977).

62. Landfield, P. W. and Lynch, G. Impaired monosynaptic potentiation in vitro hippocampal slices from aged, memory-deficient rats. *J. Gerontol.* **32**: 523–533 (1977).

63. Landfield, P. W., Waymire, J. C. and Lynch, G. Hippocampal aging and adrenocorticoids: Quantitative correlations. *Science* **202**: 1098–1102 (1978).

64. Greenough, W. T., West, R. W. and DeVoogd, T. J. Subsynaptic plate perforations: Changes with age and experience in the rat. *Science,* **202**: 1096–1098 (1978).

65. Hall, T. C., Miller, A. K. H. and Corsellis, J. A. N. Variations in the human Purkinje cell population according to age and sex. *Neuropathol. Appl. Neurobiol.* **1**: 267–292 (1975).

66. Hodge, C. F. Changes in ganglion cells from birth to senile death. Observations on man and honey bee. *J. Physiol.* **17**: 129–134 (1894).

67. Archambault, LaS. Parenchymatous atrophy of the cerebellum. *J. Nervous Mental Disease* **48**: 273 (1918).

68. Ellis, R. S. A preliminary quantitative study of Purkinje cells in normal, subnormal and senescent human cerebella. *J. Comp. Neurol.* **30**: 229–252 (1919).

69. Ellis, R. S. Norms for some structural changes in the human cerebellum from birth to old age. *J. Comp. Neurol.* **32**: 1–33 (1920).

70. Harms, J. W. Alterscheinungen in Hirn von Affen und Menschen. *Zool. Anz.* **74**: 249–256 (1927).

71. Inukai, T. On the loss of Purkinje cells with advancing age from cerebellar cortex of Albino rat. *J. Comp. Neurol.* **45**: 1–31 (1928).

72. Delorenzi, E. Constanza numerica delle cellule del Purkinje in individui di varia eta. *Bull. Soc. Ital. Biol. Sper.* **6**: 80–82 (1931).

73. Wilcox, H. H. A quantitative study of Purkinje cells in guinea pigs. *J. Geronol.* **11**: 442 (1956).

74. Van Buskirk, C. The seventh nerve complex. *J. Comp. Neurol.* **82**: 303–333 (1945).

75. Konigsmark, B. W. and Murphy, E. A. Neuronal populations in the human brain. *Nature,* **299**: 1335 (1970).

76. Vijayashankar, N. and Brody, H. Aging in the human brain stem. A study of the nucleus of the trochlear nerve. *Acta Anat.* **99**: 169–172 (1977).

77. Vijayashankar, N. and Brody, H. A study of aging in the human abducens nucleus. *J. Comp. Neurol.* **173**: 433–437 (1977).

78. McGeer, P. L., McGeer, E. G. and Suzuki, J. S. Aging and extrapyramidal function. *Arch. Neurol.* **34**: 33–35 (1977).

79. Vijayashankar, N. and Brody, H. A quantitative study of the pigmented neurons in the nuclei locus coeruleus and subcoeruleus in man as related to aging. *J. Neuropathol. and Exp. Neurol.* (1979). (in press)

80. Bugiani, O., Salvarani, S., Perdelli, F., Mancardi, G. L. and Leonardi, A. Nerve cell loss with aging in the putamen. *Eur. Neurol.* **17**: 286–291 (1978).

81. Gajdusek, D. C. and Zigas, V. Degenerative disease of the central nervous system in New Guinea: The endemic occurrence of "kuru" in the native population. *N. Engl. J. Med.* **257**: 30:974–978 (1957).

82. Gajdusek, D. C. and Zigas, V. Kuru: clinical, pathological and epidemiological study of an acute progressive degenerative disease of the central nervous system among natives of the eastern highlands of New Guinea. *Am. J. Med.,* **26**: 442–469 (1959).

83. Gajdusek, D. C. Slow virus infections of the nervous system. *N. Engl. J. Med.* **276:** 392–400 (1967).

84. Gajdusek, D. C. and Gibbs, C. J. Jr. Slow, latent and temporate virus infections of the central nervous system. *Res. Publ. Assoc. Rev. Nerv. Ment. Dis.* **44:** 254–280 (1968).

85. Sigurdsson, B. Observations on three slow infections of sheep: Reprint of three papers. *Bird. Vet. J.* **110:** 255–270; 307–322; 341–354 (1954).

86. Lewis, A. J. *Mechanisms of Neurological Disease.* Boston: Little Brown, 1st ed., 1976.

87. Katzman, R., Terry, R. D. and Bick, K. L. Recommendations of the Nosology, Epidemiology, and Etiology and Pathophysiology Commissions of the Workshop-Conference on Alzheimer's Disease-Senile Dementia and Related Disorders. In R. Katzman, R. D. Terry, and K. L. Bick (eds.). New York: Raven Press, 1978.

88. Tower, D. B. Alzheimer's disease-senile dementia and related disorders: Neurobiological status. In R. Katzman, R. B. Terry and K. L. Bick (eds.) *Alzheimer's Disease: Senile Dementia and Related Disorders.* New York:Raven Press, 1978.

89. Larsson, T., Sjögren, T. and Jacobson, G. Senile dementia. *Acta Psychiatr., Scand (Suppl. 167)* **39:** 3–259 (1963).

90. Katzman, R. The prevalance and malignancy of Alzheimer disease. *Arch. Neurol.* **33:** 217–218 (1976).

91. Sjögren, T., Sjögren, H. and Lindgren, A. Morbus Alzheimer and Morbus Pick. Genetic, chemical and patho-anatomical study. *Acta psychiat et neurol. Scand. supp. 82* (1952).

92. Huntington, G. On chorea. *Medical and Surgical Reporter* **26:** 317–321 (1872).

93. Hornykiewicz, O. Neurochemical pathology and pharmacology of brain dopamine and acetylcholine: Rational basis for the current drug treatment of Parkinsonism. In F. Plum (ed.) *Recent Advances in Neurology.* Philadelphia:Davis, 1970.

94. Lewy, F. H. Zur pathölogischen Anatomie der Paralysis agitans. *Deutsche Zeits für Nervenheil.* **50:** 50–55 (1913).

95. Wernicke, C. *Lehrbuch der Gehirukrankheiten, Band 2.* Kassel: Fischer, 1881.

96. Adams, R. D. and Victor, M. *Principles of Neurology.* New York: McGraw-Hill, 1977.

97. Hachinski, V. C., Lassen, N. A. and Marshall J. Multi-infarct dementia: A cause of mental deterioration in the elderly. *Lancet* **2:** 207–210 (1974).

98. O'Brien, M. D. and Mallett, B. L. Cerebral cortex perfusion rates in dementia. *J. Neurol. Neurosurg., Psychiat.* **33:** 497–500 (1970).

99. Hachinski, V. C., Iliff, L. D., Zilhka, E., Dubouky, G. H., McAllister, V. L., Marshall, J., Russell, R. W. R. and Symon, L. Cerebral blood flow in dementia. *Arch. Neurol.* **32:** 632–637 (1975).

100. Adams, R. D. and Vander Eecken, H. M. Vascular diseases of the brain. *Ann. Rev. Med.* **4:** 213–252 (1953).

101. Fisher, C. M. The arterial lesions underlying lacunes. *Acta Neuropathol.* **12:** 1–15 (1969).

102. Fisher, C. M. Lacunes: Small, deep cerebral infarcts. *Neurology* **15:** 774–784 (1965).

Chapter 3
Brain Physiology of Aging

T. Samorajski, Ph.D.
and
James Hartford, M. D.
Texas Research Institute of Mental Sciences

INTRODUCTION

The central role of the nervous and endocrine systems in regulating physiologic processes throughout the body has been established after many years of research. How these systems respond to aging is therefore an important question. Within recent years, extracellular factors such as hormones and neurotransmitter substances have been implicated as important regulators of cellular activities. The individual steps in many essential metabolic pathways have been identified and elaborated.[1] In contrast, little is known about the homeostatic mechanism by which complex organisms coordinate the metabolic and physiological activities of a number of organ systems. Actually, aging may be more a function of the breakdown in integrative mechanisms than of changes at the cellular level of organization.[2] Since uniformity of internal environment is achieved through the interaction of neural and endocrine systems, attention is now focused on brain regions which may be critical for homeostasis. This chapter will examine the effects of aging on some of the integrative processes involved.

Numerous studies[3,4] have provided evidence that the integration between neurotransmitters, hormones and other regulatory substances takes place in the hypothalamus. As presently conceived, hypothalamic neurons sensitive to changes in regulatory substances activate the pituitary and other endocrine glands which collectively play an important role in coordinating internal homeostatic mechanism. It is possible, therefore, that regulatory hormonal agents and afferent projections from other regions of the brain affecting target cells in the hypothalamus also regulate the sequence and chronology of many cellular events throughout the body during aging.[4,5,6,7,8]

More specifically, the significance of the hypothalamus as an aging clock is based on the possibility that age-associated changes in neurons may alter homeostatic systems in such a way that a pathologic process may develop resulting in illness and ultimately death. In this sense, structural and functional changes in the hypothalamus may have consequences far beyond those normally associated with cell disease or cell death in other regions of the brain or body.

THE PYRAMIDAL AND EXTRAPYRAMIDAL SYSTEMS

Morphological and biochemical changes in the old nervous system often appear localized or restricted to specific regions of the brain.[9] The following areas are among the more susceptible: the corpus striatum (caudate nucleus, putamen and globus pallidus), the limbic system (hippocampus, amygdala, septal area, cingulate gyrus, anterior thalamic nuclei, fornix, and mammillary nuclei of the hypothalamus), the hypothalamus, and a number of brain stem structures including the locus caeruleus, the substantia nigra, the center median of the thalamus, the dorsal nucleus of the vagus, the inferior olive and dentate nucleus and the basal nucleus of Reichert.[10]

Anatomically, the basal ganglia and certain other subcortical structures make up the extrapyramidal system which exists in parallel to the pyramidal (corticospinal) system. Together, they coordinate involuntary and voluntary motor activity. Both systems are influenced by subcortical nuclear structures which include the striatum, the subthalamic nuclei, the substantia nigra, and possibly, the neocerebellum.[11] Thus, deterioration of any of these structures may result in movement disorders.

With advancing age, certain neurologic disorders occur so often that they are considered to be part of the normal pattern of aging. Changes in motor phenomena are fairly common; there is a slowness and hesitancy of many movements.[10] Fine tremors, often accompanied by facial grimaces resembling some aspects of tardive dyskinesia, are seen in many individuals. Signs of rigidity, hypokinesia, and flexed posture may also become evident. Parkinson's disease, which is more common and more severe with advancing age, presents many of the same symptoms although the magnitude of these changes is greater in parkinsonism than would be expected of an individual of the same age without the disease. All of these symptoms have been linked to dysfunction of the extrapyramidal system[10,11,12] and they point to involvement of the basal ganglia in the development of senescence. The role of various neurotransmitters in the regulation of neuronal activity in the basal ganglia has been described in reviews by Roth and Bunney[13] and van Woert.[14]

There are other age-susceptible areas that deserve attention. The following examples may be illustrative of the involutional processes involved either during normal aging or in the presence of functional impairments that occur during the life span: damage to the olive and dentate nucleus may result in intention tremor and ataxia; the locus caeruleus and centromedian nucleus of the thalamus are involved in sleep regulation; and the substantia nigra and some regions of the basal ganglia may be associated with initiation of movement and speed of motor ability.[10] Involvement of the hippocampus is believed by some to be related to deficits in spatial memory.[15] The nucleus of Reichert is believed to be involved in emotionality, attention span, and difficulties in decision making.[16] It is of interest that several areas of the brain stem (substantia nigra, locus caeruleus and dorsal nucleus of the vagus) have a high content of neuromelanin and, as will be seen later, are also involved in the synthesis and regulation of specific monoaminergic fiber systems. Many of the fibers of these systems terminate in the hypothalamus.

THE HYPOTHALAMUS

There are at least three main morphologic features to consider in the aging hypothalamus: changes in number and metabolic efficiency of neurons and glia; changes in the blood vascular system; and pathologic processes such as amyloidosis and other immunological features related to aging. Since one of the most fundamental manifestations of aging is a decline in cell number, most investigators of the aging brain emphasize neuronal loss as an important feature. This article also will consider cellular changes in the hypothalamus as an important aspect of the aging process, but in addition, will examine other tissue constituents since changes in one may affect the others.

Neuronal-Glial Morphology

The aging hypothalamus has been the subject of several physiologic and morphologic studies, including analysis of its secretory and chemical function. Frolkis, Bezrukov, Duplenko and Genis[17] noted that there was a reduction of neurosecretory activity in the neurons of the hypothalamohypophysial system of old rats. It is known that hypothalamic secretory mechanisms are of vital importance in coordinating endocrine response to stress. Observations on Golgi-impregnated neurons from the hypothalamus of aging mice revealed a remarkable series of deteriorative changes.[18] In the early stages of aging, many neurons were observed with irregularities of the somato-dendritic profile and a decrease in the number of spinelike processes. Later, the appearance of these neurons was characterized by a further loss of dendritic processes and the presence of swollen or severely distorted somata. This spectrum of changes was most frequently observed in rostral hypothalamic neurons. In this same area, Frolkis, Bezrukov, Duplenko and Genis[17] often observed many degenerated neurons of an elongated and irregular shape with poorly outlined pyknotic nuclei.

The reaction of neuroglial cells to aging changes in the hypothalamus has not been examined in detail. If we can extrapolate from results found in other regions of the brain[19,20] to the hypothalamus, we might expect to find a proliferation of glial cells with age. In a recent study of neuroglial cells in the rat auditory cortex, Vaughan and Peters[21] found little change in the population of astrocytes and oligodendrocytes, while the number of microglial cells in-

creased by about 65% in the same animals between the ages of 3 and 27 months. In addition, microglial cells showed a striking accumulation of inclusion material which was most obvious in the oldest animals. Accumulation of inclusion material was regarded as an indication of phagocytic activity. From these findings it may be anticipated that similar increases in neuroglial cells might occur in the hypothalamus in response to age-associated neuronal degeneration. An increase in glia may reflect a compensatory process of the brain to overcome neuronal loss or changes in neuronal functions with age.[22]

Electron microscopic examination of the neurons of the rostral hypothalamus of the aging guinea pig by Hasan, Glees, and El-Ghazzawi,[23] revealed a significant accumulation of lipofuscin pigment. The number and size of the granules increased with advancing age. Further, the morphology of aging in the anterior hypothalamus differed significantly from that described for the mammillary nuclei of the posterior hypothalamus.[24] In view of the increasing accumulation of intraneuronal lipofuscin—presumably at the expense of cell volume—and the progessive loss of dendritic surfaces with age, it is likely that neurons of the anterior hypothalamus may become increasingly unable to respond adequately even to minimal environmental challenge. This condition may be aggravated even further by age-related changes in other regions of the brain with an afferent input into an already impoverished hypothalamic neuropile.

From the morphologic evidence presented, it appears that individual hypothalamic nuclei age in different ways and at different rates. Such findings are in agreement with physiologic studies by Frolkis, Bezrukov, Duplenko and Genis.[17] They found that with age, sensitivity to electrical stimulation increased in some areas of the hypothalamus and decreased in others. The sensitivity of various hypothalamic structures to direct injections of neurotransmitter substances was also variable with increasing age. This unequal distribution of structural changes and physiologic responses in the aging hypothalamus led Frolkis to suggest that disregulation at the hypothalamic level may accelerate aging throughout the body and cause an early onset of age-related pathology. Another equally plausible hypothesis has been advanced by Dilman[25] who suggested that age-associated changes at the molecular level may produce an increase in the threshold of sensitivity of hypothalamic neurons to feedback control. It seems probable that a change in hypothalamic threshold could have far reaching consequences for homeostatic mechanisms. While convincing evidence has not as yet been presented to substantiate either theory, they remain as attractive hypotheses for further experimentation.

Autoimmunity

Two theories have been advanced concerning the nature of physiologic decrements associated with aging. One theory proposes that aging is a genetically controlled cellular process resulting from a loss of fidelity in protein biosynthesis i.e., a process of misspecification resulting in synthesis of "not self" protein.[26,27,28] In this regard, Hayflick[29] suggested that functional losses within cells play key roles in senescence and that changes in nondividing (postmitotic) cells may exert the most significant effects. A second theory proposes that aging is a consequence of detrimental changes in the immune system which may result in a variety of autoimmune disorders.[30] Altered proteins may no longer be recognized by the immune system as "self" and antibody formation (autoantibody) against these may take place. Fernandes, Good and Yunis[31] associated age-related immunodeficiency characterized by thymic and immunologic involution at sexual maturity with autoimmune disorders of old age.

Blumenthal[32] proposed that a combination of protein misspecification at the cellular level, and changes in the immune system, may be the cause of the physiologic decrements associated with aging (the error-autoimmune theory). He also suggested that aging neurons, just as other cells, may be susceptible to misspecification and that abnormal changes in cell nuclei (dyskaryosis) may be a manifestation of a nuclear DNA-RNA disorder. Further, the failure of fidelity of synthesis derived from DNA-RNA may result in a change in cell membrane characteristics which would have the effect of interference with neuroendocrine mechanisms as well as impluse transmission between neurons. In the hypothalamus this may involve an alteration of membrane receptor sensitivity to hormones and transmitter substances. A further consequence of an altered neuronal sensitivity may be a change in the endocrine system which may result in failure of the immune and circulatory systems.[33]

Immunological factors have been associated with the aging process in the brain by several investigators.[32,34,35] An increase in serum immunoglobulin (gamma globulin) and a decrease of albumen with age is a characteristic of many species including man. Ingram, Phegan and Blumenthal[36] reported an increase with age in neuron-binding gamma globulin in human serum. Nandy[34] reported that brain-reactive antibody increased progressively with age in mouse serum. More recently, Miller and Blumenthal[37] reported the presence of a neuron-binding autoantibody in rat serum. Nandy[35] injected radio-labeled gamma globulin into mice and compared the levels of radioactivity present in various organs. While a lower level of radioactivity was consistently noted in the brain compared to other organs, the hypothalamus showed a significantly higher level of isotope than samples of cerebrum and cerebellum. Whether individual hypothalamic nuclei differ in binding brain-reactive antibody is unclear at the present time.

Vascularity

Vascular factors are often involved in producing softening of, or focal hemorrhagic lesions in, the human brain in old age. It is not clear, however, what part the cerebro-vascular factor plays in the genesis of senility. Machado-Salas, Scheibel and Scheibel[18] made a comparison of vascularity of the hypothalamus of mice at different ages. Their preliminary impression was that of a disruption of vascular architecture as well as a decrease in the number of branches, especially in the magnocellular nucleus. Such changes might produce an impairment of the blood-brain barrier.

Vessels of the pituitary-portal system differ from most of the other blood vessels of the brain by their relatively greater permeability to blood constituents and the presence of a basement membrane surrounded by connective tissue in place of the usual astrocytic end-feet. Connective tissue bound blood vessels of other organs such as the kidney, retina and muscle frequently reveal a thickening of the capillary basement membrane with age.[38] A thickening of the capillary basement membrane in pituitary-portal vessels during aging could have consequences for the transport of "releasing" factors from the hypothalamus to the anterior pituitary. Hunziker and associates[39] conducted morphometric studies of aging human cortex and reported an increased capillary density with age. Apparently, the capillary network of the aging brain is able to adapt to changing metabolic needs. Whether capillary alterations in the hypothalamus with age are significant in hypothalamic function remains to be determined.

NEUROENDOCRINOLOGY

The rate at which programmed changes develop can be influenced by a variety of environmental factors such as food intake,[40,41] temperature,[42,43] stress[44,45] and ionizing radiation.[46] The effect appears to be mediated through the hypothalamic-pituitary axis.[47] Hypothalamic biogenic amines have a major role in regulating pituitary function. Recent work on the localization of neurotransmitter substances in different regions of the brain has demonstrated that their concentration and turnover can change in response to different exteroceptive and interoceptive stimuli.[48] Endocrine stimuli alter anterior pituitary release by some kind of competition between the number of available molecules in the pituitary and turnover of one or more of the amines in the hypothalamus.[4] Presumably, the three biogenic amines dopamine (DA), norepinephrine (NE) and 5-hydroxytryptamine (5-HT, serotonin), influence anterior pituitary hormone secretion by the release of peptidergic releasing or inhibiting factors from nerve terminals in the hypothalamus into the portal circulation (Fig. 3–1). There is as yet only limited evidence as to which neurotransmitter(s) is involved in the release of a particular anterior pituitary hormone. Also, other putative neurotransmitters such as acetycholine (ACh), gamma-amino-butyric acid (GABA), glycine and others may act on DA, NE and 5-HT neurons, and in turn may be influenced by them. The strongest support for the argument that hypothalamic neurotransmitter substances control anterior pituitary function has been provided by studies of male and female reproductive senescence in rodents.

Reproduction (LH, FSH, and Prolactin)

Recent evidence suggests that depressed catecholamine and enhanced serotonin metabolism may underlie the cessation of cyclic gonadotropin production in female rats.[49] Controversy remains, however, as to whether they inhibit or stimulate release of LH and FSH.[50] Only one gonadotropin releasing hormone (LRH or GnRH) has been isolated from the anterior hypothalamus that has been associated with the release of both LH and FSH.[51] The administration of L-dopa, epinephrine or iproniazide, a monoamine oxidase inhibitor which increases brain catecholamine[52] was able to reinitiate estrous cycles of senescent female rats.[53,54] Further, the atropic ovaries of old

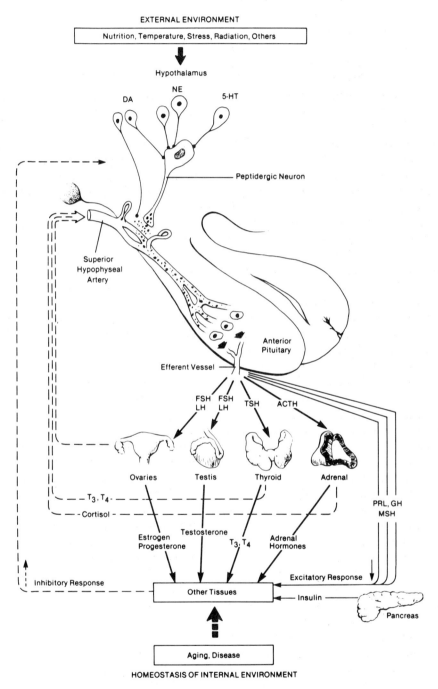

EXTERNAL ENVIRONMENT

Nutrition, Temperature, Stress, Radiation, Others

Hypothalamus

NE

DA   5-HT

Peptidergic Neuron

Superior
Hypophyseal
Artery

Anterior
Pituitary

Efferent Vessel

FSH FSH   TSH   ACTH
LH   LH

Ovaries   Testis   Thyroid   Adrenal

PRL, GH
MSH

T₃, T₄

Cortisol

Estrogen   Testosterone   Adrenal
Progesterone   T₃, T₄   Hormones

Excitatory Response

Inhibitory Response   Other Tissues   Insulin

Pancreas

Aging, Disease

HOMEOSTASIS OF INTERNAL ENVIRONMENT

Fig. 3–1. Diagrammatic illustration of external and internal environmental factors mediated by hypothalamic neurotransmitter and anterior pituitary and peripheral endocrine gland hormones. Various releasing or inhibitory factors and biogenic amines reach the anterior pituitary through the pituitary portal system.

female rats could be made functional with appropriate stimulation by gonadotropic hormones.[55] There are, however, some major differences between neuroendocrine mechanisms which control ovarian cycles in rodents and those which control ovarian function of the higher primates.[55] The ovaries of aging women, for example, tend to become fibrotic and nonresponsive to gonadotropic hormone stimulation.

Aging male rats also show a decline in fertility. Serum luteinizing hormone (LH) is lower and prolactin is higher in old than in young male rats.[56] Also, there is a decrease in spermatogenesis.[57] As in aging female rats, there is a decrease in hypothalamic catecholamine activity and an increase in serotonin activity.[4] These changes in brain biogenic amine or other hormonally sensitive molecules are believed to account for some of the reproductive decline in aging.

Probably more is known about the secretion of prolactin than any other hormone of the anterior pituitary. Agents in the hypothalamus that regulate prolactin release include a prolactin inhibitory factor (PIF), dopamine which can depress prolactin release, and acetylcholine which may act by stimulating dopaminergic pathways. The hypothalamus also contains substances that can promote prolactin release including a presumed polypeptide prolactin releasing factor (PRF), serotonin, and a tripeptide thyrotropic releasing factor (TRH) which can release both prolactin and thyroid stimulating hormone.[4]

In aging humans, as in the aging rat, deficiencies begin to occur in each of the reproductive organs but the primary fault appears to lie in the hypothalamus which becomes less responsive to stimuli that control the release of LH, FSH, and prolactin. There is some evidence in aging humans of a decrease in brain catecholamines[58] and an increase in monoamine oxidase[59] but the relationship of these changes to reproductive senescence is not clear. As yet, little is known about the responsiveness of the hypothalamus-pituitary system in aging humans to stimuli controlling the release of gonadotropins and other hormones. To this end, the rat has served as a useful model for providing guidelines for the study of reproductive aging in man.

Growth Hormone (GH)

Growth hormone release is regulated by a dual system of hypothalamic hormone factors, one inhibitory (GIF) and the other excitatory (GRF). Release of these hormones is, in turn, regulated by monoaminergic neurons. Pharmacologic studies of specific receptor agonists and antagonists indicate that GH secretion in man is facilitated by both dopaminergic and noradrenergic α-receptor stimulation, and inhibited by noradrenergic ß-receptor stimulation. Certain species differences seem to exist with respect to GH response to 5-HT. Oral administration of L-tryptophan or 5-hydroxytryptophan causes a slight increase of GH release in man and monkey and a decrease in rat.[4]

Other studies have examined the effects of melatonin on GH secretion. Administration of melatonin is reported both to stimulate GH release and to block release from insulin hypoglycemia due to differences in the time course of action of melatonin. It appears, therefore, that DA and noradrenergic ß-receptor stimulation promotes the release of GH and noradrenergic ß-receptor stimulation inhibits the release of GH. The role of 5-HT and melatonin in growth hormone release remains to be clarified.

The results of studies on growth hormone physiology in relation to aging in the human are difficult to interpret. The effects of aging are complicated by sex differences, the influence of obesity, and the fact that very few healthy older subjects have been investigated.[60] Such data as are available for mammals indicate that basal plasma levels of growth hormone remain unchanged with aging.[61] Also, the human pituitary content of GH is relatively constant with age.[62] However, some middle aged humans do not secrete GH during sleep as do younger individuals.[63] Other studies indicate that morning growth hormone secretion of women is lost after menopause.[64] Finch[61] has interpreted these findings as evidence that aging effects central neuronal mechanisms more than the pituitary production of GH.

Thyroid Stimulating Hormone (TSH)

The hypothalamus is believed to release a thyritropine-releasing hormone (TRH) from peptidergic neurons into the portal vessels of the median eminence and thereby stimulate release of TSH from the anterior pituitary. Norepinephrine appears to stimulate the release of TSH and DA, presumably, exerts an inhibitory effect on TSH secretion. The role of 5-HT in the control of TSH secretion is uncertain.[4]

The plasma TSH content of humans[65] and C57BL/6J male mice[61] does not change with age. However, pituitary response to administration of synthetic thyrotropin-releasing hormone (TRH) is reduced in aged men[66] but not in aged women.[67] Whether these differences are due to hypothalamic rather than pituitary deficiencies remains to be clarified.

Adrenocorticotropic Hormone (ACTH)

Release of ACTH from the anterior pituitary may be mediated directly by release of corticotropic releasing factor (CRF) from the hypothalamus and indirectly through the peripheral nervous systems. Norepinephrine appears to be the main central inhibitor of ACTH release. GABA and melatonin also inhibit ACTH release via NE stimulation. Both serotonin and ACh increase ACTH release, presumably by inducing CRF release in the hypothalamus.[4]

The pituitary content and basal plasma levels of ACTH do not appear to change with age in humans.[68,69] A generally adequate response to minimal levels of ACTH and a relatively intact negative feedback effect of plasma cortical levels in elderly individuals indicate that there is no obvious deficit in the hypothalamus-pituitary-adrenal axis with age.[60]

Comments

At the present time there is evidence for the existence of five "releasing" factors and two "inhibitory" factors in the hypothalamus which control the release of six different hormones from the anterior pituitary gland. Some of these hypothalamic hormones have now been isolated and synthesized and are proving to be of great importance in the treatment of many diseases and disorders of the hypothalamus. The release of the peptidergic factors or hormones from their nerve terminals in the hypothalamus into the portal circulation is in turn influenced by NE, DA, 5-HT and other centrally acting putative neurotransmitters. The possible actions of NE, DA and 5-HT on release of each anterior pituitary hormone have been summarized by Meites, Simpkins, Bruni and Advis[4] and are shown in Figure 3–2. Some monoaminergic systems may be particularly sensitive to aging.[3,61] Thus, losses of biogenic amines and changes in enzymes and metabolites of brain monoamines may be critical for hormonally regulated cell function throughout the body. Finch[5] has proposed that catecholamines containing neurons of the hypothalamus may serve as pacemakers of aging by controlling interactions between extrinsic factors and target cells with feedback interrelationships.

NEUROTRANSMITTER SUBSTANCES

Synthesis and Metabolism

To better understand how neurotransmitters may function in the hypothalamic regulation of aging, we will review briefly some general aspects of their synthesis and metabolism. The process of synthesis, release, receptor-effector response and inactivation requires precursors and various enzymes. Fig. 3–3 lists the major transmitters in the CNS and the enzymes associated with their synthesis and metabolism.

Acetylcholine (AcCh) is synthesized in the presynaptic component of the cholinergic neuron by the transfer of an acetyl group

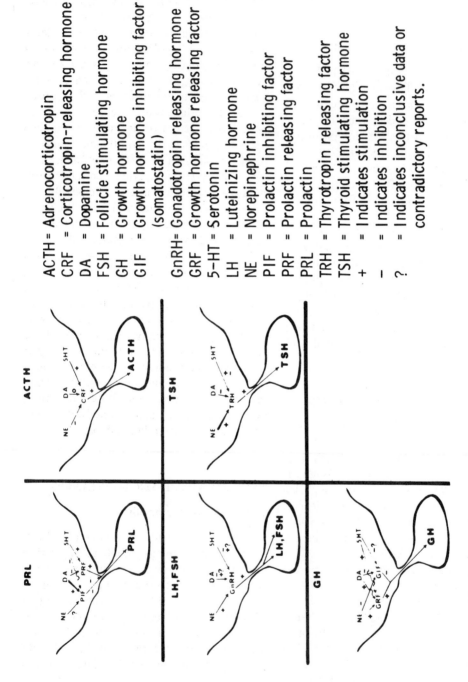

ACTH = Adrenocorticotropin
CRF = Corticotropin-releasing hormone
DA   = Dopamine
FSH = Follicle stimulating hormone
GH   = Growth hormone
GIF = Growth hormone inhibiting factor
       (somatostatin)
GnRH = Gonadotropin releasing hormone
GRF = Growth hormone releasing factor
5-HT = Serotonin
LH   = Luteinizing hormone
NE   = Norepinephrine
PIF = Prolactin inhibiting factor
PRF = Prolactin releasing factor
PRL = Prolactin
TRH = Thyrotropin releasing factor
TSH = Thyroid stimulating hormone
+   = Indicates stimulation
−   = Indicates inhibition
?   = Indicates inconclusive data or
       contradictory reports.

Fig. 3–2.   Possible actions of NE, DA and 5–HT on release of anterior pituitary hormones via hypothalamic pep-tidergic hormones. Not shown are the possible interactions of these amines with each other or with other neurotransmitters. (With permission of Meites, Simpkins, Bruni and Advis,[4] and the IRCS Journal of Medical Science).

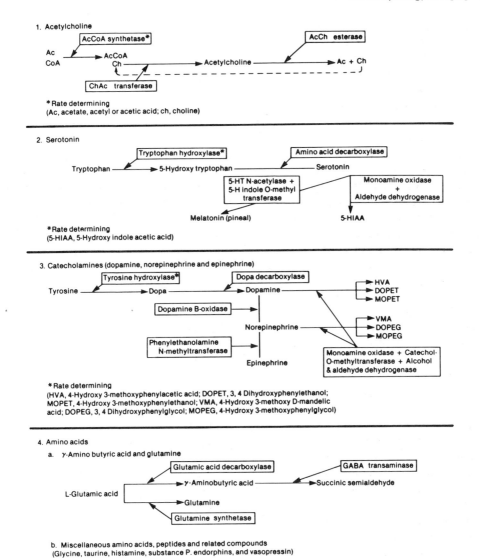

1. Acetylcholine

AcCoA synthetase*

Ac CoA → AcCoA
Ch → Acetylcholine → Ac + Ch

AcCh esterase

ChAc transferase

*Rate determining
(Ac, acetate, acetyl or acetic acid; ch, choline)

2. Serotonin

Tryptophan hydroxylase*

Tryptophan → 5-Hydroxy tryptophan → Serotonin

Amino acid decarboxylase

5-HT N-acetylase +
5-H indole O-methyl
transferase

Monoamine oxidase
+
Aldehyde dehydrogenase

Melatonin (pineal)   5-HIAA

*Rate determining
(5-HIAA, 5-Hydroxy indole acetic acid)

3. Catecholamines (dopamine, norepinephrine and epinephrine)

Tyrosine hydroxylase*   Dopa decarboxylase

Tyrosine → Dopa → Dopamine → HVA
DOPET
MOPET

Dopamine B-oxidase

Norepinephrine → VMA
DOPEG
MOPEG

Phenylethanolamine
N-methyltransferase

Epinephrine

Monoamine oxidase + Catechol-
O-methyltransferase + Alcohol
& aldehyde dehydrogenase

*Rate determining
(HVA, 4-Hydroxy 3-methoxyphenylacetic acid; DOPET, 3, 4 Dihydroxyphenylethanol;
MOPET, 4-Hydroxy 3-methoxyphenylethanol; VMA, 4-Hydroxy 3-methoxy D-mandelic
acid; DOPEG, 3, 4 Dihydroxyphenylglycol; MOPEG, 4-Hydroxy 3-methoxyphenylglycol)

4. Amino acids

a. γ-Amino butyric acid and glutamine

Glutamic acid decarboxylase   GABA transaminase

L-Glutamic acid → γ-Aminobutyric acid → Succinic semialdehyde

→ Glutamine

Glutamine synthetase

b. Miscellaneous amino acids, peptides and related compounds
(Glycine, taurine, histamine, substance P. endorphins, and vasopressin)

Fig. 3-3. Neurotransmitters in the mammalian brain, their associated enzymes and major brain metabolites. (Reprinted with permission of the Journal of the American Geriatrics Society).

from acetyl-coenzyme A (CoA) to choline. The enzyme choline acetyltransferase (CAT) is an essential catalyst for the reaction. Once synthesized, AcCh is stored within microvesicles in nerve terminals where it is released by a nerve impulse to activate postsynaptic receptors. Acetylcholine is then hydrolysed by acetylcholinesterase (ACE) and the choline is recaptured by the presynaptic component via a sodium dependent, high affinity active transport process.[70,71,72] Transport of choline and choline containing compounds from plasma into extracellular and intracellular compartments may also occur by a low affinity active transport process.[73,74,75] Most of the choline used in the synthesis of AcCh, however, is the recaptured metabolite of acetylcholine.[76,77]

Relatively little is known of the mechanism by which nerve impulses arriving at the axon terminal cause the release of monoamines. Considerably more is known about how the monoamines are formed and metabolized. The primary substrate for the synthesis of serotonin (5-HT) in the brain is tryptophan which enters the brain from the plasma by an active uptake process. Plasma tryptophan levels can be profoundly influenced by the diet. Tryptophan is hydroxylated to 5-hydroxytryptophan (5-HTP) by the rate-determining enzyme tryptophan hydroxylase. This enzyme occurs in low concentrations in most tissues, including the brain.[78] Following its synthesis, 5-HTP is almost immediately dehydroxylated to yield serotonin by the enzyme amino acid decarboxylase. Serotonin is then deaminated by the enzyme monoamine oxidase to produce 5-hydroxyindoleacetic acid (5-HIAA).

Tyrosine is the precursor for both dopamine (DA) and norepinephrine (NE). Tyrosine is taken up from the blood stream and concentrated within the brain by an active transport mechanism. Once inside the neuron, tryosine is converted to dihydroxyphenylalanine (Dopa) by the rate-limiting enzyme tyrosine hydroxylase. The next enzyme involved in catecholamine biosynthesis is Dopa-decarboxylase which transforms Dopa to Dopamine. The enzyme responsible for the conversion of dopamine into norepinephrine is dopamine ß-oxidase, In the adrenal medulla and some areas of the brain, norepinephrine is N-methylated by the enzyme phenylethanolamine-N-methyltransferase to form epinephrine. The mammalian enzymes of importance in the metabolic degradation of catecholamines are monoamine oxidase (MAO) and catechol-O-methyltransferase (COMT).

Knowledge of the role of GABA, and glycine in the central nervous system is speculative. They supposedly function as inhibitory transmitters in nerve endings to muscle and in the mammalian spinal cord, respectively. GABA is formed primarily from L-glutamic acid by the enzyme glutamic acid decarboxylase (GAD). GABA is metabolized by GABA-transaminase to succinic semialdehyde for entry into the Krebs cycle. The amino acids glycine, glutamic acid and others appear in high concentrations in some areas of the brain and seem to exert powerful effects on neuronal activity. Their status as neurotransmitters, however, is uncertain and knowledge of

their metabolism in nerve tissue is still minimal.[79]

Comments

From the outlined presented, one may discern a number of ways by which transmitter function may be altered. Changes in the amount of rate-limiting enzyme could be one factor. Another possibility is the replacement of the usual transmitter by structurally similar but noneffective (false) transmitter. An accumulation of metabolites may be yet another means of inhibiting transmitter release. A decrease in the number of synaptic processes or receptor sites per synapse might also alter the sensitivity of the postsynaptic cells to transmitter substances. The number of cell surface ß-adrenergic receptors in crude membrane fractions of mononuclear cells from human subjects is known to be reduced during aging.[80] The apparent number of ß-adrenergic receptor sites in erythrocyte ghost membranes prepared from the blood of rat also diminished with age.[81] There was, however, no age-related change in the number of ß-adrenergic receptors in membranes from the brains of the same animals. Consequently, the relationship between ß-adrenergic receptor sites and adrenergic responsiveness in the intact aging mammal is uncertain.

Neurotransmitter Pathways

To understand the range of possibilities concerning changes in neurotransmitter substances as modulators of hypothalamic function, it is important to consider the chemical pathways of known and suspected transmitter systems in the brain. A variety of histochemical and autoradiographic techniques have been developed to visualize selectively the neurons and fibers that contain particular transmitter substances or their associated enzymes. Flourescent methods developed largely by Scandinavian workers[48] have been used in many laboratories to visualize neurons containing NE,

DA, and 5-HT. The distribution of monoaminergic neuronal networks has been plotted in great detail in rat brain. From studies of human material, it appears that the basic distribution of the monoamine system of the rat is present also in man.[82] Ascending NA, 5-HT and DA systems as well as descending NA and 5-HT systems reaching nearly all areas of the brain and spinal cord have been described. Ascending adrenalin containing neurons in rat brain have also been shown.[83] A schematic representation of the mono-aminergic systems in man based on the data of Andén, Dahlström, Fuxe *et al.,*[84] and Ungerstedt,[85] is shown in Fig. 3–4.

There is no direct procedure for visualizing AcCh, and knowledge of its distribution rests largely on the use of histochemical staining techniques and biochemical assay. Shute and Lewis[86] used a combination of placing selective lesion in the brain with enzyme-staining techniques for a detailed mapping of cholinergic neurons in rat brain. A schematic representation of constituent

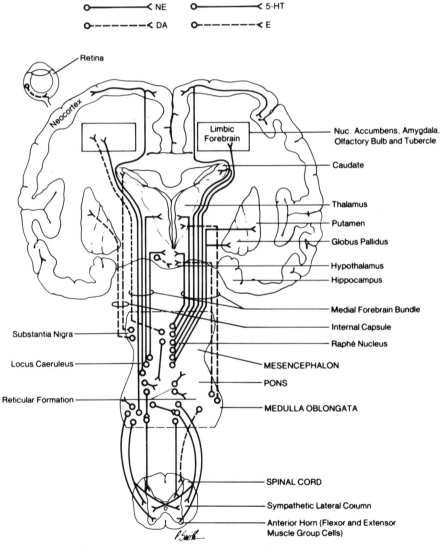

Fig. 3–4. Schematic representation of the noradrenergic, dopaminergic, serotonergic and adrenergic systems in the brain. (Adapted from Andén, Dahlström, Fuxe *et al.,*[84] and Ungerstedt,[85] reprinted with permission of the Journal of the American Geriatrics Society).

nuclei and ascending fibers of the cholinergic system as it might appear in the human brain based on findings for the rat is shown in Fig. 3–5.

Relatively high levels of GABA and GAD have been found in the globus pallidus and substantia nigra. McGeer, McGeer, Wada and Jung[87] have proposed that a GABA-containing neuronal system connects these two structures. There is some morphological and biochemical evidence for the presence of GABA[88,89] and glycine rich[90] inhibitory interneurons in the spinal cord. Other amine containing networks with a neurotransmitter role probably exist in the brain, but there are no adequate maps of the CNS distribution of these neurons. A schematic representation of the GABA and glycine containing networks are also shown in Fig. 3–5.

Subcellular Localization of Neurotransmitter Systems

The exact nature of the subcellular forms of many of the neurotransmitter systems is not always known because of the inherent difficulty in obtaining pure subcellular fractions. It is also evident that the majority of neurotransmitter substances exist in several different pools with widely different activation properties. Moreover, stimulation of nervous pathways tends to produce immediate and rapid transfer of neurotransmitters from one pool to another and changes in synthesis and metabolism may occur as a consequence. In addition, most of the information available pertains to studies done on peripheral nerves. In spite of these limitations, considerable information is available concerning the subcellular distribution of the major neurotransmitter substances in the brain.

Acetylcholine

Acetyl coenzyme A is primarily synthesized in mitochondria from citrate and glucose.[78] Most of the choline acetyltransferase (CAT) and acetylcholinesterase (ACT) originates in the perikaryon and travels out to the axon terminal by the process of axoplasmic flow. Choline acetyltransferase is found in the cytoplasm of nerve endings; acetylcholinesterase is associated with membranes of both neuronal and glial origin. Acetylcholine (ACh) is found in cell bodies, axons, and nerve terminals. In the nerve terminal, about half the ACh is localized in synaptic vesicles.[72]

Serotonin

Tryptophan hydroxylase, the enzyme responsible for the hydroxylation of tryptophan to form 5-hydroxytryptophan (5-HTP) in the brain appears as a soluble cytoplasmic enzyme[91] possibly, as a particulate enzyme associated with serotonin containing synapses.[92,93] As a second step, 5-HTP is rapidly decarboxylated to serotonin by a decarboxylase enzyme that is associated with a soluble synaptosomal fraction. Serotonin is presumably stored in granules located in the nerve terminal. Firing of a serotonergic neuron causes the release of serotonin from storage sites in the vesicles. Serotonin present in the free state can be deaminated to 5-hydroxyindoleacetic acid (5-HIAA) by the enzyme monoamine oxidase (MAO). This enzyme is localized largely in the outer membrane of mitochondria. However, both intraneuronal and oxtraneuronal distribution of MAO has been described.[78] Data has been obtained which indicates that more than one monoamine oxidase isoenzyme may exist in the brain.[94]

Dopamine (DA), Norepinephrine (NE), and Epinephrine (E)

A series of chemical transformations results in the conversion of tyrosine to DA, NE and E depending on the availability of synaptosomal tyrosine hydroxylase and other enzymes. A large portion of intraneuronal catecholamine is stored in specialized subcellular granules. Dopa decarboxylase, the second enzyme involved in catecholamine biosynthesis is associated primarily with the

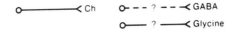

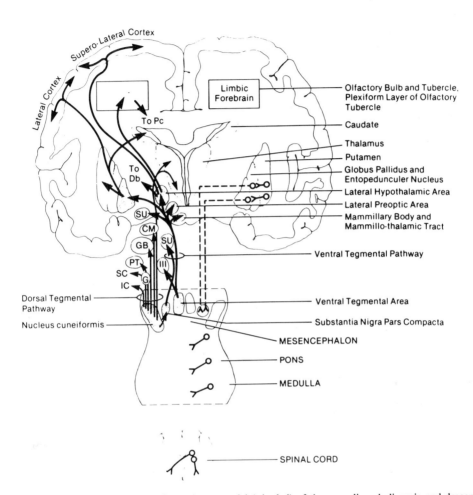

Fig. 3–5. Schematic representation of constituent nuclei (stippled) of the ascending cholinergic and descending GABA aminergic systems in the human brain. Abbreviations: CM, centromedian (parafascicular) nucleus; DB, diagonal band; G, stratum griseum intermediale of superior colliculus; GB, medial and lateral geniculate bodies; IC, inferior colliculus; III, oculomotor nucleus; PC, precallosal cells; PT, pretectal nuclei; SC, superior colliculus; SO, supraoptic nucleus; SU, subthalamus; (Adapted from Shute and Lewis,[86] McGeer and McGeer,[79] and Aprison, Davidoff and Werman.[90]

supernatant fraction of brain although some activity may be associated with synaptosomes.[78] Dopamine-ß oxidase is localized primarily in the membrane of amine storage granules. Phenylethanolamine-N-methyl transferase appears in the supernatant of brain homogenate.

Nerve impulses arriving at a nerve terminal cause a release of norepinephrine or such other catecholamine as may be stored in the granules. Norepinephrine (and probably other catecholamines) exists in more than one pool.[95] Newly synthesized norepinephrine in the granular pool is released preferentially. Norepinephrine (or dopamine) present in the free state within the nerve ending can be degraded by monoamine oxidase (MAO) located on the outer mitochondrial membrane. Free norepinephrine can also be deactivated by catechol-

O-methyltransferase (COMT) which is believed to be localized outside of the neuron. Fig. 3–6 shows some examples of neurotransmitter constituents and their subcellular localization in cholinergic, serotoninergic and noradrenergic neurons.

hypothalamic hormones that control pituitary secretions. Also, diseases such as parkinsonism, Huntington's chorea and Alzheimer's disease may be linked with disorders of neurotransmitter systems. Parkinson's disease, which usually occurs late in life, is characterized by a marked decrease in the concentration of DA in the nigro-striato-pallidal system.[98] The symptoms of Huntington's chorea seem to be associated with a reduction in the number of GABA-containing inhibitory neurons and an uneven degeneration of cholinergic fibers in the basal ganglia.[99] Other evidence shows that Alzheimer's disease, a gradually pro-

NEUROTRANSMITTER SUBSTANCES AND AGING

The hypothalamus stores large amounts of norepinephrine, dopamine and serotonin.[96,97] We have already seen that these monoamines are involved in the release of

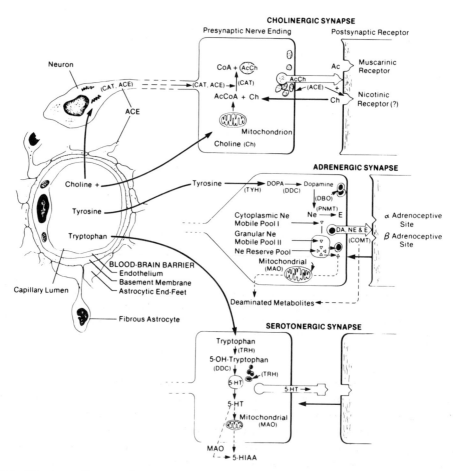

Fig. 3–6. Neurotransmitter constituents and their subcellular localization. Abbreviations: acetylcholinesterase (ACE), choline (Ch), choline acetyltransferase (CAT), Tyrosine hydroxylase (TYH), dopa decarboxylase (DDC) dopamine ß-oxidase (DBO), phenylethanolamine N-methyltransferase (PNMT), monoamine oxidase (MAO), catechol-O-methyltransferase (COMT), tryptophan hydroxylase (TRH), amino acid decarboxylase (DDC), 5-hydroxyindoleacetic acid (5-HIAA).

gressive dementia occurring in middle to late life, may result from a breakdown in the cholinergic systems.[100] However, quantitative assessments after death of biochemical changes in pathologic human brain present many difficulties.

Studies on the biochemical pathology of human material are often complicated by premortem conditions, postmortem delay, drugs, disease, nutritional state and genetic differences between individuals.[101] The use of experimental animals such as rodents eliminates some of the problems but extrapolating from rodent studies to man may be misleading in some instances.[102] The use of nonhuman primates as an animal model for human aging is obvious but, unfortunately, only limited data is available for life-span changes in neurochemistry.[102,103] Nonetheless, by examining information available for rodents in the light of the more limited human and subhuman primate data, some general principles concerning neurochemical changes and aging seem to emerge.

Of all the substances measured in brain, the catecholaminergic systems seems to be the most vulnerable to aging. In mice and rats the steady state concentration of dopamine and norepinephrine in the hypothalamus and striatum were significantly lower in old than in young animals.[5,49,104] Dopamine and norepinephrine depletion rates (catabolism) were also lower in some regions of the hypothalamus.[5,49] In contrast, the steady state concentrations of serotonin were the same in young and old rats but there was greater turnover of 5-HT in the hypothalamus of old than of young rats.[49]

An examination of life-span changes in brain norepinephrine and serotonin has been reported for the rhesus monkey. Small but significant decline in NE occurred in the hypothalamus and brain stem.[102,103] Ordy[103] reported that serotonin declined significantly in the hypothalamus after 20 years of age. Benetato, Uluitu, Suhaciu and Iordache[105] analyzed serotonin content in the hypothalamus and rhinencephalon of rat and found that serotonin increased during maturation, peaked in the adult and de-

creased in old age. A limited number of human brain samples have also been studied for life-span changes. Bertler,[58] reported a decline in the DA content of the caudate nucleus and putamen at senescence (over 70 years of age) compared to maturity (43 to 60 years). In a more recent study of a larger sample of human brain, Carlsson and Winblad,[106] also found an age-related decrease in DA content of the caudate nucleus and putamen. A small but statistically significant decline in NE has also been reported in human hindbrain (rhombencephalon).[107,108,109] Hindbrain 5-HT and 5-HIAA content, however, did not vary in relation to age. Some of these results are illustrated in Table 3-1.

Enzyme systems involved in neurotransmitter synthesis and degradation in human brain have been studied more extensively than have the neurotransmitters themselves because the enzymes are more stable, less likely to diffuse, and more easily measured. A change in enzyme activity may also be rate determining for neurotransmitter synthesis and metabolism. Enzymes involved in the catabolism of catecholamines, principally of norepinephrine, are currently the focus of interest because of the possible link between altered amine metabolism and neuropsychiatric disorders. Robinson, Davis, Nies et al.,[107] showed that there was a marked increase in MAO levels with age in human brain, blood platelets and plasma. Interestingly, hindbrain norepinephrine concentration correlated negatively with MAO levels.[107] Women were found to have a significantly higher mean platelet and plasma MAO activity than men of comparable age.[108] It has been possible to associate this change with a depressive state accompanying old age, especially in women after menopause.[110,111] Megna and Giacomo,[112] and Samorajski and Rolsten,[102] also found an age-related increase in MAO activity in several different regions of the human brain. Gottfries, Oreland, Wiberg and Winblad,[113] reported that there was a relation between low MAO activity in the brain and suicidal behavior among alcoholics. These studies suggest that aging processes may sig-

Table 3-1.   Effect of Age On Distribution of NE, 5-HT and DA in Brain of Rodent, Rhesus Monkey and Human.

	SPECIES	AGE	CHANGE	REF.
A. Norepinephrine				
1. Hypothalamus	Mouse	12 vs 28 mo	0	a
2. Hypothalamus	Rat	(3–4) vs (21) mo	–32%	b
3. Hypothalamus	Rhesus	(6–10) vs (12–18) yr	–10%	c
4. Hypothalamus	Rhesus	10 vs 20 yr	–53%	d
5. Brain Stem	Rhesus	(6–10) vs (12–18) yr	–34%	c
B. Serotonin				
1. Forebrain	Mouse	8 vs 21 mo	0	c
2. Hypothalamus	Rat	Adult (150g) vs 20 mo	–46%	d
3. Hypothalamus	Rhesus	(6–10) vs (12–18) yr	0	c
4. Hypothalamus	Rhesus	10 vs 20 yr	–43%	e
5. Hindbrain	Human	45 vs 70+ yr	0	f
C. Dopamine				
1. Neostriatum (caudate and putamen	Mouse	12 vs 28 mo	–20%	a
2. Hypothalamus	Rat	(3–4) vs 21 mo	–45%	b
3. Caudate	Human	(52–60) vs (74–87) yr	–25%	h
4. Neostriatum	Human	60 vs 80 yr	–40%	i

a. Finch[5]
b. Simpkins *et al.*,[49]
c. Samorajski and Rolsten[102]
d. Benetato *et al.*,[105]
e. Ordy[103]
f. Nies *et al.*,[59]
g. Hollander and Barrows[229]
h. Bertler[58]
i. Carlsson and Winblad[106]

nificantly affect monoamine mechanisms and be a predisposing factor in the development of clinical diseases in man e.g., depression, and other disorders of CNS homeostasis.

The influence of age on enzymes involved in the catabolism of norepinephrine have also been studied in animal tissues. Samorajski and Rolsten[102] found an increased level of MAO activity in the frontal cortex and caudate of rhesus monkey between the periods of late development and maturity, but not between maturity and old age. An increase in MAO activity, however, was demonstrated in three different brain regions of old mice.[102] In contrast, Prange, White, Lipton and Kinkead,[114] reported that the activity of both MAO and COMT in rat brain was constant across all age groups.

Recently, Anisimov, Pozdeev, Dmitrievskaya, Gratcheva, Ilin and Dilman,[115] reported that hypothalmic norepinephrine decreased in rats between 2 to 36 months of age. It will be recalled that depressed norepinephrine levels in the brain was associated with increased MAO activity.[107]

It has now been demonstrated that there are at least two types of MAO in the brain and other tissues of most mammalian species and that the ratios between the two types vary from region to region and across species. Differences are most apparent when synaptosomal fractions rather than tissue homogenates are compared.[116] Further, it has been shown that the distribution of the multiple forms of MAO change during development and possibly in old age as well.[117] Thus, while the correlation between age and MAO levels in the brain and other organs is not always apparent, there is reason to believe that age-related changes in MAO activity is a general biological phenomena.

Relatively little change is seen in brain catechol-O-methyltransferase (COMT) activity with age. Robinson, Sourkes, Nies et al.,[111] measured COMT levels in nine different areas of human brain obtained at autopsy and reported that there was no consistent age-associated pattern of change. An analysis of some mouse, rhesus monkey and human brain regions by Samorajski and Rolsten[102] likewise failed to reveal any significant changes in COMT activity with age. Prange, White, Lipton and Kinkead,[114] reported that COMT activity in the brain of rat was constant across all age groups studied. Since MAO increases with age in animal and human brain and COMT activity apparently remains constant, it may be concluded that oxidative deamination rather than methylation is increasingly the predominant pathway for amine degradation in the central nervous system of aging animals and humans.

Bowen and associates[101,118,119] examined a large number of chemical and morphological variables in the temporal lobe of the human brain in relation to normal aging, the presence of psychiatric or neurologic disease and the influence of ante- and postmortem factors. The temporal lobe was chosen because it is particularly affected in senile dementia.[120] Age-related differences in temporal lobe constituents were relatively minor in comparison with the affects of disease and differences in agonal state and postmortem handling. Of the biochemical constituents chosen as markers of possible cell loss, only GAD showed a significant decrease with age.

McGeer and McGeer[79,121,122] have studied enzymes associated with the metabolism of catecholamines, acetylcholine and GABA in many areas of human brain obtained at autopsy. With increasing age, the enzymes declined in some areas and not in others.

They reported that Dopa decarboxylase (DDC) and tyrosine hydroxylase (TYH) were the enzymes most severely affected by age in the putamen, globus pallidus and amygdala, the decline typically following a curvilinear pattern. A slight decline in choline acetyltransferase (CAT) occurred in the caudate nucleus and cortical areas of the brain. A small age-associated decline in glutamate decarboxylase (GAD) was found in the thalamic areas. These results were interpreted by McGeer and McGeer as indication that some areas of the brain were more age resistant than others.

Perry, Perry, Blessed, and Tomlinson,[123] investigated CAT levels in autopsy brain tissue obtained from mentally normal and abnormal elderly hospital patients. A substantial loss of CAT activity occurred over the age range of 63 to 94 years in the hippocampus, and to a lesser extent in the temporal cortex and caudate of mentally normal subjects. Secondly, an even greater loss of CAT activity was found in the cerebral cortex and hippocampus in senile dementia compared with age-matched mentally normal subjects. Decreased CAT activity has also been reported in the hippocampus of senescent mice.[124]

In many species of animals and in man, ACE levels in most regions of the brain show little change with age. Samorajski, Rolsten, and Ordy,[125] compared the levels of ACE activity in whole brain homogenates of mice and found no significant change between 3 and 21 months of age. Moudgil and Kanungo[126] found an age-associated decrease in the ACE activity in the cerebral hemisphere of rats, but no change in the cerebellum. An analysis of some rhesus monkey and human brain regions failed to reveal any significant change in ACE activity with age.[102] From the evidence presented, it is apparent that CAT levels are more sensitive to aging than ACE in regions of the brain with high cholinergic activity. The influence of age on some neurotransmitter enzymes of human brain are shown in Table 3-2.

Table 3-2.   Changes in Neurotransmitter Enzymes of Human Brain Associated with Aging.

ENZYME	TYPE OF CHANGE	REFERENCE
MAO	Increase in brain, platelets and plasma	Robinson et al.,[108] Megna and Giacomo,[112] Samorajski and Rolsten,[102]
COMT	No Change	Robinson et al.,[111]
GAD	Decrease in temporal lobe and thalamus	Bowen et al.,[101,230] McGeer and McGeer,[121,122]
DDC & TH	Decrease in putamen, globus pallidus and amygdala	McGeer and McGeer,[121,122]
CAT	Slight decrease in caudate and cortical areas	McGeer and McGeer,[79,121,122]
CAT	Decrease in caudate, temporal cortex and hippocampus	Perry, Gibson, Blessed, et al.,[162]
ACE	No change	Samorajski and Rolsten,[102]

MODULATING AGING WITH AGENTS AFFECTING NEUROTRANSMITTER LEVELS

Since nerve cells communicate primarily by releasing neurotransmitters at synaptic junctions, it follows that anything that alters neurotransmitter function at the synapse will disrupt normal cell communication and alter behavior. For example, many aged individuals may reveal marked changes in motor phenomena which are similar to those observed in Parkinson's disease, or tardive dyskinesia resulting from prolonged administration of antipsychotic drugs. Dysfunction of dopamine receptors in the extrapyramidal system is the common feature of these conditions.[10] In the case of parkinsonism, dramatic improvements have been achieved by the oral administration of levo-dihydroxyphenylalanine (L-dopa). L-dopa is converted to dopamine in the brain which acts as an agonist to stimulate dopamine receptors in the basal ganglia. By making up for the lack of native dopamine in the brain, the administration of L-dopa is able to reverse some symptoms of the disease.

In view of the fact that increasing old age seemingly involves a progressive imbalance between various neurotransmitters in the hypothalamus and other areas of the brain, it is an interesting question as to whether changes might be imposed on the rate of ag-

ing through drug administration or other means of intervention. Of the many ways in which investigators have attempted to alter the rate of aging in the past, caloric restriction has produced the most convincing results.[40,41,127] Recently, investigators have begun developing more precise techniques by which the role of neurotransmitters in the aging process could be explored in the laboratory. Segal and Timiras[128] have shown that tryptophan deficiency delayed growth, development and maturation of the cerebral nervous system of femal rats. In parallel experiments, these investigators also demonstrated that chronic treatment with d, l-parachlorphenylalanine, an inhibitor of serotonin synthesis, inhibited growth and delayed sexual maturation. Cotzias, Miller, Tang and Papavasiliou,[129] have shown that long-term administration of high concentration of L-dopa to mice in their diet enhanced fertility and increased the mean life span by about 50%. These findings support the hypothesis that neurotransmitter substances can have an influence on growth, maturation and aging.

To better understand the role of neurotransmitters in aging, we have conducted a series of experiments with mice to determine whether long-term administration of drugs acting on neuroreceptor sites or drugs affecting the level of neurotransmitter available to the receptor might affect physiological, biochemical or behavioral changes in relation to the probability of death at any chronologic age. Chlorpromazine (CPZ) was chosen for the initial experiments because of its frequent use in emotionally disturbed patients and for controlling a wide range of anxiety symptoms.[130] A major effect of CPZ is to hinder the binding of dopamine to its receptor. Treatment of mice with 5 and 10 mg/kg of CPZ compared to drug vehicle treated controls, resulted in a mean loss of body weight of about 10 to 20% respectively, a shortening of life span, and an accelerated decline in locomotor activity and barbital narcosis. Surprisingly, the concentration of lipofuscin age pigment (whose presence is often associated with aging)[131] decreased in the neurons of CPZ-treated animals compared to the controls.[132,133]

In another series of experiments, we chose to test the long-term effects of gerovital H₃ (GH3), a specially formulated preparation of procaine hydrochloride which reportedly is a reversible, fully competitive inhibitor of MAO.[134] The testing of a MAO inhibitor was considered to be important in light of the association that has been shown between aging and increased levels of activity of brain stem MAO and decreased levels of brain norepinephrine.[109] Long-term treatment of mice orally with 25 and 50λ of GH_3 per subject resulted in some significant changes compared to vehicle treated controls, especially at the higher dose level. Locomotor activity and uptake of radiolabeled norepinephrine and Na-K AT-Pase activity in nerve ending fractions of brain were higher in the GH_3 groups compared to the controls. These results with GH_3 were interpreted as an indication of improved physiologic state. Barbital narcosis and lipofuscin age pigment concentration did not differ between GH_3 treatment and control mice.[133] Evidently, GH_3 produced alterations in the brain that, quantitatively, may be correlated with some biochemical and behavioral changes associated with aging in mice.

Another study was conducted to deter-mine the extent to which the ergot drug, dihydroergotoxine mesylate (Hydergine^R) might affect organ functions impaired by aging, or brain damage induced by chronic administration of alcohol. Exposure of animals to alcohol is considered to be a useful experimental means of inducing disturbances in behavior and decrements in learning conditions[135] often associated with old age in humans. Hydergine is of particular interest because it has been shown to augment electroencephalic energy in the brain of animals damaged by ischemia or anoxia.[136] Recent experimental evidence suggests that the beneficial effects of Hydergine may result from its affinity for central norepinephrine receptors.[137] The change in conformation achieved by receptor binding of Hydergine presumably activates adenyl cyclase, a membrane-bound enzyme within the cell which synthesizes AMP from ATP. Cyclic AMP then acts as a control system for intracellular processes.[138] We found that concomitant treatment of mice with alcohol combined with Hydergine prevented the physiological and neurochemical changes caused by alcohol and, in some cases, Hydergine administered alone. We found, however, that the age of the animals undergoing treatment had an important bearing on the outcome. The benefits derived by administering Hydergine with alcohol were generally greater in the younger mice.[139]

Our findings and those of other investigators suggest that most treatments of adult rodents with drugs affecting behavior via action at the receptor level do not alter maximum species longevity, but rather produce significant delays of age-related physiologic decrements, possibly associated with the onset of disease. It is, of course, possible also to produce the opposite effects, often with the same drugs at higher dose levels. Inasmuch as drugs affecting behavior work in various ways at the receptor level, it remains to determine whether their effects on various aging parameters result from direct action on neuronal regulatory processes or indirectly through general effects on hormone or neurotransmitter release and the subsequent activation of adenylate cyclase and other systems involved in cell function. Age-related changes in the sensitivity of dopamine-stimulated adenylate cyclase has been described for some areas of the rat brain.[140] It is still an open question, however, of which particular neurotransmitter, hormone or site of action is primarily involved in the aging process.

Finch[61] has pointed out that if aging is a sequence of interlinked neuronal and endocrine transitions without intrinsic degenerative changes, then it should be possible to control the processes involved through drugs or hormones. There may, however, be a critical period for intervention in adults. In our experiments with a highly inbred strain of mice maintained under carefully controlled environmental conditions, the first major signs of physiologic decline in both male and female subjects appeared at about 18 months. Thus, it would be necessary to intervene earlier than 18 months if relatively irreversible changes were involved. On the other hand, changes in the genome may be accessible to intervention only after they occur. At the present time, the development of more precise techniques by which aging decrements can be delayed in mammals is primarily a laboratory exercise. By such efforts, however, some measure of control might be developed and imposed on the process of aging in the brain, thus enabling the individual to function optimally for a greater portion of its life span.

NEUROTRANSMITTER SUBSTANCES AND AGE-RELATED DISEASES

Parkinson's Disease

The role of catecholamines has been examined more extensively in parkinsonism than in any other neurologic disease. Ideopathic degeneration of the basal ganglia is the most common cause of parkinsonism with degeneration secondary to vascular disease, encephalitis, or manganese poisoning occurring less frequently. Neuroleptic drugs may also produce parkinson-like symptoms by either reducing the amount of dopamine available for binding (e.g., alphamethylparatyrosine) or by blocking the dopamine receptor (e.g., chlorpromazine).[141]

The major neurochemical finding in the brain is a decreased concentration of dopamine in the basal ganglia[98,142] secondary to cellular loss.[122] Homovanillic acid (HVA) concentrations in cerebralspinal fluid[143] and brain[144] may also be decreased, but urinary HVA levels are usually normal except in the presence of severe akinesia and rigidity.[145]

In some cases serum levels of dopamine-ß-oxidase may be low, indicating that noradrenergic systems may also be involved in this disease.[146] The cholinergic enzymes, choline acetyltransferase and acetylcholinesterase activities are high in the striatum, the area of the brain most involved in modulating extrapyramidal activity.[14] AcCh may act as an excitatory neurotransmitter in the striatum, stimulating neurons projecting to the globus pallidus. ACh stimulation in the presence of diminished dopamine induced inhibition may produce tremor and/or rigidity.[14] L-dopa and a number of other drugs effective in the therapy of Parkinson's disease presumably act by restoring neurotransmitter balance. There is, however, a decreasing response of parkinsonian patients to L-dopa with long-term treatment, presumably due to a progressive loss of dopaminergic receptors in the caudate nucleus.[147] Efforts to block the effects of ACh by drugs have not been as successful, due to undesirable side effects.

Huntington's Chorea

Huntington's chorea is a heredity disorder of unknown etiology in which changes in neurotransmitter substances have also been reported in the basal ganglia.[99] The disease is inherited as an autosomal dominant trait with complete penetrance. Morphologically, it is characterized by degeneration of small neurons in the caudate and putamen.[148] Of the various transmitters and related enzymes measured in brain removed at autopsy, only

GABA and its associated enzyme GAD were consistently reduced. The concentration of dopamine was normal except in the Westphal variant type which is prevalent among younger age groups. A characteristic feature of this condition is rigidity and increased dopamine levels in the basal ganglia.[14,149] The enzyme CAT is slightly reduced in the caudate in some cases, and markedly reduced in the putamen.[77,99] It may be that the key feature of Huntington's chorea is a general loss of GABA-containing inhibitory neurons and an uneven degeneration of cholinergic fibers in the basal ganglia which might cause an over stimulation of the dopaminergic system. The most effective therapy at the present time is dopamine receptor blockade with butyrophenones or tetrabenazine.

Creutzfeld-Jakob Disease

Creutzfeld-Jakob disease is a type of dementia that was once thought to be associated with aging. It is now recognized, however, that a transmissable slow virus is the cause of the disease.[150] The disease is characterized by a nonspecific loss of neurons in the cortex, caudate, and putamen[151] and a marked reduction of C_{20}-sphingosine in the gangliosides of brain lipids.[152]

Pick Disease

Pick disease is relatively rare and also the least well understood of the dementias. In some cases, it may be differentiated from Alzheimer disease by a lack of parietal lobe signs and by the presence of argentophilic intraneuronal inclusions (Pick bodies). There are no clear biochemical differences between Pick and Alzheimer disease. Most American neurologists do not differentiate between the two.[153]

Alzheimer's Disease

Alzheimer's disease (presenile dementia) is the most important of the dementias in terms of the number of people involved. In such cases, there is a characteristic pattern of nerve cell loss in the substantia nigra, basal ganglia and cortex and an excess of senile plaques, neurofibrillary degeneration and granulovacular change in the cortex.[153] The condition is known as presenile dementia or Alzheimer's disease if it occurs before 65 years; after that age it has been called senile dementia. Thus, both diseases presumably share a common pathology which characterizes aging in the brain except that these losses occur earlier and may be magnified in Alzheimer's disease. Genetic[154,155,156] and/or vascular conditions[157,158,159,160,161] have been implicated as causal factors in this disorder.

Reduction of glutamic acid decarboxylase (GAD) and choline acetyltransferase (CAT) in brain were recently found in dementias of various origins, including Alzheimer's type presenile dementia.[118,162] It was unclear, however, whether the finding of a reduced cortical GAD or CAT activity accurately reflected preterminal state or the effects of terminal coma and various postmortem conditions previously cited. In an attempt to resolve these problems, Spillane, White, Goodhardt et al.,[163] examined cortical biopsies removed at craniotomy. They found that CAT activity was reduced by over 50% while GAD activity was unaffected in the same Alzheimer's cases compared to cases of non-Alzheimer's age matched controls. These investigators were also able to determine that GAD activity in the brain could be affected by the agonal state wheras CAT activity was relatively unaffected.

Choline acetyltransferase activity (presynaptic cholinergic system) and high affinity binding of cholinergic antagonists (postsynaptic cholinergic system) were measured in brain tissue removed after death from both mentally normal and demented old people. Perry, Gibson, Blessed, Perry and Tomlinson,[162] found that a substantial loss of cortical CAT occurred with increasing age in mentally normal people and was most pronounced in the hippocampus. Even greater reductions of enzyme activity were found in the hippocampus of the group with senile dementia compared to an age-matched mentally normal group. Moreover, White, Hiley, Goodhardt et al.,[164] found that the number of muscarinic receptor binding sites in the frontal cortex decreased with advancing years only in people without appreciable morphological evidence of senile dementia. These data suggest that Alzheimer disease is associated with the presynaptic cholinergic component whereas normal aging is characterized by postsynaptic cholinergic decline. Data concerning cholinergic neurons in elderly people are of great interest because there is strong evidence that changes in memory and cognitive functions may be associated with interference of cholinergic transmission.[165]

ACE might be expected to show a similar correlation in spite of the fact that its presence is not limited to the postsynaptic membrane. Recently, Op Den Velde and Stam[166] found a decrease in ACE activity in the temporal lobe of gray matter of moderately to severely affected cases of Alzheimer's disease with respect to controls. Milyutin, Okun, Aksentsev, Arinchin and Konev,[167] were able to show that the ability of d-tubocararine and procaine to inhibit membrane bound acetylcholinesterase in rat brain homogenates was affected by normal aging.

Attempts to treat presenile and senile dementia by correcting cholinergic deficits have been unsuccessful. Most of the choline needed by the presynaptic portion of the neuron is recycled for use from the action of ACE on AcCh at the synaptic junction or from free or bound choline supplied by the bloodstream. There is no evidence of amelioration of presenile dementia during treatment with L-dopa.[168]

Depression

Alterations of neurotransmitter substances are a feature of aging which may relate directly to the high incidence of depression in persons over 65. Depressive illnesses occur about twice as often in women as in men and the period of risk extends primarily from age 40 onward.[169] Women consistently have higher levels of monoamine oxidase in the blood and brain than do men of comparable age, which may be related to the higher incidence of depressive illness in women.[108,170] The marked prevalence for women, however, peaks in the fifth decade after which the rates for women are only slightly higher than those of men.[171,172]

A large amount of evidence suggests that depressive illness is associated with changes in circulating hormones and a depletion of NE and possibly of 5-HT in the hypothalamus.[173] Less accumulation of 5-HIAA and HVA has been found in the spinal fluid of some depressed patients than in normal subjects.[174,175] It will be recalled that there is an age-related increase in the brain MAO, which metabolizes NE and 5-HT to 5-HIAA and HVA, respectively.[59,109] In certain types of depression urinary levels of 3-methoxyphenylglycol (MHPG) a metabolite of NE derived largely from the brain,[176,177,178] are lower than those found in nondepressed controls.[179,180,181] Differences in the excretion of MHPG in patients with affective disorders have provided biochemical criteria for classifying patients with different types of depressive diseases and possibly also for predicting differential responses to various antidepressant drugs.[182] Drugs with marked antidepressant properties inhibit the enzyme monoamine oxidase, or prevent the reuptake of discharged NE and 5-HT by the nerve endings; this would prevent the breakdown of these neurotransmitters by the elevated levels of MAO contained both inside and outside the neuron.

Since measures of the levels of circulating neurotransmitter substances and their associated enzymes and metabolites may provide some index of the integrity of neurons and their synapses, investigation of the constituents in body fluids may be of practical significance. Averbukh and Shabalova[183] compared blood and urine catecholamines and histamine levels between demented and age-matched control groups and, in some cases, found lower levels in the demented group. They also reported that there was a tendency toward normalization in the blood content of catecholamines and histamines with clinical improvement of the patients. Gottfries and associates[184] reported that levels of HVA (a metabolite of Dopamine) and 5-HIAA (a metabolite of serotonin) in cerebral spinal fluid were highest in a group of healthy volunteers and lower for patients with senile dementia, presenile dementia and parkinsonism, in that order. A study by Fisher[185] showed that urinary excretion of HVA was low in a group of demented patients compared with mentally alert controls. Such findings provide support for the concept that measures of neurotransmitters and related substances in biological fluids may provide important guidelines for the diagnosis and treatment of these dementias. Changes in neurotransmitter substances of human brain and biologic fluids associated with age-related diseases are shown in Table 3–3.

Table 3-3. Effect of Age-related Diseases On Neurotransmitter Metabolism.

DISORDER	NEUROTRANSMITTER SUBSTANCE	DISEASE-RELATED CHANGE	REFERENCE
Parkinson's disease	DA	Reduced in basal ganglia	Hornykiewicz,[98]
	HVA	Reduced in brain and CSF, normal urine levels in most cases	Bernheimer et al.,[143,144] Barbeau,[145]
	DBO	Reduced serum levels	Lieberman et al.,[146]
	CAT, ACE	Increased activity in striatum	van Woert,[14]
Huntington's chorea	GABA	Reduced in caudate and putamen	Bruyn,[148] Bird and Iversen,[99]
	DA	Increased in striatum in Westphal variety	Hayden et al.,[149]
	CAT	Reduced in caudate and putamen	Bird and Iversen,[99]
Alzheimer's dementia	CAT	Reduced in brain, especially hippocampus	Bowen et al.,[118] Spillane et al.,[163] Perry, Perry et al.,[123]
	GAD, GABA	No change	Bowen et al.,[118] Spillane et al.,[163]
	5-HIAA	Reduced in CSF	Goodwin et al.,[175]
	HVA	Reduced in brain and CSF	Gottfries et al.,[184] Fisher,[185]
Depressive illness	MHPG	Reduced in urine	Maas,[179] Deleon-Jones et al.,[181] van Praag,[180]
	MAO	Increased in brain and blood	Robinson et al.,[108] Robinson,[109]
	5-HIAA	May be reduced in CSF	Goodwin et al.,[175]
	cAMP	Reduced in urine	Abdulla and Hamadah,[231] Ramsden,[234]
	COMT	Reduced blood levels in females	Davidson et al.,[232]
	ACh	May be increased in brain (physostigmine reverses mania; all effective antidepressants are anticholinergic)	Davis,[233]

BEHAVIOR

Some progress has been made in recent years in correlating changes in behavior with neurotransmitter substances in specific areas of the brain through drug and lesion studies of animals and post-mortem surveys of human brain. Results from these studies provided the following correlations: feeding, drinking, and exercise may be regulated primarily by hypothalamic NE; sleep-wake cycles may be associated with changes in hippocampal 5-HT and DA and cortical ACh; and aggression and possibly some aspects of arousal appear to be related to changes in the concentration of ACh in the limbic system, cortex, ascending reticular system and thalamic nuclei.[186] Learning and memory may be mediated by interdependent cholinergic and noradrenergic systems, and sexual functions related to dopaminergic influences in the basal ganglia.[187,188] In some cases, a single neurotransmitter may mediate specific function at a localized site in the brain. In other instances, interacting neurochemical systems may function more generally as the substrate for behavioral control. Some of the relationships between behavior, neurotransmitter processes and the region of the brain primarily involved are summarized in Table 3–4. The following

Table 3-4.   Principle Action of NE, 5-HT, DA and ACh On Behavior.

BEHAVIOR	NEUROTRANSMITTER	PRINCIPAL ACTION	REFERENCE
Feeding and drinking	NE	α Receptors stimulate appetite	Robinson et al.,[107] Antelman and Caggiula,[191]
		β Receptors inhibit appetite	
	DA	Essential to feeding drive	Antelman and Caggiula,[191] Biggio et al.,[192]
	5-HT	May function in regulation	Nies et al.,[59] Coscina and Stancer,[190]
Aggression	NE	Stimulates predatory behavior	Goldstein,[198] Eichelman,[195]
	5-HT	Inhibits aggressive behavior	Sheard and Davis,[199]
Sex	NE	Controls erection and ejaculation (autonomic function)	Kent,[200]
	DA, 5-HT	May increase sexual drive	Doust and Huszka,[201] Shapiro,[187] Hyyppää et al.,[188]
Sleep-Wake	5-HT	Sleep induction	Jouvet,[204] Sitaram et al.,[235]
	NE	Sleep maintenance	Feinberg,[208]
	ACh, 5-HT	Regulates dreams	Hobson et al.,[207]
	ACh	Arousal from sleep	Moruzzi,[196]
Exercise	NE	Exercise increases brain NE	Prout,[211] Brown and van Huss,[216]
Memory Short term	ACh	Mediates recall	Safer and Allen,[236] Drachman and Leavitt,[224]
Long term	NE	Memory transfer and storage	Hamburg and Fulton,[237] Hamburg and Cohen,[238] McGaugh et al.,[239]

discussion provides a more detailed outline of the findings that implicate neurotransmitter substances in some age-related behavioral alterations.

Feeding and Drinking

The role of neurotransmitter substances in regulating feeding and drinking has been the subject of intensive research in recent years. Norepinephrine is considered to be the primary regulating neurotransmitter.[189] Injection of NE into the hypothalamus of the rat will provoke feeding and drinking behavior. There is evidence also that serotonergic[190] and dopaminergic[191,192] systems may be involved.

Antelman and Caggiula,[191] in reviewing current evidence, have theorized that the most likely basis for regulation of feeding and drinking behavior is an interaction between the noradrenergic and dopaminergic systems. According to these investigators, reduced DA activity precipitates aphagia and adipsia; reduced NE activity intensifies feeding.[192,193] It will be recalled that both NE and DA are reduced with advancing old age.[109] The fact that old people normally eat less most probably relates to decreased physical activity, but it also raises the possibility of an age-associated change in monoamine mechanisms controlling the ingestion of food and intake of water.

Aggression and Arousal

Studies of the neurotransmitter pathways associated with aggression and arousal have not produced uniform results. What is clear is that previous concepts of aggression have been overly simplified. Terms like arousal, aggression, and alertness do not represent a continuum of behavior and there may even be several subsets within each component. For exanple, there may be "predatory" aggression and "affective" aggression, and even different types of predatory aggression, each dependent on its own specific transmitter subsystem.[194,195]

Cholinergic mechanisms seem to play a major role in most aspects of arousal and aggression.[186,196] There may, however, be a variable degree of involvement depending on state achieved. For example, predatory aggression may involve primarily the NE system but changes in ACh may be an important modulating influence.[197,198] Little is known of the role of serotonin in aggression. There is some evidence that serotonin has an inhibitory role in aggressive behavior.[199] The relation between aggressive behavior and changes in neurotransmitter systems in the aging brain is an unresolved problem.

Sexual Function

Normal sexual function depends on an intact autonomic system and adequate levels of dopamine and serotonin in the brain.[200] Exaggerated sexual behavior may occur in men receiving L-Dopa for parkinsonism[187,188] and in schizophrenic women being treated with tryptophan, a precursor for serotonin.[201] While other influences ranging from social mores to altered hormonal levels of gonadotrophic hormones may influence sexual behavior, there may also be a relation between declining sexual function in the elderly and changes in the neurotransmitter system in the brain.

Sleep-Wake Cycles

Dement and Kleitman[202] defined five electroencephalographic (EEG) stages of sleep. Stage 1 is characterized by desynchronized EEG activity as the subject proceeds from wakefulness to sleep. This stage is often accompanied by episodic rapid eye movements, or stage 1-REM sleep. Since most dreams occur during stage 1-REM sleep, this period is often referred to as dream sleep. Stages 2 through 4 (nonrapid eye movement) represent a progressive deepening of sleep characterized by synchronized slow wave EEG activity. During normal sleep, adults generally experience 4–6 sleep cycles per night in which there is a regular progression from stage 1-REM to slow wave sleep. Each cycle is approximately 90 to 100 minutes long with progressively shorter cycles toward the end of the sleep period.[203] In the early phases of normal sleep, stages 3 and 4 predominate, whereas REM periods increase in frequency and duration as the sleep night progresses.

States of sleep have been correlated with changes in levels of brain biogenic amines. Jouvet[204,205] demonstrated that synchronized slow wave sleep results from a reduction of the ascending reticular activating system which is functionally linked to the serotonergic system. Kovačević and Radulovački[206] recently found that the metabolism of 5-HT and DA increased in the hippocampus and that the metabolism of DA decreased in the striatum and thalamus during slow wave sleep. They suggested that the progessive increase of DA in the hippocampus during slow-wave sleep may be related to a subsequent appearance of REM sleep. There is other evidence that paradoxical sleep is also under the influence of noradrenergic activity emanating from neurons located in the locus caeruleus.[207] Cortical arousal linked with awakening has been associated with the cholinergic system.[196]

Significant life-span changes have been noted in EEG patterns in the normal elderly.[208] Compared to young adults, elderly subjects show an increased number of awakenings, in the percentage of time in bed spent awake and a total decline in stage 1–REM sleep. Unfortunately, too few biochemical data are available to draw inferences concerning the role of the underlying neurotransmitter processes associated with sleep patterns of the elderly.

Exercise

The relationship between physical exercise and longevity has been approached in several ways including investigations of experimental animal subjects and epidemiologic comparisons of human subpopulations including follow-up studies of outstanding athletes. Most data are compatible with the concept that physical exercise contributes to an increased longevity, presumably due to cardiovascular benefits. Studies of animals[209,210] and humans[211,212] have demonstrated that some form of exercise may increase mean life span by 10% in animals or an extra year for each decade of exercise in man. There is evidence, however, that there may be an age threshold for exercise benefits in relation to increased longevity.[213] Several investigators have shown that the mean life span of male rats given an opportunity to mate was significantly longer than that of their unmated litter mates.[214] In a more recent study, however, Drori and Folman,[210] showed that the significant factor in prolonging life of male rats was not sexual mating, but rather, the associated exercise.

Rats exposed to acute exercise show an increased synthesis of norepinephrine in heart, spleen, and brain, due primarily to increased sympathetic stimulation.[215] Results for levels of brain catecholamines in response to exercise are conflicting. Gordon, Spector, Sjoerdsma and Undenfriend[215] found no change in the levels of NE in heart, spleen and brain following acute exposure to exercise. Brown and van Huss[216] found higher NE concentrations in the brains of rats exposed to an exercise training program of 8 weeks duration compared to sedentary controls. Tiplady[217] found that the incorporation of (^{3}H) lysine into cerebral cortex acid insoluble material in rats subjected to forced exercise was lower then in a matched groups of nonexercised controls. This result may indicate a change in the rate of protein metabolism in response to differences in motor activity, but does not rule out the possibility that stress, arousal or some other factor might be involved.

In general, activity studies conducted on noninstitutionalized[218,219] and institutionalized[220] elderly individuals have reflected the favorable effects of exercise in producing improved function. Data on individuals who have engaged in regular exercise throughout life indicate that a higher level of physiological functioning and motor capacity are maintained in later years.[221,222,223] It is possible therefore, that a program of exercise may offset some effects of aging and thereby influence mean life span. Conversely, inactivity may reduce demand on the sympathetic system resulting in lower brain catecholamines which may have consequences for late-life.

Learning and Memory

Behavioral studies have shown that many elderly people show some loss of learning and memory capacity.[165,224] Unfortunately, the levels and limits for processing information in the brain are poorly understood and consequently, efforts to establish precise neurochemical correlates have been largely unsuccessful. Pharmacological studies during the last few years have increasingly supported the behavioral impression that the cholinergic and noradrenergic neurons of the brain are involved in memory and learning.

Recent studies suggest that age-dependent impairments on learning and short-term memory may be associated not only with cell loss in the cerebral cortex[225] but also with loss of synaptic contact[226, 227] and their associated neurotransmitter substances. White, Hiley, Goodhardt et al.,[164] noted that the number of muscarine acetylcholine binding sites in the frontal cortex decreased with advancing old age. A comparison of cognitive deficits induced by scopolamine (which blocks the muscarinic type of acetylcholine receptor) with the performance of aged subjects revealed a striking behavioral similarity.[224] The cognitive and memory disturbances occurring with scopolamine and aging seemingly reflect a common disorder of cholinergic neurotransmitter even though the impairment may be temporary in the former situation and permanent in the latter.

Although the memory processing networks in the brain are not known, there is evidence that at least the frontal cortex, the entorhinal cortex, and the hippocampus may be involved in recent memory.[228] Cell loss or early degeneration in a component of the cholinergic or other interacting systems may cause a permanent deficiency in learning and memory. Age-related decline in learning and memory may also be affected indirectly by feedback deficiencies, either to a change at the neurotransmitter level or to a decrease in the number of receptor sites responsive to the neurotransmitter. As yet, it is not clear what changes at the neuronal level may be associated with decrements in learning and memory.

CONCLUDING REMARKS

The evidence discussed above suggest that there is a fundamental relationship between aging processes and changes in neurotransmitter substances in the brain and probably other regions of the body. Environmental influences and genetic factors may be imposed at any time during development, maturity and senescence which may alter the rate of the aging processes and affect the time at which an age-related pathology may appear. Many phenomena of aging may ultimately be traced to neuroendocrine factors or anatomic loci in the brain. Disregulation at the hypothalamic level may be the key to regulating aging throughout the body. There is evidence that there may be causal association between age-related changes in neurotransmitter substances in the brain and alterations in behavior. There is other evidence from studies of human brain that some age-related diseases may be associated with decreases in neurotransmitter substances. Little is known, however, of the relative contributions of aging and disease processes to hypothalamic regulation of homeostasis. A great deal more needs to be learned to determine the importance of the neurotransmitter substances to aging and the degree of control that might be developed and imposed by their manipulation.

ACKNOWLEDGEMENTS

The collaborative effect of Danielle Miller-Soule and Dr. Joseph Meites are gratefully acknowledged. The skilled assistance of Carolyn Rolsten, Les Goekler, Darci Volpendesta, Marcia Tibbets, and Phyliss Roberts in preparation of this chapter is especially appreciated.

REFERENCES

1. Greengard, P. 1978. Phosphorylated proteins as physiological effectors. *Science,* 199, 146–152.
2. Shock, N. W. 1977. Systems integration. In C. E. Finch and L. Hayflick (eds.) *Handbook of the Biology of Aging,* pp. 639–665. New York: Van Nostrand Reinhold.
3. Samorajski, T., Strong, J. R., and Sun, A. 1977. Dihydroergotoxine (Hydergine®) and alcohol-induced variations in young and old mice. *J. Geront.,* 32, 145–152.
4. Meites, J., Simpkins, J., Bruni, J., and Advis, J. 1977. Role of biogenic amines in control of anterior pituitary hormones. *IRCS Med. Sci.,* 5, 1–7.
5. Finch, C. E. 1973. Catecholamine metabolism in the brains of aging male mice. *Brain Res,* 52, 261–276.
6. Finch, C. E. 1975a. Aging and the regulation of hormones: a view in October 1974. *Adv. Exper. Med. Biol.,* 61, 229–238.
7. Finch, C. E. 1975b. Neuroendocrinology of aging: a view of an emerging area. *Bioscience,* 25, 645–650.
8. Finch, C. E. 1977. Neuroendocrine and autonomic aspects of aging. In C. E. Finch and L. Hayflick (eds.) *Handbook of the Biology of Aging.* pp. 262–280. New York: Van Nostrand Reinhold.
9. Samorajski, T. 1976. How the human brain responds to aging. *J. Am. Geriatrics Soc.,* 24, 4–11.
10. Barbeau, A. 1973. Aging and the extrapyramidal system. *J. Am. Geriatrics Soc.,* 21, 145–149.
11. Beasley, B. A. L. and Ford, D. H. 1976. Aging and the extrapyramidal system. *Med. Clin. N. Amer.,* 60, 1315–1324.
12. McGeer, P. L., McGeer, E. G., and Suzuki, J. S. 1977. Aging and extrapyramidal function. *Arch. Neurol.,* 34, 33–35.
13. Roth, R. H. and Bunney, B. S. 1976. Interaction of cholinergic neurons with other chemically defined neuronal systems in the CNS. In A. M. Goldberg and I. Hanin (eds.) *Biology of Cholinergic Function,* pp. 379–394. New York: Raven Press.
14. van Woert, M. H. 1976. Parkinson's disease, tardive dyskinesia, and Huntington's chorea. In A. M. Goldberg and I. Hanin (eds.) *Biology of Cholinergic Function,* pp. 583–601. New York: Raven Press.
15. Olton, D. S. 1977. Spatial memory. *Scientific American,* 236, 82–96.
16. Hassler, R. 1965. Extrapyramidal control of the speed of behavior and its change by primary age processes. In A. T. Welford and J. E. Birren (eds.), *Behavior, Aging and the Nervous System,* pp. 284–306. Springfield, Illinois: Charles C. Thomas.
17. Frolkis, V. V., Bezrukov, V. V., Duplenko, Y. K., and Genis, E. D. 1972. The hypothalamus in aging. *Exp. Geront.,* 7, 169–184.
18. Machado-Salas, J., Scheibel, M. E., and Scheibel, A. B. 1977. Morphologic changes in the hypothalamus of the old mouse. *Exp. Neurol.,* 57, 102–111.
19. Ravens, J. R. and Calvo, W. 1965. Neuroglial changes in the senile brain. In *Proceedings of the Fifth International Congress of Neuropathology, Internat. Congr. Ser. No. 100,* pp. 506–513. New York: Excerpta Medica Fdn.
20. Brizzee, K. R., Sherwood, N., and Timiras, P. S. 1968. A comparison of cell populations at various depth levels in cerebral cortex of young adult and aged Long-Evans rats. *J. Geront.,* 23, 289–297.
21. Vaughan, D. W. and Peters, A. 1974. Neuroglial cells in the cerebral cortex of rats from young adulthood to old age: an electron microscope study. *J. Neurocytology,* 3, 405–429.
22. Vernadakis, A. 1975. Neuronal-glial interactions during development and aging. In G. J. Thorbecke (ed.) *Biology of Aging and Development,* pp. 173–188. New York: Plenum.
23. Hasan, M., Glees, P., and El-Ghazzawi, E. 1974. Age associated changes in the hypothalamus of the guinea pig: effect of dimenthyaminoethyl p-chlorophenoxyacetate. An electron microscopic and histochemical study. *Exp. Geront.,* 9, 153–159.
24. Glees, P. and Hasan, M. 1976. Lipofuscin in neuronal aging and diseases. In *Normale und Pathologische Anatomie, Vol. 32,* 1–61.
25. Dilman, V. M. 1971. Age-associated elevation of hypothalamic threshold to feedback control and its role in development, ageing and disease. *Lancet,* 1, 1211–1219.
26. Blumenthal, H. T. and Berns, A. 1964. Autoimmunity and aging. In, B. L. Strehler (ed.) *Advances in Gerontological Research, Vol. 1,* pp. 289–342. New York: Academic Press.
27. Burnet, Sir M. 1974. *Intrinsic Mutagenesis. A Genetic Approach to Aging.* New York: Wiley.
28. Medvedev, Z. A. 1975. Aging and longevity. New approaches and new perspectives. *Gerontologist,* 15, 196–201.

29. Hayflick, L. 1976. The cell biology of human aging. *New Eng. J. Med., 295*, 1302–1308.

30. Walford, R. L. 1969. *The Immunologic Theory of Aging.* Copenhagen: Munsgaard.

31. Fernandez, G., Good, R. A., and Yunis, E. J. 1977. Attempts to correct age-related immunodeficiency and autoimmunity by cellular and dietary manipulation in inbred mice. In T. Makinodan and E. Yunis (eds.), *Immunology and Aging,* pp. 111–133. New York: Plenum Publ. Corp.

32. Blumenthal, H. T. 1976. Immunological aspects of the aging brain. In R. D. Terry and S. Gershon (eds.) *Neurobiology of Aging,* pp. 313–334. New York: Raven Press.

33. Denckla, W. D. 1974. A time to die. *Life Sci., 16,* 31–44.

34. Nandy, K. 1972. Brain-reactive antibodies in mouse serum as a function of age. *J. Geront., 27,* 173–177.

35. Nandy, K. 1975. Significance of brain-reactive antibodies in serum of aged mice. *J. Geront., 30,* 412–416.

36. Ingram, C. R., Phegan, K. J., and Blumenthal, H. T. 1974. Significance of an aging-linked neuron binding gamma globulin fraction of human sera. *J. Geront., 29,* 20–27.

37. Miller, D. I. and Blumenthal, H. T. 1978. Neuron-thymic lymphocyte binding by serum IgG of 90-and 500-day-old female Wistar albino rats. *J. Geront.* 33: 329–336.

38. Beauchemin, M. L., Antille, G., and Leuenberger, P. M. 1975. Capillary basement membrane thickness: a comparison of two morphometric methods for its estimation. *Microvasc. Res., 10,* 76–82.

39. Hunziker, O., Abdel' Al, S., Frey, H., Veteau, M. J., and Meier-Ruge, W. 1978. Quantitative studies in the cerebral cortex of aging humans. *Gerontology, 24,* 27–31.

40. McCay, C. M. 1942. Chemical aspects and the effect of diet upon aging. In E. V. Cowdry (ed.) *Problems of Ageing, Second Edition,* pp. 680–727. Baltimore: Williams and Wilkins.

41. Ross, M. H. 1972. Length of life and caloric intake. *Am. J. Clin Nutr., 25,* 834–838.

42. Héroux, O. and Campbell, J. S. 1960. A study of the pathology and life span of 6° C- and 30° C- acclimated rats. *Lab. Invest., 1,* 205–315.

43. Johnson, H. D., Kintner, L. D., and Kibler, H. H. 1963. Effect of 48°F (8.9°C) and 83°F (28.4°C) on longevity and pathology of male rats. *J. Geront., 18,* 29–36.

44. Ordy, J. M., Rolsten, C., Samorajski, T., and Collins, R. L. 1964. Environmental stress and biological ageing. *Nature, 204,* 724–727.

45. Ordy, J. M., Samorajski, T., Zeman, W., and Curtis, H. J. 1967. Interaction effects of environmental stress and deuteron irradiation of the brain on mortality and longevity of C57BL/10 mice. *Proc. Soc. Exp. Bio. Med., 126,* 184–190.

46. Samorajski, T. 1975. Ionizing irradiation and aging. In J. M. Ordy and K. R. Brizzee (eds.) *Neurobiology of Aging,* pp. 521–543. New York: Plenum Press.

47. Everitt, A. V. 1973. The hypothalamic-pituitary control of ageing and age-related pathology. *Exp. Geront., 8,* 265–277.

48. Hökfelt, T., Elde, R., Fuxe, K., Johansson, O., Ljungdahl, Goldstein, M., Luft, R., Efendic, S., Nilsson, G., Terenius, L., Ganten, D., Jeffcoate, L., Rehfeld, J., Said, S., Perez de la Mora, M., Possani, L., Tapia, R., Teran, L., and Palacios, R. 1978. Aminergic and peptidergic pathways in the nervous system with special reference to the hypothalamus. In S. Reichlin, R. J. Baldessarini and J. B. Martin (eds.) *The Hypothalamus,* pp. 69–136. New York: Raven Press.

49. Simpkins, J. W., Mueller, G. P., Huang, H. H., and Meites, J. 1977. Evidence for depressed catecholamine and enhanced serotonin metabolism in aging male rats: possible relation to gonadotropin secretion. *Endocrinology, 100,* 1672–1678.

50. Sawyer, C. H. 1975. First Goeffrey Harris Memorial Lecture. Some recent developments in brain-pituitary-ovarian physiology. *Neuroendocrinology, 17,* 97–124.

51. Schally, A. V., Arimura, A., and Kastim, A. J. 1973. Hypothalamic regulatory hormones. *Science, 179,* 341–350.

52. Spector, S., Prockop, D., Shore, P. A., and Brodie, B. B. 1957. Effect of iproniazid on brain levels of norepinephrine and serotonin. *Science, 127,* 704.

53. Clemens, J. A., Amenomori, Y., Jenkins, T., and Meites, J. 1969. Effects of hypothalamic stimulation, hormones and drugs on ovarian function in old female rats. *Proc. Soc. Exp. Biol. Med., 132,* 561–563.

54. Quadri, S. K., Kledzik, G. S., and Meites, J. 1973. Reinitiation of estrous cycles in old constant estrous rats by central acting drugs. *Neuroendocrinology, 11,* 807–811.

55. Meites, J., Huang, H. H., and Simpkins, J. W. 1978. Recent studies on neuroendocrine control of reproductive senescence in rats. In E. L. Schneider (ed.) *The Aging Reproductive System* (Aging, Volume 4), pp. 213–235. New York: Raven Press.

56. Shaar, C. J., Euker, J. S., Riegle, G. D., and Meites, J. 1975. Effects of castration and gonadal steriods on serum luteinizing hormone and prolactin in old and young rats. *J. Endocrinol., 66,* 45–51.

57. Hafez, E. S. E. and Evans, T. 1963. Reproductive life cycle. In E. S. E. Hafez and T. N. Evans (eds.) *Human Reproduction,* pp. 157–200. Hagerstown: Harper & Row.

58. Bertler, A. 1961. Occurrence and localization of catecholamines in the human brain. *Acta. Physiol. Scandinav.,* **51,** 97–107.

59. Nies, A., Robinson, D. S., Davis, J. M., and Ravaris, C. L. 1973. Changes in monoamine oxidase with aging. In C. Eisdorfer and W. E. Fann (eds.) *Psychopharmacology and Aging,* pp. 41–54. New York: Plenum Press.

60. Andres, R., and Tobin, J. D. 1977. Endocrine systems. In C. E. Finch and L. Hayflick (eds.) *Handbook of the Biology of Aging,* pp. 357–378. New York: Van Nostrand Reinhold.

61. Finch, C. E. 1976. The regulation of physiological changes during mammalian aging. *Quart. Rev. Biol.,* **52,** 49–83.

62. Gershberg, H. 1957. Growth hormone content and metabolic actions of human pituitary glands. *Endocrinology,* **61,** 160–165.

63. Carlson, H. E., Gillin, J. C., Gorden, P., and Snyder, F. 1972. Absence of sleep-related growth hormone peaks in aged normal subjects and in acromegly. *J. Clin. Endocrinol. Metab.,* **34,** 1102–1105.

64. Frantz, A. G., and Rabkin, M. T. 1965. Effects of estrogen and sex difference on secretion of human growth hormone. *J. Clin. Endocrinol.,* **25,** 1470–1480.

65. Mayberry, W. E., Gharib, H., Bilstad, J. M., and Sizemore, G. W. 1971. Radioimmunoassay for human thyrotrophin. *Ann. Internal Med.,* **74,** 471–480.

66. Snyder, P. J. and Utiger, R. D. 1972. Response to thyrotropin releasing hormone (TRH) in normal man. *J. Clin. Endocrinol.,* **34,** 380–385.

67. Azizi, F., Vagenakis, A. G., Portnay, G. F., Rapoport, B., Ingbar, S. H., and Braverman, L. E. 1975. Pituitary-thyroid, responsiveness to intra-muscular thyrotropin-releasing hormone based on analysis of serum thyroxine, triiodothyronine and thyrotropin concentrations. *New Engl. J. Med.,* **292,** 273–277.

68. Verzar, F. 1966. Anterior pituitary function in age. In B. T. Donovan and G. W. Harris (eds.) *The Pituitary Gland, Vol. 2,* pp. 444–459. Berkeley: University of California Press.

69. Jensen, H. K. and Blichert-Toft, M. 1971. Serum corticotrophin, plasma cortisol and urinary excretion of 17-ketogenic steroids in the elderly (age group: 66–94 years). *Acta Endocrinol.,* **66,** 25–34.

70. Haga, T. and Noda, H. 1973. Choline uptake systems of rat brain synaptosomes. *Biochem. Biophys. Acta,* **291,** 564–575.

71. Yamamura, H. and Snyder, S. H. 1973. High affinity transport of choline into synaptosomes of rat brain. *J. Neurochem.,* **21,** 1355–1374.

72. Barker, L. A. 1976. Subcellular aspects of acetylcholine metabolism. In A. M. Goldberg and I. Hanin (eds.) *Biology of Cholinergic Functions.* pp. 203–238. New York: Raven Press.

73. Clark, D. E., Estel, R. J., Ouyang, F., and Franke, F. R. 1972. Choline uptake in myocardial cell cultures. *Life Sci.,* **11,** 269–275.

74. Fonnum, F. and Malthe-Snorenssen, D. 1972. Molecular properties of choline acetyltransferase and their importance for the compartmentation of acetylcholine synthesis. *Prog. Brain Res.,* **36,** 13–27.

75. Pert, C. B. and Snyder, S. H. 1974. High affinity transport of choline into the mysenteric plexus of guinea pig intestine. *J. Pharmacol. Exp. Ther.,* **191,** 102–108.

76. Browning, E. T. 1976. Acetylocholine synthesis: substrate availability and the synthetic reaction. In A. M. Goldberg and I. Harin (eds.) *Biology of Cholinergic Functions* pp. 187–202. New York: Raven Press.

77. Eckernäs, S. A. 1977. Plasma choline and cholinergic mechanisms in the brain: methods, function, and role in Huntington's chorea. *Acta Physiol. Scand.,* Supp. 449.

78. Cooper, J. R., Bloom, F. E., and Roth, R. H. 1974. *The Biochemical Basis of Neuropharmacology,* pp. 1–272. New York: Oxford University Press.

79. McGeer, P. L. and McGeer, E. G. 1973. Neurotransmitter synthetic enzymes. In G. A. Kerkut and J. W. Phillips (eds.) *Progress in Neurobiology, Vol. 2,* pp. 69–117. New York: Pergamon Press.

80. Schocken, D. D. and Roth, G. S. 1977. Reduced β-adrenergic receptor concentrations in ageing man. *Nature,* **267,** 856–858.

81. Bylund, D. B., Tellez-Iñon, M. T., and Hollenberg, M. D. 1977. Age-related parallel decline in beta-adrenergic receptors, adenylate cyclase and phosphodiesterase activity in rat erythrocyte membranes. *Life Sci.,* **21,** 403–410.

82. Olson, L. 1974. Post-mortem fluorescence histochemistry of monoamine neuron systems in the human brain: A new approach in the search for a neuropathology of schizophrenia. *J. Psychiat. Res.,* **11,** 199–203.

83. Hökfelt, T., Fuxe, K., Goldstein, M., and Johansson, O. 1974. Immunohistochemical evidence for the existence of adrenaline neurons in the rat brain. *Brain Res.,* **66,** 235–251.

84. Andén, N. E., Dahlström, A., Fuxe, K., Larsson, K., Olson, L., and Ungerstedt, U. 1966. Ascending monoamine neurons to the telencephalon and diencephalon. *Acta Physiol. Scand.,* **67,** 313–326.

85. Ungerstedt, V. 1971. Stereotaxic mapping of the monoamine pathways in the rat brain. *Acta Physiol. Scand.,* **367,** 1–48.

86. Shute, C. C. D. and Lewis, P. R. 1967. The ascending cholinergic reticular system: neocortical olfactory and subcortical projections. *Brain,* **90,** 497–520.

87. McGeer, P. L., McGeer, E. G., Wada, J. A., and Jung, E. 1971. Effects of globus pallidus lesions and Parkinson's disease on brain glutamic acid decarboxylase. *Brain Res., 32,* 425–431.

88. Huffman, R. D. and McFadin, L. S. 1972. Suppression of presynaptic inhibition and cerebellar disfacilitation by bicuculline. *Life Sci., 11,* 113–121.

89. Iversen, L. L. and Bloom, F. E. 1972. Studies of the uptake of ³H-gaba and ³H-glycine in slices and homogenates of rat brain and spinal cord by electron microscopic autoradiography. *Brain Res., 41,* 131–143.

90. Aprison, M. H., Davidoff, R. A., and Werman, R. 1970. Glycine: its metabolic and possible roles in nervous tissue. In A. Lajtha (ed.) *Handbook of Neurochemistry, Vol. 3,* pp. 381–397. New York: Plenum Press.

91. Deguchi, T. and Barchas, J. 1972. Regional distribution and developmental change of tryptophan hydroxylase activity in rat brain. *J. Neurochem., 19,* 927–929.

92. Grahame-Smith, D. G. 1967. The biosynthesis of 5-hydroxytryptamine in brain. *Biochem. J., 105,* 351–360.

93. Peters, D. A. V., McGeer, P. L., and McGeer, E. G. 1968. The distribution of tryptophan hydroxylase in cat brain. *J. Neurochem., 15,* 1431–1435.

94. Shih, J. C. 1975. Multiple forms of monoamine oxidase and aging. In H. Brody, D. Harmon, and J. M. Ordy (eds.) *Aging. Volume 1,* pp. 191–197. New York: Raven Press.

95. Koelle, G. B. 1975. Neurohumoral transmission and the autonomic nervous system. In L. S. Goodman and A. Gilman (eds.) *The Pharmacological Basis of Therapeutics* (5th Ed.), pp. 404–444. New York: Macmillan.

96. Palkovits, M., Brownstein, M., Saavedra, J., and Axelrod, J. 1974. Norepinephrine and dopamine content of hypothalamic nuclei of the rat. *Brain Res., 77,* 137–149.

97. Page, I. H. and Carlsson, A. 1970. Serotonin. In A. Lajtha (ed.) *Handbook of Neurochemistry, Vol. 4,* pp. 251–262. New York: Plenum Press.

98. Hornykiewicz, O. 1973. Metabolism of dopamine and L-dopa in human brain. In E. Usdin and S. H. Snyder (eds.) *Frontiers in Catecholamine Research.* pp. 1101–1107. New York: Pergamon Press.

99. Bird, E. D. and Iverson, L. L. 1974. Huntington's chorea: Post-mortem measurement of glutamic acid decarboxylase, choline acetyltransferase and dopamine in basal ganglia. *Brain, 97,* 457–472.

100. Davies, P. and Maloney, A. J. F. 1976. Selective loss of central cholinergic neurons in Alzheimer's disease. *Lancet, 2,* 1403.

101. Bowen, D. M., Smith, C. B., White, P., Goodhardt, M. J., Spillane, A., Flack, R. H. A. and Davison, A. N. 1977b. Chemical pathology of the organic dementias part I. Validity of biochemical measurements on human post-mortem brain specimens. *Brain, 100,* 397–426.

102. Samorajski, T. and Rolsten, C. 1973. Age and regional differences in the chemical composition of brains of mice, monkeys and humans. In D. H. Ford (ed.) *Progress in Brain Research, Vol. 40,* pp. 253–265. New York: Elsevier.

103. Ordy, J. M. 1975. Neurobiology and aging in nonhuman primates. In J. M. Ordy and K. R. Brizzee (eds.) *Neurobiology of Aging,* pp. 575–597. New York: Plenum Press.

104. Miller, A. E., Shaar, C. J. and Riegle, G. D. 1976. Aging effects on hypothalamic dopamine and norepinephrine content in the male rat. *Exp. Aging Res., 2,* 475–480.

105. Benetato, G. R., Uluitu, M., Suhaciu, G. H. and Iordache, S. 1967. Variatiile serotoninei din hipotalamus si rinencefal in raport cu vîrsta la sobolani. *Fiziologia Normala Si Patologica, 13,* 245–251.

106. Carlsson, A. and Winblad, B. 1976. Influence of age and time interval between death and autopsy on dopamine and 3-methoxytyramine levels in human basal ganglia. *J. Neural Trans., 38,* 271–276.

107. Robinson, D. S., Davis, J. M., Nies, A., Colburn, R. W., Davis, J. N., Bourne, H. R., Bunney, W. E., Shaw, D. M., and Coppen, A. J. 1972. Ageing monoamines, and monoamine-oxidase levels. *Lancet, 1,* 290–291.

108. Robinson, D. S., Davis, J. M., Nies, A., Ravaris, C. L. and Sylwester, D. 1971. Relation of sex and aging to monoamine oxidase activity of human brain, plasma, and platelets. *Arch. Gen. Psychiat., 24,* 536–539.

109. Robinson, D. S. 1975. Changes in monoamine oxidase and monoamines with human development and aging. *Fed. Proc., 34,* 103–107.

110. MacFarlane, M. D. 1972. Ageing, monoamines and monoamine oxidase blood levels. *Lancet, 2,* 337.

111. Robinson, D. S., Sourkes, T. L., Nies, A., Harris, L. S., Spector, S., Bartlett, D. L. and Kaye, I. S. 1977. Monoamine metabolism in human brain. *Arch. Gen. Psychiat., 34,* 89–92.

112. Megna, G. and Giacomo, P. De. 1973. Le attivitá delle mònoaminossidasi cerebrali nell'uomo: rilievi in relazione ad etá, sesso a páthologie mentali. *Acta Neurol., 28,* 459–465.

113. Gottfries, C. G., Oreland, L., Wiberg, A., and Winblad, B. 1975. Lowered monoamine oxidase activity in brains from alcoholic suicides. *J. Neurochem., 25,* 667–673.

114. Prange, A. J. Jr., White, J. E., Lipton, M. A., and Kinkead, A. M. 1967. Influence of age on monoamine oxidase and catechol-O-methyltransferase in rat tissues. *Life Sci., 6,* 581–586.

115. Anisimov, V. N., Pozdeev, V. K., Dmitrievskaya, A. Y., Gratcheva, G. M., Ilin, A. P., and Dilman, V. M. 1977. Age-related changes of the biogenic amines level in the rat brain. *Sechenov. Physiol. J. U.S.S.R.,* **63**, 353–358.

116. Edwards, D. J. and Malsbury, C. W. 1977. Distribution of types A and B monoamine oxidases in discrete brain regions, pineal and pituitary glands of the golden hamster. *Life Sci.,* **21**, 1009–1014.

117. Youdim, M. B. H., Grahame-Smith, D. G. and Holzbauer, M. 1975. Effect of age on the development and properties of brain monoamine oxidase. *Biochem. Soc. Trans.,* **3**, 702–704.

118. Bowen, D. M., Smith, C. B., White, P., and Davison, A. N. 1976. Neuro-transmitter-related enzymes and indices of hypoxia in senile dementia and other abiotrophies. *Brain,* **99**, 459–496.

119. Bowen, D. M. 1977. Biochemistry of dementia. *Proc. Roy. Soc. Med.,* **70**, 351–353.

120. Tomlinson, B. E., Blessed, G., and Roth, M. 1970. Observations on the brains of demented old people. *J. Neurol. Sci.,* **11**, 205–242.

121. McGeer, E. G. and McGeer, P. L. 1975. Age changes in the human for some enzymes associated with metabolism of catecholamines, GABA and acetylcholine. In J. M. Ordy and K. R. Brizzee (eds.) *Neurobiology of Aging,* pp. 287–305. New York: Plenum Press.

122. McGeer, P. L. and McGeer, E. G., 1976. Enzymes associated with the metabolism of catecholamines, acetylcholine and GABA in human controls and patients with Parkinson's disease and Huntington's chorea. *J. Neurochem.,* **26**, 65–76.

123. Perry, E. K., Perry, R. H., Blessed, G., and Tomlinson, B. E. 1977. Necropsy evidence of central cholinergic deficits in senile dementia. *Lancet,* **1**, 189.

124. Vijayan, V. K. 1977. Cholinergic enzymes in the cerebellum and the hippocampus of the senescent mouse. *Exp. Geront.,* **12**, 7–11.

125. Samorajski, T., Rolsten, C., and Ordy, J. M. 1971. Changes in behavior, brain, and neuroendocrine chemistry with age and stress in C57B1/10 male mice. *J. Geront.,* **26**, 168–175.

126. Moudgil, V. K. and Kanungo, M. S. 1973. Induction of acetylcholinesterase by 17-estradiol in brains of rats of various ages. *Biochem Biophys. Res. Commun.,* **52**, 725–730.

127. Berg, B. N. and Simms, H. S. 1960. Nutrition and longevity in the rat. II. Longevity and onset of disease with different levels of food intake. *J. Nutr.,* **71**, 255–263.

128. Segall, P. E. and Timiras, P. S. 1976. Pathophysiologic findings after chronic tryptophan deficiency in rats: a model for delayed growth and aging. *Mech. Ageing Dev.,* **5**, 109–124.

129. Cotzias, G. C., Miller, S. T., Tang, L. C., and Papavasiliou, P. S. 1977. Levodopa, fertility, and longevity. *Science,* **196**, 549–551.

130. Carr, C. J. 1974. The search for a relationship between phenothiazine drug metabolism and clinical effectiveness. In I. S. Forrest, C. J. Carr, and E. Usdin (eds.) *Advances in Biochemical Psychopharmacology, Vol. 9,* pp. 1–3. New York: Raven Press.

131. Brizzee, K. R., Kaach, B., and Klara, P. 1975. Lipofuscin: inter- and extraneuronal accumulation and regional distribution. In J. M. Ordy and K. R. Brizzee (eds.) *Neurobiology of Aging,* pp. 463–484. New York: Plenum Press.

132. Samorajski, T. and Rolsten, C. 1976. Chlorpromazine and aging in the brain. *Exp. Geront.,* **11**, 141–147.

133. Samorajski, T., Sun, A. and Rolsten, C. 1977. Effects of chronic dosage with chlorpromazine and Gerovital H₃ in the aging brain. In K. Nandy and I. Sherwin (eds.) *The Aging Brain and Senile Dementia,* pp. 141–156. New York: Plenum Press.

134. MacFarlane, M. D. and Besbris, H. 1974. Procaine (Gerovital H₃) therapy: mechanism of inhibition of monoamine oxidase. *J. Geriatrics Soc.,* **22**, 365–371.

135. Tewari, S., Fleming, W., and Noble, E. P. 1975. Alterations in brain RNA metabolism following chronic ethanol ingestion. *J. Neurochem.,* **24**, 561–569.

136. Meier-Ruge, W., Enz, A., Gygax, P., Hunziker, O., Iwangoff, P., and Reichlmeier, K. 1975. Experimental pathology in basic research of the aging brain. In S. Gershon and A. Raskin (eds.) *Aging, Vol. 2,* pp. 55–126. New York: Raven Press.

137. Markstein, R. and Wagner, H. 1975. The effect of dihydroergotoxine, phentolamine and pindolol on catecholamine-stimulated adenylcyclase in rat cerebral cortex. *FEBS Letters,* **55**, 275–277.

138. Enz, A., Iwangoof, P., Markstein, R., and Wagner, H. 1975. The effect of Hydergine® on the enzymes involved in cAMP turnover in the brain. *Triangle,* **14**, 90–92.

139. Samorajski, T., Strong, J. R., Sun, G. Y., Sun, A. Y. and Seaman, R. 1978. Dihydroergotoxine and ethanol: physiological and neurochemical variables in male mice. *Gerontology,* **24**, Suppl. 1, pp. 43–54.

140. Govoni, S., Loddo, P., Spano, P. F. and Trabucchi, M. 1977. Dopamine receptor sensitivity in brain and retina of rats during aging. *Brain Res.,* **138**, 565–570.

141. Nathanson, J. A. and Greengard, P. 1977. "Secondary messengers" in the brain. *Scientific American,* **237**, 108–119.

142. Ehringer, H. and Hornykiewicz, O. 1960. Verteilung von noradrenalin und dopamine (3-Hydroxytryptamin) im Gehirn des menschen und ihr verhabten be: erkrankungen des ex-

trapyramidalen systems. *Klin. Wchnschr.,* **15,** 1236–1239.

143. Bernheimer, H., Birkmayer, W., and Hornykiewicz, O. 1966. Homovanillinsäure in liquor cerebrospinalis: untersuchungen beim Parkinson-Syndrome und anderen erenkrankungen des ZNS. *Wien. Klin. Wchnschr.,* **78,** 417–419.

144. Bernheimer, H., Birkmayer, W., Hornykiewicz, O., Jellinger, K., and Seitelberger, F. 1973. Brain dopamine and the syndromes of Parkinson's and Huntington's. Clinical, morphological, and neurochemical correlations. *J. Neurol. Sci.,* **20** 415–455.

145. Barbeau, A. 1968. Effect of phenothiazines on dopamine metabolism and biochemistry of Parkinson's disease. *Agressologie,* **9,** 195–200.

146. Lieberman, A. N., Freedman, L. S., and Goldstein, M. 1972. Serum dopamine-beta-hydroxylase activity in patients with Huntington's chorea and Parkinson's disease. *Lancet,* **1,** 153–154.

147. Reisine, T. D., Fields, J. Z., Yamamura, H. I., Bird, E. D., Spokes, E., Schreiner, P. S. and Enna, S. J. 1977. Neurotransmitter receptor alterations in Parkinson's disease. *Life Sci.,* **21,** 335–344.

148. Bruyn, G. W., 1968. Huntington's chorea: historical, clinical, and laboratory synopsis. In P. J. Vinken and G. W. Bruyn (eds.) *Handbook of Clinical Neurology, Diseases of Basal Ganglia, Vol. 6,* pp. 298–377. Amsterdam: North Holland.

149. Hayden, M. R., Vinik, A. I., Paul, M., and Beighton, P. 1977. Impaired prolactin release in Huntington's chorea: evidence for dopaminergic excess. *Lancet,* **2,** 423–426.

150. Gajdusek, D. C., Gibbs, C. J. Jr., and Alpers, M. 1966. Experimental transmission of a Kuru-like syndrome to chimpanzees. *Nature,* **209,** 794–796.

151. Berry, R. G. 1975. Pathology of dementia. In J. G. Howells (ed.) *Modern Perspectives in the Psychiatry of Old Age,* pp. 51–83. New York: Brunner-Mazel.

152. Tamai, Y., Kojima, H., Ikuta, F. and Kumanishi, T. 1978. Alterations in the composition of brain lipids in patients with Creutzfeldt-Jakob disease. *J. Neurol. Sci.,* **35,** 59–76.

153. Terry, R. D. 1976. Dementia. *Arch. Neurol.,* **33,** 1–4.

154. Larsson, T., Sjogren, T., and Jacobson, G. 1963. Senile dementia: a clinical, sociomedical and genetic study. *Acta Psychiat. Scand.,* **39** (suppl. 167), 1–259.

155. Feldman, R. G., Chandler, K. A. and Levy, L. L. 1968. Familial Alzheimer's disease. *Neurology* (Minneap.), **12,** 811–824.

156. Carter, C. O. 1969. Genetics of common disorders. *Br. Med. Bull.,* **25,** 52–57.

157. Ingvar, D. H. and Gustafson, L. 1970. Regional cerebral blood flow in organic dementia with early onset. *Acta Neurol. Scand.,* **46,** Suppl. 43, 42–73.

158. Ingvar, D. H., Risberg, J., and Schwartz, M. S. 1975. Evidence of subnormal function of association cortex in presenile dementia. *Neurology,* **25,** 964–974.

159. Hagberg, B. and Ingvar, D. H. 1976. Cognition reduction in presenile dementia related to regional abnormalities of the cerebral blood flow. *Br. J. Psychiat.,* **128,** 209–222.

160. Goodhardt, M. J., Strong, A. J., Bowen, D. M., White, P., Branston, N. M., Symon, L., and Davison, A. N. 1977. The effects of middle-cerebral-artery occlusion on neurotransmitter metabolism in baboons. *Biochem. Soc. Trans.,* **5,** 160–163.

161. Strong, A. J., Goodhardt, M. J., Branston, N. M., and Symon, L. 1977. A comparison of the effects of ischemia on tissue flow, electrical activity and extracellular potassium ion concentration in cerebral cortex of baboons. *Biochem. Soc. Trans.,* **5,** 158–160.

162. Perry, E. K., Gibson, P. H., Blessed, G., Perry, R. H., and Tomlinson, B. E. 1977. Neurotransmitter enzyme abnormalities in senile dementia. *J. Neurol. Sci.,* **34,** 247–265.

163. Spillane, J. A., White, P., Goodhardt, M. J., Flack, R. H. A., Bowen, D. M., and Davison, A. N. 1977. Selective vulnerability of neurons in organic dementia. *Nature,* **266,** 558–559.

164. White, P., Hiley, C. R., Goodhardt, M. J., Carrasco, L. H., Keet, J. R., Williams, I. E. I., and Bowen, D. M. 1977. Neocortical cholinergic neurons in elderly people. *Lancet,* **1,** 668–669.

165. Drachman, D. A. 1977. Memory and cognitive function in man: does the cholinergic system have a specific role? *Neurol.,* **27,** 783–790.

166. Op Den Velde, W. and Stam, F. C. 1976. Some cerebral proteins in Alzheimer's presenile and senile dementia. *J. Am. Geriatrics Soc.,* **24,** 12–16

167. Milyutin, A. A., Okun, I. M., Aksentsev, S. L., Arinchin, N. I., and Konev, S. V. 1976. On age-dependent allosteric properties of the brin acetylcholinesterase. *Biofizika,* **21(b),** 1120–1122.

168. Kristensen, V. 1976. Ekstrapyramidal og praesenil demens. *Ugeskr. Laeg.,* **138,** 2047–2050.

169. Sachar, E. J. 1974. The concept and phenomenology of depression with special reference to the aged: some clinical and biological considerations in depressive illness. *J. Geriat. Psychiat.,* **7,** 55–69.

170. Cohn, C. K., Dunner, D. L., Axelrod, J. 1970. Reduced catechol-O-methyltransferase activity in red blood cells of women with primary affective disorders. *Science,* **170,** 1323–1324.

171. Essen-Möller, E. and Hagnell, O. 1961. The frequency and risk of depression within a rural population group in Scandia. *Acta Psychiat. Scand.,* Supp. **162,** 28–32.

172. Wing, J. K. and Hailey, A. M. 1972. *Evaluating a Community Psychiatric Service: The Camberwell*

Register 1964-1971. New York: Oxford Univ. Press.

173. Samorajski, T. 1977. Central neurotransmitter substances and aging: a review. *J. Am. Geriatrics Soc.,* **25,** 337-348.

174. van Praag, H. M. and Korf, J. 1973. Monoamine metabolism in depression: clinical application of the probenecid test. In J. D. Barchas and E. Usdin (eds.) *Serotonin and Behavior,* pp. 457-468. New York: Academic Press.

175. Goodwin, F. K., Post, R. M., Dunner, D. L., and Gordon, E. K. 1973. Cerebrospinal fluid amine metabolites in affective illness: the probenecid technique. *Am. J. Psychiat.,* **130,** 73-79.

176. Maas, J. W., Landis, D. H. 1968. In vivo studies of the metabolism of norephinephine in the central nervous system. *J. Pharmacol. Exp. Ther.,* **163,** 147-162.

177. Sharman, D. F. 1969. Glycol metabolites of noradrenalin in brain tissue. *Br. J. Pharmacol.,* **26,** 523-534.

178. Sjoquist, B. 1975. Mass fragmentographic determination of 4-hydroxy-3 methoxymandelic acid in human urine, cerebrospinal fluid, brain and serum using a deuterium-labelled internal standard. *J. Neurochem.,* **24,** 199-201.

179. Maas, J. W. 1975. Biogenic amines and depression: Biochemical and pharmacological separation of two types of depression. *Arch. Gen. Psychiat.,* **32,** 1357-1361.

180. van Praag, H. M. 1977. Significance of biochemical parameters in the diagnosis, treatment, and prevention of depressive disorders. *Biol. Psychiat.,* **12,** 101-131.

181. Deleon-Jones, F., Maas, J. W., Dekirmenjian, H. and Sanchez, J. 1975. Diagnostic subgroups of affective disorders and their urinary excretion of catecholamine metabolites. *Am. J. Psychiat.,* **132,** 1141-1148.

182. Schildkraut, J. J. 1974. Biochemical criteria for classifying depressive disorders and predicting responses to pharmacotherapy: preliminary findings from studies of norepinephrine metabolism. Contributions to biochemistry. *Parmakopsychiatr. Neuropsychopharmakol.,* **7,** 98-107.

183. Averbukh, E. S. and Shabalova, A. A. 1970. The catecholamine and histamine blood and urine content in patients with senile psychosis. *ZH. Nevropatol Psikkiatr.,* **70(b),** 888-891.

184. Gottfries, C. G., Gottfries, I., and Ross, B. E. 1969. Homovanillic acid and 5-hydroxyindoleacetic acid in the cerebrospinal fluid of patients with senile dementia, presenile dementia and Parkinsonism. *J. Neurochem.,* **16,** 1341-1345.

185. Fisher, R. H. 1972. The urinary excretion of homovanillic acid and 4-hydroxy 3-methoxy mandelic acid in the elderly demented. *Geront. Clin.,* **14,** 172-175.

186. Iversen, S. D. and Iversen, L. L. 1975. Central neurotransmitters and the regulation of behavior. In M. S. Gazzaniga and C. Blakemore (eds.) *Handbook of Psychobiology.* pp. 158-200. New York: Academic Press.

187. Shapiro, S. K. 1973. Hypersexual behavior complicating levodopa (L-dopa) therapy. *Min. Med.,* **56,** 58-59.

188. Hyyppä, M. T., Falck, S. C., and Rinne, V. K. 1975. Is L-dopa an aphrodisiac in patients with Parkinson's disease? In M. Sander and G. L. Gessa (eds.) *Sexual Behavior: Pharmacology and Biochemistry,* pp. 315-328. New York: Raven Press.

189. Van der Gugten, J., De Kloet, E. R., Versteeg, D. H. G., and Slangen, J. L. 1977. Regional hypothalamic catecholamine metabolism and food intake regulation in the rat. *Brain Res.,* **135,** 325-336.

190. Coscina, D. V. and Stancer, H. C. 1977. Selective blockage of hypothalamic hyperphagia and obesity in rats by serotonin-depleting midbrain lesions. *Science,* **195,** 416-419.

191. Antelman, S. M. and Caggiula, A. R. 1977. Norepinephrine-dopamine interactions and behavior. *Science,* **195,** 646-653.

192. Biggio, G., Porceddu, M. L., Fratta, W., Gessa, G. L. 1977. Changes in dopamine metabolism associated with fasting and satiation. In E. Costa and G. L. Gessa (eds.) *Advances in Biochemical Psychopharmacology.* pp. 337-380. New York: Raven Press.

193. Alheid, G. F., McDermott, L., Kelly, J., Halaris, A., and Grossman, S. P. 1977. Deficits in food and water intake after knife cuts that deplete striatal DA or hypothalamic NE in rats. *Pharmacol. Biochem. Behav.,* **6,** 273-287.

194. Malick, J. B. and Barnett, A. 1976. The role of serotonergic pathways in isolation-induced aggression in mice. *Pharmacol. Biochem. Behav.,* **5,** 55-61.

195. Eichelman, B. 1977. Neurochemical studies of aggression in animals. *Psychopharm. Bull.,* **13,** 17-19.

196. Moruzzi, G. 1972. The sleep-waking cycle. *Ergebnisse Physiol. Biol. Chem. Exp. Pharmakol.,* **64,** 1-165.

197. Eichelman, B. and Thoa, N. B. 1973. The aggressive monoamines. *Biol. Psychiat.,* **6,** 143-164.

198. Goldstein, M. 1974. Brain research and violent behavior. *Arch. Neurol.* (Chicago), **30,** 1-34.

199. Sheard, M. H. and Davis, M. 1976. Shock elicited fighting in rats: importance of intershock interval upon the effect of *p*-chlorophenylalanine (PCPA). *Brain Res.,* **111,** 433-437.

200. Kent, S. 1976. Neurotransmitters may be the weak link in the aging brain's communication network. *Geriatrics,* **31,** 105-111.

201. Doust, J. W. L. and Huszka, L. 1972. Amines

and aphrodisiacs in chronic schizophrenia. *J. Nerv. Met. Dis.,* **155,** 261–264.

202. Dement, W. C. and Kleitman, N. 1957. Cyclic variations in EEG during sleep and their relation to eye movements, body mobility and dreaming. *Electroencephalogr. Clin. Neurophysiol.,* **9,** 673–690.

203. Boyar, R. M. 1978. Sleep-related endocrine rhythms. In S. Reichlin, R. J. Baldessarini and J. B. Martin (eds.) *The Hypothalamus,* pp. 373–385. New York: Raven Press.

204. Jouvet, M. 1969. Biogenic amines and the states of sleep. *Science,* **163,** 32–41.

205. Jouvet, M. 1975. The function of dreaming: a neurophysiologist's point of view. In M. S. Gazzaniga and C. Blakemore (eds.) *Handbook of Psychobiology,* pp. 499–527. New York: Academic Press.

206. Kovačević, R. and Radulovački, M. 1976. Monoamine changes in the brain of cats during slow-wave sleep. *Science,* **193,** 1025–1027.

207. Hobson, J. A., McCarley, R. W., and Wyzinski, P. W. 1975. Sleep cycle oscillation: reciprocal discharge by two brainstem neuronal groups. *Science,* **189,** 55–58.

208. Feinberg, I. 1976. Functional implications of changes in sleep physiology with age. In R. D. Terry and S. Gershon (eds.) *Neurobiology of Aging, Vol. 3,* pp. 23–41. New York: Raven Press

209. Retzlaff, E. and Fontaine, J. 1965. Functional and structural changes in motor neurons with age. In A. T. Welford and J. E. Birren (eds.) *Behavior, Aging, and the Nervous System,* pp. 340–352. Springfield, Ill.: Charles C. Thomas.

210. Drori, D. and Folman, Y. 1975. Environmental effects on longevity in the male rat: exercise, mating, castration and restricted feeding. *Exp. Geront.,* **11,** 25–32.

211. Prout, C. 1972. Life expectancy of college oarsmen. *JAMA,* **220,** 1709–1711.

212. Karvonen, M. J., Klemola, H., Virkajärvi, J., and Kekkonen, A. 1974. Longevity of endurance skiers. *Med. Sci. Sports,* **6,** 49–51.

213. Edington, D. W., Cosmas, A. C., and McCafferty, W. B. 1972. Exercise and longevity: evidence for a threshold age. *J. Geront.,* **27,** 341–343.

214. Drori, D. and Folman, Y. 1969. The effect of mating on the longevity of male rats. *Exp. Geront.,* **4,** 263–266.

215. Gordon, R., Spector, S., Sjoerdsma, A., and Udenfriend, S. 1966. Increased synthesis of norepinephrine and epinephrine in the intact rat during exercise and exposure to cold. *J. Pharmacol. Exp. Ther.,* **153,** 440–447.

216. Brown, B. S. and van Huss, W. 1973. Exercise and rat brain catecholamine. *J. Applied Physiol.,* **34,** 664–669.

217. Tiplady, B. 1972. Brain protein metabolism and environmental stimulation, effects of forced exercise. *Brain Res.,* **43,** 215–225.

218. deVries, H. A. 1970. Physiological effects of an exercise training regimen upon men aged 52–88. *J. Geront.,* **25,** 325–336.

219. deVries, H. A. 1971. Exercise intensity threshold for improvement of cardiovascular-respiratory function in older men. *Geriatrics,* **26,** 94–101.

220. Clark, B. A., Wade, M. G., Massey, B. H., and Van Dyke, R. 1975. Response of institutionalized geriatric mental patients to a twelve-week program of regular physical activity. *J. Geront.,* **30,** 565–573.

221. Fischer, A., Parizkova, J., and Roth, Z. 1965. The effect of systematic physical activity on maximal performance and functional capacity in senescent men. *Internationale Zeitschrift für Angernandte Physiologie,* **21,** 269–304.

222. Szewczuk, W. 1966. Rehabilitation of the aged by means of new forms of activity. *Gerontologist,* **6,** 93–94.

223. Espenschade, A. S. 1969. Role of exercise in the well-being of women 35–80 years of age. *J. Geront.,* **24,** 86–89.

224. Drachman, D. A. and Leavitt, J. 1974. Human memory and the cholinergic system. A relationship to aging? *Arch. Neurol.,* **30,** 113–121.

225. Shefer, V. F. 1973. Absolute number of neurons and thickness of the cerebral cortex during aging, senile and vascular dementia and Pick's and Alzheimer's disease. *Neurosci. Beh. Physiol.,* **6,** 319–324.

226. Scheibel, M. E. and Scheibel, A. B. 1975. Structural changes in the aging brain. In H. Brody, D. Harman, and J. M. Ordy (eds.) *Aging, Vol. 1.* pp. 11–37. New York: Raven Press.

227. Feldman, M. L. and Dowd, C. 1975. Loss of dendritic spines in aging cerebral cortex. *Anat. Embryol.,* **148,** 279–301.

228. Diamond, M. C. 1978. The aging brain: some enlightening and optimistic results. *Am. Scientist,* **66,** 66–71.

229. Hollander, J. and Barrows, C. H. 1968. Enzymatic studies in senescent rodent brain. *J. Geront.,* **23,** 174–179.

230. Bowen, D. M., Smith, C. B., White, P., Flack, R. H. A., Carrasco, L. H., Gedye, J. L., and Davison, A. N. 1977a. Chemical pathology of the organic dementias part II. Quantitative estimation of cellular changes in postmortem brains. *Brain,* **100,** 427–453.

231. Abdula, Y. H. and Hamadah, K. 1970. 3', 5' Cyclic adenosine monophosphate in depression and mania. *Lancet,* **1,** 378–381.

232. Davidson, J. R. T., McLeod, M. N., White, H. L., and Raft, D. 1976. Red blood cell catechol-O-methyltransferase and response to imipramine in unipolar depressive women. *Am. J. Psychiat.,* **133,** 952–955.

233. Davis, J. M., 1975. Critique of single amine theories: evidence of a cholinergic influence in the major mental illnesses. In D. Freedman (ed.) *Biology of the Major Psychoses. Res. Publ. Assoc. Res. Nerv. Ment. Dis., Vol. 54,* pp. 333–342. New York: Raven Press.

234. Ramsden, E. N. 1970. Cyclic AMP in depression and mania. *Lancet,* **1,** 108.

235. Sitaram, N., Wyatt, R. J. Dawson, S., and Gillin, J. C. 1976. REM sleep induction by physostigmine infusion during sleep. *Science,* **191,** 1281–1283.

236. Safer, D. J. and Allen, R. P. 1971. The central effects of scopolamine in man. *Biol. Psychiat.,* **3,** 347–355.

237. Hamburg, M. D. and Fulton, D. R. 1972. Influence of recall on an anticholinesterase induced retrograde amnesia. *Physiol. Behav.,* **9,** 409–418.

238. Hamburg, M. D. and Cohen, R. P. 1973. Memory access pathway: role of adrenergic versus cholinergic neurons. *Pharm. Biochem. Behav.,* **1,** 295–300.

239. McGaugh, J. L., Gold, P. E., van Buskirk, R., and Haycock, J. 1975. Modulating influences of hormones and catecholamines on memory storage process. *Prog. Brain Res.,* **42,** 151–162.

Chapter 4
Cerebral Blood Flow and EEG Changes Associated with Aging and Dementia

Walter D. Obrist, Ph.D.
University of Pennsylvania

A full understanding of senescent behavioral changes requires information from *in vivo* physiologic studies, including both the electroencephalogram (EEG) and cerebral blood flow (CBF). The present paper summarizes the available findings from such studies in both normal aging and dementia.

ELECTROENCEPHALOGRAPHIC CHANGES

The human electroencephalogram undergoes progressive changes with age from birth through senescence.[1] Following a period of rapid development associated with physical growth, EEG patterns become stabilized in early maturity, but then undergo further alterations in the senium. Outstanding among the age-related changes are shifts in the frequency spectrum. Relative to young adult standards, the average senescent EEG is shifted to the slow side, so that its frequency content resembles that of childhood. Specifically, there is a decrease in frequency of the dominant alpha rhythm (8 to 12 cycles per second), accom-

panied by an increase in the abundance of slower theta (4 to 7 c/s) and delta (1 to 3 c/s) waves. This regression of EEG frequency to an earlier level follows the general trend of many growth curves, including those for brain weight and intellectual function.

Individuals differ widely in the degree to which their EEGs manifest senescent changes, so that some subjects over age 80 have tracings indistinguishable from young adults, whereas others only 60 years old show pronounced deviations. Fig. 4–1 illustrates two such EEGs from subjects of approximately the same age. The upper one has a mean alpha frequency of 10.2 c/s, the average for young adults, while the lower record shows an alpha rhythm of only 7.3 c/s mixed with occasional 6 to 7 c/s theta waves. Because of the appearance of slow alpha and theta activity in all leads, the latter tracing is said to show mild diffuse slowing.

Both longitudinal and cross-sectional studies suggest that health is a critical variable related to the occurrence and rate of EEG changes.[1] Elderly subjects who live

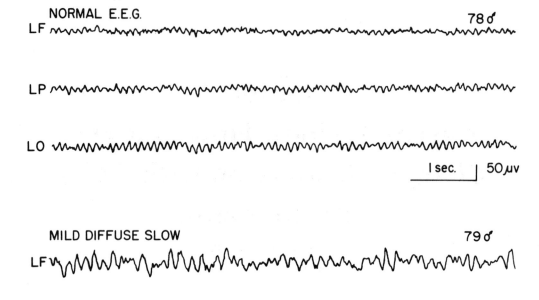

Fig. 4–1.   EEG recordings from two elderly community volunteers. Upper tracing: A 10 c/s alpha rhythm in a healthy 78-year-old man. Lower tracing: Mixed alpha and theta activity in a 79-year-old man with severe heart disease. LF, LP, LO = left frontal, parietal and occipital areas, respectively. All leads are referred to the homolateral ear.

in the community and maintain good health continue to reveal tracings that deviate only slightly from young adult standards, while patients suffering from illnesses that directly or indirectly affect the nervous system undergo more pronounced alterations. Thus, characterization of specific EEG changes and their relationship to other variables will depend on the particular population of elderly persons studied.

Dominant Alpha Rhythm

The most common age-related EEG change in senescence is a slowing down of the dominant alpha rhythm, the magnitude of which is related to health status, longevity and intellectual function. In comparison with the young adult average of 10.0 to 10.5 c/s, the mean alpha frequency of mentally normal old subjects is significantly lower, reaching 9.0 to 9.5 c/s around age 70 and 8.5 to 9.0 c/s after age 80.[2-5] The decline is greater among aged patients with cerebrovascular disease[4] or psychiatric disorders,[6] where the frequency is often 8 c/s or less. An even slower alpha rhythm is found in demented patients, the majority of whom have frequencies of 7 c/s.[7]

Although the etiology of alpha slowing in old age is obscure, there is some suggestion that vascular disease is a contributing factor. Obrist and Bissell[8] compared age-matched groups of normal and nondemented arteriosclerotic subjects. The latter were observed to have significantly lower alpha frequencies, regardless of whether the vascular disease was clinically manifest in the heart or brain. Patients with abnormal electrocardiograms and/or cardiac enlargement could be differentiated from normals on the basis of their alpha frequency. Even subjects with asymptomatic arteriosclerosis, detectable only by extensive laboratory and physical examinations, have been found to have reliably slower rhythms than healthy controls.[9] Fig. 4-1 illustrates the difference between a normal subject who remained in good health over the next 11 years (upper tracing) and a patient with severe, but com-pensated heart disease who died 18 months following his EEG (lower tracing).

Given the relationship between alpha slowing and vascular disease, it is not sur-prising that EEG findings are related to longevity. Fig. 4-2 plots alpha frequency changes in a mentally normal group[2] stud-ied longitudinally by the author with C.

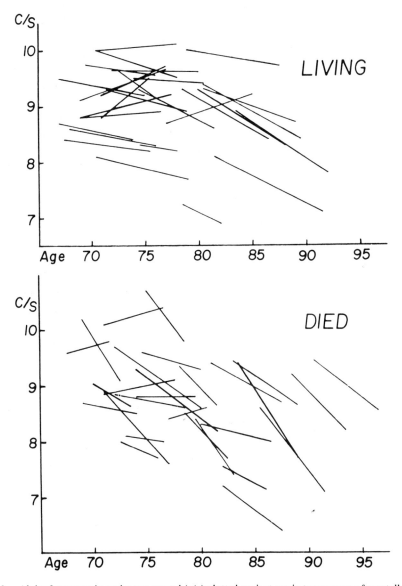

Fig. 4-2. Alpha frequency in cycles per second (c/s) plotted against age in two groups of mentally normal sub-jects studied longitudinally over a 5-to 7-year period. Upper graph: Subjects who continued to live 3 years after their last EEG. Lower graph: Subjects who died within 3 years of their last EEG (mean survival = 18 months). See text for further details.

E. Henry and W. A. Justiss (unpublished). Twenty-eight subjects who remained alive 3 years after their final EEG are compared with 28 cases who died during the same period of time (mean survival = 18 months). Whereas the survivors showed an average decline in frequency of 0.3 c/s over 7.3 years, those who died had a significantly greater decline of 0.6 c/s over a span of only 5.1 years ($p < .01$). This result has recently been confirmed by Wang and Busse[10] and by Müller and coworkers.[11] The selective drop-out of subjects with slower alpha rhythms may well explain the apparent leveling-off of frequency changes in extreme old age.[12]

Although intellectual impairment is associated with a slow alpha rhythm in aged psychiatric patients,[6,7] such a relationship is not found in relatively healthy old people where mental function is well preserved and alpha frequency remains moderately high. Thus, Obrist et al.[13] obtained no relationship between alpha frequency and intelligence test performance in community volunteers, but did find significant correlations in institutionalized subjects where both variables underwent appreciable decline. Data from the latter study are presented in Table 4–1, where a comparison is made between subjects in whom vascular disease was diagnosed as either absent or present. It was considered present if there was unequivocal evidence of cardiac or cerebrovascular involvement. As shown in Table 4–1, the patients with vascular disease yielded higher correlations between alpha frequency and scores on the Wechsler Intelligence Scale than did those with negative physical and laboratory findings. These results suggest that pathological factors are primarily responsible for the relationship between EEG and intellectual function in old age.

A more subtle relationship may exist between age changes in alpha frequency and motor response speed. In a group of community volunteers ranging from 28 to 99 years, Surwillo[14] found a correlation of 0.72 between simple auditory reaction time and average duration of alpha waves in the stimulus-response interval. Since he also found a significant correlation across responses within the individual, it was concluded that speed of information processing is dependent on brain wave frequency. This interesting hypothesis deserves further investigation.

Focal Alterations

The term focal alterations is employed here to designate localized EEG patterns that clinical electroencephalographers generally regard as abnormal. These consist of focal slow activity (theta or delta waves), amplitude asymmetries, and localized sharp waves or spikes. The foci may be unilateral or bilateral, the latter being distinguished

Table 4-1. Product-moment Correlations Between Alpha Frequency and Intelligence Test Scores in Elderly Subjects.

	VASCULAR DISEASE	
	ABSENT	PRESENT
Retirement Home (N = 32)		
Verbal Scale	−.16	.20
Performance Scale	.03	.58*
Full Scale	−.08	.41
Psychiatric Hospital (N = 30)		
Verbal Scale	−.15	.43
Performance Scale	.23	.61*
Full Scale	−.01	.56#

Significantly different from zero: * $p < .02$, # $p < .05$
Data were obtained from Obrist et al.[13]

from diffuse abnormalities by their restriction to a limited brain region.

Silverman and coworkers[15] were the first to report a high incidence of focal slow activity in elderly people. They found slow wave foci in 30–40% of community volunteers over age 60, predominantly from the left anterior temporal area. Three-quarters of the focal alterations were either lateralized to the left hemisphere or had a left-sided emphasis, while 80% appeared maximally over the anterior portion of the temporal lobe. Amplitude asymmetries and random spiking were also noted, usually in association with the slow waves. These findings were later replicated on a different community sample.[3] In both studies, some of the most prominent foci occurred among neurologically and mentally normal old people who were making adequate social adjustments. Such subjects, however, rarely showed foci outside of the temporal region. Fig. 4–3 illustrates a delta wave focus from the left anterior temporal area of a healthy 66-year-old woman. The slow waves are episodic, being interspersed by runs of normal alpha activity.

Temporal lobe foci first appear to a significant degree during middle age. In a systematic study of "temporal transients," Kooi et al.[16] observed a pronounced increase in episodic theta and delta activity after age 40. Thorough medical examinations could not elicit a cause for the foci. These findings were substantiated by Busse and Obrist,[17] who found temporal slow waves in approximately 20% of normal subjects between ages 40 and 60, in contrast to less than 5% under 40 years. The incidence rose to 35% after age 60.

Although temporal slow activity is more prevalent among patients with cerebrovascular disease,[18] where it may exceed 60% following an acute stroke,[19] a temporal focus *per se* cannot be considered pathognomonic of a neurological or psychological deficit in the average old person. In a study by Obrist and Davis,[20] 13

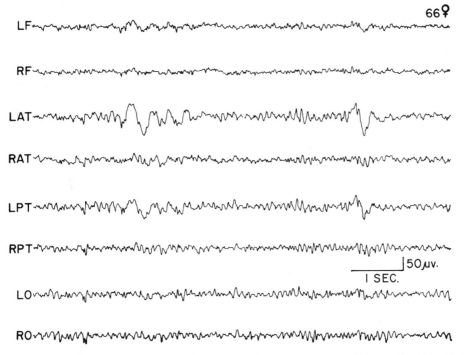

Fig. 4–3. A left anterior temporal delta wave focus in a 66-year-old woman who is in good health and living in the community. L = left, R = right, F = frontal, AT = anterior temporal, PT = posterior temporal, O = occipital. From Busse and Obrist.[17]

elderly community volunteers with severe anterior temporal foci (delta waves) were compared with 13 age- and education-matched subjects having normal EEGs. Neurological findings were negative in all subjects except one in each group who had minimal evidence of cerebrovascular disease. The focal and normal EEG groups were essentially identical in learning ability, immediate memory, 48-hour recall, and intelligence test performance. A follow-up study 12 years later revealed that the two groups were similar with respect to health and longevity. Six and eight subjects, respectively, survived to a mean age of 80 years.

The fact that temporal EEG foci in the elderly are highly circumscribed topographically, can occur in healthy people, and are unaccompanied by psychological deficit, suggests that the underlying pathology is restricted to a small behaviorally "silent" region of the brain. Recently, Tomlinson and Henderson[21] described a relatively high incidence of neuronal loss, gliosis and senile plaques in the anterior temporal lobe which, in demented patients, was usually widespread and gross. Among nondemented subjects, however, neurofibrillary tangles were confined almost exclusively to the anterior temporal lobe, being absent in other cortical areas. The possibility that this region undergoes early pathological changes may explain the appearance of temporal foci in mentally normal old people. Because the electrical disturbance is more prevalent in the left hemisphere, it would be interesting to learn whether there is a corresponding asymmetry in pathological findings.

Diffuse Slow Activity

Diffuse slow activity consists of theta and delta waves that have a generalized as opposed to focal distribution, involving the anterior as well as posterior regions of both hemispheres. In its milder form diffuse slowing is contiguous in frequency with a slow alpha rhythm, from which it may be difficult to distinguish. Only tracings with a considerable amount of activity below 7 c/s will be regarded as diffusely slow in the present discussion.

In contrast to other age-related EEG characteristics, diffuse slow activity is relatively rare among mentally normal subjects during early senescence, but increases progressively with advancing age, reaching approximately 20% after 80 years.[3,15] Both the incidence and severity of such slowing, however, do not approach that obtained in aged psychiatric patients, where it occurs in almost half of the cases.[15,22]

Diffuse slow activity, more than any other EEG variable, is related to senile intellectual deterioration. As in the case of alpha frequency, the magnitude of the correlation between EEG and mental function varies with the sample studied. Little or no relationship is found in healthy community volunteers where the slowing is mild and there is minimal intellectual impairment.[9] On the other hand, institutionalized subjects who display more pronounced EEG and intellectual alterations have correlations as high as 0.50 between diffuse slow activity and tests of cognitive function.[13] Studies employing psychological tests are necessarily limited to cases with mild deterioration because of the cooperation required by the examination. Using a psychiatric rating scale, McAdam and Robinson[23] were able to assess a greater range of intellectual deficit. They obtained a rank-order correlation of 0.79 between ratings of dementia and quantitative estimates of theta and delta activity in elderly mental patients.

Fig. 4–4 compares the EEG frequency spectra obtained from two groups of aged subjects: healthy controls and patients with organic brain syndrome. As can be seen, the patients have a lower peak frequency and a significantly greater proportion of delta and theta waves. Fast activity, on the other hand, is more prevalent in the healthy controls. The entire frequency spectrum appears shifted toward the slow side in the group with organic brain syndrome.

If EEG slowing is quantitatively related to intellectual deterioration, it is not surprising

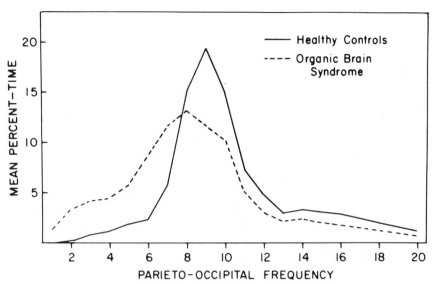

Fig. 4–4.   Mean EEG frequency spectra from two groups of elderly subjects: 47 healthy community volunteers (average age = 71), and 45 hospitalized patients with organic brain syndrome (average age = 76). The curves indicate the percentage of time that waves of a given frequency are present in the parieto-occipital tracing as determined by manual analysis. Taken from Obrist.[1]

that diffuse slow activity has been used to differentiate functional from organic mental disorders in old age. This distinction was first emphasized by Luce and Rothschild,[6] and reiterated by Frey and Sjögren[7] and by Obrist and Henry[22] in their studies on psychiatric patients. In the latter investigation, 79% of cases with diffuse slow activity were found to have organic brain syndrome, while 88% of those with normal EEGs had functional disorders, consisting primarily of depressions and paranoid reactions.

Diffuse slow activity is related not only to psychiatric diagnosis, but also to prognosis and life expectancy. Obrist and Henry[22] found that a majority of elderly patients with diffuse slow activity either remained hospitalized or died within a year after their EEG. Patients with normal tracings or purely focal abnormalities, on the other hand, tended to be discharged or transferred to convalescent homes. According to Cahan and Yeager,[24] a normal EEG in aged psychiatric patients carries twice the prognostic advantage for survival and subsequent hospital release than an abnormal tracing. Similar findings have been obtained by Müller and coworkers,[11] who argue for

the use of EEG as a prognostic indicator in geriatric psychiatry.

Focal slow waves also occur in aged psychiatric patients where, in demented cases, they are frequently seen as a localized accentuation of diffuse slow activity.[15] In contrast to community volunteers, the foci usually extend over a much wider region, involving the adjacent frontal as well as temporal lobes bilaterally.[22] The involvement of large areas in both hemispheres is compatible with intellectual deterioration.

EEG Sleep Patterns

Among the more sensitive age-related physiologic variables are changes in all-night EEG sleep patterns. In normal aging[25-28] the sleep patterns become fragmented, so that awakenings are both longer and more frequent than in young adults. This is associated with a marked reduction in stage-4 sleep (high voltage delta waves) and a moderate decrease in the amount of time occupied by rapid eye movement (REM) sleep. In addition, there is a significant decline in the number of 12–14 c/s spindle bursts, which are replaced by lower frequency spindle-like rhythms.[25] The decrease in REM sleep is of particular interest, since it is correlated with impairment on intelligence and memory tests.[26,27] Furthermore, the decline in REM sleep is consistent with age-related pathological changes observed in the locus coeruleus,[29] a brain stem structure that is believed to modulate REM activity.

Among elderly patients with organic dementia, EEG sleep patterns undergo similar but more pronounced alterations than observed in normal aging. In the only definitive study, Feinberg et al.[25] found longer and more numerous periods of wakefulness, greater reductions in both stage-4 sleep and amount of spindle activity, and a striking decrease in REM sleep. Again, the latter variable was significantly correlated with impaired intelligence test performance, as was the reduction in number of spindles. These correlations led Feinberg[26] to propose a common pathophysiologic mechanism underlying sleep alterations and disturbances in cognition.

The general nature of the sleep changes in aging and dementia are such that differences between sleep stages become progressively less as one proceeds from young adulthood to normal aging and dementia. Thus, there is an increasing homogeneity of EEG patterns across the night, marked by a significant reduction in their distinguishing characteristics; i.e., spindles, high voltage delta waves, and rapid eye movements. In demented patients, there is the additional tendency for sleep and waking patterns to become similar in that both are dominated by irregular diffuse slow activity. Although the magnitude of EEG sleep changes is correlated with the degree of intellectual deterioration, it remains to be determined whether differences exist between the several etiologic categories of dementia.

EEG Activation

Activation techniques, specifically hyperventilation, photic stimulation and drowsiness, have been widely used to elicit EEG changes in clinical electroencephalography. Induction of slow waves by hyperventilation is significantly reduced in senescence,[2,30] the major reduction occurring before age 40.[31] Although the inability of elderly people to alter their arterial pCO_2 may be responsible for the decreased response, diminished cerebrovascular reactivity is another factor that should be considered, particularly in patients with vascular disease.

Both the alpha blocking response to light and the photic driving response to intermittent stimulation undergo changes in senescence. With increasing age, fewer individuals show alpha blocking,[30] and the response latency is prolonged.[5] Photic driving responses are also significantly reduced.[5,31]

Drowsiness has been found to accentuate temporal lobe amplitude asymmetries and sharp waves, both of which increase with advancing age.[3,16,31] Recently, Hughes and Cayaffa[31] reported that elderly females have a much higher incidence of drowsiness-induced temporal sharp waves than males. This finding is consistent with the greater prevalence of fast (beta) rhythms in senescent females,[17] which are associated with temporal lobe transients.[16]

Neuropathological Studies

Until recently, there has been a general paucity of data on the neuropathologic correlates of EEG findings in demented patients. The earlier studies, which dealt primarily with presenile dementia, relied on in vivo neuroradiologic findings and biopsy confirmation. Gordon and Sim[32] review this work, including a large series of their own. They conclude that diffuse slow activity without localizing features, plus a general absence of alpha rhythm, is characteristic of most presenile dementias, especially Alzheimer's disease. An exception is the relatively normal tracings found in Pick's disease. They also note that the extent of cerebral atrophy, as determined by pneumoencephalography, is roughly correlated with the severity of EEG findings.

Two recent studies, based on fairly extensive autopsy material, are concerned mainly with the dementias of old age. Both studies attempt to differentiate between a vascular etiology and senile degeneration of the Alzheimer type. Constantinidis and co-workers[33] compared 32 cases of cerebro-vascular disease with 40 cases of Alzheimer's disease and 25 mixed cases (both etiologies). In contrast to Alzheimer's disease where there was a general absence of alpha activity, patients with cerebrovascular pathology usually had well-preserved rhythms in the 7-8 c/s range. On the other hand, there was a much higher incidence of focal theta and delta activity in cerebrovascular disease, in contrast to the diffuse slowing found in patients with an Alzheimer etiology.

These findings were confirmed by Müller and Schwartz,[34] who emphasized the occurrence of intermittent lateralized slow waves in cerebrovascular pathology, and the association of diffuse slow activity with Alzheimer's disease. The latter authors concluded that the EEG is useful in discriminating the two types of dementia, especially when combined with clinical information. A full assessment of the contribution of EEG to the differential diagnosis of dementia awaits further quantitative pathological studies of the type recently introduced.[21]

Cerebral Circulatory Studies

In 1963, Obrist and coworkers[35] reported a significant correlation between EEG frequency and both cerebral blood flow (CBF) and cerebral metabolic rate for oxygen (CMRO$_2$) in elderly patients with organic dementia. Table 4-2 presents the results of this study. EEG spectral analysis was carried out, as illustrated in Fig. 4-4. Both peak frequency (modal point of the frequency spectrum) and %-slow activity (the proportion of waves below 7 c/s) were analyzed in relation to cerebral circulatory variables.

As indicated by the signs in Table 4-2, increased EEG slowing was associated with greater circulatory impairment in the demented patients. The fact that no relationship was found in healthy controls suggested that the correlation depended upon the existence of pathology. Since patients with focal neurological signs were excluded from the study, it seemed unlikely that circulatory insufficiency due to cerebrovascular disease was responsible for the observed relationship. On the other hand, the higher correlations obtained with CMRO$_2$ suggested that diminished metabolic rate, rather than blood flow, was the primary variable.

Correlations between CBF and EEG have subsequently been reported by Sulg and coworkers[36] in patients with cardiac pacemakers and by Wang and Busse[37] in elderly communtity volunteers. Together, the several studies indicate the sensitivity of EEG to underlying cerebral hemodynamic and metabolic events. Further discussion of these relationships may be found in the following section.

CEREBRAL BLOOD FLOW CHANGES

Cerebral blood flow undergoes a decline with aging, the magnitude of which is a function of health status. As described

Table 4-2. Product-moment Correlations Between EEG and Cerebral Circulatory Variables in Elderly Subjects.

	HEALTHY CONTROLS		ORGANIC BRAIN SYNDROME	
	PEAK EEG FREQ. (N = 24)	% - SLOW ACTIVITY (N = 27)	PEAK EEG FREQ. (N = 17)	% - SLOW ACTIVITY (N = 20)
CBF	+ .02	− .01	+ .47	− .57*
CMRO$_2$	.00	+ .14	+ .74#	− .78#

Significantly different from zero: * $p < .01$, # $p < .001$
Data were obtained from Obrist et al.[35]

below, reductions in CBF are correlated with intellectual deterioration and are paralleled by decreases in cerebral metabolic rate.

Normal Aging

In 1956, Kety[38] reviewed the existing literature based on the nitrous oxide technique, and concluded that cerebral blood flow progressively decreases with age. Fig. 4-5 presents the relationship between age and CBF as illustrated by Kety. Although care was taken to exclude individuals with neurological and circulatory disorders, the older groups nevertheless included hospital patients with various chronic illnesses.

In a subsequent study, Dastur et al.[39] attempted to rule out the effects of disease by selecting elderly subjects who were in excellent health. The large circle in Fig. 4-5 represents this select healthy group, who had a mean CBF equal to young control subjects. From this, Dastur and coworkers argued that age per se cannot account for the decline in cerebral blood flow. Since they also found a significantly lower CBF in

elderly subjects with mild asymptomatic disease, these authors concluded that pathology is primarily responsible for the decreased CBF in old age. It is interesting to note that the dependence of CBF on health status is similar to that described above for EEG.

Organic Dementia

Following the pioneer study of Freyhan et al.,[40] it is now generally accepted that CBF is significantly reduced in patients with organic dementia. Lassen and coworkers[41,42] were the first to show that this reduction is correlated with performance on psychological tests. Correlation coefficients ranging from 0.40 to 0.70 were obtained between intelligence test scores and measurements of global cerebral blood flow.

With the introduction of radioisotope methods it became possible to study cerebral blood flow on a regional basis. Fig. 4-6 illustrates the type of information derived from regional CBF studies. In patients with senile dementia, Obrist et al.[43] found that the prefrontal and anterior temporal regions

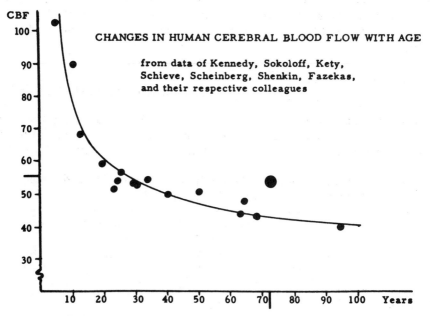

Fig. 4–5.   Cerebral blood flow in ml/100g/min plotted against age, as shown by Kety.[38] Each dot represents the mean of a separate group. The large circle has been added to indicate the mean for a select healthy aged sample.[39]

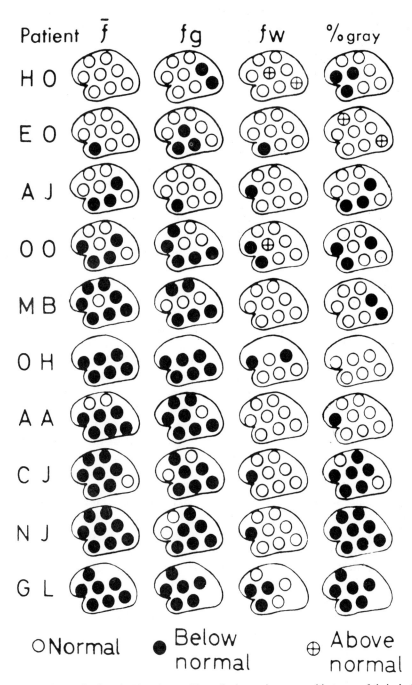

Fig. 4-6.   Regional CBF findings in 10 patients with senile dementia expressed in terms of their deviation from young control values. Each circle represents an extracranial detector which monitored isotope clearance from the brain following an intracarotid injection of Xe^{133}. A two-compartment analysis was performed that yielded separate blood flow estimates for gray and white matter. $\bar{f}$ = mean CBF for the two tissue compartments, f_g = CBF for the fast clearing "gray matter" compartment, f_w = CBF for the slow clearing "white matter" compartment, f_{gray} = the relative size of the fast compartment. The patients are listed in descending order of their $\bar{f}$ values, which were significantly correlated with the severity of dementia. Taken from Obrist et al.[43]

underwent greater blood flow reductions than other cortical areas. These findings were subsequently extended[44] and confirmed.[45] They are consistent with the increasing incidence of EEG abnormalities in the fronto-temporal region with advancing age.

Recently, Baer and coworkers[46] reported a significant relationship between regional CBF measurements and a battery of psychological tests in elderly patients with dementia. The frontal and temporal areas gave consistently higher correlations than the parietal and occipital areas, again suggesting greater pathological involvement of these regions.

Aging versus Dementia

The use of a noninvasive method for measuring cerebral blood flow has permitted comparisons between hospitalized patients and normal volunteers living in the community. Table 4-3 presents data obtained by the Xe^{133} inhalation method from studies by Obrist et al.[47] and by Wang and Busse.[37] CBF values are shown for the fast clearing compartment (F_1), which was derived from a two compartment analysis of the clearance curves. Because of differing detector locations, comparisons were limited to the parietal region, where F_1 values from the left and right sides were averaged.

As shown in Table 4-3, the normal aged group had a significantly lower blood flow than the young controls ($p < .01$). Unlike the study of Dastur and coworkers described above, the elderly volunteers were not preselected for good health, although they did function quite normally in their home environment. It is therefore of interest that the 28% reduction in CBF at age 80 agrees with the decrease predicted by the curve in Fig. 4-5.

Table 4-3 also reveals a significant blood flow reduction in demented patients. The decrease was even greater than obtained for the normal aged group, in spite of the fact that the patients were 20 years younger. A similar difference between normal aging and dementia has been reported by Lavy and coworkers.[67] From a purely hemodynamic point of view, it might be argued that aging and dementia lie along a continuum, the two being qualitatively similar but quantitatively different. Whereas blood flow declines significantly in the average (unselected) old person, the reduction occurs earlier and is of greater magnitude when accompanied by intellectual deterioration.

This hypothesis is supported by the findings in Table 4-4, where a comparison is made between blood flow levels within the normal aged sample itself. The subjects were divided into two groups according to whether their CBF was above or below the median value of the sample. The groups differed significantly, both in performance on the Wechsler Adult Intelligence Scale (WAIS) and in dominant EEG frequency (alpha rhythm). Of special interest is the fact that the WAIS Performance Scale, as opposed to the Verbal Scale, was more impaired in the low CBF group, a finding consistent with higher Deterioration Quotients in these subjects. Again, the CBF and EEG findings run parallel, there being a slower alpha frequency in subjects with reduced blood flow.

Table 4-3.   Fast Compartment CBF (Parietal Region).

	NO. CASES	AGE MEAN ± S.D.	F_1 (ML/100G/MIN) MEAN ± S.D.
Normal Young	35	23 ± 3	66.4* ± 8.7
Normal Aged	48	80 ± 7	47.4 ± 10.2
Dementia	20	60 ± 9	40.9 ± 9.8

* Equivalent to 72.6 ml/100g/min at a $PaCO_2$ of 40 mm Hg.
Data were obtained from Obrist et al.[47] and from Wang and Busse.[37]

Table 4-4.   Normal Aged Subjects with High and Low CBF.

	HIGH FLOW (N = 24) MEAN ± S.D.	LOW FLOW (N = 24) MEAN ± S.D.
WAIS		
Scaled Scores		
Verbal	60 ± 21	52 ± 21
Performance	32 ± 14*	24 ± 11*
Full	92 ± 34	77 ± 32
Deterioration		
Quotient	.19 ± .11#	.30 ± .16#
EEG Frequency (c/s)	9.3 ± 0.6#	8.5 ± 0.7#

Significant differences: * $p < .05$, # $p < .01$.

Data were obtained from Wang and Busse.[37]

Neuropathological Findings

Some insight into senescent CBF and intellectual changes is provided by recent neuropathological findings. In very careful quantitative studies, Tomlinson and coworkers[21,48] have identified two distinct etiologies underlying dementia in old age: (1) vascular disease, characterized by large, usually multiple areas of ischemic brain softening, and (2) Alzheimer's disease, characterized by numerous widespread senile plaques and neurofibrillary tangles. Contrary to the traditional view that cerebral arteriosclerosis is the primary cause of senile mental deterioration, Alzheimer's disease was found to be twice as prevalent as the vascular etiology. Taken together, they accounted for 80–85% of the observed dementias, there being a number of cases in which the two conditions coexisted.

Other factors undoubtedly play an important role in the intellectual decline of the elderly. Scheibel and coworkers[49] reported an extensive loss of dendritic spines, particularly in cortical pyramidal cells, which clearly involved a reduction in number of synapses. Confirming the earlier work of Brody,[50] Tomlinson and Henderson[21] found a progressive loss of neurons in nondemented elderly subjects that gave a correlation of 0.60 with age. The latter authors emphasize that the neuronal loss (approximately 50% of large cortical cells at age 90) may be even greater, since their method did not take into account reductions in total brain volume. Although gross cerebral atrophy is prevalent in dementia,[48] recent evidence from computerized tomography reveals a significant shrinkage of the brain in normal individuals over 70 years.[51]

In discussing the causes of senile dementia, Tomlinson and Henderson[21] argue that simple cell loss is not sufficient to explain intellectual deterioration, since cell counts in normal and demented individuals are frequently similar. They propose a multifactorial hypothesis in which the probability of dementia increases when Alzheimer changes and/or ischemic lesions are superimposed upon an already reduced neuronal population. It remains to be seen, however, whether the more subtle behavioral changes in normal old people can be accounted for by the simple loss of synapses and neurons.

Certainly, the decrease in cerebral blood flow, both in normal senescence and in dementia, is consistent with the magnitude of the observed pathological changes. The reduction in cells, the loss of dendritic spines, the presence of senile plaques (representing degenerated axon terminals), as well as gross areas of ischemic infarction, are each capable of impairing the brain's functional activity and thereby lowering its metabolism. Indeed, most of the blood flow changes are probably secondary to a decline in cerebral metabolic rate. The fact that the anterior temporal lobe is particularly vulnerable to neuronal loss and Alzheimer changes[21] may well explain the lower CBF found in this region.

Differential Diagnosis of Dementia

The recent neuropathological findings have had considerable impact on the clinical diagnosis of dementia. It is now recognized that ischemic lesions occur in only 30–40% of the dementias in old age, while Alzheimer-type degenerative changes are present in 60–70%. Furthermore, cerebrovascular disease *per se* is probably not a sufficient cause of dementia unless it results in widespread multiple areas of infarction. This lead Hachinski and coworkers[52] to propose the term "multi-infarct dementia" to distinguish such pathology from the less clearly defined and often erroneously inferred "cerebral arteriosclerosis."

The possibility that cerebral blood flow might differentiate the two types of dementia has been the subject of several investigations. O'Brien and Mallett[53] and Hachinski *et al.*[54] found significantly lower CBFs in demented patients with clinical evidence of cerebrovascular disease than in patients with primary neuronal degeneration; in fact, the latter tended to have normal flows. On the other hand, Ingvar and Gustafson[44] were unable to distinguish Alzheimer's disease from a vascular etiology, the two types having equally low CBFs. The latter agrees with the 20 patients studied by Obrist *et al.*[47] described in Table 4-3. Seven of these cases had a clearcut history of stroke, but their blood flow was not different from the 13 patients with presumed Alzheimer's disease.

The discrepancy between the two sets of findings can probably be attributed to differences in the severity of the underlying pathology. The studies by O'Brien and Mallett and by Hachinski *et al.* both involved early stages of dementia, where blood flow reductions due to degenerative changes were probably less than those associated with cerebral ischemia. On the other hand, the studies by Ingvar and Gustafson and by Obrist *et al.* involved more advanced stages of Alzheimer's disease, where blood flow reductions comparable to those of ischemia might be expected. Given the wide range of blood flow in demented patients, even among those with the same etiology, it seems unlikely that a differential diagnosis could be based on CBF measurements.

Responsiveness to Arterial pCO$_2$

A potentially more sensitive method for discriminating the two types of dementia is the responsiveness of CBF to alterations in arterial pCO$_2$. In 1953, Novack and coworkers[55] proposed that CO$_2$ inhalation might be used to identify individuals with cerebrovascular disease, since in their experience such patients had diminished blood flow responses. Based on preliminary findings, Schieve and Wilson[56] suggested that CBF responses to CO$_2$ might differentiate dementias of vascular etiology from primary neuronal degeneration. Unfortunately, subsequent investigations have contributed little to an understanding of this problem, due either to the smallness and mixed etiology of the samples[41,45] or to ambiguities in classifying dementia.[57,58]

In one of the more definitive studies, Hachinski and coworkers[54] found a small (nonsignificant) decrease in CBF responsiveness to hyperventilation among patients with multi-infarct dementia. These authors were careful to note, however, that the vasoconstrictor response to hypocapnia may not be as discriminating as the vasodilator response to hypercapnia. Recently, Yamaguchi *et al.*[59] reported a clearcut difference between patients with Alzheimer's disease and multi-infarct dementia during 5% CO$_2$ inhalation. Whereas patients with Alzheimer's disease had normal or even elevated CBF responses, those with multi-infarct dementia were only one-third as reactive.

Assuming that the latter findings can be confirmed, the difference in responsiveness to hypo- and hypercapnia requires explanation. One possibility is that in cerebrovascular disease, the normal reactive portions of the vascular bed are already maximally dilated due to ischemia in the more diseased portions. Thus, hypercapnia may be unable to increase CBF beyond existing levels in the dilated vessels, although the same vessels might still be capable of constricting appropriately to hypocapnia. In interpreting CBF responses to CO_2, allowance should be made for changes in systemic blood pressure which, as described in the next section, could influence cerebral blood flow. For this reason, cerebrovascular resistance (ratio of perfusion pressure to blood flow) is probably a better index of CO_2 effects.

Influence of Systemic Blood Pressure

In their normal aging study, Wang and Busse[37] observed a correlation between CBF and mean arterial blood pressure (MABP). Table 4-5 presents these findings, which show a significant rise in CBF with increasing blood pressure. Similar findings were obtained by Hedlund and coworkers[60] in patients with cerebrovascular disease and dementia, where a correlation of 0.60 was obtained between CBF and MABP.

On the surface, these observations suggest impairment of CBF autoregulation. However, because blood pressure was not manipulated in the individual subject, a firm conclusion cannot be drawn. Two possibilities exist that could explain the above results: (1) CBF autoregulation to blood pressure changes may actually be impaired, similar to that found in long-term diabetics,[61] or (2) the lower limit of autoregulation (i.e., the blood pressure at which CBF begins to fall) may be shifted to higher MABP levels, as in the case of severe hypertensive disease.[62] Because of its relevance to the maintenance of adequate blood flow in old age, further investigation of this problem is clearly indicated.

Cerebrovascular Insufficiency

A promising area of aging research is the relationship between cerebral hemodynamic and metabolic variables. In 1956, Kety[38] suggested that information about arteriovenous oxygen differences might shed light on cerebral blood flow alterations in senescence. Because the arteriovenous oxygen difference represents the ratio of oxygen utilization to blood flow, it can be used to indicate adequacy of the circulation. Rearrangement of the Fick equation for oxygen uptake in the brain yields: $CMRO_2/CBF = (A-V)O_2$, where $CMRO_2$ is the cerebral metabolic rate for oxygen, and $(A-V)O_2$ is the difference in oxygen content between arterial and jugular venous blood. When CBF decreases in response to a fall in $CMRO_2$ (as with anesthesia or coma), the A-V difference is essentially unchanged, indicating an adjustment of blood flow to the lesser metabolic demands of the tissue. However, when CBF declines because of ischemia, $(A-V)O_2$ increases, indicating that the brain is extracting more oxygen per unit of blood. Up to a point, a widened A-V difference can compensate for a reduction in blood flow, thereby maintaining a stable $CMRO_2$. Failure of the compensatory mechanism occurs, however, when venous

Table 4-5.   CBF at Different Mean Arterial Blood Pressures.

MABP (mm Hg)	≤ 94	95–114	≥ 115
No. Cases	10	29	9
F₁ (ml/100g/min)			
Mean	42.3*	47.5	52.5*
S.D.	4.4	10.0	11.5

* Significant difference: $p < .02$.

Data were obtained from Wang and Busse.[37]

pO_2 reaches a lower limit (about 20–25 mm Hg), thus forcing $CMRO_2$ to decline. It is at this point that circulatory insufficiency results in tissue hypoxia. Even when $CMRO_2$ is not depressed, a widened A-V difference can serve as a clue to impending or incipient cerebral hypoxia, the threshold of which may be crossed during minor hemodynamic disturbances. In cerebrovascular disease, inhomogeneous perfusion may result in some brain regions being affected earlier and to a greater degree than others.

A series of studies carried out by Dastur and coworkers[39] offers some insight into $(A\text{-}V)O_2$ changes associated with normal aging, vascular disease and dementia. Table 4-6 summarizes these findings. Whereas CBF, $(A\text{-}V)O_2$ and $CMRO_2$ were essentially the same in the normal young and elderly groups, subjects with mild, asymptomatic vascular disease showed a significant reduction in CBF that was associated with a rise in $(A\text{-}V)O_2$. Since the two variables tended to offset each other, $CMRO_2$ was unchanged. In the case of organic dementia, however, the decline in CBF was not associated with an increase in $(A\text{-}V)O_2$, but was correlated with a reduction in $CMRO_2$. Sokoloff[63] interpreted these results to indicate that in the early stages of vascular disease, reductions in cerebral blood flow are indicative of circulatory insufficiency, while in the later stages of the disease (after tissue damage has

occurred), reduced blood flow is secondary to a depression of cerebral metabolic rate.

The above findings are consistent with previous investigations by Scheinberg[64] and by Heyman *et al.*[65] on patients with cerebrovascular disease. In these studies, reduced CBF and widened A-V oxygen differences were observed following acute cerebrovascular episodes, usually with only minimal alterations in $CMRO_2$. However, in cases with long-standing cerebrovascular disease, particularly those with progressive mental deterioration, the A-V differences were not as great and cerebral blood flow tended to parallel decreases in oxygen uptake. Further confirmation of these findings is provided by Géraud *et al.*,[57] who studied three groups of patients with vascular disease of different severity. When compared with normal controls and patients with negative neurological findings, subjects who had clinically evident cerebral ischemia showed increased A-V differences. Mentally deteriorated patients, on the other hand, revealed a normal or slightly reduced $(A\text{-}V)O_2$.

The several studies cited above lend support to the notion that increased arterio-venous oxygen differences occur during the early ischemic stages of a circulatory disorder, and that $(A\text{-}V)O_2$ is essentially normal in the later stages after extensive pathological changes have occurred. They do not,

Table 4-6.   Relation of Cerebral Circulatory and Metabolic Variables to Age, Vascular Disease and Mental Status.

	NO. CASES	MEAN AGE	MEAN AND STANDARD ERROR		
			CBF (ML/100G/MIN)	$(A\text{-}V)O_2$ (VOL-%)	$CMRO_2$ (ML/100G/MIN)
From Dastur et al.[39]					
Young Controls	15	21	62.1 ±2.9	5.70 ±.30	3.51 ±.21
Normal Elderly	26	71	57.9 ±2.1	5.88 ±.17	3.33 ±.08
Asymptomatic Vascular Disease	15	73	50.8* ±2.7	6.79* ±.45	3.34 ±.14
Organic Dementia	10	72	48.5* ±3.8	5.69 ±.23	2.72* ±.18

* Significantly different from Young Controls: $p < .05$

however, indicate whether the later neuronal damage is caused by the preceding circulatory insufficiency. The interesting hypothesis that elderly persons may experience chronic cerebral hypoxia that ultimately leads to degenerative changes and dementia is difficult to support by available evidence. A-V differences of the magnitude reported are considerably below the threshold for hypoxia. Given a normal arterial O_2 content, $CMRO_2$ does not decline until $(A-V)O_2$ exceeds 9.0 vol-%.[66] Although it is possible that A-V differences of this size might occur on a regional or local level due to inhomogeneous perfusion, or that they might occur intermittently on a global level due to systemic hemodynamic disturbances, there is no reason to believe that the accompanying decrease in metabolic rate will lead to structural changes of sufficient magnitude to cause dementia. In any event, it seems unlikely that the extensive cerebral softening associated with dementia, or the occurrence of Alzheimer changes, can be produced by this mechanism.

The possibility still remains, however, that intermittent or chronic circulatory insufficiency might cause subtle changes in the neuropil which, although not producing dementia, may be responsible for the less severe intellectual impairment found in the average old person. The fact is that normal aging involves both intellectual decline and neuronal changes on the cellular level. Whether these two phenomena are related and whether circulatory insufficiency contributes to them remains a challenging question for future research.

REFERENCES

1. Obrist, W. D. Problems of aging. In A. Remond (ed.) *Handbook of Electroencephalography and Clinical Neurophysiology, Vol. 6, Part A.* Amsterdam: Elsevier Publ. Co., pp. 275–292, 1976.
2. Obrist, W. D. The electroencephalogram of normal aged adults. *Electroenceph. clin. Neurophysiol.* **6:** 235–244 (1954).
3. Obrist, W. D. and Busse, E. W. The electroencephalogram in old age. In W. P. Wilson (ed.) *Applications of Electroencephalography in Psychiatry.* Durham, N.C.: Duke University Press, pp. 185–205, 1965.
4. Otomo, E. Electroencephalography in old age: Dominant alpha pattern. *Electroenceph. clin. Neurophysiol.* **21:** 489–491 (1966).
5. Mankovsky, N. B. and Belonog, R. P. Aging of the human nervous system in the electroencephalographic aspect. *Geriatrics* **26:** 100–116 (1971).
6. Luce, R. A. and Rothschild, D. The correlation of electroencephalographic and clinical observations in psychiatric patients over 65. *J. Geront.* **8:** 167–172 (1953).
7. Frey, T. S. and Sjögren, H. The electroencephalogram in elderly persons suffering from neuropsychiatric disorders. *Acta psychiat. Scan.* **34:** 438–450 (1959).
8. Obrist, W. D. and Bissell, L. F. The electroencephalogram of aged patients with cardiac and cerebral vascular disease. *J. Geront.* **10:** 315–330 (1955).
9. Obrist, W. D. The electroencephalogram of healthy aged males. In J. E. Birren, R. N. Butler, S. W. Greenhouse, L. Sokoloff and M. R. Yarrow (eds.) *Human Aging: A Biological and Behavioral Study.* Washington: PHS Publication No. 986, U.S. Govt. Printing Office, pp. 79–93, 1963.
10. Wang, H. S. and Busse, E. W. Brain impairment and longevity. In E. Palmore (ed.) *Normal Aging II.* Durham, N.C.: Duke University Press, pp. 263–268, 1974.
11. Müller, H. F., Grad, B. and Engelsmann, F. Biological and psychological predictors of survival in a psychogeriatric population. *J. Geront.* **30:** 47–52 (1975).
12. Hubbard, O., Sunde, D. and Goldensohn, E. S. The EEG in centenarians. *Electroenceph. clin. Neurophysiol.* **40:** 407–417 (1976).
13. Obrist, W. D., Busse, E. W., Eisdorfer, C. and Kleemeier, R. W. Relation of the electroencephalogram to intellectual function in senescence. *J. Geront.* **17:** 197–206 (1962).
14. Surwillo, W. W. The relation of simple response time to brain wave frequency and the effects of age. *Electroenceph. clin. Neurophysiol.* **15:** 105–114 (1963).
15. Silverman, A. J., Busse, E. W. and Barnes, R. H. Studies in the processes of aging: Electroencephalographic findings in 400 elderly subjects. *Electroenceph. clin. Neurophysiol.* **7:** 67–74 (1955).
16. Kooi, K. A., Güvener, A. M., Tupper, C. J. and Bagchi, B. K. Electroencephalographic patterns of the temporal region in normal adults. *Neurology* **14:** 1029–1035 (1964).
17. Busse, E. W. and Obrist, W. D. Pre-senescent electroencephalographic changes in normal subjects. *J. Geront.* **20:** 315–320 (1965).
18. Bruens, J. H., Gastaut, H. and Giove, G. Electroencephalographic study of the signs of chronic vascular insufficiency of the sylvian region in aged people. *Electroenceph. clin. Neurophysiol.* **12:** 283–295 (1960).

19. Frantzen, E. and Lennox-Buchthal, M. Correlation of clinical electroencephalographic and arteriographic findings in patients with cerebral vascular accident. *Acta psychiat. Scand.* **36**, *Suppl. 150:* 133-134 (1961).

20. Obrist, W. D. Cerebral physiology of the aged: Relation to psychological function. In N. Burch and H. L. Altshuler (eds.) *Behavior and Brain Electrical Activity.* New York: Plenum, pp. 421-430, 1975.

21. Tomlinson, B. E. and Henderson, G. Some quantitative cerebral findings in normal and demented old people. In R. D. Terry and S. Gershon (eds.) *Neurobiology of Aging.* New York: Raven Press, pp. 183-204, 1976.

22. Obrist, W. D. and Henry, C. E. Electroencephalographic findings in aged psychiatric patients. *J. nerv. ment. Dis.* **126**: 254-267 (1958).

23. McAdam, W. and Robinson, R. A. Senile intellectual deterioration and the electroencephalogram: A quantitative correlation. *J. ment. Sci.* **102**: 819-825 (1956).

24. Cahan, R. B. and Yeager, C. L. Admission EEG as a predictor of mortality and discharge for aged state hospital patients. *J. Geront.* **21**: 248-256 (1966).

25. Feinberg, I., Koresko, R. L. and Heller, N. EEG sleep patterns as a function of normal and pathological aging in man. *J. psychiat. Res.* **5**: 107-144 (1967).

26. Feinberg, I. Functional implications of changes in sleep physiology with age. In R. D. Terry and S. Gershon (eds.) *Neurobiology of Aging.* New York: Raven Press, pp. 23-41, 1976.

27. Prinz, P. N. Sleep patterns in the healthy aged: Relationship with intellectual function. *J. Geront.* **32**: 179-186 (1977).

28. Brezinová, V. The number and duration of the episodes of the various EEG stages of sleep in young and older people. *Electroenceph. clin. Neurophysiol.* **39**: 273-278 (1975).

29. Brody, H. An examination of cerebral cortex and brainstem aging. In R. D. Terry and S. Gershon (eds.) *Neurobiology of Aging.* New York: Raven Press, pp. 177-181, 1976.

30. Otomo, E. and Tsubaki, T. Electroencephalography in subjects sixty years and over. *Electroenceph. clin. Neurophysiol.* **20**: 77-82 (1966).

31. Hughes, J. R. and Cayaffa, J. J. The EEG in patients at different ages without organic cerebral disease. *Electroenceph. clin. Neurophysiol.* **42**: 776-784 (1977).

32. Gordon, E. B. and Sim, M. The EEG in presenile dementia. *J. Neurol. Neurosurg. Psychiat.* **30**: 285-291 (1967).

33. Constantinidis, J., Krassoievitch, M. and Tissot, R. Corrélations entre les perturbations électroencéphalographiques et les lésions anatomohistologiques dans les démences. *L'Encéphale* **58**: 19-52 (1969).

34. Müller, H. F. and Schwartz, G. Electroencephalograms and autopsy findings in geropsychiatry. *J. Geront.* **33**: 504-513 (1978).

35. Obrist, W. D., Sokoloff, L., Lassen, N. A., Lane, M. H., Butler, R. N. and Feinberg, I. Relation of EEG to cerebral blood flow and metabolism in old age. *Electroenceph. clin. Neurophysiol.* **15**: 610-619 (1963).

36. Sulg, I. A., Cronqvist, S., Schüller, H. and Ingvar, D. H. The effect of intracardial pacemaker therapy on cerebral blood flow and electroencephalogram in patients with complete atrioventricular block. *Circulation* **39**: 487-494 (1969).

37. Wang, H. S. and Busse, E. W. Correlates of regional cerebral blood flow in elderly community residents. In A. M. Harper, W. B. Jennett, J. D. Miller and J. O. Rowan (eds.) *Blood Flow and Metabolism in the Brain.* London: Churchill Livingstone, pp. 8.17-8.18, 1975.

38. Kety, S. S. Human cerebral blood flow and oxygen consumption as related to aging. *Res. Publ. Ass. nerv. ment. Dis.* **35**: 31-45 (1956).

39. Dastur, D. K., Lane, M. H., Hansen, D. B., Kety, S. S., Butler, R. N., Perlin, S. and Sokoloff, L. Effects of aging on cerebral circulation and metabolism in man. In J. E. Birren, R. N. Butler, S. W. Greenhouse, L. Sokoloff and M. R. Yarrow (eds.) *Human Aging: A Biological and Behavioral Study.* Washington: PHS Publication No. 986, U.S. Govt. Printing Office, pp. 57-76, 1963.

40. Freyhan, F. A., Woodford, R. B. and Kety, S. S. Cerebral blood flow and metabolism in psychoses of senility. *J. nerv. ment. Dis.* **113**: 449-456 (1951).

41. Lassen, N. A., Munck, O. and Tottey, E. R. Mental function and cerebral oxygen consumption in organic dementia. *Arch. Neurol. Psychiat.* **77**: 126-133 (1957).

42. Lassen, N. A., Feinberg, I. and Lane, M. H. Bilateral studies of cerebral oxygen uptake in young and aged normal subjects and in patients with organic dementia. *J. clin. Invest.* **39**: 491-500 (1960).

43. Obrist, W. D., Chivian, E., Cronqvist, S. and Ingvar, D. H. Regional cerebral blood flow in senile and presenile dementia. *Neurology* **20**: 315-322 (1970).

44. Ingvar, D. H. and Gustafson, L. Regional cerebral blood flow in organic dementia with early onset. *Acta neurol. Scand.* **43**: 42-73 (1970).

45. Simard, D., Olesen, J., Paulson, O. B., Lassen, N. A. and Skinhøj, E. Regional cerebral blood flow and its regulation in dementia. *Brain* **94**: 273-288 (1971).

46. Baer, P. E., Faibish, G. M., Meyer, J. S., Mathew, N. A. and Skinhøj, E. Regional cerebral blood correlates of hemispheric and regional cerebral flow in dementia. In J. S. Meyer, H. Lechner and M Reivich (eds.) *Cerebral Vascular Disease: 7th International Conference Salzburg.* Stuttgart: Georg Thieme, pp. 100-106, 1976.

47. Obrist, W. D., Thompson, H. K., Jr., Wang, H. S. and Wilkinson, W. E. Regional cerebral blood flow estimated by[133] xenon inhalation. *Stroke* **6**: 245–256 (1975).

48. Tomlinson, B. E., Blessed, G. and Roth, M. Observations on the brains of demented old people. *J. neurol. Sci.* **11**: 205–242 (1970).

49. Scheibel, M. E., Lindsay, R. D., Tomiyasu, U. and Scheibel, A. B. Progressive dendritic changes in aging human cortex. *Exp. Neurol.* **47**: 392–403 (1975).

50. Brody, H. Structural changes in the aging nervous system. *Interdiscipl. Topics Geront.* **7**: 9–21 (1970).

51. Barron, S. A., Jacobs, L. and Kinkel, W. R. Changes in size of normal lateral ventricles during aging determined by computerized tomography. *Neurology* **26**: 1011–1013 (1976).

52. Hachinski, V. C., Lassen, N. A. and Marshall, J. Multi-infarct dementia: A cause of mental deterioration in the elderly. *Lancet* **2**: 207–210 (1974).

53. O'Brien, M.D. and Mallett, B. L. Cerebral cortex perfusion rates in dementia. *J. Neurol. Neurosurg. Psychiat.* **33**: 497–500 (1970).

54. Hachinski, V. C., Iliff, L. D., Zilhka, E., DuBoulay, G. H., McAllister, V. L., Marshall, J., Russell, R. W. R. and Symon, L. Cerebral blood flow in dementia. *Arch. Neurol.* **32**: 632–637 (1975).

55. Novack, P., Shenkin, H. A., Bortin, L., Goluboff, B. and Soffe, A. M. The effects of carbon dioxide inhalation upon the cerebral blood flow and cerebral oxygen consumption in vascular disease. *J. clin. Invest.* **32**: 696–702 (1953).

56. Schieve, J. F. and Wilson, W. P. The influence of age, anesthesia and cerebral arteriosclerosis on cerebral vascular activity to CO_2. *Amer. J. Med.* **15**: 171–174 (1953).

57. Géraud, J., Bes, A., Delpla, M. and Marc-Vergnes, J. P. Cerebral arteriovenous oxygen differences: Reappraisal of their significance for evaluation of brain function. In J. S. Meyer, H. Lechner and O. Eichhorn (eds.) *Research on the Cerebral Circulation.* Springfield, Ill.: Charles C. Thomas, pp. 209–222, 1969.

58. Dekoninck, W. J., Collard, M. and Jacquy, J. Comparative study of cerebral vasoactivity in vascular sclerosis of the brain in elderly men. *Stroke* **6**: 673–677 (1975).

59. Yamaguchi, F., Meyer, J. S., Sakai, F. and Yamamoto, M. Behavioral activation testing in the dementias. In J. S. Meyer, H. Lechner, M. Reivich and E. Ott (eds.) *Cerebral Vascular Disease: 9th International Conference Salzburg.* Amsterdam: Excerpta Medica, (in press), 1979.

60. Hedlund, S., Köhler, V., Nylin, G., Olsson, R., Regnström, O., Rothström, E. and Aström, K. E. Cerebral blood circulation in dementia. *Acta psychiat. Scand.* **40**: 77–106 (1964).

61. Bentsen, N., Larsen, B. and Lassen, N. Chronically impaired autoregulation of cerebral blood flow in long-term diabetics. *Stroke* **6**: 497–502 (1975).

62. Strandgaard, S., Olesen, J., Skinhøj, E. and Lassen, N. A. Autoregulation of brain circulation in severe arterial hypertension. *Brit. med. J.* **1**: 507–510 (1973).

63. Sokoloff, L. Cerebral circulatory and metabolic changes associated with aging. *Res. Publ. Ass. nerv. ment. Dis.* **41**: 237–254 (1966).

64. Scheinberg, P. Cerebral blood flow in vascular disease of the brain. *Amer. J. Med.* **8**: 139–147 (1950).

65. Heyman, A., Patterson, J. L., Duke, T. W. and Battey, L. L. The cerebral circulation and metabolism in arteriosclerotic and hypertensive cerebrovascular disease. *New Eng. J. Med.* **249**: 223–229 (1953).

66. Finnerty, F. A., Witkin, L. and Fazekas, J. F. Cerebral hemodynamics during cerebral ischemia induced by acute hypotension. *J. clin. Invest.* **33**: 1227–1232 (1954).

67. Lavy, S., Melamed, M., Bentin, S., Cooper, G. and Rinot, Y. Bihemispheric decreases of regional cerebral blood flow in dementia: Correlation with aged-matched normal controls. *Ann. Neurol.* **4**: 445–450 (1978).

Chapter 5

Neuropharmacology of Aging

J. Ingram Walker, M.D.
and
H. Keith H. Brodie, M.D.

Duke University Medical Center

INTRODUCTION

It is estimated that almost one-third of the 20 million U.S. citizens over 60 years of age receive a psychotropic medication during the course of a year.[1] A survey conducted at Duke University Medical Center[2] showed that 28% of the elderly living in Durham County were on psychoactive medications. This figure jumped to 65% in those who were residents of extended care facilities. Prien and his associates[3] conducted a survey of all patients over 60 years of age at 12 Veterans Administration hospitals. Seventy per cent of those patients with a diagnosis of mental illness received a psychoactive drug, while 23% with a diagnosis of no mental disorder received some type of psychoactive drug. The most commonly prescribed psychoactive drugs were thioridizine (Mellaril), 21% of the drug orders: chlorpromazine (Thorazine), 16%; diazepam (Valium), 7%; dihydroergotoxine (Hydergine), 7%; amitriptyline (Elavil), 5%; and trifluoperazine (Stelazine), 5%. Twenty-eight drugs comprised the remaining 39% of the orders. In 1974, HEW[4] randomly sampled 288 long-term care facilities participating in Medicare-Medicaid programs. Of the 3458 residents surveyed, 78% of the patients were 65 years of age or older. There were 1,731,360 prescriptions written—6.1 per patient. Sixty per cent of the patients had prescriptions for cathartics; 51.3% for analgesics; and 46.9% for tranquilizers. Thioridizine (given to 26% of the population) was the sixth most frequently prescribed drug in skilled nursing facilities, led only by aspirin, magnesium hydroxide, multiple vitamins, digoxin, and propoxyphene. Chlordiazepoxide was tenth (23%) and diazepam was twelfth (18%); 5.67% of the population were on prochlorperazine, and 5.57% were on haloperidol.

Despite tremendous advances in psychopharmacology over the past 25 years (hundreds of double blind studies have been done on chlorpromazine alone)[5] and an ever-increasing geriatric population (Currently 10% of the U.S. population is over 65 years of age, and this figure is estimated to grow 40% by the year 2000.),[6] there is an alarming paucity of psychopharmacological studies involving the elderly. The choice of drug seems to be related more to conjecture and physician prescribing habits rather than to sound scientific study. Because of the lack of well-controlled studies on the effectiveness of psychotropic medications in the elderly, it will be necessary to extrapolate by relating what is known about psychopharmacology in the general population to the elderly.

After discussing the general effect of aging on the activity of drugs, this chapter will address the use of specific psychotropic agents for the elderly including indications, contraindications, and therapeutic outcome.

EFFECT OF AGING ON THE ACTIVITY OF PSYCHOTROPIC MEDICATION

Physiologic changes with aging alter the activity of psychotropic medication considerably. Decreased absorption of drugs in the elderly can result from a reduction in digestive enzymes, a smaller intestinal absorbing surface, impaired epithelial transport systems, and reduced mensenteric blood flow.[7] Transportation of drugs decreases with age, due in part to decreased cardiac output. Bender[8] found that cardiac output declines approximately 1% a year from age 19 to 86, with a proportionately larger blood flow to the brain and coronaries than to the liver and kidneys. The redistribution of blood flow can cause an increase in drug potency in the brain and heart with a decrease in drug elimination. A decreased cardiac output, vasoconstriction of renal vasculature, and a decline of renal tubular mass causes a 55% reduction in renal clearance from age 40 to 89. Body fat increases with age while protein decreases. Highly lipid-soluble drugs are reabsorbed by the renal tubule and remain in the circulation longer. Increased total body fat in the elderly prolongs the duration of action of highly lipid-soluble drugs while decreased enzyme activity and increased liver disease in the elderly result in a slower drug metabolism. The decrease in protein-binding

capacity increases the concentration of the active drug.[9]

Altered drug activity in the elderly may occur despite normal psychoactive drug blood levels due to a decrease in the number of receptors and concentration of neurotransmitters as well as structural changes in the responsive tissues. Dopamine, norepinephrine, serotonin concentrations, and the activity of tyrosine hydroxylase and cholinesterase in brain, all decrease with age.[10] The activity of monamine oxidase (MAO), which metabolizes norepinephrine, dopamine, and serotonin, increases with age, particularly in the fifth, sixth, and seventh decades.[11]

TREATMENT OF SCHIZOPHRENIA AND FUNCTIONAL PARANOID DISORDERS

Schizophrenia usually begins during the patient's early life while paranoid disorders may develop as a reaction to the changes resulting from aging.

The elderly are susceptible to paranoid disorders because of a tendency toward social isolation and increased visual and hearing difficulties that occur with advancing age.[7] Paranoid disorders include persecutory or grandiose delusions in which organic dementia or primary affective illness cannot explain the symptoms.

Though schizophrenia usually persists into old age, the clinical picture may change considerably: hallucinations often become less frequent, delusions are modified, and the elderly schizophrenic generally becomes more withdrawn and isolated.[7] Young schizophrenic patients when taken off their antipsychotic medication generally relapse.[12] These findings correlate well with both the dopamine hypothesis of schizophrenia which suggests that schizophrenia may be associated with a relative increase of dopamine at the postsynaptic receptor sites and the findings that brain concentrations of dopamine decrease with age.[7]

The mode of action of the antipsychotic agents in the treatment of schizophrenia and paranoid states is believed to be related to the blockade of dopaminergic receptor sites. There are five major classes of antipsychotic medications: (1) the phenothiazines consisting of aliphatics with a straight chain of carbon atoms attached to a tricyclic nucleus containing two benzine rings and a central ring containing a sulfa and a nitrogen atom, the piperidines which have a cyclic structure as part of the side chain, and the piperazines with variations in the cyclic side chain that increase their potency; (2) the butyrophenones which were developed from meperidine (Demerol) in the search for a non-addicting analgesic; (3) the thioxanthenes with a substitution of a carbon atom for a nitrogen atom in the central phenothiazine ring; (4) the dibenzoxazepine (5) the indoles.[13] The three latter classes have rarely been used in the elderly (Table 5-1).

Since the selection of an antipsychotic depends on the drug's pharmacological properties and side effects, it is useful to divide the antipsychotic agents into low and high potency groups. The high potency drugs are powerful blockers of dopamine receptors and require a lower dose to produce the same effects as the low potency antipsychotics which are weaker blockers of dopamine receptors. Chlorpromazine (an aliphatic phenothiazine), and thioridizine (a piperidine phenothiazine), are the low potency antipsychotics most frequently used in the elderly. They have strong sedative effects (due to alpha adrenergic blocking properties), marked anticholinergic effects, and a low incidence of extrapyramidal reactions. The high potency compounds used in the elderly—acetophenazine fluphenazine, perphenazine, and trifluoperazine (piperazine phenothiazines), and haloperidol (a butyrophenone)—have less sedative and anticholinergic effects, but a greater tendency to produce extrapyramidal side effects.[14]

While there is a large variety of available antipsychotics that appear to have equal efficacy when given in adequate dosage, the

Table 5-1. Equivalent Doses of Commonly used Antipsychotic Agents in the Elderly by Chemical Type.

GENERIC NAME	TRADE NAME	APPROXIMATE EQUIVALENT DAILY DOSE (MG)
Phenothiazines		
Aliphatic		
Chlorpromazine	Thorazine, etc. (generic)	100
Piperidines		
Thioridazine	Mellaril	95
Piperazines		
Acetophenazine	Tindal	20
Fluphenazine	Prolixin, Permitil	2
Periphenazine	Trilafon	10
Trifluoperazine	Stelazine	5
Thioxanthenes		
Aliphatic		
Chlorprothixene	Taractan	65
Piperazine		
Thiothixene	Navane	5
Butyrophenones		
Haloperidol	Haldol	2

From Baldessarini, R. J. *Chemotherapy in Psychiatry*. Cambridge: Harvard University Press, 1977.

evaluation of several parameters can be helpful in selecting an antipsychotic medication. The patient's response to medication and physical condition are important considerations. For example, an insomniac might respond best to the sedative effects of chlorpromazine, while a malnourished elderly patient might suffer from this drug's hypotensive side effects.

Antipsychotic drugs are rapidly absorbed into the bloodstream—5–10 minutes after IM injection, and 30–60 minutes after oral administration—and readily cross the blood brain barrier. They are highly lipid-soluble and are slowly metabolized because of tissue binding. The hepatic microsomal enzymes break down the antipsychotics into water soluble products that are excreted in the bile and urine.[13]

In initiating antipsychotic medication in the elderly, a small test dose is recommended after which, if no major side effects develop, the dose may be increased until therapeutic benefits or toxicity develop. The maintenance dose should be the lowest possible that can sustain the patient at an acceptable level of improvement. Occasionally, after an adequate trial of 2–3 weeks, a patient will fail to respond to a particular antipsychotic. If this occurs, the patient should be switched to an antipsychotic of a different class. Generally, however, the most common cause of drug failure is patient noncompliance.

Because of the long half-life of the antipsychotics, the medication can be given in single nighttime doses if this does not result in orthostatic hypotensive effects. To lessen the chance of long-term side effects, especially tardive dyskinesia, drug-free holidays are advocated. Most patients can skip their medications for two or three days weekly without exacerbation of symptoms. Patients who have been on low doses of antipsychotics for many years without fluctuation in clinical course probably do not need to continue their medications.[12] Gardos and Cole,[15] in a review of outpatient drug withdrawal studies, concluded that as many

as 50% of chronic schizophrenics may not need to be on antipsychotic medication at all. Prien and his associates found that older schizophrenics receiving doses equivalent to less than 250 mg. chlorpromazine can tolerate discontinuation of the drug without relapse.[16]

Thioridazine is the most commonly used antipsychotic in the elderly. Its anticholinergic properties can lead to cardiac arrhythmias and toxic delirium but these properties protect against extrapyramidal side effects, minimizing the tendency for drug-induced movement disorders.[13] Branchey[17] et al. found electrocardiographic changes, weight gain, and decreased blood pressure in 27 of 30 elderly schizophrenic patients treated with thioridazine. Pigmentary retinopathy develops in patients who are maintained on doses of thioridazine greater than 800 mg. Thioridizine has alphaadrenergic blocking properties resulting in sedation equal to that produced by chlorpromazine but more profound than that produced by haloperidol. For reasons that have not been completely explained, thioridizine causes more frequent inhibition of ejaculation than drugs with stronger alpha-adrenergic blocking properties.[13] In the elderly patient already concerned about his deteriorating physical condition, inhibition of ejaculation could have serious psychological consequences.

In a survey conducted at 12 Veterans Administration hospitals, chlorpromazine was used in 22% of the elderly schizophrenic patients.[16] Since chlorpromazine has a tendency to produce hypotensive crises in debilitated patients, supine and standing blood pressure measurements should be done in the elderly before and after a test dose of chlorpromazine prior to routine administration of the drug. Several studies have shown the efficacy of chlorpromazine in treating elderly psychotic patients with dosages ranging from 50–300 mg. daily.[18]

The piperazine, trifluoperazine (Stelazine), was used in 8% of schizophrenics in the VA study.[16] Trifluoperazine has a high potential for acute dystonic muscle spasms, motor restlessness, and parkinsonian-like side effects. In most clinical studies, the effective dosage ranged from 2 mg. to 20 mg. daily.[18]

Branchey et al.,[17] in a crossover study, compared fluphenazine hydrochloride (dose range, 1.5 mg. to 5.0 mg. daily) with thioridizene hydrochloride (dose range, 84 mg. to 285 mg.) in 30 elderly schizophrenics. They concluded that the clinical efficacy of the two medications was similar, but the side effects of fluphenazine were less severe.

The long-acting parenteral piperazines, fluphenazine enanthate (with a duration of action of 10–14 days) and fluphenazine decanoate (with a duration of 14–21 days), can be used if the patient is not reliable enough to take his oral medication or if it is suspected that the medication is poorly absorbed when given orally. Approximately 25 mg. of enanthate or decanoate given every other week is equal to 5 mg. of oral fluphenazine administered once daily.[19]

A relatively mild acting piperazine, acetophenazine (Tindal), has few extrapyramidal side effects and is apparently well tolerated in the elderly.[18]

Haloperidol, a butyrophenone, has minimal anticholinergic and alpha-adrenergic blocking properties, thus producing fewer electrocardiographic, hypotensive and sedative effects than the low potency antipsychotics, but this drug produces a high frequency of extrapyramidal side effects. Haloperidol has been found to be effective in treating excitement, hostility, hallucinatory behavior, suspiciousness, grandiosity, withdrawal, uncooperativeness, and paranoid symptomatology in the elderly, with an average dose of 2 mg. daily.[18] The geriatric patient should receive 0.5 mg. daily as a starting dose to lessen the chances of extrapyramidal side effects.

Evidence has accumulated that the more potent antipsychotics are the most powerful blockers of dopamine resulting in a greater tendency to produce extrapyramidal symptoms (EPS). There are three dopamine pathways in the CNS: the nigro-striatal, the mesolimbic, and the tubo-infundibular.[20] Dopamine blockade in the mesolimbic terminals is believed to reverse psychotic thought, while dopamine blockade in the nigro-striatal results in EPS.[21] It has been estimated that extrapyramidal symptoms occur in 50% of all patients on antipsychotics between the ages of 60 and 80; 90% of these reactions occur within the first two months of therapy.[9] It has been noted that younger patients tend toward dyskinesia, patients between age 40 and 50 toward akathesia, and the elderly have a greater likelihood of a parkinsonian-like syndrome.[9]

Acute dystonic reactions usually occur within the first hour to five days of the onset of treatment and are characterized by acute spasms of the trunkal, nuchal, buccal, and oculomotor muscle groups. Acute dystonias can be reversed dramatically with benztropine (Congentin) 0.5–2.0 mg. IV or 25–50 mg. IV diphenhydramine (Benadryl).[19]

Akathesia—motor restlessness with an inability to sit still—usually develops within 5 to 40 days after treatment is started. It can be misdiagnosed as agitation, resulting in a tendency for the physician to increase the dose of antipsychotic medication. Increasing the dosage will only make the akathesia patient more restless or lead to sedation and rigidity. The correct treatment for this side effect is to discontinue or decrease the dosage of the antipsychotic. Alternatively, IV benztropine or diphenhydramine will generally reduce the symptoms in a few minutes.[19]

A parkinsonian-like syndrome associated with antipsychotic administration produces bradykinesia, resting tremor, masked faces, rigidity, and occasional drooling. This syndrome is more common in the elderly than dyskinesia or akathesia. This complication generally occurs within a few weeks after initiation of antipsychotic therapy and may cause the patient to appear depressed. Instead of adding an antidepressant, the physician should prescribe an antiparkinsonian medication. Either benztropine (Congentin), 0.5–2.0 mg. p.o. daily or trihexyphenadryl (Artane), 2–8 mg. p.o., given in daily divided doses would be reasonable choices.[19] These anticholinergic drugs are effective because they restore the cholinergic/dopaminergic balance in the caudate nucleus. When dopaminergic activity is blocked by the antipsychotics, cholinergic activity dominates, resulting in EPS. When an anticholinergic is added, cholinergic activity is decreased, restoring the balance and thus relieving the extrapyramidal symptoms.[21]

Antiparkinsonian medications should be given only when extrapyramidal symptoms develop for several reasons: (1) There is some evidence that the antiparkinsonian agents decrease the effectiveness of antipsychotics by causing a relative increase in dopaminergic activity; (2) Antiparkinsonian drugs may decrease the absorption of antipsychotics; (3) Antiparkinsonian drugs exacerbate tardive dyskinesia; (4) The antiparkinsonian drugs may produce an acute brain syndrome, decreased bladder or bowel function, prostatic hypertrophy, cardiac arrhythmias, or aggravation of glaucoma secondary to their potent anticholinergic properties.[23] In those patients who develop extrapyramidal signs, the antiparkinsonian drugs may be discontinued after two or three months because extrapyramidal signs tend to dissipate within a few months of dopaminergic blockade with antipsychotics[13] (probably due to tolerance to the dopaminergic blockade in the caudate nucleus).[22]

Prolonged dopaminergic blockage results in a state of hypersensitivity of the dopamine receptors in the nigro-striatal area.[21] Eventually small amounts of dopamine that escape blockade stimulate their receptors resulting in tardive dyskinesia, a syndrome characterized by ticlike choreiform movements that occasionally have an athetotic or dystonic component and typically involve the face, tongue, and neck muscles, and rarely the extremities.[13]

Reports of tardive dyskinesia in association with antipsychotic administration vary from 3-6% in a mixed psychiatric population to 40% in elderly, chronically hospitalized patients.[22] Elderly patients are prone to develop this disorder after relatively brief periods of antipsychotic treatment.[24] The more potent dopamine blockers induce tardive dyskinesia more frequently.[22]

To prevent tardive dyskinesia, every effort should be made to achieve therapeutic benefits with the least amount of medication and intermittent therapy (drug holidays) should be used whenever possible. Every patient should be examined at least quarterly for early signs of tardive dyskinesia. Early dyskinesia is exhibited by rhythmical vermiform movements of the tongue and the floor of the mouth. The inability to protrude the tongue for more than a few seconds is also indicative. Early digital dyskinesia is characterized by small involuntary movements of the fingers.[13] If the antipsychotic medication is discontinued when early signs of tardive dyskinesia begin to appear, it is usually possible to reverse the condition completely.

There is no treatment for tardive dyskinesia, although several methods have been tried. The disorder can be temporarily suppressed by increasing the dose of antipsychotic, but there soon will be a breakthrough (escape) and the medication will be needed in ever-increasing doses, eventually failing completely. Several uncontrolled studies suggest that deanol acetamidobenzoate, a postulated acetylcholine precursor, may be an effective treatment.[22] In a double-blind crossover study involving 14 patients, 2mg. of deanol given daily for four weeks was found to be no more effective than placebo in the treatment of tardive dyskinesia.[25] In another study, oral choline in doses of 150–200 mg/kg decreased choreic movements in 9 of 20 patients with tardive dyskinesia.[26] Physostigmine[27] and low dose apomorphine[28] have been reported to be effective in a few experimental studies using a small patient sample. Apomorphine decreases dopamine synthesis at the presynaptic neuron in low doses but is a dopamine agonist at the postsynaptic receptor in higher doses. Antiparkinsonian drugs are contraindicated because they increase dopamine dominance and there is some evidence that prophylactic use of antiparkinsonian drugs increases the possibility of later development of tardive dyskinesia.[29]

Withdrawal dyskinesia can result from the rapid discontinuation of large doses of antipsychotic medications. To avoid acute choreoathetotic reactions, the dose of antipsychotics should be decreased gradually.[13]

A rather common problem in the elderly is a central anticholinergic syndrome, which is especially frequent with thioridizine and chlorpromazine, as well as with tricyclic antidepressants, because of their high anticholinergic side effects. The incidence varies from 16% to 35% of elderly patients receiving psychoactive medications.[12/30] Signs include agitation, anxiety, restlessness, dilirium, disorientation, impaired recent memory, hallucinations and slurred speech. Peripheral signs include cardiac arrhythmias, dilated pupils which react slowly to light, warm dry skin, decreased mucosal secretions, and urinary retention. Treatment consists of 1–2 mg. IV of physostigmine given slowly which may be repeated as needed every 15–30 minutes. Physostigmine may cause the *opposite* peripheral signs of atropine toxicity in addition to confusion, seizures, nausea, and hallucinations. Treatment of physostigmine-induced cholinergic excess is atropine given subcutaneously, 0.5 mg. for every mg. of physostigmine previous given.[13]

Older patients are particularly prone to the peripheral anticholinergic effects of the antipsychotics such as urinary retention, blurred vision, paralytic ileus, and dry mouth. Twenty-five mg. of bethanechol (Urecholine) given three times daily may be helpful in preventing annoying anticholinergic side effects.[13] Xerostomia and subsequent parotid infections secondary to dry mouth can occur in the elderly. Hydration, good oral hygiene, chewing gum, and candy sucking (especially butterscotch) can be helpful.[13] A saliva substitute—VA/oral tube—has recently been found effective for xerostomia in psychiatric patients receiving psychoactive medications.[31] Undiagnosed glaucoma occurs in approximately 2½% of persons over 40 and is aggravated by the anticholinergic properties of the antipsychotics.[9] The patient who is maintained on cholinomimetic eyedrops for chronic glaucoma can receive antipsychotic medications. An acute attack of glaucoma that is precipitated by psychotropic medications requires immediate ophthalmological consultation.[13]

A cholestatic-type jaundice occurs in approximately 1% of patients treated with antipsychotic medication,[32] particularly chlorpromazine, and is believed to be a hypersensitivity reaction which results in small bile duct obstruction; most patients recover spontaneously a few weeks after the medication is discontinued. Apparently the incidence of chlorpromazine jaundice is decreasing, probably due to a greater purity in the manufacture of the drug.[32]

Agranulocytosis, a life-threatening side effect of antipsychotic medications, usually occurs in the first 2 months of treatment and is almost always associated with low potency antipsychotic administration. One in 200 elderly patients have drug-induced agranulocytosis, compared to one in 6,000 of the general population; 75% of all agranulocytosis occurs in patients over 50 years of age.[9]

Approximately 4% of the elderly have photosensitivity rashes secondary to antipsychotic administration. A chronic blue-gray discoloration of the skin can result from long-term antipsychotic medication. Low potency phenothiazines can also cause deposition of pigment in the cornea, lens, and retina.[33]

Low potency phenothiazines may have a tendency to increase seizures in epileptic patients. Patients with seizures respond best to the high potency piperazines and haloperidol.[13]

The alpha-adrenergic blocking properties of the low potency antipsychotics correlate with their sedative effects and their tendency to produce orthostatic hypotension. The risk of cardiovascular toxicity secondary to the antipsychotics is rare although sudden death presumably due to ventricular tachyarrhythmias have been reported. Prolonged ventricular repolarization can occur with the low potency antipsychotics, especially thioridizine. In addition, thioridazine can produce electrocardiographic changes resembling hypokalemia. One study demonstrated EKG changes in 90% of elderly patients treated with thioridizine.[17]

The ratio of toxic dose to effective dose (therapeutic index) is very high in antipsychotic agents. Respiratory depression, coma, and death is extremely uncommon. However, it should be remembered that the antipsychotic agents are not easily dialyzable because of their protein and lipid-binding properties.[13]

TREATMENT OF AFFECTIVE ILLNESS

The affective disorders include primary mood disturbances and are divided into three groups as defined in DSM-III:[34] (1) Episodic affective disorders characterized by a mood disturbance in which there is a sustained disturbance clearly distinguished from previous functioning; (2) Chronic affective disorders characterized by an illness of two years or more without a clear onset; (3) Atypical affective disorders characterized by a disturbance of mood that cannot be classified as episodic, chronic, or an adjustment disorder (Table 5-2).

The present biological theories of affective illness include the catecholamine (dopamine and norepinephrine) and the idoleamine (serotonin) hypotheses. These hypotheses suggest that the functional turnover of catecholamines is increased at specific central synapses in mania and decreased in depression.[35] The indoleamine hypothesis posits a deficit of serotonin turnover in both mania and depression, with a greater decrease of serotonin in depression.[35] In addition, cholinergic mechanisms may play a role in the etiology of affective disorders.

Treatment of mania and bipolar disorders

Lithium is indicated for the treatment of acute manic attacks, to prevent the recurrence of manic attacks, and to modify bipolar mood swings. Despite numerous controlled trials suggesting that lithium is prophylactic against recurrent depressions, the FDA has yet to approve it for this use.[36]

Although acute episodes of mania or hypomania occur infrequently for the first time in old age, many patients begun on lithium earlier in their life will need to be maintained on the medication for decades to prevent recurrent attacks.

Since lithium is not an innocuous drug, the physician should use clinical judgment as to whether the patient's abnormal mood swings are significant enough to merit continued long-term treatment risk. Any disease that would impair lithium excretion is an

Table 5-2. Recommended Treatments for Affective Disorders

TYPE OF AFFECTIVE DISORDER	TREATMENT OF FIRST CHOICE
Adjustment disorder with depressed mood	Psychotherapy
Recurrent depressive disorder	Tricyclic antidepressant during acute phase; Lithium for prophylaxis if there is a history of hypomania.
Bipolar affective disorder	Lithium
Episodes of recurrent manic attacks	Lithium
Depressive disorder, single episode	Tricyclic antidepressants
Intermittent depressive disorder	Psychotherapy; Tricyclic antidepressants if symptoms severe.
Psychotic depression	Antipsychotics; if no response, ECT.
Atypical depression	MAO inhibitors

absolute contraindication to lithium administration. Suicidal or impulsive patients are poor candidates for therapy because of the danger of lithium overdose which can be fatal. In patients with heart disease or on treatment programs that require diuretics or sodium restriction, lithium may be indicated if the risks of therapy are less than the benefits, and the patient can be followed closely. Since lithium use can affect thyroid function and white cell count, these parameters should be assessed periodically. Thus, an annual evaluation of patients on maintenance lithium should include a thorough physical examination, complete blood count, urinalysis, electrocardiogram, blood urea nitrogen, serum creatinine, and serum thyroxine. (Table 5-3)

Over 99% of a single oral dose of lithium is easily absorbed with serum levels reaching a peak in one to three hours. Lithium is not bound to plasma proteins and is excreted unchanged in the urine at the rate of approximately one-fifth of the creatinine clearance. Excretion varies considerably with age, the half-life ranging from 18 hours in young adults to 36 hours in the elderly.[36]

Since sodium and lithium compete for reabsorption at the proximal renal tubule, a deficit in sodium results in an increase in lithium reabsorption. A fall in total body sodium resulting from salt restriction, dehydration, increased sweating, or diuretic medication leads to lithium retention.

The ease of determining the concentration

Table 5-3.   Recommended Evaluation Prior to Beginning Lithium Therapy.*

1. Physical Examination
2. Complete Blood Count
3. Urinalysis
4. T-4 (Mean-Free Thyroxin)
5. Electrocardiogram
6. Electrolytes
7. Blood-Urea-Nitrogen
8. Creatinine

* Adapted from Cain, N. N., & R. M., "A Compendium of Psychiatric Drugs, Part II", *Drug Therapy*, 1975. p. 82.

of lithium in serum reported in mEq/1, measured by atomic absorption assay or flame photometry, has contributed tremendously to the reliability and safety of its use. To provide a reliable measure of the lithium level, the blood sample should be drawn 12 hours after the last lithium dose when absorption is complete and excretion less erratic.[36]

Occasionally an episode of acute manic behavior will occur in an elderly patient who is not on lithium, but who has a history of an affective disorder that would justify a trial of lithium. Since the onset of action of lithium is 7–10 days, it is probably best to begin the patient on an antipsychotic such as haloperidol or chlorpromazine concurrently with lithium. As the manic behavior comes under control, the antipsychotic can be discontinued and the patient continued on lithium alone.[37]

The dose of lithium depends on the severity of the illness, the patient's age, weight, physical condition, and kidney function. Since elderly patients excrete lithium slowly, they require less medication to reach therapeutic blood levels. While a younger manic patient may require 1200–1800 mg. of lithium carbonate daily in divided doses to reach a lithium level in the therapeutic range of 1.0 to 1.5 mEq/1, an elderly manic patient may require only 600–900 mg. daily. Blood levels should be followed every second or third day until the manic level subsides.

After the manic episode has been controlled, the initial dose of lithium should be reduced to maintain a lithium level of between .8–1.2 mEq/1. Although there may be considerable variation in dosage and the elderly may require a much lower dose than would generally be expected, the usual maintenance dose ranges from between 600–1800 mg. per day and most frequently is 300 mg. three times a day. After the patient has been discharged from the hospital, it is judicious to monitor serum levels once a week for four weeks and then once a month for 12 months. Once a certain dose has been established, it can often be maintained in a particular patient for many years; however, serum levels should be determined frequently enough to insure compliance and safety. Signs of a manic or depressive episode, an intercurrent disease, a significant change in salt intake, the institution of or symptoms of intoxication require more frequent monitoring of the lithium level.

Mild symptoms of lithium toxicity generally begin at a blood level of 1.5 mEq/1. At 2.0 mEq/1 symptoms of toxicity become serious and lithium levels greater than 3.0 mEq/1 are life-threatening. It should be kept in mind that elderly patients are prone to severe toxic symptoms despite a serum lithium level in the maintenance range; thus, clinical judgment should be the final determining factor in evaluating a patient with possible lithium toxicity. The earliest toxic signs include nausea, vomiting, lethargy, slurred speech, and an exaggerated coarse tremor of the hands. Electrocardiographic changes may include flattening and inversion of the T-wave. As intoxication increases, neurological symptoms become prominent with fasciculations, clonic movements, EEG changes, progressing to seizures, stupor, and finally coma. Fatalities are usually secondary to pulmonary complications resulting from coma.[36]

If lithium toxicity develops, the drug should be stopped immediately and the patient monitored with daily or more frequent lithium levels, electrolytes, and electrocardiograms. Electrolytes should be replaced as needed. Lithium excretion is enhanced by increasing the fluid intake to 5–6 liters a day. Twenty grams of urea, given IV two times daily, or manitol, 50–100 grams IV daily, also increases lithium diuresis. Aminophyline, 500 mg., given by slow IV push every 6 hours, suppresses tubular reabsorption of lithium in addition to increasing blood flow through the tubules. One ampule of sodium lactate can be given as a bolus IV or added to each IV bottle. This increases lithium excretion by alkalyzing the urine. Hemodialysis may be necessary for refractory lithium toxicity.[36]

Chronic side effects unrelated to blood levels occur infrequently and are reversible when lithium is discontinued. The initial sodium diuresis is common during the first few weeks of lithium treatment but may persist as a chronic polyuria in some patients. Rarely, polyuria develops into a nephrogenic diabetes insipidus-like syndrome characterized by excessive intake of fluids, constant thirst, and a large output of very dilute urine. A benign diffuse enlargement of the thyroid gland occurs in approximately 3% of patients on chronic lithium therapy. These patients are usually euthyroid and the goiters disappear when lithium is discontinued. Rarely, localized edema, skin rashes, or ulcerations may develop. Patients with these side effects may benefit from topical steroids or oral antihistamines. An insignificant leucocytosis without a left shift found in infection may develop in patients on lithium treatment.[36]

Although the mechanism of action of lithium is unknown, lithium may affect neuronal membrane potential by displacing sodium ions. Lithium also prevents the release of norepinephrine and dopamine at CNS synapses, increases catecholamine uptake and turnover, and inhibits serotonin turnover.[37]

Treatment of depression

Depression, easily confused with organic brain syndrome (dementia) or hypochondriasis, is a global term that encompasses several distinct clinical entities as defined in DSM-III:[34]

Adjustment disorder with depressed mood is a maladaptive reaction to a psychosocial stress that gradually remits when the stress ceases. Uncomplicated bereavement is an expected reaction to loss of a loved one and is not considered an adjustment disorder.

Recurrent depressive disorders are characterized by episodes with the biological signs of depression, including decreased appetite, decreased libido, terminal sleep disturbance, diurnal mood variation, as well as apathy and anergy. These episodes of depression are separated by periods of normal mood.

Depressive disorder, single episode can also be described as an agitated depression, retarded depression or unresolved grief depending on the presenting symptomatology.[38] An agitated depressive syndrome characterized by pacing, hand wringing, paranoid ideation, and feelings of guilt commonly occur in patients 45 years of age and was formerly known as involutional depression. Retarded depression, characterized by slowed speech and decreased psychomotor activity, is common in the elderly. Unresolved grief is a single episode of depression related to a loss that persists beyond eight weeks, generally requiring medical treatment for resolution.

Bipolar affective disorder is characterized by episodes of depression alternating with periods of mania.

Chronic depressive disorder, previously known as chronic characterological depressive disorder, neurotic depressive disorder, or depressive character disorder, applies to patients with life-long depressive behavior that may be separated by periods of normal mood lasting no more than two months.

Psychotic depression can include any of the above depressions if they are severe enough to lead to loss of contact with reality and the inability to function. Persecutory and somatic delusions and hallucinations are common.

Atypical depression is a depressive disorder that fits none of the above categories. There is a predominance of phobic anxiety in the depressive symptomatology with emotional lability, histrionic attention-seeking, and demanding behavior.[38]

Since their development in the late 1950s, the tricyclic antidepressants have become the treatment of first choice for patients with biological signs of depression. There are currently six tricyclic compounds marketed in the U.S., the tertiary amines—imipramine, amitriptyline, and doxepin, and their demethylated metabolites—desipiramine, nortriptyline, and protriptyline.[39] The tertiary amines appear to block the reuptake inactivation of biogenic amines principally serotonin at the CNS synaptic junction, the secondary amines principally block reuptake inactivation of norepinephrine.[40] By blocking reuptake of the monoamines, the tricyclic antidepressants elevate the concentration of the neurotransmitter at the synaptic junction. The tricyclics also appear to weakly inhibit MAO and are powerful anticholinergic agents as well.[39]

The six tricyclic compounds have a common structure, consisting of two benzene rings between a seven member central ring containing a side chain. They differ chemically from each other by minor changes in the central ring and the side chain.[39] These chemical changes result in a difference in their clinical effects; thus, imipramine and desipramine are less sedating than amitiptyline, doxepin, and nortriptyline, while protriptyline is a stimulating agent.[40]

The tricyclic antidepressants (TCA) are rapidly absorbed after oral administration. In middle-aged adults, only 10% of the drug is found in the bloodstream in the active, unbound form;[39] thus in the elderly who have less protein, there is a tendency to have higher levels of unbound tricyclics resulting in a higher incidence of side effects than in the population under age 60.[7]

The rate of metabolism for the TCA decreases with advancing age probably due to a loss of liver mass in relation to body size as well as a gradual decrease in liver enzymes. Recently, Nies and his associates[41] studied the plasma levels of imipramine, desipramine and amitriptyline in older depressed patients. They found that patients over 65 years of age had higher amitriptyline, imipramine and desipramine plasma levels than a group of younger patients, despite the fact that the older age group received a lower daily dose of the drugs. In addition, elderly patients did not achieve a steady state plasma level for two-three weeks, while the steady state in the average adult was achieved in five-ten days. It took twice as long for desipramine to be eliminated in the older group as compared with the younger age group.

From this study the authors concluded that imipramine and amitriptyline dosage should be started at 25 mg. daily and gradually increased every four to seven days to a maximum limit of 100 mg. daily, or until troublesome side effects develop, whichever comes first. Generally, the average dose should be 1 mg./kg. Because there is a lag period from the time to reach a steady state and the onset of antidepressant effect, the therapeutic trial period for antidepressants in the elderly may be as long as six weeks, as opposed to three weeks in the normal aged adult.

Friedel and Raskin[42] studied plasma levels of doxepin in 15 depressed patients 60 years of age or older. The daily dose ranged from 50-300 mg. daily. Seven patients who responded had a mean steady state plasma concentration of doxepin and its metabolite desmethyldoxepin of 111 mg./ml.; those who did not respond had mean plasma concentrations of 60 mg./ml. The responders had an average daily dose of 164 mg. without adverse side effects. From this very limited study it would appear that the elderly can tolerate higher doses of doxepin than the other tricyclics and that the therapeutic plasma level correlates more closely with levels found in younger depressed patients. In addition to having anxiolytic properties, doxepin has the fewest anticholinergic properties and does not produce EKG changes, so that it may be the antidepressant of choice in the elderly.

Amitriptyline, the most sedating of the tricyclics, may be the drug of first choice in patients with marked insomnia, although it is also the TCA with the most anticholinergic properties. Imipramine may cause transient insomnia.[43] Nortriptyline, pro-triptyline, desipramine have not been used extensively in the elderly, so that data is not available concerning their efficacy in the geriatric population.

Determination of tricyclic plasma levels are becoming increasingly more important as an aid in evaluating therapeutic dose ranges, especially in the elderly, where a small change in dose might cause a marked alteration in the plasma level. These should be ordered whenever there appears to be a lack of response to therapy, unexpected or serious side effects occur, or there is a suspicion of noncompliance.[44] Because there is a lag of steady state plasma TCA levels of 5-10 days in the general population and up to 2-3 weeks in the elderly,[44] the assay should not be carried out earlier than the eighth to fourteenth day of treatment.[45] Blood should be collected from the fasting patient before the morning dose in containers containing no anticoagulants. Caffeine interferes with these determinations and should not be ingested 12 hours before the sample is taken.

There appears to be a curvilinear relationship between plasma levels of the secondary amine tricyclic antidepressants and therapeutic effect while the tertiary amines have a linear or sigmoid relationship.[44]

Once there has been a complete remission of symptoms, the dose of TCA may be reduced gradually at a rate of about 25 mg. every 14 days to approximately one-half the therapeutic dose. Generally, patients should be asymptomatic for a total of 6 months until the medicine is completely discontinued.[38] Since depressions usually last longer in aged persons—sometimes up to 2 years—low dose maintenance therapy should be considered for longer than 6 months in the elderly.[46]

Contraindications to tricyclics include cerebrovascular disease, prostatitis, and glaucoma. Tricyclics directly suppress the contractility of the myocardium and increase the risk of left ventricular hypertrophy, cardiac arrhythmias and congestive heart failure. TCAs worsen tardive dyskinesia and other choreas. They can also precipitate a manic attack in patients with episodes of recurrent depressions alternated with episodes of hypomania.[13]

The most common side effects of TCAs are due to their anticholinergic properties and include dry mouth, sweating, blurred vision, urinary retention, and paralytic ileus.[13] Confusional states resembling atropine poisoning (central anticholinergic syndrome) have been reported in 35% of patients over 40 years of age receiving TCAs.[30] Amitriptyline is the most potent anticholinergic, doxepin the least.[47] Various skin reactions have been reported and rarely an allergic obstructive type jaundice occurs with tricyclic administration.[13] Although agranulocytosis is rare, the incidence increases with age.[33] In addition, the seizure threshold is lowered by the tricyclics.[13]

Because the elderly take large numbers of prescription and nonprescription drugs, it is important to delineate drug-drug interactions between TCA's and other drugs consumed by the elderly. Tricyclics prolong CNS depression associated with alcohol, the barbiturates, and the antipsychotics. The anticholinergic activity of tricyclics can also be increased by antipsychotics which also have anticholinergic properties. The tricyclics interfere with the antihypertensive effects of guanethidine (Ismelin) by blocking its uptake in the postganglionic receptor sites.[13] Doxepin is said to have the least guanethidine blocking properties.[48] The antihypertensives, reserpine and alpha-methyldopa (Aldomet) can exacerbate depression, probably secondary to their central adrenergic properties. Diuretics can be safely used with the tricyclic antidepressants for the treatment of hypertension. Propranolol (Inderal) in combination with hydralazine (Apresoline) is also safe to use with antidepressants, although high doses of propranolol may cause enough sedation to exacerbate depressive symptomatology.[13]

In agitated depressed patients, especially those with somatic delusions and paranoid ideation, antipsychotic medicine should be considered. Several studies have showed that delusional depressions do not respond to tricyclics.[46] A high potency antipsychotic agent may be preferred to avoid cardiovascular side effects and excessive sedation. After the delusions and paranoid ideation have cleared, it will probably be necessary to add a tricyclic to treat the depression. Thioridizine has also been recommended for the treatment of depression characterized by agitation and anxiety without psychotic manifestations.[7]

MAO inhibitors increase the amounts of norepinephrine, dopamine, and serotonin at the central receptor sites in the brain by preventing their deamination.[7] As a class, the MAOI seem inferior to the effects of TCA or ECT in the treatment of depression; overall, the MAOI produced results significantly better than placebo in 38% of clinical trials compared to 80% for TCA and nearly 90% of ECT.[13] Indications for MAOI include: (1) atypical depression; (2) lack of response to tricyclics; (3) previous response to MAOIs.[46/49] If sympathomimetic agents can be avoided, MAOI lack the cardiotoxic effects of the tricyclic agents and offer a relative advantage in patients with heart disease and hypertension, provided these patients can be closely monitored.[13] (Table 5-4)

Hypertensive crises associated with the ingestion of MAOIs and tyramine-containing foods (cheese, wine, yeast, pickled products, etc.) have produced unwarranted hesitation to use the MAOIs. It is estimated that only 2% of patients being treated with MAOI will develop headaches and 0.5% hypertensive crises. The death rate of MAOI-treated patients is approximately 1 per 20,000,[32] compared to 1 death in 10,000 cases treated with ECT,[49] and a much higher frequency with the tricyclic antidepressants. Of 119 patients with cardiovascular disease who were treated with amitriptyline for a concomitant depression, 13 died suddenly compared to 3 sudden deaths in the matched control group.[50]

There are two classes of MAOIs availa-

Table 5-4.   General Characteristics of MAO Inhibitors.

PRECAUTIONS	CONTRAINDICATIONS	DRUG INTERACTIONS
Warn patient to: Report headache or unusual symptoms immediately Avoid self-medication (including over-the-counter drugs like cold and sinus drugs and analgesics) Avoid tyramine-containing foods—cheese, wine (especially sherry and Chianti), beer, pickled herring, yeast extracts, chicken liver, cream, chocolate, fava beans Avoid excess amount of caffeine Also avoid: Marmite, Bovril, yogurt, bee stings Use analgesics in lower doses if needed Taper off when stopping Safe use in pregnancy not yet established	Tricyclic drugs (concurrent use) Stop MAO inhibitor a minimum of 14 days before beginning tricyclic Amphetamines Sympathomimetic amines Hypertension Cardiovascular disease Headaches Pheochromocytoma Liver or advanced renal disease Quiescent schizophrenia Avoid combination with: dopa, amphetamines, hypoglycemics, alcohol, narcotics, diuretics, levodopa, meperidine; methyldopa, barbiturates, antiparkinsonian agents, insulin, guanethidine, sympathomimetic amines, reserpine, anticholinergics, antihypertensives, antihistaminics, hypnotics, other MAO inhibitors, anesthetics, phenothiazines	Alcohol: inhibits MAO inhibitor (possible hypertensive crisis if beverage contains tyramine) Amphetamine: potentiates amphetamine, risk of hypertensive crisis Anesthetics: increase CNS depression Anticholinergics: effect increased Antiparkinsonian agents; potentiated Barbiturates: potentiated Chloral hydrate: potentiated Cocaine: potentiated hypertensive crisis Curare: effect increased Foods with tyramine: hypertensive crisis Meperidine: hypotension potentiated; may inhibit MAO inhibitor Methyldopa (Aldomet®); hypertension, excitation; Minor tranquilizers: potentiated Other MAO inhibitors: additive Phenothiazines: potentiated; may inhibit MAO inhibitor Sympathomimetic: potentiate; extreme hypertension Thiazide diuretics: hypotension; potentiate MAO inhibitor Tricyclic antidepressants: potentiated both

From Goldstein, Burton J. Drug therapy for the depressed patient. *Hospital Formulary*. December, 1977.

ble in the U.S., the hydrazines—phenelzine (Nardil) and isocarboxazide (Marplan), and the nonhydrazines—tranylcypramine (Parnate) and pargyline (Eutonyl). The hydrazines are somewhat safer, while the nonhydrazines, due to their amphetamine-like actions, are effective faster and are associated with more hypertensive crises.[51]

Tranylcypramine is the most potent MAOI available for clinical use and causes severe adverse effects. The recommended starting dose is 10 mg. bid and improvement should be seen in 48 hours. If no response occurs after three days, the dose may be increased to 30 mg. daily. If after a week no improvement occurs, then the medication is not likely to be beneficial.

Pargyline, marketed as an antihypertensive, is useful in depressed patients with a history of hypertension. The initial daily dose in the elderly should be 10–25 mg. The dosage should be increased by 10 mg. increments until the desired response is obtained. Because it may take four days to three weeks to produce complete therapeutic effects, the dosage should not be increased more frequently than once a week.

Isocarboxazide is a weak but useful drug in patients with mild degrees of depression. The usual starting dose in the elderly is two to three 10 mg. tablets, given in single or divided doses. Adverse effects increase at dosages larger than 30 mg. daily.

Phenelzine, starting at 15 mg. tid and gradually increased to 60 mg. daily has been found particularly effective for patients with mild depression associated with anxiety and agitation. Many patients do not show a response until four weeks after initiation of treatment.

Both minor and serious side effects can be encountered with MAOIs. Hypotension may become serious in the elderly who are at high risk for stroke or myocardial infarction. MAOIs are contraindicated in chronic liver disease and parenchymal hepatotoxic reactions occur frequently enough to justify regular serum bilirubin determinations. CNS toxicity can include insomnia, agitation, and exacerbation of functional psychosis. In addition to tyramine-containing foods, medicines containing sympathomametics such as ephidrine, phenylephrine (Neosynephrine), the amphetamines and alpha-methyl-dopa (Aldomet) can potentiate a hypertensive crisis in combination with MAOIs. If hypertensive reactions occur, 5 mg. IV of phentolamine (Regitine), a potent alpha adrenergic blocking agent, is the antidote. Thorazine 50–100 mg. IM can also be used.[13]

If a patient is being switched from a TCA, there should be a delay of at least seven to ten days before beginning a MAOI to prevent severe interactions. Combined tricyclic and MAOI therapy requires further investigation before it can be recommended for use in the elderly.[46]

GH-3 (Gerovital), a 2% solution of procaine hydrochloride buffered to a pH of 3.3 has been suggested as an effective antidepressant for the elderly because of its mild MAO inhibiting properties. Ostfeld and his associates,[52] after reviewing the world literature on the use of procaine which included data on 10,000 patients, could not state unequivocally that GH-3 was an effective antidepressant.

The Stimulant Drugs, amphetamine, methamphetamine, and methylphenadate, have been proved ineffective as antidepressants in controlled studies.[13] Some clinicians feel that in low doses the stimulants might be helpful as a psychomotor activator; but because of their high risk of abuse and their tendency to induce paranoid psychosis, agitation, confusion, and depression on withdrawal, they should be used sparingly in low doses to treat mild anergy and never to treat depression.[53]

The Benzodiazepines have been found to be of some benefit in patients diagnosed as anxious neurotic depressives,[54] but the development of tolerance to the euphorant and antianxiety effects of these drugs make them questionable as an effective long-term antidepressant. In addition, these medications have a potential to cause confusion in the elderly.[53]

Electroconvulsive Therapy is safe and more effective than antidepressant medication. Approximately 66% of depressed patients respond to the tricyclics,[55] 78% to ECT,[56] and morbidity and mortality rates are higher with drugs;[57] but because of recent legal and ethical considerations and the possibility of increased confusion with ECT in the elderly, convulsive therapy is not recommended unless the patient is so severely depressed that he is "not taking adequate food or fluids or the risk of suicide is high and the use of drug therapy will take an unacceptably long period to manifest a therapeutic response".[57]

The incidence of death in ECT is approximately 1 per 10,000[49] patients treated, with the major cause of death being cardiac complications, yet ECT is safer in elderly patients with heart disease than TCA.[57] ECT may be used following a myocardial infarction once cardiac enzymes and EKG have stabilized.[58] Likewise, patients with chronic heart disease requiring maintenance digitalization tolerate ECT if the usual precautions are taken. Peptic ulcer, substernal hematoma, aortic aneurysm, and other conditions that might lead to hemorrhage do not represent a contraindication when muscle relaxation is used.[59] In certain patients, ECT can be beneficial in depressed patients with a brain tumor if intracranial pressure is normal. The only definite contraindication to ECT is increased intracranial pressure.[60]

Before administering ECT, the following laboratory procedures should be performed: (1) EKG; (2) chest X-ray; (3) EEG [to rule out brain tumor]; (4) X-rays of the spine, pelvis, and hips [to assess the degree of osteoporosis]; and (5) liver function studies [to evaluate the patient's ability to metabolize drugs used in conjunction with ECT].[43] Since there is some evidence that antipsychotic or antidepressive medicine augments the cardiovascular complications of ECT, this medication should be discontinued for a few days prior to convulsive therapy; if this is impossible, the dose prior to treatment should be withheld.[58]

In general, approximately 15 minutes prior to ECT, the patient is given 0.6–1.0 mg. of atropine IM to block the vagal stimulating effects of ECT and to decrease secretions. Just prior to shock, the patient is anesthetized with 30–100 mg. of sodium methohexital (Brevital) IV. Since the motor aspects of a cerebral seizure are not essential, peripheral seizure movements can be modified by administration of 30–80 mg. of succinylcholine IV (.75–1.5 mg./kg.) after the patient is asleep. A few seconds later, muscle fasiculations will begin at the head and move caudally. During this time, it is recommended that the patient receive preoxygenation with 100% O_2. Seventy to 130 volts for .1–.5 seconds is usually required for a cerebral seizure; generally older people have a higher seizure threshold than younger patients. Ideally, with a modified convulsion, the only indication of a seizure will be a slight plantar flexion, minimal finger and toe movements, or the appearance of gooseflesh (autonomic evidence).[59] If none of these manifestations is seen after 90 seconds, an additional stimulus should be given.

It is wise to administer treatments twice weekly in the elderly to decrease the possibility of post-ECT confusion and memory impairment.[7] A complete course generally consists of six to eight seizures, but treatment should be kept to a minimum and with the first signs of improvement, the older patient can be switched to an antidepressant to minimize the possibility of memory loss. Unilateral ECT with the electrodes placed over the nondominant hemisphere is recommended by some clinicians because this procedure reduces memory loss without diminishing, or minimally diminishing, the efficacy of the treatment.[61]

In patients with a recent history of cardiac arrhythmias or myocardial infarction, pretreatment with lidocaine may be necessary. The patient should be monitored with an electrocardiogram during treatment, and it is a good idea to have a cardiologist available to assist patients with severe heart disease. To avoid cardiovascular and pulmonary complications that are more frequent with ECT modified by barbiturates, a subconvulsive stimulus to render the patient unconscious can be given instead of barbiturates just prior to the time the patient begins to experience respiratory distress from the succinylcholine.[59] It may be necessary to replace pretreatment atropine with 5 mg. of diazepam given slowly IV in hypertensive patients. Elderly patients may require less barbiturate anesthesia to prevent prolonged sleep following ECT.[43]

Increased succinylcholine dosage for patients with susceptibility to fractures is recommended. Doses up to 150 mg. can be given without prolonged respiratory depression as long as the patient does not have a deficiency of pseudocholinesterase. Liver disease, a genetic abnormality, or cholinesterase inhibitors such as echothiophate (used to treat glaucoma), can cause a lack of pseudocholinesterase.[57] A deficiency even in small amounts of succinylcholine will result in prolonged apnea. If apnea occurs, it will be necessary to oxygenate the patient until the succinylcholine is gradually metabolized.

When ECT is used properly it is rapid, safe and effective in relieving the symptoms of severe depression.

TREATMENT OF ORGANIC BRAIN SYNDROME

Loss of brain tissue functioning results in organic brain syndrome, characterized by a decrease in intellectual ability, memory loss, disorientation, and impaired judgment. In contrast to acute organic brain syndrome, which is reversible when the precipitating cause is removed, chronic organic brain syndrome is insidious, the treatment empirical.

Many cases of depressive equivalents characterized by social withdrawal, loss of energy and somatic symptomatology as well as impairment of cognitive function are misdiagnosed as organic brain syndrome; at other times the patient's depression can be a reaction to his knowledge that he has a deteriorating mental condition. If depression is suspected, a therapeutic trial of antidepressants is indicated and may reverse cognitive deficiencies.[62]

Poor nutrition contributes to impaired cognition in the elderly. The plasma lipids play a major role in the development of organic brain syndrome secondary to atherosclerosis so that serum cholesterol should not exceed 220 mg. % and the triglyceride level should not be greater than 150 mg. %.[63] A prudent diet is one containing less than 300 mg. of cholesterol a day with no more than 30% of the daily calories as fat.[63] Saturated animal fats should be eliminated as much as possible and foods should be cooked only with polyunsaturated vegetable oils when necessary. There is no convincing data to indicate that exercise decreases atherosclerosis, but steady physical activity is desirable in a program of prevention management because it may improve sympathetic tone and general circulation. A decrease in cigarette smoking and control of high blood pressure are also recommended. Cholestyramine (Questran) 4 g. qid, clofibrate (Atromid-S) .5 g. bid, and niacin 1/2–3 g. tid have been used to control the five major genetic abnormalities of lipid metabolism.[63]

Decreased absorption secondary to aging or drugs, such as mineral oil and phenobarbitol, as well as a failure to eat properly, all contribute to poor nutrition. Whanger and Wang[64] found that 70% of elderly hospital patients were on inadequate diets; 50% of these had low levels of folic acid and 12% low levels of B_{12}, both of which are associated with dementia. Thiamine (B_1) deficiency causes beri-beri, characterized by intellectual deterioration, nystagmus, opthalmoplegia, and cerebellar ataxia. Niacin deficiency produces pellagra; B_{12} deficiency, pernicious anemia; and folic acid deficiency, macrocytic anemia—all of which can cause CNS symptomatology with impaired memory and orientation as well as neurological disorders. It may take up to 1 year for vitamin therapy to reverse the symptoms of these disorders.[7] Since it is estimated that 10% of the total geriatric population have vitamin deficiencies, it is wise to administer a daily multiple vitamin preparation to all patients over 65.[7]

The stimulants dextroamphetamine, methylphenydate (Ritalin), deanolacetamdobenzoate (Deaner), pentylenetetrazol (Metrazol), pipradol (Meretran), ethamivan (Emivan) are believed to increase attention span and motivation for new learning. Most adequately controlled studies of the stimulants do not substantiate the rationale for their use.[65] Though they may tend to produce transient mild increases in some intellectual functioning, the risk of drug dependency, accelerated heart rate, hypertension, anorexia, irritability, and paranoid reactions supercede the benefits of the medications. Controlled studies of magnesium pemoline (Cylert), a mild CNS stimulant, which increases RNA synthesis, have thus far proved the drug to be ineffective in organic brain syndrome.[62]

The experimental drug, piracetam (Nootropil), a cyclic GABA derivative, is believed to increase the polyribosome/ ribosome ration. In a double-blind placebo-controlled study with 196 geriatric patients diagnosed as having organic brain syndrome, patients on 2400 mg. of piracetam daily showed significant improvement in their general mental condition.[65]

No well-controlled trials of the cerebral dilators—papaverine (Pavabid), 150 mg. Q12h, cyclandelate (Cyclospasmol) 800–1200 mg. daily, and nicotinic acid, 1/2–3 g. daily—have shown they improve cognitive function in the elderly.[7] Although these drugs might be useful in the early stages of mild organicity, because atherosclerotic vessels cannot dilate in severe disease, there is a possibility of increased blood flow only to the healthy vessels resulting in an additional compromise of blood flow to the damage areas.[62] Side effects include nausea, rash, dizziness, headaches, flushing, and hypotension.[66]

Anticoagulant therapy is not indicated in the elderly for the treatment of psychopathology unless there is clear evidence of thrombosis.[62]

The commercial products, Hydergine and Deapril-ST, are dihydrogenated ergot alkaloids that have been shown to have a primary effect on ganglion cell metabolism. Changes in the lactate/pyruvate ratio have been found in experimental animals treated with dihyroergotoxine, indicating improved oxygenation in the cells. This is thought to lead to a decrease in local edema with secondary improvement in microcirculation. Double-blind controlled clinical investigations have demonstrated improvement in mood, confusion, unsociability, dizziness, and levels of performance of self-care in the elderly treated with dihydroergotoxine.[67] The usual dose is 2.5 mg. tablets sublingually three times daily. It is still uncertain how much drug is absorbed when it is taken orally instead of sublingually, and failure to take the drug properly could cause it to be ineffective in certain patients. There are very few side effects; sinus bradycardia, nausea and vomiting are rare complications. Because of the drug's slow onset of action, it

should be given for at least 3 months before being deemed ineffective.[67]

G-H3 (Gerovital) has inconsistently been reported to improve memory, mobility, concentration, attention span, skin texture and hair color; but most of these studies were poorly controlled. In the clinical trials where there is evidence of improved physical and cognitive changes, these are thought to be due to the effect of the drug on mood secondary to its mild MAO inhibiting properties.[68] It is alarming that G-H3 has been dropped from clinical evaluation in the United States in the light of the possible benefits.

More than 100 patients with organic brain syndrome have been treated with hyperbaric O_2 since 1969 when it was first suggested by Jacobs as a treatment for dementia. In Jacobs' initial study, 13 patients were treated twice daily for 15 days with 100% O_2 at 2.5 atmospheres absolute for 90 minutes. Beneficial results seemed to occur in patients with the least impairment and persisted for only a week to ten days following a course of treatment. Subsequent studies have failed to replicate the initial positive findings.[69]

Estrogen, testosterone, corticosteroids, and thyroid preparations should not be given to patients with dementia unless there is proven hormone deficiency. Improper administration of thyroid medication can lead to thyrotoxic psychosis, or, more commonly in the elderly, "apathetic hyperthyroidism" manifested by apathy and depression. Corticosteroids can cause an initial euphoria followed by depression. Testosterone can produce liver toxicity while estogens may contribute to the development of endometrial carcinoma.[7]

Acute episodes of agitation, confusion and restlessness associated with organic brain syndrome can be controlled with the judicious use of antipsychotics.[43] Since the low potency antipsychotics have a greater tendency to produce a toxic psychosis, haloperidol, having the fewest anticholinergic side effects, is probably the drug or choice. The starting dose of 0.5 mg. once or twice daily can gradually be increased to control the symptomatology.

TREATMENT OF ANXIETY AND DISORDERS OF SLEEP

The barbiturates, benzodiazepenes, propanediols, glycerol derivatives and some antihistamines have been used to treat anxiety and sleep disturbances in the elderly.

Although the barbiturates are widely used in the general population, they are not recommended in elderly patients because of their potential for intoxication and lethal overdosage and their propensity to produce paradoxical agitation. The barbiturates increase liver enzyme activity resulting in increased metabolism of coumadin, steroids, and the tricyclic antidepressants.[13]

The propanediols, meprobamate and tybamate, like the barbiturates, produce psychological and physical dependence and induce hepatic enzymes. They too are contraindicated in the elderly. Meprobamate is particularly dangerous because the addicting dose overlaps the therapeutic dose.[13]

The benzodiazepines—chloridazepoxide (Librium and others), diazepam (Valium), oxazepam (Serax), flurzaepam (Dalmane), and chlorazepate (Tranxene)—selectively depress the limbic system, sparing the cerebral cortex and the reticular activating system at low doses so there are less sedating side effects than with the barbiturates. The benzodiazepines are rapidly absorbed after oral administration, and except for oxazepam, are converted to active metabolites in the liver. Because of the tendency to accumulate in tissues, IM absorption can be slow and incomplete.[70] Diazepam has a marked tendency to accumulate in the fat tissues and has an elimination half-life of 20–50 hours. Chlordiazepoxide has a half-life of 24 hours in the general population, but preliminary studies indicate that its half-life may be more prolonged in the elderly. Chlorazepate has a half-life of 30–60 hours in the general population.[71] Because oxazepam is rapidly absorbed after oral administration and has no active metabolites or tendency to accumulate in the tissues, it

may be safer for use in the elderly, although few patients over age 65 have been studied. The half-life of oxazepam is 5–20 hours.[71]

Recently Reidenberg and his associates[72] found that the dose of diazepam and the resulting plasma level were inversely correlated with age and that the elderly are more sensitive to the depressant effects of diazepam. A reasonable starting dose of the benzodiazepines in the elderly would be: 2 mg. at bedtime for diazepam, 3.75 mg. for chlorazepate, 5 mg. for chlorazepate, and 10 mg. two or three times daily for oxazepam.

The major side effects of the benzodiazepenes are ataxia, drowsiness, headache, and lethargy. Paradoxical reactions are common in the elderly and include agitation, hullucinations, insomnia, and rage. In addition, alcohol, sedatives, hypnotics, antipsychotics, and antidepressants mutually potentiate the benzodiazepines. In contrast to the barbiturates and meprobamate, large amounts of the benzodiazepines can be taken without fatal results, but in rare cases overdoses equivalent to a two-week supply have resulted in death, especially when they have been combined with some other medication.[13] Withdrawal from large doses of benzodiazepines results in the symptoms similar to barbiturate withdrawal. The benzodiazepines are metabolized more slowly in patients with hepatic dysfunction; patients with cirrhosis show a more than twofold prolongation in the half-life of diazepam.[73]

Propranolol (Inderal) 10 mg. tid, a β-adrenergic blocking agent, is effective in the treatment of anxiety, although it has not been approved by the FDA for this use and is contraindicated in patients with decreased cardiac output, obstructive pulmonary disease, and asthma.[74]

The elderly frequently complain of insomnia; they normally have less REM sleep, more difficulty getting to sleep, wake faster, have less stage 4 sleep, and have less total sleep.[7] Before prescribing a hypnotic, the physician should make certain that the patient is not suffering from depression or psychosis and the hypnotic should only be used for short-term treatment of situational insomnia. Flurazepam (Dalmane) 15–30 mg.

at bedtime is the drug of choice. According to most studies, REM sleep is relatively unimpaired in doses lower than 30 mg. daily[48] but has the side effects of the other benzodiazepines. The antihistimines, diphenylhydramine (Benadryl) 25–30 mg. and hydroxyzine (Atarax) 10–25 mg. at bedtime, have sedative properties with addictive potential and can cause acute toxic delusions secondary to their anticholinergic properties. Chloral hydrate 500 mg.–1g. is a gastric irritant that can inflame peptic ulcer disease. It also protentiates the effects of coumadin, and some studies suggest that it depresses REM sleep. The hypnotics, glutethimide (Doriden), ethylcholorynol (Placidyl), methaqualone (Qualude and others) in addition to having the potential for habituation and abuse, can cause confusional reactions and depress cardiac and respirator functions. In addition, glutethimide and methaqualone depress REM.[48]

Sedative-hypnotic withdrawal is generally treated with phenobarbital or pentobarbital. For a patient who is experiencing withdrawal, a 200 mg. test dose of pentobarbital is given orally and changes in the neurological exam are evaluated one hour later. If an hour after the test dose the patient is asleep, no withdrawal treatment is required; if the patient is drowsy with slurred speech and ataxia, the 24-hour pentobarbital requirement is 400–600 mg. daily; if lateral nystagmus is the only sign of intoxication, 800 mg. is required; and if the patient shows no signs of drug effects 1000–1200 mg. or more is required. After the withdrawal dosage has been determined, pentobarbital is divided into four equal doses and given orally every six hours. If phenobarbital is used, the dose is 30 mg. for each 100 mg. of pentobarbital. Because of the long duration of action, the dose of phenobarbital can be given every eight hours. The starting dose of pentobarbital or phenobarbital is reduced at a rate of one-tenth the starting dose each day until the drug is completely withdrawn.[75]

In contrast to abstinence from sedative hypnotics, opioid withdrawal, though uncomfortable, rarely causes convulsions and is not lethal. Mild withdrawal signs include lacrimation, rhinorrhea, piloerection, tremor, and anorexia. Disabling signs such as abdominal cramps, vomiting, diarrhea, and tachycardia are treated with 10–20 mg. of methadone given in divided doses; this is reduced by 20% each day for complete withdrawal in 7–10 days. For severe addicts, the methadone maintenance dose ranges from 40–100 mg. daily.[76] Opioid abuse is not rare in the elderly—about 1% of the methadone treatment population is over age 60.[77]

Overdose of narcotics is characterized by pinpoint pupils, loss of consciousness, hypotension, and pulmonary edema. The opioid antagonist, naloxone (Narcan), O.4 mg. IV, quickly reverses the respiratory depression of narcotic overdose. If two-three doses given at three-minute intervals do not reverse the syndrome, then other causes of coma should be considered. The effects of naloxone last only 30 minutes to 2 hours so that repeat injections are sometimes necessary.[76]

In the elderly, alcoholism accounts for 12% of male[77] and 4% of female admissions[78] to inpatient psychiatric facilities and occurs much more frequently in outpatient facilities. Treatment of alcohol withdrawal includes:

1. Thiamine 100 mg. IM or IV initially, then 100 mg. orally or parentally for at least 1 week.
2. Folic acid, 1–5 mg. PO or IM for at least 1 week.
3. One multiple vitamin tablet daily.
4. Diazepam 5–10 mg. twice daily, chlordiazepoxide 25–50 mg. twice daily, or oxazepam 10 mg. three times daily.
5. 2–4 cc of 50 percent magnesium sulfate intramuscularly every 8 hours for 3 doses.
6. Correction of electrolyte and fluid deficits.

Prophylactic anticonvulsants should be given only to those patients who are known to have grand mal seizures with alcohol withdrawal. Since starting maintenance therapy without a loading dose produces inadequate anticonvulsant blood levels for 4–5 days, a patient with known seizures who has not been on maintenance anticonvulsants for five days prior to admission requires a loading dose of diphenylhydantoin (Dilantin). One gram of Dilantin should be added to 500 cc of 5% D5W and given over a four-hour period. After the loading dose, most patients require 300–400 mg. of Dilantin daily to maintain effective serum concentrations of 10–20 mcg./ml. Dilantin is incompletely absorbed when given IM. Because antipsychotics can lower the seizure threshold, they should be used with extreme caution and given only if necessary to control agitation, hallucinations or frightening delusions.[79]

The physician who prudently applies his general knowledge of psychopharmacology can avoid the common mistakes of overtreatment, polypharmacy, and the indiscriminate use of drugs, enabling him to better assist the elderly patient adjust to the psychiatric problems of older life.

REFERENCES

1. Eisdorfer, C. and Fann, W. (eds.) *Psychopharmacology and Aging.* New York: Plenum Press, 1973.
2. Maddox, G. et al. *Report to the Community on Durham's Elderly* by the Older Americans Resources and Services Program. (unpublished material).
3. Prien, R. F. A survey of psychoactive drug use in the aged at Veterans Administration hospitals. *Aging,* Vol. 2. Gershon and Raskin (eds.) New York: Raven Press, pp. 143–154, 1975.
4. Physicians drug prescribing patterns in the skilled nursing facilities: Long-term facility campaign. *Monograph, No. 2.* DHEW Publication No. 76–50050. U.S. Gov't Printing Office. Washington, DC., June, 1976.
5. Davis, J. M. Efficacy of tranquilizing and antidepressant drugs. *Archives of General Psychiatry* **13:** 552 (1965).
6. Wynder, E. and Kristein, M. Suppose we die young late in life. *JAMA* **238:** 1507 (1977).
7. Verwoerdt, A. *Clinical Geropsychiatry.* Baltimore: Williams & Wilkins, 1976.
8. Bender, Douglas. The effect of increasing age on the distribution of peripheral blood flow in man. *J. Amer. Geriatric Soc.* **13:** 192–198 (1965).
9. Holloway, D. Drug problems in the geriatric patient. *Drug Intelligence and Clinical Pharmacy* **8:** 632–642 (1974).
10. Meier-Ruge, W., et al. Experimental pathology in the aging brain. *Aging,* Vol. 2. Gershon and Raskin (eds.) New York: Raven Press, pp. 55–126, 1975.
11. Nies, A. et al. Changes in monoamine oxidase with aging. *Psychopharmacology and Aging.* Eisdorfer and Fann (eds.) New York: Plenum Press, pp. 41–54, 1973.
12. Davis, J. et al. Clinical problems in treating the aged with psychotropic drugs. *Psychopharmacology and Aging.* Eisdorfer and Fann (eds.) New York: Plenum Press, pp. 111–128, 1973.
13. Baldessarini, R. J. *Chemotherapy in Psychiatry.* Cambridge: Harvard University Press, 1977.
14. Salzman, C., Shader, R. and van der Kolk, B. Clinical psychopharmacology in the elderly patient. *New York State Journal of Medicine.* **76:** 71–77 (1976).
15. Gardos, G. and Cole, J. O. Maintenance antipsychotic therapy: Is the cure worse than the disease? *Am. J. Psychiatry* **133:** 32–36 (1976).
16. Prien, R. F., Haber, P. A. and Caffey, E. M. The use of psychoactive drugs in elderly patients with psychiatric disorders: Survey conducted in 12 Veterans Administration hospitals. *J. Amer. Geriatric Soc.* **23:** 104–112 (1975).
17. Branchey, M. H. et al. High and low potency neuroleptics in elderly psychiatric patients. *JAMA* **239:** 1860–1867 (1978).
18. Stotsky, B. Psychoactive drugs for geriatric patients with psychiatric disorders. *Aging,* Vol. 2. Gershon and Raskin (eds.). New York: Raven Press, pp. 229–253, 1975.
19. Shader, R. and Jackson, A. Approaches to schizophrenia. *Manual of Psychiatric Therapeutics.* R. Shader (ed.) Boston: Little, Brown, pp. 63–101, 1975.
20. Friedel, R. Norepinephrine, dopamine and serotonin: CNS distribution, biosynthesis and metabolism. *Psychopharmacology and Aging.* Eisdorfer and Fann (eds.). New York: Plenum Press, pp. 11–16, 1973.
21. Eadie, M. J. Tardive dyskinesia. *The Medical Journal of Australia* **1:** 682–683 (1977).
22. Kobarjashi, R. M. Drug therapy of tardive dyskinesia. *NEJM* **296:** 257–260 (1977).
23. DiMascio, A. and Sovner, R. Neuroleptic-induced extrapyramidal side effects. *Drug Therapy* **6:** 99–103 (1976).
24. Gulevich, G. Psychopharmacological treatment of the aged. *Psychopharmacology, From Theory To Practice.* Barchas, Berger, Ciaranello, Elliott (eds.). New York: Oxford University Press, pp. 448–465, 1977.
25. Penovich, P. et al. Double-blind evaluation of deanol in tardive dyskinesia. *JAMA* **239:** 1997–1998 (1978).
26. Growdan, J. H. et al. Oral choline administration to patients with tardive dyskinesia. *NEJM* **297:** 524–527 (1977).

27. Tamminga, C. Cholinergic influences in tardive dyskinesia. *Am. J. Psych.* **134:** 769–774 (1977).

28. Carroll, B. *et al.* Paradoxical response to dopamine agonist in tardive dyskinesia. *Am. J. Psych.* **134:** 785–789 (1977).

29. Fann, W. *et al.* Attempts at pharmacological management of tardive dyskinesia. *Psychopharmacology and Aging.* Eisdorfer and Fann (eds.). New York: Plenum Press, pp. 89–96, 1973.

30. Davies, R. K. *et al.* Confusional episodes and antidepressant medication. *Am. J. Psych.* **128:** 95–99 (1971).

31. Fann, W. and Shannon, I. A treatment for dry mouth in psychiatric patients. *Am. J. Psych.* **135:** 251–252 (1978).

32. Klein, D. F. and Davis, J. M. *Diagnosis and Drug Treatment of Psychiatric Disorders.* Baltimore: Williams & Wilkins, 1969.

33. Leroyd, B. Psychotropic drugs in the aging patient. *Med. J. of Australia* **1:** 1131 (1973).

34. The Task Force on Nomenclature and Statistics of the APA. *Diagnostic and Statistical Manual of Mental Disorders,* 3rd Ed. New York: New York, 1978.

35. Shopsin, B. and Gershon, B. The current status of lithium in psychiatry. *Am. J. of Med. Sciences* **268:** 311 (1974).

36. Walker, J. I. and Brodie, H. K. H. Current concepts of lithium treatment and prophylaxis. *J. of Cont. Ed. in Psych.* **39:** 19–30 (1978).

37. Gershon, S. Lithium. *American Handbook of Psychiatry,* 2nd ed., Vol. 1. Arieti, S. (ed.). New York: Basic Books, pp. 490–513, 1975.

38. Shildkraut, J. and Klein, D. The classification and treatment of depressive disorders. *Manual of Psychiatric Therapeutics.* Shader (ed.). Boston: Little, Brown, pp. 39–61, 1975.

39. Hollister, L. E. Clinical use of psychotherapeutic drugs 11: Antidepressant and anti-anxiety drugs and special problems in the use of psychotherapeutic drugs. *Drugs* **4:** 361–410 (1972).

40. Prange, A. J. Antidepressants. *American Handbook of Psychiatry,* 2nd ed., Vol. 5. Freedman and Dyrud (eds.). New York: Basic Books, pp. 476–489, 1975.

41. Nies, A. Relationship between age and tricyclic antidepressant plasma levels. *Am. J. Psych.* **134:** 790–793 (1977).

42. Friedel, R. and Raskin, D. Relationship of blood levels of sinequan to clinical effects in the treatment of depression in the aged patients. Mendels (ed.). *Sinequan: A Monograph of Recent Clinical Studies.* pp. 51–53.

43. Salzman, C., van der Kolk, B. and Shader, R. I. Psychopharmacology and the geriatric patient. *Manual of Psychiatric Therapeutics.* Shader (ed.). Boston, Little, Brown, pp. 171–184, 1975.

44. Taska, R. Clinical laboratory aids in the treatment of depression: Tricyclic antidepressant plasma levels and urinary MHPG. *Comprehensive Psychiatry* **3:** 12–20 (1977).

45. Alexanderson, B. Pharmocokinetics in nortriptyline in man after single and multiple oral doses: The predictability of steady state plasma concentrations from single-dose plasma level data. *European J. of Clin. Pharmacology* **4:** 82–91 (1972).

46. Bielski, R. and Friedel, R. Subtypes of depression—diagnosis and medical management. *The Western J. of Med.* **126:** 347–352 (1977).

47. Prange, A. Use of antidepressant drugs in the elderly patient. *Psychopharmacology and Aging.* Eisdorfer and Fann (eds.). New York: Plenum Press, pp. 225–238, 1973.

48. Greenblatt, D. and Shader, R. Psychotropic drugs in the general hospital. *Manual of Psychiatric Therapeutics.* Shader (ed.). Boston: Little, Brown & Co., pp. 1–26, 1975.

49. Cole, J. and Davis, J. Antidepressant drugs. *Comprehensive Textbook of Psychiatry,* 2nd ed., Vol. 2. Freedman, Kaplan, Sadoch (eds.). Baltimore: Williams & Wilkins, pp. 1941–1956, 1978.

50. Jefferson, J. W. A review of the cardiovascular effects and toxicity of the tricyclic antidepressants. *Psychosomatic Med.* **37:** 160–170 (1975).

51. Friend, D. G. Antidepressant drug therapy. *Clin. Pharmacology and Therapeutics* **6:** 805–814 (1965).

52. Ostfeld, A., Smith, D. and Stotsky, B. A systemic use of procane in the treatment of the elderly: A review. *J. Amer. Geriatric Soc.* **15:** 1–19 (1977).

53. Fann, W. and Wheless, J. Depression in elderly patients. *Southern Med. J.* **68:** 468–473 (1975).

54. Rosenthal, S. and Bowden, C. A double-blind comparison of thioridizine versus diazepam in patients with chronic mixed anxiety and depressive symptoms. *Current Therapeutic Research* **15:** 261–267 (1973).

55. Morris, J. B. and Beck, A. T. The efficacy of antidepressant drugs: A review of research, 1958–1972. *Arch. Gen. Psych.* **30:** 667–674 (1974).

56. Greenblatt, M., Grosser, G. H. and Wechsler, H. Differential response of hospitalized depressed patients to somatic therapy. *Am. J. Psych.* **120:** 935–943 (1964).

57. Frankel, F. H. *et al.* American Psychiatric Association Task Force Report on *Electroconvulsive Therapy.* August, 1977 (unpublished material).

58. Salzman, C. Electroconvulsive therapy. *Manual of Psychiatric Therapeutics.* Shader (ed.). Boston: Little, Brown & Co., pp. 115–124, 1975.

59. Kalinowsky, L. B. The convulsive therapies. *Comprehensive Textbook of Psychiatry,* 2nd ed., Vol. 3. Freedman, Kaplan, Sadock (eds.). Baltimore: Williams & Wilkins, pp. 1969–1976, 1975.

60. Dressler, D. and Folk, J. The treatment of depression with ECT in the presence of brain tumor. *Am. J. Psych.* **132:** 1320–1321 (1975).

61. Squire, L. ECT and memory loss. *Am. J. Psych.* **134:** 997–1001 (1977).

62. Hollister, L. E. Drugs for mental disorders of old age. *JAMA* **234:** 195-198 (1975).

63. Fredrickson, D. Atherosclerosis and other forms of arteriosclerosis. *Principles of Internal Medicine,* 7th ed. Wintrobe *et al* (eds). New York: McGraw-Hill Pub. Co., pp. 1225-1236, 1974.

64. Whanger, A. D. and Wang, H. S. Vitamin B$_{12}$ deficiency in normal aged and psychiatric patients. *Normal Aging,* Vol. 2. Palmore (ed.) Durham: Duke University Press, pp. 63-73, 1974.

65. Lehmann, H. and Ban, T. Central nervous system stimulants and anabolic substances in geropsychiatric therapy. *Aging,* Vol. 2. Gershon and Raskin (eds.). New York: Raven Press, pp. 179-197, 1975.

66. DiMascio, A. and Goldberg, H. Managing disturbed geriatric patients with chemotherapy. *Hospital Physician* pp. 35-48 (June 1975).

67. Gaitz, C. M., Varner, R. V. and Overall, J. E. Pharmacotherapy for organic brain syndrome in late life. *Arch. Gen. Psych.* **34:** 839-845 (1977).

68. Jarvik, L. F. and Milne, J. F. Gerovital-H3: A review of the literature. *Aging,* Vol. 2. Gershon and Raskin (eds.) New York: Raven Press, pp. 203-223, 1975.

69. Thompson, L. Effects of hyperbaric oxygen on behavioral functioning in elderly persons with intellectual impairment. *Aging,* Vol. 2. Gershon and Raskin (eds.). New York: Raven Press, pp. 169-177, 1975.

70. Greenblatt, D. J. *et al.* Slow absorption of intramuscular chlordiazepoxide. *NEJM* **291:** 1116-1118 (1974.

71. Shader, R. and Greenblatt, D. J. Clinical implications benzodiazepine pharmacokinetics. *Am. J. Psych.* **134:** 652-656 (1977).

72. Reidenberg, M. M. *et al.* Relationship between diazepam dose, plasma level, age, and central nervous system depression. *Clin. Pharmacology and Therapeutics* **23:** 371-374 (1978).

73. Klotz, U. *et al.* The effects of age and liver disease on the disposition and elimination of diazepam in adult man. *J. Clin. Invest.* **55:** 347-359 (1975).

74. Shader, R. and Greenblatt, D. J. Psychopharmacological treatment of anxiety states. *Manual of Psychiatric Therapeutics.* Shader (ed.). Boston: Little, Brown, pp. 27-38, 1975.

75. Shader, R., Caine, E. and Meyer, R. Treatment of dependence on barbiturates and sedative/hypnotics. *Manual of Psychiatric Therapeutics.* Shader (ed.). Boston: Little, Brown, pp. 195-202, 1975.

76. Green, A., Meyer, R. and Shader, R. Heroin and methodone abuse: Acute and chronic management. *Manual of Psychiatric Therapeutics.* Shader (ed.). Boston: Little, Brown, pp. 203-210, 1975.

77. Bozzetti, L. P. and MacMurray, J. P. Drug misuse among the elderly: A hidden menace. *Psychiatric Annals* **7:** 95-107 (1977).

78. Pascarelli, E. F. Drug dependence: An age-old problem compounded by old age. *Geriatrics* **29:** 109-114 (1974).

79. Greenblatt, D. and Shader, R. Treatment of alcohol withdrawal syndrome. *Manual of Psychiatric Therapeutics.* Shader (ed.). Boston: Little, Brown, pp. 211-236, 1975.

Chapter 6
Bodily Changes With Aging

Isadore Rossman, Ph.D., M.D.
Montefiore Hospital and Medical Center

The clinician who is objective in his evaluation of aging changes should be as impressed by individuality and variability as he is by their universality. Time of onset, rate of progression, and clinical import of aging processes are strikingly variable and should be kept in mind lest the patient fall victim to inaccurate generalization and symbolic reactivity by the practitioner. This is despite the fact that true aging processes have been defined as possessing the characteristics of universality, progressiveness, irreversibility, and being essentially detrimental. Evaluation problems are compounded because age changes can be classified as (a) anatomical, which includes alterations such as loss of stature or that loss of cells from any tissues somewhat pejoratively referred to as "senile atrophy"; (b) functional, such as declines in cardiac output, vital capacity, renal excretion, nerve conduction velocity, etc.; (c) pathological, of which common examples would be arthritic changes in many joints, sclerotic changes in arteries, cataract formation, and the like. Some of these alterations, for example the arcus senilis, are so common as to elicit little or no comment on many records of physical examinations. In Western society, at least, such also would be the case for mild to moderate degrees of atherosclerosis even with diminutions in blood flow to some important organs.

Though expected and accepted, there are hopeful implications in the fact that most of the pathologic or other changes observed in older patients are not universal and thus may not be true aging changes.[1] Therefore, therapeutic programs and prophylactic regimes may serve to diminish and perhaps prevent many of them. Better understanding of the impact of such factors as diet (salt, fats, fiber, total calories, calcium intakes) may make great inroads on hypertensive cardiovascular disease, several serious colonic diseases, atherosclerosis, and osteoporosis, all common in old age. The effect of smoking and the other variables elicited in the Framingham longitudinal study marked a historical milestone in our approach to the atherosclerosis of the elderly.[2] Consideration of another group of common aging changes such as osteoarthritis further exemplifies the problems of classification and orientation. Narrowing of intervertebral discs and osteoarthritic changes of the vertebrae have a linear relationship both to age and, quite clearly, to use.[3,4] The major osteoarthritic changes in the vertebral spine occur in the regions of greatest mobility, at the cervical and lumbar levels. These use-related changes are universal and have sometimes been referred to as "wear and tear changes." To the extent that they are hypertrophic changes, they may seem to fall into a different grouping than the many atrophic changes characteristic of aging tissues. Thus in the hip, a functionally very important area, osteoarthritis is extremely variable and the factors that increase the degree of degenerative change, sometimes to the point of warranting operative intervention, are mostly unknown. In short, aging human beings typically present so variable a mix of morphologic and functional modifications, not all "true" aging changes, that one should be cautious not to have generalized expectations with any given patient. Classification systems which dwell on inevitability, progressiveness, and irreversibility can be taken with a grain of salt, and may have less validity than anticipated in an ongoing clinical setting.

Changes in Stature and Posture

Old people tend to be short, and even the seasoned geriatrician may be surprised when a patient initially encountered bedridden, becomes ambulatory and turns out to be well under 5 feet in height. A number of factors contribute to this. Older patients were born at a time when average heights were less by several inches than is currently the case. Increase in height during the 20th century is regarded by physical anthropologists as a secular trend ascribable to better environments, which now seems to be plateauing, as least in better nourished populations. An example would be the intergenerational jump of over 2 inches in Italo-Americans

noted by Damon.[5] Thus shortness in our elderly is in part due to shortness at maturity. However, a lifetime loss of 1 to 2 inches has been demonstrated in longitudinal studies. The decrement in height appears to start in the fifth decade and is progressive thereafter.[6,7] Initial losses are ascribed to shrinkage in the intervertebral discs followed by declines in height of vertebrae. Thus loss of height with aging is primarily due to shrinkage in trunk length, and indeed the length of the long bones in general is unaltered. The influence of environment both on height attained and the rate of decline with aging was well brought out in the study by Miall et al.[8] In comparing a group in a Welsh mining area with an economically more favored group, they showed that both males and females in the mining area had a shorter height and experienced more rapid decrease with aging (Fig. 6-1).

In females, the loss of height is commonly aggravated by osteoporosis, with a bone loss which is particularly manifest in vertebrae. As osteoporotic vertebrae narrow, particularly in the thoracic spin, characteristic bowing with marked loss of stature results. This is more common and severe in white females of northern European extraction with initially lighter builds. Osteoporotic collapse may add markedly to the age-related decrement in height. Of interest, however, is that it virtually never produces spinal cord compression syndromes. However, it may necessitate hyperextension of the neck to avoid a literally downcast look and often contributes to chronic pain syndromes. Shrinkage in height and deformity, needless to say, has an impact on the self-image. Women complain of getting smaller, of "dowager's hump," and of the ugliness of the round back deformity. There is some reason to believe that preventive measures such as long continued calcium supplementation, perhaps with the addition of fluoride, may some day resolve the osteoporosis problem, but until then the aggravation of loss in height and deformity

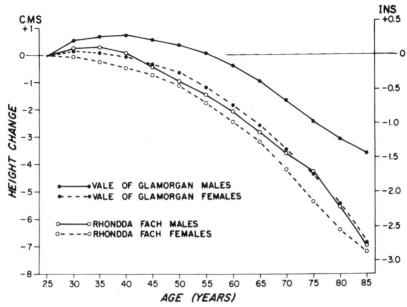

Fig. 6–1. Decrements in stature for two groups in Wales based on remeasurements. An age-related decline appears somewhat earlier and is more marked in the Rhonda Fach (mining area) group, presumably reflecting a less favorable environment.

will continue to be widespread and irreversible.

Other Contour Changes

Redistribution in the fat and subcutaneous tissue possesses a life history of its own. Its shifting about accounts for many of the contour changes seen in the progression from youth to old age. In general, one might characterize the shift by contrasting the firm and fully packed roundness of youth to the sagging asymmetry and deepening hollows seen in the aged. This is not to disregard the importance of constitutional factors such as degrees of endomorphy and mesomorphy and weight fluctuations due to calorie intake. In most individuals a loss of fat from depots in the extremities and the face becomes apparent past age 50. This has been demonstrated for the upper part of the tibial area by Garn,[9] and for the hand by Ryckewaert.[10] This loss of fat can be obvious despite a gain in weight in preferred depots such as the upper arm, scapular area and abdomen. Differences between the sexes

are also apparent. For example, the upper arm in women possesses a thicker skinfold which is preserved longer than in males. In males with aging, the triceps skinfold may begin to shrink while the subscapular skinfold concurrently shows increased deposition (Fig. 6-2). Deposition of periumbilical and buttock fat in both the sexes becomes increasingly manifest past the sixth decade. This, too, is more marked in the female, sometimes standing in marked contrast to the loss of fat in the hands and forearms. Attenuation of fat in the subcutaneous tissue of the face is cosmetically important. With its loss increased wrinkling and the more haggard "older" appearance ensues. Ethnic differences partly attributable to pigment protection play some part in this, as it is a matter of everyday observation that shrinkage and wrinkling of the face occurs at a lesser rate in blacks and Asians than in lighter skinned whites. Decrements in facial fat may act as an inhibition (or excuse) against weight reduction programs, since the fat loss component increases the aged look. It is the part of medical wisdom to warn

Physique and age—selected variables
White veterans, Normative Aging Study
(N=2,015)

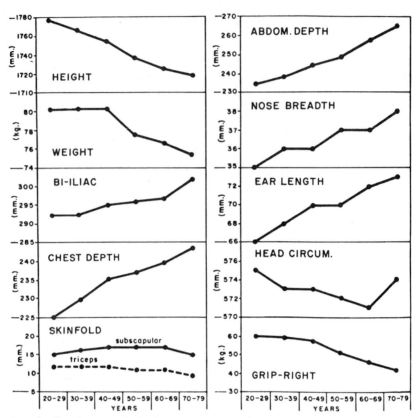

Fig. 6-2. Age-related anthropemetric findings in Boston veterans. Though derived from cross-sectional data, they are in agreement with longitudinal measurements.

older patients where weight reduction programs are being discussed to anticipate appearing older and more wrinkled and offset this by emphasizing the overriding health values.

Despite the apparent loss of fat in subcutaneous fatty depots it often comes as a surprise to learn that the fat content of the human body reaches a maximum in the older years, higher than in infancy, childhood or middle age.[11,12] The rising fat content is notable in several sites: in muscle, increasing numbers of fat cells appear between muscle fibers and larger muscle groupings. Thus Frantzell and Ingelmark[13] demonstrated by both roentgenographic methods and biopsies that there was a rising content of fat in the calf muscles, starting in the forties. No such alteration was initially occurring in the arm muscles of the same subjects. The transformation can perhaps be grossly likened to that which occurs from veal to beef. In addition, "internalized fat," fat in the viscera, between the organs, including also the constituent parts of the organs, also rises. As a result of absolute rise in fat content, the specific gravity of the aging human body decreases (Fig. 6-3), since fat is the only constituent with a specific gravity of less than 1.

Muscle

A bodily decline in muscle mass, and, therefore, in strength, seems to be characteristic of the aging process. It is not, as is some-

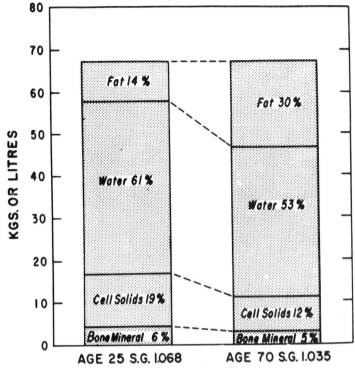

Fig. 6–3. Aging changes in major body components contrasting "reference males" ages 25 and 70. Due to rising fat content, specific gravity falls. Diminished water and cell solids reflects loss in lean body mass (From Fryer, J. H. pp. 59–78 in N. W. Shock (Ed.) Biological Aspects of Aging, 1962. N.Y. Columbia University Press)

times thought, a disuse atrophy. Smaller upper extremity muscles are noted in older working longshoremen, and shrinkage occurs in the eye and laryngeal muscles, muscles used continually into old age. Involutionary changes result in disappearance of some muscle fibers with shrinkage and fragmentation of other muscle fibers along with the above mentioned fat infiltration. All the changes are quite clear in aging laboratory animals (Review in Gutmann '77).[14] A noninvasive investigational tool for analysis of this process has been furnished by the technology of whole body counting. Although the techniques vary somewhat, the principle is to count the total radioactivity of the body, essentially attributable to the naturally occurring isotope of potassium, ^{40}k. Since potassium is almost wholly an intracellular ion with only relatively minute amounts in the extracellular fluids, or in fat cells, whole body counting essentially measures the potassium of the lean body

mass, and chiefly the very large reservoir of potassium found in muscle. Both cross-sectional and longitudinal studies have clearly documented an age-related decline in bodily radioactivity, quite distinct from weight fluctuations (Fig. 6-4). Sex differences related to the larger muscle mass of the male are obvious. Of interest also is the earlier onset of this decline in the male. This decline is evidenced by the thirties and parallels the decrement in muscle strength that also begins at this time. The regression continues in the ensuing decades and accelerates late in life. In contrast, the female with a lesser initial muscle mass has a steady state through the fourth and fifth decades; the decline in the muscle mass of the female thus appears later. The rate of decline is steeper in both the sexes past 60. Though an exercise program in a sedentary middle-aged individual with involuted muscles may produce a measurable rise in his radioactive potassium, remeasurements of these individ-

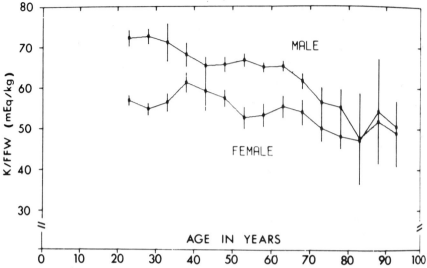

Fig. 6-4.   Decline in lean body mass with aging as indicated by decreased total 40^K. The decline is greater and appears earlier in the male, probably reflecting the proportionately greater shrinkage in muscle.

uals as the years go by still shows the inevitable nature of this phenomenon.[15] There is thus a clear anatomical basis for the complaints of older people of increasing weakness in carrying out their usual tasks. Why muscle cells degenerate and muscle mass declines with aging remains a mystery. However, the facts of involution are to be kept in mind in the interpretation of similar regression of other important tissues, such as that which occurs in the brain.

Bone and Joint Changes

Change in the bony skeleton is complicated by the existence of hypertrophic and anabolic processes simultaneously with catabolic ones. The bone is a unique tissue in simultaneously being an arena in which mineral deposition by osteoblasts and resorption by osteoclasts are concurrent. With age, overall bone loss triumphs. However, it is now well established that bony growth can and does go on in the middle and late years. Increments in growth of the bone, such as rib, metacarpal, and the femoral cortex have been demonstrated by various investigators.[16,17,18] Finding of an approximately 3.5% increase in the width of the pelvis in both sexes that goes on into old

age has modified earlier thoughts that dimensions of the bony pelvis were fixed after maturity. The skull thickens into advanced old age, with some sutures such as the masto-occipital and parietomastoid not closing over until ages 70 to 80.[19] In many long bones deposition on the surface may be occurring simultaneously with resorption from the endosteum. In the case of the femur this leads to a slightly wider bone with a wider marrow cavity and, therefore, structurally weaker.[20]

Of more significance in the bony weakening is the usually slow progressive loss of osteoid tissue generally. This is the phenomenon of osteoporosis, already noted above in relationship to statural shortening due to vertebral osteoporosis. The gradual demineralization of bone is the background to that most important fracture in old age, that of the femur. The risk factors for osteoporosis are being female, having a low calcium intake for many years, and being white of northern European extraction with a delicate build to start with. Clinical osteoporosis and femoral fractures are both less marked in blacks.[21] Some clinicians believe osteoporosis to be an involutionary process affecting the bone in much the same way as similar involutionary processes affect subcutaneous fatty depots, muscle, and other organs. According to this concept, loss of osteoid tissue would be an inevitable age-related decline with the degree of osteoporosis attained at any given age dependent on how well calcified the bone was initially. Nonetheless, clinical evidence also suggests the importance of other controllable factors such as lack of adequate calcium or Vitamin D, variations in fluoride, exercise. The two common fractures of old age, of the wrist, and femoral, are ascribable to the increased tendency to fall, impaired balancing reflexes and poor perception, plus the long preceding stealthy loss of osteoid tissue so that the osteoporotic bone gives way.

Changes in joints are generally ascribed to use and stress of weight bearing, multiplied by a time factor. But here too, other variables are involved. Thickening of the distal interphalangeal joints (Heberden's nodes) appears earlier and is more severe in females than in males and has a hereditary component. Obvious thickening appears as early as the thirties with gross distortions taking place over the next decade or two. There is no evidence that use or abuse plays a significant role, and such osteoarthritic changes in the fingers are not correlated to changes elsewhere.

Though seldom more than a cosmetic disorder, some pain may be complained of. The thickening and distortion of the fingers may also serve as a daily early warning signal to the person of the uncontrollable nature of age-related changes. Among the most common and predictable joint changes are those that occur in the spine. Such vertebral changes are sufficiently time-related as to be of value to the physical anthropologist in estimating age. In addition to narrowing of discs, the characteristic changes are the bony proliferations known as osteophytes. These occur on both the anterior and posterior aspects of vertebrae. In the neck, the maximum changes are seen at the C5-C6 level, which has been shown radiologically to be the site of the greatest motion in flexion-extension movements of the neck.

The bony proliferation and disc regression may produce impingement on nerves with resulting radiculopathies and the familiar well-nigh universal symptoms of stiffness with pain, steady or recurrent.

Studies of the knees have documented the early onset and age-related progression of change.[22] Microscopic changes in the knee cartilages are visible during the second decade of life. The originally smooth glistening cartilage progressively thereafter shows fibrillar degeneration, fragmentation and irregularity. As this proceeds through the middle years, hypertrophic changes may take place and the end result may be a more or less complete loss of cartilage with eburnation of the bony surfaces and variable degrees of osteophyte formation. Osteoarthritic changes in the knees, like those of vertebrae, thus seem inevitable. Often, there is no significant disability and even where the disorder is well established, evidence of effusion and pain may be episodic and respond to appropriate therapies. Earlier onset seems to be characteristic of overweight middle-aged women. What has been said of the knee seems to be true also for the hip, another important joint from the rheumatologist's viewpoint. Severe change in this joint may lead to such profound disability as to warrant hip replacement. Oddly, the ankle more or less escapes osteoarthritic change, despite its location and weight-bearing function.

Anthropometric changes with aging have long been an area of interest to the physical anthropologist. Some of this literature is discussed elsewhere, and illustrated in Fig. 6-2. As can be seen, in the male veterans lengthening and broadening of the nose, lengthening of the ears, decline in grip strength as an index to muscle regression, increasing bi-iliac and antero-posterior chest measures are some of the characteristic age-related changes. Over all, similar changes occur in females, the greatest sex-related variable perhaps being differences in redistribution of fat in the skin folds. Shrinking muscle mass is relatively greater in the male, and in the aging male the decline in hemoglobin is also relatively more marked. This is attributed to decline in androgens, so that the male-female difference in red blood cell mass diminishes. By this and other parameters (e.g. muscle, body hair) the two sexes become more alike in old age.

Ectodermal Changes

On inspection of the aged individual, it is obvious that most of what one sees are ectodermal changes. One observes wrinkling, decrease in hair with graying, atrophy of subcutaneous tissue, or the arcus senilis and these chiefly contribute to our estimate of age and our reaction. Hair loss with aging is universal although subject to a great deal of variability and having an important sex-related component. Patterns of baldness in the male have important genetic determinants, being transmitted from mother to son and unfolding under the influence of androgens. Ensuing patterns of baldness are a matter of every day observation: when severe in the male, almost all of the head hair may be lost except at the periphery. Such peripheral hairs when transplanted into the formerly bald areas continued to thrive, thus pointing up some of the unknowns in the hair loss process. Even in the absence of this hereditary component, thinning of scalp hair does occur in progressive fashion in middle-aged and older males and at a lesser rate in most females. Many women note a distressing amount of hair loss post menopausally, and it is unclear as to why this affects some women earlier and to a greater degree than others. In addition to hair loss, hairs that remain tend to be finer, so that the thinning is both quantitative and qualitative. Also, body hair tends to be lost especially past age 50. Very old men and women have very little body hair.[23] In part, this seems to be an atrophy much like the atrophy of other components of the subcutaneous tissue. Striking degrees of hair loss in the axilla may occur in women. Here the loss is from the periphery to the center and thus occurs in the reverse

manner to that seen during puberty. Japanese women have virtually no axillary hair 10 years post menopause and aging Caucasian women exhibit fewer and fewer axillary hairs. Pubic hairs also become sparse. Graying of the hair has traditionally and symbolically been recognized as an aging parameter. It begins in the twenties, tends to progress thereafter, but does show considerable variability. Damon et al.[24] found that of many parameters, the one that best correlated with biologic aging was the extent of graying.

Wrinkling of the skin of the face is well known to be worsened by solar exposure. However, even in the most sun-protected individuals, use lines proceed linearly with aging. These are the predictable indentations of the skin produced by the action of the muscles of facial expression. They result in the familiar parallel wrinkles of the forehead, the fan-shaped groups at the corners of the eyes, the radial wrinkles around the mouth, all of which are more marked in older persons. A wrinkle of considerable clinical interest, since it is not use-related, is the somewhat oblique crease of the ear lobe seldom seen before the fifth or sixth decades. This tends to deepen once it appears, and has been referred to as the "coronary crease" because of studies relating it to an increased incidence of coronary events and coronary artery disease.[25,26] How portentous this crease is, is far from clear in view of the relatively small number of case reports in the literature. Similar grave implications were once thought to be true of the arcus senilis. This is an infiltrate at the corneal limbus due to localized deposition of fat in the cells in that location. The arcus initially appears as small segments of the final ring and continued deposition finally produces a complete white ringing of the corneal periphery. Some degree of arcus is exceedingly common in the elderly. There is little doubt that it appears earlier in life in familial hypercholesterolemia. However, it also appears early in life in blacks, having been found by Macaraeg et al.[27] in blacks in their twenties. Though once linked to ECG abnormalities and coronary artery disease, this implication of the arcus senilis has been considerably de-emphasized in recent years.

Despite computer generated correlates such as those linking graying and age, there is considerable question as to whether we have any quantitative ectodermal change that is a simple parameter to the aging process. There is no reason to doubt that the many changes in the skin described above may have some positive correlate with age-related changes in deeper tissues and even the brain. On the basis of present knowledge, it would be difficult to assess the clinical value or validity of the correlations in a great body of aging data. Gray hairs may be more a sign of experiential wisdom, as has often been thought in some societies, than an indicator of aging decline, as has been implied by some investigators.

Arterial Changes

Elongation, sometimes associated with increasing tortuosity, occurs in many of the larger arteries with aging. In part, it is thought to reflect the loss of the elastic tissue and increased stiffness of connective tissue in the arterial wall, changes which are characteristic of collagen in other parts of the body. The process is certainly abetted by hypertension. On chest x-ray, widening of the aorta and elongation are commonly observed in the older patient especially if blood pressures are elevated. Below the diaphragm, a similar elongation and bowing in the abdominal aorta may simulate early abdominal aneurysm. A serpentine tortuosity of the brachial artery in the subcutaneous tissue of the arm is easily seen in some older persons. Variable degrees of coiling and kinking are found in carotid angiography and initially were also thought related to aging changes. However, some kinking has been found in cerebral angiograms in every decade from the 1st to the 8th, and Weibel and Fields[28] in reviewing the carotid angiograms of almost 1500 patients concluded that tortuosity and coiling of the internal carotid artery was a con-

genital condition which could worsen with aging of the artery but that kinking was an acquired condition which occurred later in life.

Shrinkage in Organs

As can be seen from Fig. 6-5, weights of most organs diminish in old age. However, the difficulties posed by data derived from cross-sectional rather than longitudinal study are inherent in this and most of the human studies reported in the literature. Some of the pitfalls in interpreting data of this sort are discussed by Calloway.[29] As mentioned earlier, the secular increase in size in the past century makes it likely that these larger individuals have a related increase in organ size and weight. Conversely, the very old persons in our midst, smaller initially, would have smaller and lighter viscera. An example of this relationship is implicit in the data reported by Sato, Miwa and Tauchi.[30] They reported the mean liver weight in Japanese males, age 50, to be around 1200 gms. as compared to approximately 1800 gms. in Caucasian males. Insofar as could be judged from such cross-sectional studies, liver size and weight did decrease with aging, if anything relatively more in the Japanese.

Presumptively, a decrease in cellular mass in the liver is a paradigm for shrinkage in vital organs elsewhere. In fact, the degree of loss seems quite variable in different tissues, as is also clear in the figure. The kidneys suffer a greater degree of shrinkage than such organs as the thyroid or the brain or pancreas. Shrinkage in brain size and weight has generally been thought to be a characteristic aspect of aging with estimates of 90–100 gm. given for the life span (discussion in Brody '77[31]). There has been widespread circulation of a calculation which estimated that 100,000 brain cells drop out daily starting after the first 25 years of life. There is not reliable evidence that cell attrition occurs in a steady fashion, and the "daily drop out" conception was a calculation based on estimates of loss in brain weight over the life

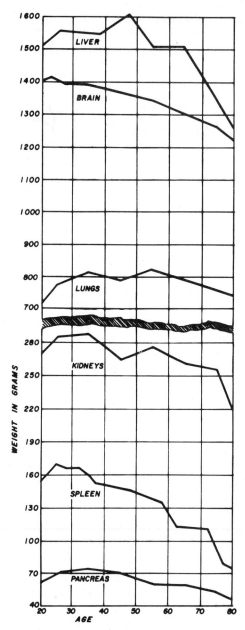

Fig. 6-5. The decrease in weight of body organs with aging is apparent for most organs, lung, prostate and perhaps heart being exceptions. (Redrawn from Rossle and Roulet, 1032 Zahl and Mass in Pathologie from Rossman, I., The Anatomy of Aging in Rossman, I. (Ed.) Clinical Geriatrics 2nd ed. 1979, Philadelphia, Lippincott.

that cell loss is regional.[33] Loss of cells is demonstrable in the precentral gyrus, the superior frontal and superior temporal gyri, but not in the post central gyrus or in a typical brain stem nucleus such as the abducens. In addition to the variability true of any aging process, the interrelation of aging and pathology again emerges in the interpretation of data on the brain. It is possible that the more marked shrinkage in brain weight in some individuals is a step on the pathway to dementia, a common disorder. For the present, the evidence favors the conception that as with other organs, such as muscle, a significant degree of cell loss in the brain is an accompaniment of the aging process. Besides cell loss, cellular change may be of equal if not greater importance, as in the loss of dendritic connections in extant cells reported by Scheibel and Scheibel.[34]

However, there are tissues and organs which may enlarge with aging. Reference has already been made to the continued deposition of new bone in various parts of the skeleton over the lifetime. The lung appears grossly to maintain its weight over the lifetime although histologically some dilation of alveoli takes place and function declines considerably. The impact of aging on the heart has been fraught with many doubts because of the widespread existence of hypertension in the population. In addition, the tendency of the systolic pressure to rise with aging in the absence of diastolic hypertension also poses difficulty since hypertension is well known to increase left ventricular thickness and cardiac weight. The most recent evidence points to an increasing thickness of the ventricle with aging in normotensives,[35] as demonstrated by echocardiography in longitudinal studies. The same phenomenon has been described in dogs. The most famous organ subject to hypertrophy is the prostate in man, with urinary obstruction as an end result; prostatic hypertrophy, though widespread in aging males, is by no means universal. Some elderly males, in fact, have juvenile prostates. It is presently thought that this hypertrophy has a hormonal base and is not a true aging process.

span. There is reason to believe that some 25% of the Purkinje cells are lost from the cerebellum, with much of the loss occurring later, past the age of 50 (Hall *et al.*'75[32]). Elsewhere in the brain, Brody has shown

Other examples can be cited to indicate the paradox of hypertrophy occurring in what is overall the atrophic scene that characterizes aging. Hyperkeratosis and areas of pigmentation ("liver spots") develop on skin which may be obviously atrophic. Hairs may develop around the chin and lips in aging females. Fibrotic nodules often with deforming contractures involving the palmar tendons may progress in the latter years (Dupuytren's contracture). Costal cartilages in the thorax thicken and calcify. Formerly inapparent veins such as those of the lip, the fingers, and the under surface of the tongue, may thicken and become prominent. Glandular tissue of the breast more or less disappears post menopausally, and loss of breast fat may be considerable, despite which the breasts become pendulous and longer due to loss of supporting tissues.

In addition to hyperplastic and hypertrophic processes, neoplasia also takes place. A frequently cited example is the development of carcinoma in the atrophic gastric mucosa of pernicious anemia. Similarly, neoplasms of the skin frequently proliferate on areas that show histological atrophy. In other areas, the problem of neoplasia becomes complex and probably multiple factors are involved. Overall, there is a strong age relationship: some carcinomas are almost exclusively characteristic of the elderly, as for example, prostatic carcinoma. The geometric increase of some neoplastic processes with age has been attributed to factors that culminate in neoplasm—and also to diminution in immunologic competency, as discussed below.

DECLINES IN ORGAN FUNCTION

Since morphologic changes are often the visible base for functional change, it comes as no surprise that decremental functioning is characteristic of aging. Despite this, homeostasis is generally preserved although adaptive capacity to stress does diminish. As an example, body temperature will still be pegged at the normal level, though it may rise and fall excessively in different environ-ments, hence an increased incidence of heat stroke and hypothermia.[36] The somatic picture is quite variable: some primitive systems such as the gastro-intestinal tract show comparatively little impairment through the life cycle, in contrast to the renal-excretory system which shows marked diminution in reserve. Similarly, cerebral cortical function is impaired far more than brain stem function. The endocrine system continues to function surprisingly well for a complex set of regulatory glands linked through the feedback of chemical messages. Some of the highlights and contrast from system to system can be seen in Fig. 6-6, and are considered in the following:

Cardiovascular System

Contrary to previous statements, it is now thought that the heart normally undergoes a physiological hypertrophy with aging in the absence of hypertension. Despite this, the resting cardiac output decreases almost linearly with aging past maturity, the decrement being on the order of 30–40% between ages 25 and 65.[37] This exceeds the decline in lean body mass, but doubtless reflects diminished physiological need. In addition, when stressed, the cardiac output cannot be pushed to the same heights as in younger years, and the exercise-induced tachycardia achieves a lower peak level. In addition to these declines in physiological capacity, there is much impairment because of the widespread silent or overt existence of coronary atherosclerosis. Coronary artery disease progresses through the decades past 60 so that an increasing percentage of older individuals may quite slowly rather than dramatically develop congestive heart failure. In some homes for the elderly even in the ambulatory group, as many as half the group may need to be digitalized. Needless to say, most elderly persons pace themselves almost unconsciously in making appropriate adjustment to cardiac limitation. There is some reason to believe that continued vigorous exercise can favorably modify the normal rate of decline in cardiac capacitance.

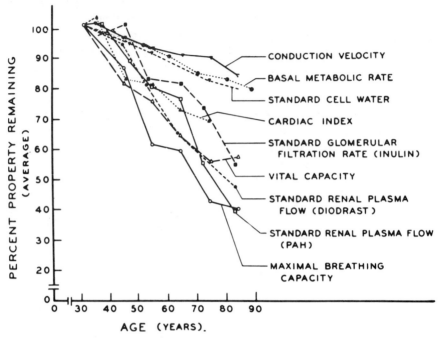

Fig. 6–6.   Decrements in various physiologic variables with aging. Renal, cardiac and pulmonary declines are prominent. (From Kohn, R. R. *Aging,* 1973, Upjohn Co., Kalamazoo, Mich.)

The connective tissue of the arteries, as is true of connective tissue elsewhere, tends to stiffen with aging. This loss of elasticity contributes to the tendency of the arteries to elongate, to diminution in elastic recoil in the aorta and increased propagation of pulse wave, and to the widening of the pulse pressure. In addition, vascular sclerosis is well nigh universal, certainly in Western society, and is regarded by some as a normal aging change, up to some levels at least. Although most prominent clinically in the coronary arteries, atherosclerosis once manifest is always generalized to some degree. A patient who has had a myocardial infarction is at substantially greater risk for manifestations of frank cerebral atherosclerosis and vice versa. Stroke may be triggered by myocardial infarction, or even an arrythymia without an MI. Peripheral vascular disease is the result of arterial circulatory impairment almost exclusively to the lower extremities, and practically never to the upper extremities. This is due to the greater degree of sclerosis in the abdominal, iliac and femoral arteries. The classic symptom is intermittent claudication, essentially an angina of the skeletal muscle of the legs, in which pain is produced by walking and relieved by resting in characteristic cyclic fashion. Atherosclerosis in the abdomino-iliac system may produce Leriche's syndrome: the claudication is experienced chiefly in the thigh and buttock muscles and because of diminution in the arterial circulation to the penis, organic impotence results.

Various vascular reconstructive procedures for improving these circulatory defects are available. Coronary bypass surgery is the most spectacular, carotid endarterectomy and prostheses for larger arteries well established. For most cases of mild peripheral disease, intervention is not indicated. In fact, intermittent claudication may improve with the passage of the years as collateral circulation is formed. The Framingham study has made clear the chief significance of peripheral arterial insufficiency is its high correlation with coronary artery disease, a far more threatening form of vascular sclerosis. When both PVD and coronary artery disease are present, cerebral vascular sclerosis is well nigh inevitable. However, with much vascular disease, both extent of clinical manifestations and disability have a somewhat capricious element. Thus intellectual functioning may be reasonably preserved despite overt cerebral atherosclerosis, transient ischemic attacks or small cerebral thromboses. Aneurysmal dilatation of the abdominal aorta, a fairly common disease in the elderly, has a rising incidence of rupture even when asymptomatic. Despite this frequent outcome, some of the patients who refuse the generally advised elective operation will escape this catastrophe. Evidence of continuing enlargement is a strong operative indication.

Pulmonary Function

The vital capacity decreases with aging although total lung capacity remains more or less unchanged. The residual capacity doubles over the life span. Anthropometric studies suggest that some deepening of the chest in the AP diameter is a normal aging change found in non-smokers and in various groups studied. In contrast, the maximum voluntary ventilation may decrease by up to 50% between 20 and 80, as do other pulmonary functional parameters such as the forced expiratory volume.[38] Some of the anatomical changes have been likened to emphysema, but it is probable that the so-called "senile emphysema" represents dilatation of alveoli without breakdown of alveolar septa or the usual chronic bronchitis and out flow obstruction seen in the typical emphysema patient. With aging there is a lowered resting arterial oxygen tension ascribed to ventilation-perfusion defects which do not, however, affect the CO_2. Decreased ventilatory capacity is generally ascribed to stiffening of the tissues of the chest wall including its musculature, to calcification of the costal cartilages with decreased rib motion and other changes that alter lung compliance. Probably the shortness of breath complained of by elderly persons as they climb stairs represents a combination of both cardiac and pulmonary factors in an interaction which will diminish the capacity for exercise or other efforts. Also, chronic bronchitis and emphysema do rise with age and in varying degrees contribute to declining pulmonary function. It has been noted that a marked drop in vital capacity precedes a steep rise in mortality in the elderly. It has been ascribed to weakness superimposed on pulmonary aging changes.

Renal Excretory System

As can be seen in Fig. 6-5, there is a sharp decline in the renal mass with aging. This anatomically reflects chiefly a continuing subtraction from the approximately 1 million nephrons present at birth. Both renal weight and number of nephrons decrease by approximately 30–40% over the life span. Loss of nephrons commences as a sclerosis of the glomeruli followed by atrophy of the afferent arterioles.[39] The atrophic nephrons are not replaced. It is known that intact nephrons can hypertrophy, a phenomenon that occurs rapidly both in the neonate and after removal of a kidney at any age. However, no compensatory hypertrophy of nephrons to make up for the loss of units with aging takes place to help maintain original renal mass and function. As a consequence the glomeruler filtration rate decreases 45% from age 20 to age 90.[40] The renal plasma flow decreases slightly more over the same span. These declines in renal excretory capacity do not ordinarily impair the capacity to excrete such metabolites as urea or creatinine. The BUN of older persons is about the same as for younger ones or but slightly higher.

However, the aged kidney responds less well to the stresses that may be caused by infusions of large amounts of fluid or salt solutions. Thus, overload of the circulation with consequent edema is not uncommon in older hospitalized patients on IV infusion such as normal saline. The diminished renal capacity is also the background to prolongation of the half life of some important drugs such as digoxin. Because of its diminished renal excretion, the daily maintenance dose is frequently half that required by a younger cardiac (0.125 mgm.). A number of important drugs resemble digoxin in this respect including the sulfonamides, lithium, and widely used antibiotics such as gentamycin and kanamycin. Vascular diseases produced by hypertension and pyelonephritis are further frequent contributors to diminished renal function. For this and other reasons the elderly are far more likely to experience adverse drug reactions. For drugs whose route of excretion is mainly by way of the kidneys, cuts in the usual dosage in the very old may be mandated.

The Bladder

The reservoir function of the bladder also undergoes change with aging. As has been emphasized by the British geriatrician, J. C. Brocklehurst, the characteristics of the geriatric bladder are: (1) A diminished capacity; (2) a higher residual volume; thus a 100 cc. residual volume is not uncommon in many older women; (3) an earlier onset of tetanic bladder contractions. The compounded effects of all these changes in both sexes is to produce increased frequency, an increased sense of urgency, and increasing nocturia.[41] Prostatic hypertrophy may further compound these findings, but these changes in bladder behavior hold for females and for males without prostate enlargement. However, the common development of prostatic hypertrophy may superimpose an often stealthy disease which has been known to result in uremia without the patient's consulting a physician. Even with the best of bladders, significant prostatic hypertrophy will generally make its presence known by marked increase in frequency day and night and weakness of the urinary stream, especially with dribbling and hesitancy on arising in the morning. Provided all these symptoms do not interfere markedly with rest and do not produce bladder infection or obstructive uropathy, it is possible to nurse many elderly men with various grades of prostatic hypertrophy through the remainder of their life span.

Sudden complete retention in a former mildly symptomatic male is a common precipitant for prostatic resection. A disease with a strong age correlation and most common past 70 is carcinoma of the prostate. It is apparently independent of benign prostatic hypertrophy. Of interest is the very low incidence of both of these disorders in Asia.[42]

Urinary incontinence is the bane of patient, family, and geriatrician alike. As a single symptom, it may tip the scale in favor of institutionalization. Overflow incontinence results from obstructive or neurogenic interference with bladder emptying. An atonic bladder fills up (it may reach the umbilicus), and empties in small dribbling amounts as it attempts to decompress itself. Diabetes is one common cause of neurogenic bladder which is potentially reversible. Rather, more common is the incontinence associated with organic brain changes. In the life history of the individual, the cerebral cortex assumes a dominant, chiefly inhibiting, role in control of bladder function in the early childhood years. Brain damage, whether due to stroke or neuronal degeneration, and rarely, other causes such as tumor, is the usual cause for uninhibited neurogenic bladder with incontinence. Incontinence can be transient or short-lived, as in association with surgical operations and anesthesia, in early phases of a stroke, a debilitating illness, or toxic delirium. With improvement, the urinary incontinence is reversed. Most of the cases the geriatrician sees in older impaired individuals carry a poor or guarded prognosis. Various devices are available for the collection of urine in such patients, the problem most often being that they will not wear them. The Kanga pouch, more widely employed in Britain, is constructed with a gelling material which absorbs up to 150 cc. of urine before the skin will be wetted. Medications designed to inhibit bladder contractions may be of value. Diphenhydramine, a soporific antihistamine with some atropine-like properties, may be useful for nocturnal incontinence and frequency.

Various regimes have been worked out for the control of incontinence and are described by Broklehurst.[43] These include an initial careful charting of the times of incontinence from which is derived a schedule for toileting the patient. Toileting before the onset of tetanic bladder contractions, combined with medications, may considerably reduce and sometimes abolish a distressing incontinence. The program requires considerable individualization and attention to detail.

Changes in the Reproductive System

Aging changes in the female are ushered in more or less abruptly with the onset of the menopause, with cessation of usual ovarian activity and loss of menses. It may or may not be accompanied by such vasomotor changes as flushes and sweats. Some of the disability is explainable by the annoyance of nocturnal sweats with awakening, perhaps with depressive reactions to the realization of one of life's passages. "Nervousness" and irritability seem to be frequent. There is a striking decrease in estrogens particularly the "true" ovarian hormone, estradiol. The drop in estrogen alters the feedback circuit to the pituitary, and as a consequence there are marked rises in pituitary gonadotropins. Marked elevations of FSH and LH, especially the former, are classic endocrine hallmarks for the postmenopausal state. The ovary is by no means reduced to a state of nonsecretion, however. Direct analyses of ovarian blood samples in postmenopausal women indicate a goodly output of androgens such as testosterone and androstenedione, with estrogen barely higher in concentration there than in the peripheral blood. The androstenedione is known to be converted by the peripheral tissues, probably the fat, to estrone. This may be the chief source of estrogen in the postmenopausal female but is not sufficient to prevent various atrophic phenomena in the reproductive tract and breasts. These progress with the passage of the years and include atrophic changes in the vagina, shrinkage of the body and cervix of the uterus, and involutionary changes in the vulva, labia, and loss of pubic hair.[44]

As atrophy continues, there is a progressive narrowing and shrinkage of the vagina readily recognizable by loss of rugae, thinning of the epithelium, and fragility. This often leads to complaints of dyspareunia. On sexual stimulation, lubrication occurs more slowly and may be considerably less abundant than in the younger female. The total amount of lubrication may be inadequate, and supplementation by the usual lubricants may be necessary. Many of these changes are reversible by the administration of estrogen. Since other involutionary changes such as osteoporosis seem synchronous with the menopause, estrogens were widely prescribed throughout the 1950s and 1960s. There seems little doubt about the value of estrogen replacement, but this widespread use declined precipitously with the demonstration that the risk of endometrial carcinoma increased in estrogen-treated females, the risk being proportionate to dose and duration of estrogenic treatment. Many geriatricians do not hesitate to prescribe them in women who have had hysterectomies. It is also possible that the addition of progesterone to the estrogenic treatment, which may reproduce the normal cycle, may lessen if not abolish, the threat of endometrial cancer. This area is under active investigation currently.

In the male reproductive system, aging changes proceed much more slowly without the sudden decline in sex hormone production seen with the menopause. Though histologic and involutionary changes may be seen in the testes past the age of 50, adequate sperm production may continue for decades thereafter, and feisty old men in their 70s can certainly become fathers. There is no significant decline in blood testosterone levels up until age 60 at least and considerable individual variability thereafter. Thus, there is no hormonal background or explanation for the declining capacity to have intercourse which occurs in most males past 30. The normal range of this capacity is certainly subject to great individual variability in older men. Probably with males past 60–65 once a week to once a month might be considered to be a median range. This is to be contrasted with the far greater sexual frequency of earlier decades. Older men take longer to reach erection and have a longer latent period following ejaculation before further erection is possible.[45] The intensity of the muscle contractions associated with orgasm is diminished, and seminal spurts are considerably lessened. Some of the data on the decrement in frequency of sexual intercourse and the rising rate of impotence are noted in Tables 6-1, and 6-2.

What is most difficult to evaluate are the complaints of diminished potency or outright impotency in aging men.[46] Diabetes, depression, thyroid disorders, falls in testosterone titers may all be co-existent, and are sometimes regarded as causal. There is even some loose talk about the "male menopause," with the possibility raised that with low testosterone titers, testosterone

Table 6-1.   Incidence of Impotence Cited by Various Authors*.

AGE	% IMPOTENCE	AGE	% IMPOTENCE
KINSEY		BOWERS	
40	1.9	60–64	28.0
45	2.6	65–69	50.0
50	6.7	70–74	61.0
55	6.7		
60	18.4	NEWMAN	
65	25.0		
70	27.0	60–64	40.0
75	55.0	65–69	37.0
80	75.0	70–74	42.0
		75 +	75.0
FINKLE		PERLMAN, KOBASHI	
55–59	31.0		
60–64	37.0	40–49	5.0
65–69	37.0	50–59	11.3
70–74	61.0	60–69	36.6
75–79	76.0	70–79	59.0
80 +	60.0	80 +	85.0

* From "Frequency of Intercourse in Males at Different Ages" by C. K. Perlman. Reprinted from *Medical Aspects of Human Sexuality.* November 1972. Hospital Publications, Inc. 1972 ALL RIGHTS RESERVED.

Table 6-2.   Prevalence of Intercourse in Males by Age Group*

AGE GROUP	25	40	55–65	65–75
MEDIAN AGE	25	40	59.9	68.5
NUMBER	85	85	49	45
MEDIAN FREQUENCY OF INTERCOURSE PER MONTH	27.6 ± 3.1	17.2 ± 1.8	3.9 ± 0.7	1.8 ± 0.3
EXTREME VALUES	1–180	1–135	0–24	0–8

* From "The Effects of Age on Male Sexual Activity" by H. Cendron and J. Vallery-Masson, *La Presse Médicale,* 1970, 78, 1975. MASSON, S.A. Paris.

replacement therapy may be the key to successful treatment. Psychological factors are often easy to note, but depression may be secondary to the realization of other losses than that of potency. The data for males suggest an age-related concurrent rising incidence of outright impotence with the lessened capacity for sexual intercourse. It is, therefore, difficult to judge whether impotence in aging males always has a pathological base, or may fall under the bell-shaped curve describing a deterioration in any biological function. Studies of some aging males complaining of erectile impotence indicate that they experience penile tumescence during REM sleep at night.[47] In the older males studied, the degree of tumescence is reduced. Further studies of this phenomenon may shed light on what is and is not pathological impotence in the male. A good deal more data from a general population basis are needed. Granting that chronic illness, fatigue, depression, and other influences frequently associated with aging are clearly operative with many individuals does not gainsay the fact that overall the capacity to have intercourse as revealed in the surveys cited in Table 6-1 undergoes a more marked decrement with aging than almost any other physiological function.

Changes in Metabolic and Endocrine Systems

Because of the decline in the lean body mass, there is a decline in total oxygen consumption with aging. The older studies using the basal metabolism technique were first interpreted as showing a decline in metabolic rate, but when this is corrected for the decline in lean body mass, it is apparent that the consumption of oxygen by individual cells is not altered in old age. Furthermore, direct studies of the blood for thyroxin (T-4) indicate no decline with aging.[48] Tri-iodo-thyronine (T-3) decreases 25–40% after the sixth decade. Thyrotropin stimulating hormone levels in the blood are unchanged indicating that the feedback mechanism from

thyroid to pituitary is stable. Radioiodine uptake by the thyroid at six hours decreases with age, but to total uptake at 24 hours still falls within the normal range. It is believed that reduced renal excretion of the radioiodine permits a longer period for the thyroid of older persons to take up the marker. Combinations of a reduced radioiodine uptake by the gland together with a normal plasma thyroxine concentration suggest that even if thyroxine secretion is decreased its rate of degradation is decreased in parallel, thus giving the unaltered serum T-4. In fact, studies of rates of hormone degradation indicate a 50% decline between ages 20 and 80. This is probably related to a slower hepatic disposal but contributes to preservation of a normal serum T-4 level.

Hypothyroidism is a disease of some importance in the elderly. It may be spontaneous or follow thyroiditis or be a late consequence of surgical or radioiodine therapy for hyperthyroidism. Because hypothyroidism may develop slowly, early symptoms are often missed or attributed to aging: fatigability, slow cerebration, mild anemia, etc. The similarity in symptomatology calls for serum thyroxine studies in the differential diagnosis of early organic mental syndrome. Hyperthyroidism may also be difficult to diagnose in the elderly, and may present atypically as so-called "apathetic hyperthyroidism" generally without exophthalmos. Generally tachycardia, hyperkinesis or nervousness and insomnia, tremor or depression, and crying spells may be noted. Only rarely is the thyroid not palpably enlarged, and direct blood determination for T-3 and T-4 are diagnostic.

Glucose Tolerance. It is well established that the glucose tolerance test levels rise with aging.[49] Usually a one-hour glucose of more than 160, with a two-hour level of more than 120 (Fajans and Conn criteria) are considered diagnostic of diabetes, at least "chemical diabetes." However, when these criteria are applied to the elderly, 25% or more may show higher figures. It thus came to be recognized that glucose intolerance increases with aging as of course does the incidence of true diabetes mellitus. Follow-up studies on older patients with glucose intolerance indicate that some show no further progression, while others become diabetic. Apart from the questions of definition, it is apparent that a number of factors present in the elderly contribute to the impaired ability to dispose of administered glucose: (1) the decrease in the lean body mass, especially muscle; (2) a delay in the output of insulin by the pancreas coupled with a delay in hepatic response; and (3) physical inactivity. A number of proposals have been made to aid in distinguishing between diabetes and glucose intolerance in the elderly. At present, it does not appear that a sharp distinction can be drawn. Indeed any alleged sharp distinction would overlook the fact that there is a rising incidence of diabetes mellitus with aging which would commence initially by evidence of glucose intolerance. The diabetes of old age is mild, tends to be nonketotic and stable, and generally does not produce management problems. The chief difficulty may be the avoidance of hypoglycemia, especially with long-acting insulin preparations and also with some of the oral hypoglycemic agents. Episodes of confusion, agitation, or nocturnal wandering in diabetics on antidiabetic therapy should be suspect for the possibility of hypoglycemia.

Sex Hormones. Throughout most of the life span, direct assays of testosterone in men indicate no significant decline. Past 60–70 the trend is down; borderline and below normal declines may be registered in some men, with normal levels present in others.[50] As previously noted there is no direct relationship between the decline in rate of male sexual performance which sets in early and testosterone levels. However, in older men with low serum levels, testosterone injections have been recommended for a possible effect on declining sexual capacity or impotence. Interpretation is rendered the more difficult because of the variably low to borderline readings found in many sexually functioning, elderly males.

Male hormone levels thus stand in contrast to the sharp drop in estrogens post menopausally.

Adrenal Hormones.   Production and degradation studies show that cortisol secretion is preserved in old age as are plasma cortisol levels.[51,52] The studies indicate that the cortisol secretion rate is diminished, but an almost parallel decrease in the degradation of cortisol results in approximately similar plasma levels. This maintenance of the norm is thus comparable to that described for the thyroid and thyroxine secretion. Both blood levels and urinary excretion of aldosterone drop about 50% over the life span. Increased urinary excretion of aldosterone following sodium depletion is around a third of the increase of young adults and the secretion of renin also shows an age-related decrease. Adrenal androgens, the largest component of adrenal steroid hormone output, decrease with aging. The 17 ketosteroid urinary excretion falls progressively to one-half of the values in youth. As has been noted, more androgens from sources such as the ovary may be found in the aged female.

In summary, then, apart from the failure of the ovary represented by the menopause, there are no very marked changes in the endocrine system with aging. Longstanding clinical experience, with the use of estrogens, androgens, and thyroid hormone in aging individuals, in the absence of an endocrinopathy, indicates that endocrine preparations of this type, whatever their symptomatic or placebo effect, are not likely to be the fountain of youth in which aging reversibility is likely to occur.

Hemopoietic System

The male-female difference in total red blood cell mass is due to androgenic stimulation of the bone marrow. In aging males with falling androgen levels significant drops in red blood cell mass may be observed. Thus the male-female RBC difference tends to diminish. Healthy elderly men and women have blood counts within the normal range. A slight falloff in the total circulating number of lymphocytes is suggested by some recent studies. Hematopoietic response to a stress such as hemorrhage may be diminished in old age, but overall the bone marrow is responsive. Thus in some benign bleeding disorders, such as hiatus hernia, courses of iron therapy may be sufficient to make up for an ongoing intermittent or low grade blood loss. Lymphomatous proliferative disease, sometimes of an autoimmune nature, rises with aging and is manifested by such disorders as chronic lymphatic leukemia, multiple myeloma, and Hodgkin's disease; the latter can be a more aggressive disease in old age than in younger groups. The same linkage to age has been observed in laboratory animals such as longlived strains of mice. In general, CBCs in elderly individuals should fall within the normal range; anemia is not a part of the aging process and thus requires the same kind of evaluation as in younger age groups.

Immune System

There has been rapid accumulation of clinical and laboratory data documenting a decline in the functional capacity of the immune system with aging.[53] The processing of lymphocytes by the thymus which turns them into T cells is a key aspect of the bodily defense mechanism against invading organisms, especially intracellular and viral ones and perhaps even tumorous. In a sense, the involution of the thymus around puberty with the somewhat later decline in the lymphoid tissue generally are anatomical markers on the path to declining immunological competence. The other great group of lymphocytes, the B cells, manufacture antibodies and are responsible for humoral immunity. It has been known for half a century that the natural isoagglutinins for the blood groups decline with aging. The level of production of antibodies on exposure to a novel antigen such as DNCB (dinitrochlorobenzene) is demon-strably less in older individuals and previously established, clinically important indices such as the tuberculin reaction may turn negative. This seems to be an important background to the reactivation of latent tuberculosis in the elderly. Individuals receiving chemotherapy that diminishes the immune responses, for example, renal transplant patients, have in some cases unwittingly received a transplant containing cancer cells from the donor. These cancers may proliferate unless chemotherapy is stopped, whereupon an upsurge in bodily defense mechanisms destroys the carcinoma. The age-related rise in cancer has been linked to a similar decline in immunological effectiveness.

The elderly show an increasing mortality from causes such as influenza, pneumonia, and meningitis. The diminished ability to mount a defense against organisms such as the pneumococcus, a frequent cause of infection and death in old age, is well documented. It is the practical base for advocating routine immunization with antipneumococcal vaccines which are derived from capsular polysaccharides of the more common types of pneumococci. Similarly, routine influenza immunization seems to be of clinical value in heightening the defense capacity of the elderly.

Digestive System

There is a gradual loss of taste with age. This may be due to age-related atrophy of the taste buds or to repeated trauma to these structures.[55] Results of such changes may include loss of appetite and subsequent weight loss. These symptoms may be mistaken for mental illness (such as depressive illness) or may complicate such conditions. Significant changes occur in the stomach with aging, leading to a decrease in mucosal thickness. A common condition in the elderly related to these gastric changes is chronic atrophic gastritis.[56] This condition definitely predisposes to the development of carcinoma of the stomach. An increase in achlorhydria associated with a definite decline in acid secretion are additional findings. Unfortunately there is little data available on the anatomical and physiological changes in the small intestine with aging.

Colonic dysfunction in the aged is typically manifested by constipation and diverticulosis. Though the evidence remains unclear, constipation in late life is likely to be caused more by lack of bulk in the diet, decreased fluid intake and the chronic abuse of laxatives, then by the chronic colonic morbidity. Diverticular disease of the colon increases with age, especially in females. Again, dietary changes to low residue food are considered important etiological factors (ie., the colonic lumen is narrowed and intraluminal pressure is increased).

There appears to be an increase in connective tissue in the liver of older persons along with a progressively diminishing liver weight, yet the evidence is conflicting. Some reduction in hepatic enzyme concentrates and response to stimuli also occurs, though the liver has a large reserve capacity.[58] Specifically, there is no distinct increase in bromsulphalein retention (BSP) with aging, but definite evidence of a relative and absolute decrease in albumin and in all the globulin fractions. The only known relationship between the gallbladder and aging is the common presence of calculi with increasing age.

Temperature Regulation and Control

At resting or basal conditions, the body temperature of an elderly person is maintained within the same limits as that of the young,[59] yet response to high or low environmental temperatures is less effective. Exposure to a cold environment may lead to the development of hypothermia, a significant cause of death in the geriatric population. All older persons may not be at risk for the development of hypothermia, however. A group of individuals who are at risk may show a fall in core body temperature when exposed to cold for more than one hour.[60] The older person living alone, who becomes depressed and therefore pays little attention to the external environment may be particularly at risk for the development of hypothermia.

CONCLUSION

As we have seen in the above, irreversible, decremental processes occur with aging. These are manifested by shrinking organ and muscle size and declining functional capacity in many organs such that the ability of the aging organism to cope with stresses diminishes. In normal circumstances and mild stress states, the aging human organism can cope adequately. In major stressful circumstances, as for example the events that might be associated with gastrointestinal bleeding and the need for surgery, the diminished functional capacity of the heart, lungs, and kidneys may be quickly manifested by a disproportionate degree of shock, organic mental syndrome, increased incidence of pneumonia, congestive heart failure and/or impairments in the excretory capacity for intravenous fluids. These declines, brought out by stress, need not produce therapeutic catastrophes but make successes more difficult to attain. The increasing success rate of major surgery, including coronary bypass operations on the very old (e.g. over 70), are indicative of the triumph over age. Indeed, our ability to compensate for the declines of the aging organism have increased to a point where the major limiting factor may not be somatic but psychiatric. Thus organic mental syndromes are often the chief obstacle in the ability to deal with stress and are a prognostic factor in limiting the life span. Older patients with severe organic mental syndrome do have shortened life spans compared to individuals of the same age with reasonable degrees of psychological functioning. A patient with organic mental syndrome may have difficulty in following directions, in carrying out therapeutic programs such as those associated with successful surgery for hip fracture, have a greater tendency to aspirate foods, and to develop bronchopneumonia.[54] Because of obtundation, a patient may lack ability to recognize bodily changes of pathological import and call them to the attention of the doctor. For these and other obvious reasons, the organic mental syndromes associated with aging have become a major problem of the geriatrician, the psychiatrist, and society as a whole.

REFERENCES

1. Rossman, I. 1977. Anatomic and body composition changes with aging, pp. 189–221. In C. E. Finch and L. Hayflick (eds.) *Handbook of the Biology of Aging,* New York: Van Nostrand Reinhold.
2. Kannel, W. B. 1976. Some lessons in cardiovascular epidemiology from Framingham. *Am. J. Cardiol.* **37:** 269.
3. Nathan, H. 1962. Osteophytes of the vertebral column. *J. Bone Joint Surg.* **44:** 243–268.
4. Howells, W. W. 1965. Age and individuality in vertebral lipping: Notes on Stewart's data. *Homenaje a Juan Comas* 2: 169–178. Mexico.
5. Damon, A. 1965b. Stature increase among Italian-Americans: Environmental, genetic, or both? *Am. J. Phys. Anthropol.* **23:** 401–408.
6. Büchi, E. C. 1950. Änderung der körperform beim erwachsenen menschen, eine untersuchung nach der Individual-Methode. *Anthrop. Forsch., Heft 1.* Anthrop, Gesel., Wien.
7. Hooton, E. A. and Dupertuis, C. W. 1951. Age changes and selective survival in Irish males. Studies in Physical Anthropology (American Association of Physical Anthropologists and Wenner-Gren Foundation). 2: 1–130.
8. Miall, W. E., Ashcroft, M. T., Lovell, H. G. and Moore, F. 1967. A longitudinal study of the decline of adult height with age in two Welsh communities. *Human Biol.* **39:** 445–454.
9. Garn, S. M. and Young, R. W. 1956. Concurrent fat loss and fat gain. *Am. J. Phys. Anthropol.* **14:** 497–504.
10. Ryckewaert, A., Parot, S., Tamisier, S. and Bourlière, F. 1967. Variations, selon l'âge et le sexe, de l'épaisseur du pli cutané mesuré au dos de la main. *Rev. Franc. Études Clin. Biol.* **12:** 803–806.
11. Brozek, J. and Keys, A. 1953. Relative body weight, age and fatness. *Geriatrics.* **8:** 70–75.
12. Fryer, J. H. 1962. Studies of body composition in men aged 60 and over. In N. W. Shock (ed.) *Biological Aspects of Aging,* New York: Columbia University Press, pp. 59–78.
13. Frantzell, A. and Ingelmark, B. E. 1951. Occurrence and distribution of fat in human muscles at various age levels. *Acta. Soc. Med. Upsalien.* **56:** 59–87.
14. Gutmann, E. 1977. Muscle. pp. 445–469 In C. E. Finch, L. Hayflick (eds.) Handbook of the Biology of Aging. New York: Van Nostrand Reinhold.
15. Forbes, G. B. and Reina, J. C. 1970. Adult lean body mass declines with age: Some longitudinal observations. *Metabolism.* **19:** 653–663.
16. Garn, S. M., Rohmann, C. G., Wagner, B. and Ascoli, W. 1967. Continuing bone growth throughout life: A general phenomenon. *Am. J. Phys. Anthropol.* **26:** 313–318.
17. Epker, B. N. and Frost, H. M. 1966. Periosteal appositional bone growth from age two to age seventy in man. A tetracycline evaluation. *Anat. Record.* **154:** 573–578.
18. Israel, H. 1973b. Age factor and the pattern of change in craniofacial structures. *Am. J. Phys. Anthropol.* **30:** 11–128.
19. Todd, T. W. and Lyons, D. W., Jr. 1924. Endocranial suture closure. Its progress and age relationship. Part 1. Adult males of white stock. *Am. J. Phys. Anthropol.* **7:** 325–384.
20. Smith, R. W., Jr. and Walker, R. R. 1964. Femoral expansion in aging women: Implications for osteoporosis and fractures. *Science.* **145:** 156–157.
21. Moldawer, M., Zimmerman, S. J. and Collins, L. C. 1965. Incidence of osteoporosis in elderly whites and elderly negroes. J. Am. Med. Assoc. **194:** 859–862.
22. Bennett, G. A., Waine, H. and Bauer, W. 1942. Changes in the Knee Joint at Various Ages. With Particular Reference to the Nature and Development of Degenerative Joint Disease. New York: The Commonwealth Fund.
23. Melick, R. and Taft, H. P. 1959. Observations on body hair in old people. *J. Clin. Endocrinol.* **19:** 1597–1607.
24. Damon, A., Seltzer, C. C., Stoudt, H. W. and Bell, B. 1972. Age and physique in healthy white veterans at Boston. *Aging and Human Development.* **3:** 202–208.
25. Lichtstein, E., Chadda, K. D., Naik, P. and Gupta, P. K. 1974. Diagonal ear-lobe crease: Prevalence and implications as a coronary risk factor. *New Engl. J. Med.* **290:** 615–616.
26. Frank, S. T. 1973. Aural sign of coronary heart disease. *N. Engl. J. Med.* **289:** 327–328.
27. Macaraeg, P. V. J., Jr., Lasagna, L. and Snyder, B. 1968. Arcus not so senilis. *Ann. Internal Med.* **68:** 345–354.
28. Weibel, J. and Fields, W. S. 1965. Tortuosity, coiling and kinking of the internal carotid artery. I. Etiology and radiographic anatomy. *Neurol.,* **15, (11):** 7–18.
29. Calloway, N. O., Foley, C. F. and Lagerbloom, P. 1965. Uncertainties in geriatric data, II. Organ size. *J. Am. Geriat. Soc.* **13:** 20–29.

30. Sato, T., Miwa, T. and Tauchi, H. 1970. Age changes in the human liver of the different races. *Gerontologia.* **16:** 368–380.

31. Brody, H., Vijayashankar, N. 1977. Anatomical Changes in the Nervous System. In C. E. Finch, L. Hayflick (eds.) *Handbook of the Biology of Aging.* New York: Van Nostrand Reinhold.

32. Hall, T. C., Miller, A. K. H. and Corsellis, J. A. N. 1975. Variations in the human Purkinje cell population according to age and sex. *Neuropathol. Appl. Neurobiol.,* 1: 267–292.

33. Brody, H. 1955. Organization of the cerebral cortex, III. A study of aging in the human cerebral cortex. *J. Comp. Neurol.,* 102: 511–556.

34. Scheibel, M. D. and Scheibel, A. B. 1975. In H. Brody, D. Harmon, J. M. Ordy (eds.) Clinical, Morphological and Neurochemical Aspects of the Aging Nervous System. New York: Raven Press.

35. Gerstenblith, G., Fredericsen, J., Yin, F. C. P., Fortuin, N. S., Lakatta, E. G. and Weisfeldt, M. L. 1977. Echocardiographic Assessment of a Normal Aging Population. Circ. **56**, pp. 273–278.

36. Agate, J. 1979. Special hazards of illness in later life. Ch. 7. In I. Rossman (ed.) *Clinical Geriatrics.* Phila.: J. B. Lippincott.

37. Brandfonbrener, M., Landowne, M. and Shock, N. W. 1955. Changes in Cardiac Output With Age. Circ. 12, p. 577.

38. Muiesan, G., Sorbini, C. A. and Grassi, V. 1971. Respiratory function in the aged. *Bull. PhysioPathol. Respir.* **7:** 973–1007.

39. Ljungqvist, A. and Lagergren, C. 1962. Normal intrarenal arterial pattern in adult and aging human kidney. A microangiographical and histological study. *J. Anat. Lond.* **96:** 285–298.

40. Davies, D. F. and Shock, N. W. 1950. Age changes in glomerular filtration rate, effective renal plasma flow and tubular excretory capacity in adult males. *J. Clin. Invest.* **29:** 496–506.

41. Brocklehurst, J. C. 1973. The bladder. In J. C. Brocklehurst (ed.) *Textbook of Geriatric Medicine and Gerontology.* Edinburgh & London-Churchill Livingstone, pp. 298–320.

42. Rotkin, I. D. 1976. Epidemiology of benign prostatic hypertrophy. In *Benign Prostatic Hyperplasia.* HEW Publ. No. NIH 76–1113.

43. Brocklehurst, J. C. and Dillane, J. B. 1967. Studies of the female bladder in old age IV. Drug effects in urinary incontinence. *Geront. Clin.* **9:** 182–191.

44. Goldfarb, A. F. 1979. Geriatric Gynecology. Ch. 17. In I. Rossman (ed.) Clinical Geriatrics. Philadelphia: J. B. Lippincott.

45. Masters, W. H. and Johnson, V. E. 1966. The aging male. Ch. 16. In *Human Sexual Response.* Boston: Little Brown. pp. 248–270.

46. Rossman, I. 1978. Sexuality and aging: An inter-

nist's perspective, In *Sexuality and Aging* (Rev. Ed. 1978) Robert L. Solnick (ed.) Andrus Gerontol. Center, Los Angeles, California University S. Calif. Press. pp. 66–77.

47. Kahn, E., Fisher, C. 1969. REM sleep and sexuality in the aged. *J. Geriat. Psychiat.* **2:** 181–199.

48. Gregerman, R. I., Gaffney, G. W., Shock, N. W. and Crowder, S. C. 1962. Thyroxine turnover in euthyroid men with special reference to changes with age. *J. Clin. Invest.* **41:** 2065.

49. Andres, R., Pozefsky, T., Swerdloff, R. S. and Tobin, J. D. 1970. Effect of aging on carbohydrate metabolism. In R. A. Camerini-Davalos and H. S. Cole (eds.) *Early Diabetes.* New York: Academic Press.

50. Vermeulen, A., Rubens, R. and Verdonck, L. 1972. Testosterone secretion and metabolism in male senescence. *J. Clin. Endocrin. Metab.* **34:** 730–735.

51. Jensen, H. K. and Blichert-Toft, M. 1971. Serum corticotrophin, plasma cortisol, and urinary excretion of 17-ketogenic steroids in the elderly (age group 66–94) years. *Acta Endocrin.* **66:** 25–34.

52. Blichert-Toft, M. 1978. The adrenal glands in old age. In R. B. Greenblatt, (ed.) *Geriatric Endocrinology.* Raven Press: New York, pp. 81–102.

53. Makinodan, T. 1977. Immunity and Aging. In C. E. Finch and L. Hayflick (eds.) *Handbook of the Biology of Aging.* New York: Van Nostrand Reinhold.

54. Rossman, I., Rodstein, M. and Bornstein, A. 1974. Undiagnosed diseases in an aging population. *Arch. Int. Med.* **133:** 366–369.

55. Arey, L. B., Tremain, M. J., Manzingo, F. L. 1935. The numerical and topographical relation of taste buds to circumvallate papillae throughout the life span. *Anat. Record.* **64:** 9.

56. Siurala, M., Isokoski, M., Varis, K., *et al.* 1968. Prevalence of gastritis in a rural population: bioptic study of subjects selected at random. *Scan. J. Gastroenterol.* **3:** 311.

57. Hughes, L. E. 1969. Postmortem survey of diverticular disease of the colon. I. Diverticulosis and diverticulitis. II. The muscle abnormality in the sigmoid colon. *Gast.* **10:** 336, 344.

58. Bhanthumnavin, K., Shuster, M. M. 1977. Aging and gastrointestinal function. In C. E. Finch, L. Hayflick (eds.), *Handbook of the Biology of Aging.* New York: Van Nostrand Reinhold, p. 709.

59. Shock, N. W. 1952. Aging of homeostatic mechanisms. In A. I. Lansing (ed.) *Cowdry's Problems of Aging.* Baltimore: Williams and Wilkins, p. 415.

60. MacMillan, A. L., Corbett, J. L., Johnson, R. H., *et al.* 1967. Temperature regulation in survivors of accidental hypothermia of the elderly. *Lancet,* 2: 165.

Chapter 7
Perceptual Changes with Aging

Gail R. Marsh, Ph.D.
Duke University Medical Center

Sensory abilities change throughout our lives. Typically these changes come upon us so slowly that they are not noticed until they interfere with everyday life. The perception of simple stimuli changes only mildly during the adult years, but may show steep declines after about the seventh or eighth decade. However, as we deal with the more complex perceptual problems of everyday life—speech, reading, or operating a machine—then changes in functional abilities with age can be detected even during the early years of the adult life span. In dealing with these more complex and meaningful stimulus situations, the cognitive abilities of the person begin to interact with what was classically defined as perception. Some experimental methods are better than others at excluding these interacting influences. Perception, however, not only reflects the ability of the senses, but also the meaning imputed to the stimuli by the person being tested. To the extent that different age groups may interpret stimuli or experimental situations differently, then these cognitive influences upon perception could become important.

Such imputation of meaning cannot be totally overcome by any experimental design, but one improvement in method must be mentioned here since it will appear several times in later pages. Since the mid-1960s a new method of observing perceptual changes has taken a strong hold. Under this method, signal detection theory (SDT), the concept of a threshold, is dropped and replaced by the concept that an observer's threshold can be altered by biases inherent in the observer or his environment. Thus the observer's responses ("yes, I perceive a stimulus" or "no, I do not perceive a stimulus") are broken down into two independent components: one reflecting perceptual sensitivity and another reflecting the observer's bias toward responding "yes" or "no" more frequently. This has allowed the study of possible sensitivity changes with age to be examined separately from possible changes in observer bias. Since changes in bias with age have been widely proposed[1]—

147

largely under the label of increased 'cautiousness' in the elderly, the use of SDT must be considered a major step forward despite its several practical and theoretical limitations.

This chapter will attempt to summarize, without extensive treatment of methods or theory, those changes which take place with age (from young adult to old age) in the way we perceive our world. For more detailed analysis of the theories or methods underlying this work the reader is referred to several excellent recent review articles.[2-12]

While perception is the focus of this chapter, the physiological and anatomical correlates of perception have been heavily studied for some of the senses and will be incorporated here as well. Each section of this chapter will start with a review of changes in physiology and anatomy that are thought to be involved in age-related perceptual changes. In some of the senses that have been less well studied, the linkage between the psychological and the physiological/anatomical mechanisms is weak and the review will be brief and will break from the more detailed format.

When possible a distinction will be made between normal aging and pathology. Such a distinction is not always easy and is sometimes impossible. However, since the reader may wish to know to what extent a sensory loss is widespread in the population, or selective following an insult, the following material will attempt to make such a distinction.

VISION

Physiological Alterations

All aspects of the eye change with age including the relationship of the eye to its supporting structures. The eye sinks more deeply into its orbit with the loss of surrounding fat, the lacrimal gland decreases its output, and the muscles lose strength and control. However the changes mentioned above have little influence on function except for the loss of muscular control of the orb, which decreases the ability to move the eye on a smooth controlled course, or to swing the eye through as wide an arc, especially in an upward direction.[13] The most important age changes in the eye occur in the tissues passing light to the retina: the cornea, the lens, the iris, and the aqueous and vitreous humor.

Cornea. The cornia flattens, thickens, and increases its horizontal diameter relative to its vertical diameter with age; all of which create astigmatic problems in the older eye. Not often appreciated is the fact that the cornea is the principal refracting surface of the eye, and thus, changes in curvature can have a significant effect on image forming ability.[14] A significant proportion of elderly persons (40% of those over 60)[15] also develop a gray ring around the outer edge of the cornea (arcus senilis) from accumulation of lipids in the membrane. The effect of this ring is to make the eye lose its youthful luster. However light transmission into the eye is not hampered, especially since the elderly eye maintains a continual miosis relative to the young adult.

Crystalline Lens. The lens is a pale yellow, oval spheroidal collection of radially oriented fibers enveloped by a membrane called the capsule (see Fig. 7-1). The lens grows continually from its outermost equator (that part facing the ciliary muscle) by laying down new fibers along its outer surface running toward the center of the lens. Nutrients for metabolism are obtained from the aqueous humor. Accommodation is accomplished by the sphincter-like contractions of the ciliary muscle which, via the zonular ligaments and the capsule, pulls the lens into a more flattened state for focusing at a greater distance. For near vision the ciliary muscle relaxes and relies upon the lens to resume its unstressed spheroid shape.

The lens undergoes three different changes over the adult years. The first to be generally noted is the loss of accommodation. The lens in youth is easily extended by the ciliary muscle, and very resilient in re-

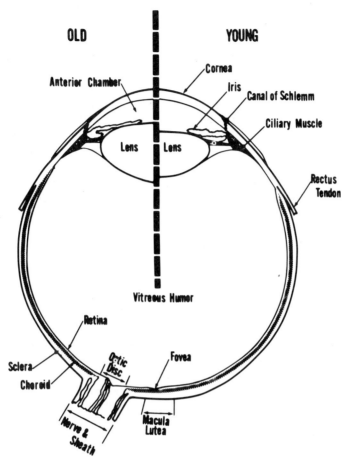

Figure 7-1. Diagram of the eye showing some of the age-related changes in the anterior portion of the eye.

turning to its original shape when the ciliary muscle forces are relaxed. The distensibility and resiliency is lost steadily over the adult years with noticeable effects after the age of 40.[16] Further adding to the loss of accommodation is the decrease in the strength of the ciliary muscle in old age. The changes in the lens are partially due to cross-linkages between the fibers of the lens. Part of the change is also due to the lens growing throughout life, doubling in diameter and causing the center cells to shrink into a hard core which not only is less resilient, but has decreased transparency and a greater refractive index.

A second change in the lens is that it becomes increasingly less transparent and more yellow in color.[17-19] As it yellows it also becomes more resistant to passage of the shorter wavelengths of light. As a result persons slowly become less able to detect the color spectrum between yellow and blue. Of course, losing sensitivity to that portion of the spectrum makes all the colors with some contribution from the yellow-blue portion of the spectrum appear somewhat different in hue.

The third and most marked effect on vision in the aged person is the development of cataract. Most cataracts requiring surgical intervention are found in persons over 60. The magnitude of the problem can be seen in that, while only about 0.2% of the population require such surgery each year, that surgery is the sixth most often performed operation in America. The mechanisms causing cataract are only partly understood. There are two types: nuclear and cortical. Nuclear cataract is characterized by the darkening of the lens core. Initially the usual pale yellow may only deepen, but with further development the core may become brown or even black. The changing color is due to the unfolding and recombining of the sulfhydryl groups both within and between protein molecules. This may be due to lack of sufficient nutrients and oxygen in the increasingly buried lens core.

Cortical cataracts form on the outermost edge of the lens and then progressively spread down the outer layers toward the center. They are typically seen as wedge shaped swellings. They may not interfere with vision until well advanced since the outer edge of the lens is rarely used unless the iris is fully retracted. Stress has been suggested as the causative agent. The stress may take several forms. Between the ages of 50 and 60 the lens becomes less pliable and the effort of the ciliary muscle to induce accommodative changes in the lens subjects the lens to considerable physical stress. After 60 the capsule surrounding the lens weakens, as does the ciliary muscle, and the stress on the hardening lens is lessened. Another model is provided by the reaction of the lens to high blood sugar levels as found in diabetics. Aldose reductase, an enzyme found in lens tissue, as well as in many other cells of the body, is only active when glucose levels are very high. Sorbitol, one of the major products of this enzyme, unfortunately is trapped in the lens, which induces high osmotic gradients leading to swelling and eventual breakdown of the tissue. As age increases, the control of blood sugar levels is reduced and high levels may be seen following meals.[20,21]

Cataracts are opacities in the lens. But, while this is true, it is an insufficient description. As may be surmised from the above, the opaque feature of a cataract is formed due to a sudden shift in refractive index between the cataract and surrounding lens tissue. Sudden shifts in refractive (index) tend to reflect rather than refract light. Thus the cataract not only blocks passage of light in a portion of the lens, but also sends scattered light throughout the lens. Such scattered light is the basis of glare, and all persons with cataract have greatly increased problems with glare.

Iris. In the normal eye the size of the pupil is kept well matched to the light level in which the eye is working. To open too widely is to invite aberrations in the periphery of the visual field. To be too small is to screen out the light necessary to form an image on the retina. The elderly eye tends to keep a rather small and somewhat fixed aperture at the pupil under all lighting conditions. Even in well-lighted conditions the elderly eye may screen out as much as 50% more light than a young adult in the same environment (it must be remembered that the amount of light varies with the area of the pupil, which varies as the square of the radius). As light levels are lowered, the older person is worse off relative to the young adult since in the young the iris retracts widely and rapidly, while in the elderly it retracts little and more slowly.[22,23]

The iris may not be physically able to retract as far in the elderly as in the young, but it is the neural input that holds the iris in its constricted state. It is not well understood how this condition arises. The constant miosis can aid those with cortical cataracts and with arcus senilis. However persons with nuclear cataracts have problems compounded by this state of affairs. In fact, lowered illumination levels help the nuclear cataract sufferer since light can then bypass the opaque core through the larger pupil.

Aqueous Humor. The anterior chamber of the eye shrinks with the continuing growth of the lens. This shrinkage has its greatest effect at the narrow-angle junction between the iris and the sclera which is the outflow point for the aqueous humor. With this narrowing of the outflow channel the chamber is more vulnerable to blockage. Such blockage may occur under full dilation of the iris. Under full retraction the narrow angle between lens and cornea can easily be filled by the iris.[3] This is especially true if the iris is no longer in close contact with the surface of the lens, which is often true in the aged eye.

Unlike the younger eye, a number of epithelial cells may be found on the inner surface of the cornea and the outer surface of the lens resulting in an increased scattering of light.

Vitreous Humor. The vitreous tends to aggregate in the older eye, which does not allow as good a flow of its aqueous portion throughout its volume. It also tends to form an aqueous pocket in its posterior portion, thus changing its strength and support characteristics. The vitreous changes its transmission characteristics by changing color slightly, and, also by increasing the number of inclusion bodies which increases the amount of light scatter in the eye. Local discoloration may result from small hemorrhages from the retina or choroid. This problem becomes more acute in very old age.

Retina. Little change in the retina has been documented as due to normal aging processes. However, Gordon[24] has estimated that 45% of vision problems in the elderly are due to loss of macular elements, seen as irregular dark patches of deterioration, which is the leading cause of blindness in the very old. The optic disc grows larger and paler with age, and the blood vessels tend to reflect arteriosclerotic changes by having a smaller cross-section and straighter course.

Perceptual Phenomena

Accommodation and Acuity. The problem of focusing on a near object has an earlier onset than that of loss of acuity. The progressive increase in the near point of vision (that point closest to the face that can be brought into sharp focus) has its onset at about age 40 and appears to progress no further after about age 55.[25] However, problems in accommodating to a moving target may continue to increase—probably due, in part, to the physical difficulty in changing the shape of the stiff crystalline lens and, in part, to CNS difficulties in calculating the range and controlling the increasingly sluggish accommodation process.[27]

Visual acuity decreases due to: decreased light input, increased scattering of light from the various media in the eye, growth of the crystalline lens, and loss of retinal elements in the macula.[26] Acuity, which is usually tested on the Snellen scale, begins to show sharp decreases after about 60 years of age. Usually these changes are progressive but are not sufficient to cause distress until 10–15 years after onset. Even then, better illumination and aids such as a magnifying lens can overcome the difficulties. The differences in acuity between young and old adults can be made artificially large by using low illumination levels during testing. Under high levels of illumination the difference between young and old will be at its lowest level. But with decreases in illumination below moderate levels, the elderly person will show much more rapid deterioration of acuity than will a younger person, due solely to the continual miosis of the elderly.

Visual Thresholds. The minimum amount of light necessary for the eye to detect its presence increases with age. The smaller pupil and lower transmittance of the ocular media (especially to violet and blue) contribute to the need for more light with increased age. Above and beyond these problems, the minimum amount of light required by the retina in order to function seems to increase with age.[28] However, no direct test of retinal sensitivity to light has been performed with the ocular media removed or with the size of pupil controlled across age groups.

One aspect of the visual system that is based on retinal function alone is dark adaptation. The data of two experiments are partially divergent.[28,29] Both studies agree that with increasing age more light is required to achieve a threshold level. However, it is uncertain whether older subjects have a slower rate of adaptation, or whether the rate is the same as that of younger persons. The data from one study are shown in Fig. 7-2 to demonstrate the magnitude of the deficit.

Brightness discrimination also is a clue to retinal function, although CNS involvement cannot be discounted. Several studies[30,31] have shown that greater differences are required before the older subject can detect a difference. These differences have not been related to known physiological changes in retina, nor have the studies excluded the possibility of retinal degeneration in their study populations. Retinal metabolism has been suggested as the cause of the changes in retinal function. However, there is no direct evidence for or against this claim thus far.

Glare. The aged eye is more susceptible to glare.[32,33] Since with increasing age all the ocular media have a greater tendency to disperse the light passing through them, the problem with glare is not surprising. Glare becomes a major change in eye function only after the age of 40.[34,35] The presence of cataracts greatly increases glare problems as was mentioned above.

Visual Field Size. The size of the visual field perimeter shrinks and the blind spot increases with age.[36,37,38] The losses are greatest in the horizontal aspects, but occur at all points, although the losses are not severe until past 60 years of age. Wolf[37] has argued that these changes are related to alterations in the retina since the changes in visual fields occur in the sixties and seventies, while the changes in the optic media occur in the forties and fifties. But some caution may be necessary. The methods used to test field size seem especially prone to possible changes in the CNS, or even changes in the psychological biases of the person being tested, as well as physiological changes in the eye.

Since motion detection is largely a non-macular function, loss of peripheral field vision with age has an adverse impact on such tasks as driving an automobile. Further, since loss of peripheral field vision with age may simply reflect lowered sensitivity in that portion of the retina,[39] the loss of peripheral vision may be much larger under low illumination conditions for the elderly than for the young adult.

Color Perception. Changes in color vision due to changes in the ocular media, principally the lens, have already been mentioned. The changes in visual field perimeters may also have impact on color vision, but this has not been studied. Deficiencies in color vision in the 40–60 age group is largely in the short wavelengths (yellow-blue). However after 60 losses are also seen in the longer wavelengths (green-red).[40] Losses in color discrimination start as early as age 30 and proceed in almost linear fashion with females performing slightly better throughout.[41] Certainly the losses in advanced old age are not due to lens changes since eyes with the lens removed still show color discrimination deficiencies.[42]

Depth Perception. The perception of depth is not fully understood but may involve both binocular and monocular cues. Loss of depth perception with age, using only monocular cues, has been reported by Jani.[43] Such judgments are thought to be based on textural cues, and thus would be poorer in those persons losing acuity, which is what was found with persons between the ages of 40–50. However, another study[44] only found a loss when both accommodation and convergence were required to per-

Figure 7-2. The top portion of the figure shows the theoretical change in visual threshold over time by the two different elements in the retina, the cones and the rods, when they are allowed to recover from light exposure by being placed in darkness. The level of initial light adaptation of the eye is marked by A. The asymptote of dark adaptation of the cone elements is indicated by B; the rod asymptote is similarly indicated by C. The bottom portion of the figure shows change in dark adaptation by 10 year increments. The first measurement was made 30 seconds after darkness was initiated. (from McFarland *et al.* 1960 29, by permission of the *Journal of Gerontology*).

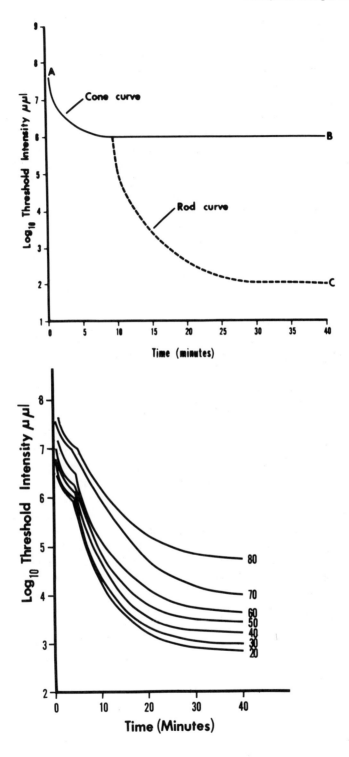

form the task. Other aspects of the testing situation could influence the results (such as illumination levels). Thus the findings above should be taken only as an estimate of ability under good viewing conditions. Since both studies report a deficit with age, the decrease in ability seems well founded, although the mechanism is not yet established.

Image Persistence. How long an image persists can be a clue to both retinal and CNS function. Critical flicker frequency (CFF) is that rate of presentation at which a rapidly flashing light is perceived to cease being constant and start flickering. Several studies of the influence of age on CFF have shown a lower CFF with increased age.[18,45-47] However, there are several influences on this phenomenon, the most important for the issue of an age differential being how much light reaches the retina. Dilating the pupil eliminates much of the difference between young and old.[18,48] Thus, once again it can be shown that it is the nonretinal portion of the eye that causes loss of function with age, especially before the age of 70.

But some of the age difference may be due to retinal or central factors. The longer persistence of an image with age has been both supported and refuted. Slower retinal metabolism or slower CNS information processing is generally cited as the likely cause. The so-called "time-intensity trade" was used as the basis of one experiment.[49] The basis of the time-intensity trade is that for brief stimuli the increased duration of a stimulus can compensate for a lowering of the illumination level. The elderly were able to integrate the light energy over a longer period than the young in order to compensate for a lower illumination level. Whether this is a retinal or central effect is not clear however. A test of after-image persistence[50] gives some clues. A negative after-image (or with color, as in this study, a complementary image) seems to be due to retinal processes, but positive after-images seem to be from central mechanisms. Immediately after a stimulus is removed, one has a brief period of a positive after-image which is then replaced for a longer period by a negative after-image. The elderly were found to have longer persistence of a complementary image of a red-green color patch, which would substantiate claims of longer retinal persistence.

Evidence based on the positive after-image, however, runs contrary to the notion of longer persistence with greater age. One study[51] presented a flashing letter that was on for only a fixed, brief time. The "off" period between flashes was increased until the letter began to be observed as flashing. If older persons have longer persistence, then the "off" period should have been longer than the young. But in fact the reverse was found. That this is a central effect, not retinal, is assured since the same results could be obtained by presenting the figure alternately to the left and right eyes rather than just to one eye. Another study[52] using somewhat similar techniques found similar results using words as stimuli.

Perceptual Masking. Another line of experimentation that deals with positive after-images and central processing of complex stimuli is that set of studies examining perceptual masking. The studies of central perceptual masking,[53,54] where a stimulus is presented to one eye and a masking stimulus is presented to the other eye, either before, during, or after the target stimulus, all seem to show one main result: that processing of a stimulus takes longer with increasing age. At what level in the nervous system this slowing occurs, or how it occurs, has not really been addressed yet, other than to point out that fewer neurons and fewer synaptic contacts per neuron are found in the old person's brain.

AUDITION

Physiological Alterations

While most of the effects of aging, especially in its early phases, are in the nonneural portion of the visual system, just the reverse is true of the auditory system. The major alterations in the auditory system are the loss of receptors from the organ of Corti and the loss of neurons in the auditory pathway.

Outer and Middle Ear. The pinnea continues to grow throughout life. However, the folds of the structure do not undergo large changes in conformation. The ear canal, likewise, does not undergo large changes in length or diameter. Whether the slight structural changes that do take place have an impact is not known. Excessive buildup of cerumen (ear wax) in the elderly is common. One report found one-third of all patients seeking aid for a hearing problem had the problem solved or markedly ameliorated by removal of cerumen from one or both ears.[55] The tympanic membrane may stiffen with age and the ossicular chain may transmit the higher frequencies less well.[56,57] However, since the ossicles tend to undergo arthritic changes[58,59] which form a solid communicating link, it is unclear how such losses would take place other than at the tympanic membrane itself. Also, such conductive hearing losses would show up as a growing difference between the thresholds for air and bone conduction. One study[60] has reported such an increase with age, but several others have not.[61-63] When hearing loss is found even in young adults the pattern of loss tends to persist throughout life, although the loss may increase in severity.[64]

Cochlea. The cochlea shows four major types of impairment with age:[10] (1) loss of elasticity in the basilar membrane; (2) atrophy of the stria vascularis; (3) loss of neurons; and (4) loss of the sensory receptor cells in the organ of Corti.

The loss of elasticity in the basilar membrane reduces the displacement the membrane would otherwise undergo in response to the acoustic input. This displacement is different in two ways: (1) it is less in amplitude, thus imparting less shearing force to the organ of Corti; and (2) when it does bend, it does so with a shallower gradient, thus stimulating a longer portion of the basilar membrane which makes it more difficult for the CNS to discern what frequency constituted the stimulus. Furthermore, since the sensory receptors for high frequency are packed very closely on a short strip of the basilar membrane, which is thicker and narrower than the low frequency portion, they receive proportionally less stimulation when the basilar membrane loses its flexibility.

Atrophy of the stria vascularis apparently reduces metabolic processes throughout the cochlea with resultant decreases in sensitivity across the entire frequency range and eventually also leads to loss of cochlear elements. The atrophy may affect the flow of endolymph and lower the usual standing potential of 80 mv generated by this structure. Persons with this difficulty show loss of hearing across all frequencies and often show loudness recruitment (see below).

Loss of neurons serving the cochlea is paralleled by losses in hearing ability. Typically the losses are heavier in the basal end which subserves high frequencies. However the losses are found throughout the cochlea and occur with the sensory receptors still intact. This degeneration seems to be mainly genetic in origin, but may also be caused by growth of the temporal bone, causing pressure on the auditory nerve.[65] Persons suffering this type of loss show greater losses for speech than they do for pure tones.

Atrophy of the organ of Corti (with subsequent loss of the associated neurons) has been observed, but is not well understood. It may be in response to injury, or to a genetic tendency toward metabolic problems in these sensory endings. Loss of receptors is noted most frequently in the basal turn and is characterized by a sharp loss of high tone sensitivity. Persons with this type of hearing problem show losses for high frequency but have little difficulty with speech or speech frequencies.

Loss of Cells in the CNS. There may be loss of cells with age in the auditory system at several points from the ganglion of nerve VIII to the cortex.[66-68] These losses have not been well correlated to function and have not been well integrated into the literature on CNS lesions.

Perceptual Phenomena

Auditory Thresholds. There is a gradual loss of sensitivity starting at least as early as the age of 20, with the bulk of the loss in the frequencies above 1000 Hz.[69,70] In fact, the loss of sensitivity, especially at 4000 Hz and above, is so common in aging that it has been given a name: presbycusis. Except in cases of accident or disease, both ears show similar deterioration with age. Men generally show a faster and greater loss in the frequencies above 1000 Hz than do women. However these losses do not predict well, on an individual basis, loss of hearing for speech unless the losses are very severe.[71]

Pitch Discrimination. The findings for pitch discrimination strongly parallel those for the sensitivity threshold. For all ages it is true that the higher the frequency the larger the change in frequency that stimulus must undergo before a person can detect the change. Also, the lower the intensity of the stimulus the larger the frequency change must be in order to be detected. Thus it is no surprise that with increased age the discriminability of frequencies deteriorates, and does so more rapidly for the higher frequencies.

Sound Localization. Loss of sensitivity makes localization more difficult, especially since for high frequencies the localization mechanism depends on intensity differences between the ears.[72,73] For the lower frequencies (below 2000 Hz) the input stimulus must be analyzed quickly since localization depends on time-of-arrival differences between the ears. Thus, it is not surprising that the elderly are less capable of sound localization. The ability to localize seems to begin to drop as early as 30 years of age.[74-76] The extent to which more complex stimuli may be more difficult to deal with in sound localization has not been explored.

Masking. The audiogram of the older person obtained by pure tone testing is often conservative in its estimate of hearing loss. One of the reasons for this low estimate is that the tests are performed under quiet conditions. With little background noise and simple stimuli the aged person is at his best. The ability to disentangle wanted signals from background noise is notably diminished with age.[77] This is especially true if the target stimuli are complex (such as speech) and the masking background noise is similar to the target sounds.

The incidence of tinnitus increases with age, up to 10% by age 65.[78] This self-generated "ringing in the ears" is at best annoying, and is often accompanied by hearing loss. Its property as a masker has not been studied.

Loudness Recruitment. A person reporting relatively normal loudness for low-intensity sounds, but reporting relatively high loudness for moderate intensities, and painful or distorted loudness for only moderately high intensities is said to be suffering from loudness recruitment. One study[79] estimated loudness recruitment as occurring in as much as 50% of the elderly population. This is very troublesome if employment of a hearing aid would otherwise be an acceptable treatment for a hearing loss, since amplification sufficient to hear the low intensity sounds will be so great as to make the moderate level sounds painfully loud and distorted.[80]

Speech Comprehension. The greatest auditory problem of the older person is understanding speech. This loss is not to be underestimated in its impact, since persons with hearing loss often show isolation stress and develop paranoid tendencies.

All the difficulties noted above can contribute to loss of speech comprehension. Loss of high frequencies is especially damaging to speech comprehension because the consonants are recognized by their high-frequency components, and the consonants

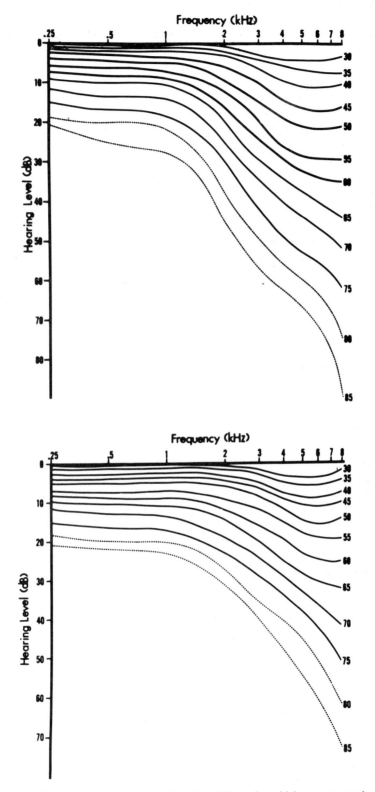

Figure 7-3. The graphs illustrate changes in hearing level (that is loss of sensitivity as compared to young normal adults of 20–25) for both males (left) and females (right) by five year increments. (from Spoor, 1967 69, by permission of *International Audiology.*)

are the differentiating aspects of most words. To add to the difficulty, consonants are also low in power, and are thus harder to hear and easier to mask. However, many of the important frequencies in speech can be expressed between 500 and 2000 Hz. Thus, obtaining the average audiogram over those frequencies gives a better prediction of speech comprehension than does any single frequency of the audiogram.

But even basing predictions on the 500–2000 Hz band does not predict all of the speech comprehension loss experienced by persons over 50 (although it does a good job for young adults).[81] It appears that changes in the CNS are responsible for a good deal of this loss. When speech is delivered at accelerated rates (by compressing the speech without changing the frequencies involved), the elderly lose comprehension very rapidly, while young persons show little loss.[81-83] Moreover, those losses in the young can be compensated for by increasing the intensity of the stimuli, but this does not aid the elderly.

One method of testing for the difficulty in speech comprehension is to give a standard list of words at increasing intensity levels until 50% of the words can be recognized. This "speech reception threshold" test[84] has been shown to require an intensity of about 22 dB SPL (with 0 dB = 0.0002 dynes/cm^2) for young adults.[85] Elderly men and women with no more than mild hearing loss, tested under the same conditions need about a 20 dB increase in intensity to achieve the same level of identification.[86,87] This test uses relatively easy words which are of two syllables receiving equal accent (e.g., baseball, railroad) and are called spondees. A list of more difficult monosyllabic words can show even greater deficits.[88]

Listening conditions which make the speech content less intelligible shows even larger differences between old and young. Speeded speech was noted above. Another study used several other means of lowering intelligibility (such as, reverberation, rapid interruption (8/sec.), listening to one speaker among several, and presenting the

500–800 Hz component of speech to one ear and the 1800–2400 Hz component to the other). All conditions affected speech comprehension more in the elderly. Unfortunately, the most profound loss was for the rapid interruption condition which produced conditions similar to those found in most modern telephone systems.[81,89]

While the above test conditions clearly implicate the CNS in the deficits, no testable mechanisms have been suggested. There is an abundance of evidence that the elderly process information more slowly. Therefore, testing comprehension at an accelerated rate gives an estimate of the top rate of processing speech information. The presentation of some speech frequencies to one ear and others to the opposite ear established the extent to which the elderly could integrate the information from both ears. The speech sounds could not be understood without integration of the information from both ears. Other such dichotic tasks used in other experiments have given competing, rather than compatible stimuli and found the elderly less able to repeat all or only part of the stimuli.[90] This has suggested some sort of registration deficit, but without a known physiological mechanism.

Since many of the higher level perceptual tests tread on cognitive ground, one study attempted to determine to what extent cognitive abilities might predict hearing loss on a pure tone test. It showed the correlations to be strong, especially so for males, and especially when only the range of normal speech frequencies were included. Another aspect of cognition that becomes important when words (especially words in sentences) are used as stimuli, is how language rules are used to comprehend speech. A series of studies[91,92] have shown that repeated repetition of a single word will be perceived by young adults as a different word every few seconds. Most often the elderly report hearing only the single stimulus word. Furthermore, if the word is only a close approximation to an English word, only the closely related English word will be heard by the elderly (never the non-

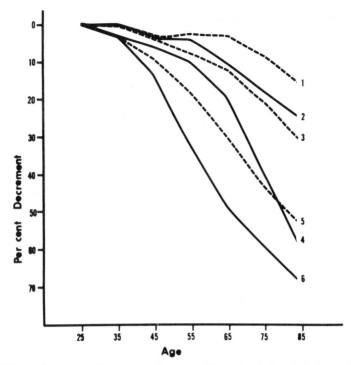

Figure 7-4. The ability to detect a spoken message decreases with age but is heavily influenced by the conditions under which the task is performed. Condition 1 was a control condition with no interference. Condition 2 was speech spoken 2½ times faster than normal. Condition 3 presented speech with the low frequency components only presented to one ear while the high frequency components were presented to the other. Condition 4 was speech presented with reverberation. Condition 5 presented a different two-part single word (e.g., overboard, downtown) to each ear, timed so that the beginning of one word in one ear overlapped the ending of the other word in the other ear. Condition 6 presented sentences which were electronically interrupted at the rate of 8 times per second. (from Bergman *et al.* 1976 (89) by permission of the *Journal of Gerontology*.)

word). Such high level aberrations suggest cortical deficits as the basis of such phenomena.

A relationship of the auditory system with cardiovascular disease has been found in several studies.[11,93,94] Whether this relationship goes beyond the subset of persons suffering from hearing loss due to problems in the stria vascularis is open to question. A study incorporating the Mabaan tribesmen in the Sudan[95-97] also reinforces the cardiovascular link since the Mabaans have low levels of cardiovascular disease. These data have also been interpreted as showing that the relatively noise-free environment was the basis of the hearing difference between Mabaans and Americans. However, this conclusion is certainly premature. Other differences such as genetic, dietary or other environmental aspects between the two cultures could as easily be the basis of the difference. In fact the studies of British subjects by Hinchcliffe[98-101] were centered on rural participants so as to avoid problems possibly accompanying a noisy urban environment. Several studies[102,103] do not support the notion of normal hearing loss with age being principally induced by noise. Particular losses can be induced by high noise exposure, but these can be differentiated from hearing loss due to age.

TASTE

Physiological Mechanisms

The number of taste buds are known to decrease with age.[104-106] The decrease apparently starts about 40–45 in women and

50–60 in men. Like their appearance, their disappearance seems to be tied to levels of gonadal hormones. Thus women start the loss earlier than men. By the time old age (75+) is reached, as many as two-thirds of the papillae have atrophied.[104,107] Additional factors such as more fissuring of the tongue and diminished salivary production with high mucus content and a neutral pH, have not been seriously studied as mechanisms affecting taste.

Detection and Recognition Capabilities

Taste has traditionally been tested for four qualities: salty, sweet, sour and bitter. These qualities are often tested in different experiments by different substances with the assumption that the differences between substances are negligible. Occasionally other substances are encountered which do not fit well into this framework. But the psychological dimensions of taste have not yet been tied closely with specific molecular structures that stimulate the receptors. However, despite the lack of theoretical structure there seems to be good agreement that taste sensitivity declines in old age. Unfortunately, little work has been done on intermediate aged groups.

The threshold for perception of salty seems to be hardest hit by age, especially in males.[108–111] Decline in the sensitivity for sweet and sour is almost as great as for salty.[110,112] With the exception of one study[110] most studies have reported that bitter sensitivity also declines in old age. There is evidence that males may suffer a greater decline than females in most taste categories.[113] However, not all studies agree on this point.

Of course, beyond ability to detect that something is present it is also crucial to recognize the flavor of that substance, if the sense of taste is to perform its function. It is this aspect of the decline in taste abilities that is most distressing to the aging person, especially the very old. Even when tested at moderately strong concentrations, elderly males make many errors at taste recognition, with the percentage of errors highest for sour.[114] Females do not show this deterioration.

Studies of food recognition (which has aspects related to both taste and smell) have shown that the elderly are poorer at identifying foods than young adults.[115] There were no differences noted between males and females. An attempt to describe how taste was perceived showed that young adults rated foods along two dimensions ('hedonic' and 'tactile'), while the elderly seemingly only used one ('hedonic'). The differences extended beyond this in that many of the tastes were linked to unpleasant qualities by the elderly. The few pleasant aspects to the taste continuum for the elderly were clustered around fruity flavors.

Improved oral hygiene has been shown to benefit taste detection and identification thresholds for salty, sour, and sweet.[116] This supports an earlier contention[110] that loss of taste abilities was accompanied by inflammation. These same authors also pointed out that dentures blocked full utilization of some of the gustatory sensory endings. Sour and bitter are best detected on the palate, while the tongue is more acute for sweet and sour. Other studies have dealt with the question by having subjects remove dentures before testing (or else have not taken note of denture wearing at all). The full extent of the wearing of dentures on taste abilities is not known. Smoking effects are not clear. Several studies were not able to show an effect of smoking on taste sensitivity,[111,117,118] while one has been able to do so.[119]

SMELL

The sense of smell has been so sparsely tested with regard to age that only the most general of statements can be made and little understanding given. Of the several substances tested, most showed a decline in sensitivity with age, with males showing lesser sensitivity than females.[120–122] One study showed no decrement with age in judging intensity of an odor.[123]

However, changes with age may depend

on what test substance is used. One study found a steady decline for one substance, but a stablization of sensitivity after about 70 years of age for another substance.[121] Moreover, health status is implied as a major determinant of olfactory sensitivity in at least one study.[122] This has led Engen[124] to conclude that age may have little effect on olfactory and gustatory sensitivity, and that health and shifting olfactory preferences may be the most important factors. Several studies[125,126] have shown changing preferences as a function of age. Also, as noted earlier, descriptions of food tastes change with age. It appears highly speculative to draw any conclusions in this area until more definitive work is carried out.

Anatomical findings are not established in this area. One study reported losses in the bulb and tract comparable to the loss of neurons in the rest of the CNS.[127] The other[128] described only atrophy of fibers and glomeruli in the majority of persons studied. These studies are not contradictory since they focused on different aspects of the CNS, but they do show that few possibilities have as yet been ruled out as causative agents in change in olfactory abilities. Certainly health has not been ruled out as a major determining factor.

SOMESTHESIS

Since somesthesis is comprised of several components which may differ in their response to aging they are considered separately.

Tactile and Temperature Sensitivity

Glabrous (nonhairy) skin of the palms of the hand and soles of the feet must be considered separately from the rest of the skin. This is due to the presence of Meissner corpuscles that act as receptors in the glabrous skin. These corpuscles tend to grow in size, but decrease in number throughout the life span. They are more numerous in the hands than the feet throughout life.[129,130] The hairy skin seems to rely more on free nerve endings in the dermis, which seem unchanged

through the life span.[129,131] However, the skin itself may change. Decreased amounts of collagen and elastin are found in the skin of aged persons,[132,133] thus allowing for easier deformation of the skin. However, one study found the skin thinner but less elastic.[134] Others, however, have failed to replicate these findings.[135,136]

The above anatomical findings might lead one to expect possible increases in sensitivity or no change with age. One report found an increase in the number of points responding on the forearm in old age.[137] However, the other studies, restricted to corneal sensitivity, either showed no change or a decreased sensitivity beginning in early old age.[138,139] Kenshalo[9] has suggested that wide variance between studies could be reflecting wide variance in the aged population such that some elderly may show large changes in skin thickness and deformability while others show little.

In fact, neuropathies may also contribute to this variance found among elderly persons. As many as one-third of the cells in the dorsal and ventral root ganglia may be lost in the very old.[140,141] While such changes are not "aging," they are certainly found with higher frequency in the aged, and are confused and confounded with normal age changes. Such pathological changes may be one of the reasons why the lower half of the body, especially the extremities, loses sensitivity much faster than does the upper half of the body.

The ability to detect temperature via the skin does not seem to change appreciably with age.[142,143] Perhaps unexpectedly, one study has also reported that the thermal comfort range for the elderly is approximately the same as that for young adults.[144] However, it should be remembered that the ability to closely regulate body core temperature is deteriorated in the elderly.[145] It is this temperature that is more likely to control perceived comfort, and also be controlled to a larger extent in the elderly by the environment rather than intrinsic homeostatic mechanisms. It is also this core temperature that is more likely to get out of control when temperature extremes, rather than normal living temperatures, are encountered.

Vibratory Sense

Testing the patient's ability to detect vibration has been a long-time favorite with the medical practitioner since it is easily tested and has become a diagnostic tool for some neurological disorders. Vibratory sense is likely a combination of several senses and is thus discussed here between tactile and kinesthetic sensibilities. The previously discussed tactile sense likely provides the sensibility for the sensitivity to frequencies up to 90 Hz. Above that point the Pacinian corpuscle, free nerve endings, and possibly the receptors on the hair follicles provide the sensibility. Thus, soft tissue responds to low frequencies, but the higher frequencies provide better response through bone where they stimulate the more deeply lying Pacinian corpuscles on tendons and ligaments.[146] The higher frequencies also test for how long the person feels the stimulation since these receptors are notably quick adapting.[147]

Loss in vibratory sensibility is a general finding among the reports of age changes.[148,149] However, the losses may be more pervasive in the higher frequencies, as one report could only find losses above 150 Hz. As previously noted, the lower extremities are less sensitive than the upper extremities, and in one study sensitivity was highly related to history of disease, not with chronological age.[147]

Underlying causes for these declines have not been specified. Among suggested causes are: changes in circulation or microcirculation,[150] loss of uniform mylination on nerves,[151] thiamin deficiency,[152] or subclinical problems with such disorders as diabetes.[148]

Kinesthesis

Reports of young and old compared on the ability to discern passive movement or posi-

tion of joints have shown only mild differences between the two groups.[147,153,154] Deficits found were confined to the lower limbs. In tests of active movement, one study[153] found that a small percentage of elderly subjects needed visual guidance to bring their finger to the tip of their nose. However, when only small percentages of a population show a particular deficiency something other than a general mechanism, such as aging, should be invoked as a possible explanation.

In a test involving judging weights,[155] young and old groups did not differ in accuracy. Thus, while it is well established that the elderly may suffer more unsteadiness or muscular weakness, none of these factors seems to intrude critically in judging body position. The combining of muscle and joint sensations with vestibular cues may be less well integrated and slower in the elderly. Appealing as this generalization may be, however, it has not been clearly established by clinical tests.

Pain

Pain is troublesome in that it is not only a sensation, but a sensation with emotional properties. Thus a person's traits and environmental cues may heavily influence what is labelled painful. To discuss pain, it is necessary to distinguish between pain tolerance (which has an obvious emotional component), and sensitivity to pain or pain detection (which attempts to treat pain as a simple sense like touch or audition). These two methods of assessing pain can give very different results.[156] Also, until recently, the measure most often employed in studies of pain detection was pain threshold, which has the possibility of being heavily influenced by emotion.

Early studies gave mixed indications of age effects on pain detection. The earliest showed no difference,[157,158] but later work showed older persons were less sensitive, with loss starting early (around 40 years of age) for the upper body (where loss was greatest overall), and later (after 60 years of age) for the lower extremities.[159] Socioeconomic status was also a factor, in that better paid and educated persons had higher thresholds.

Tolerance for pain, on the other hand, has been reported both to increase with age[160] and to decrease with age.[161,162] These conflicting results probably arise due to the impossibility of obtaining data not influenced by the person's long-term attitudes and short-term biases, as mentioned above. (See Melzack[163] for discussion of these and other problems.) The placebo effect seems to grow more potent with age. Persons reporting relief from placebos tend to be older, and also older persons tend to report greater relief from a single dose.[164-166] The nature of this suggestibility is not understood.

Recent investigations of pain detection have used the signal detection method mentioned in the introduction to this chapter. Such approaches allow sensitivity to be separated from the biases the subject has toward responding in any particular way. This approach has shown that in the 40–55 year range men are not different from young adults of either sex, but women have dropped in sensitivity.[142] Measurement of response bias indicated that older persons were less likely to label the stimulation as painful. That is, they were more cautious or conservative about calling stimuli painful. Most of the above studies were conducted with radiant heat as the stimulus source. Two recent studies used tooth pulp stimulation to avoid the problem of changes in the skin which could affect pain measurements. These studies first obtained traditional detection threshold measures, which did not differ with age, and then obtained the usual signal detection observations. The signal detection measures of sensitivity showed that both men and women were less able to detect painful stimulation.[167,168] The response bias was interesting in that the elderly were less likely than the young to label faint stimulation as painful, yet were more likely to label strong stimulation as painful. Further work is necessary before this interaction with age can be understood.

Vestibular Sense

Older individuals display a decreased response to rotation or to hot or cold stimuli which cause nystagmus (sometimes severe) in younger individuals.[169,170]

With increasing age there is an increasing number of persons reporting difficulties with the vestibular system. Schuknecht[10] has categorized the difficulties into four problems which may occur separately or in combination: (1) cupulolithiasis; (2) ampullary disequilibrium; (3) macular disequilibrium; and (4) vestibular ataxia.

The first problem is presumably caused by deposits on the cupula (which would normally only be stimulated by movement of the endolymph), which thereafter cause it to behave like the otolith (i.e. the deposit causes the cupula to bend under the force of gravity). It may be of sudden onset.

Ampullary disequilibrium is a vertigo of at least several seconds duration following a sudden head movement. While an atrophy of the sensory cells of the ampulla has been suggested as the cause, it remains only a speculation thus far.

Macular disequilibrium is similar to ampullary disequilibrium except that in the macular case only changes of the head relative to gravity will trigger off the attack of vertigo. Individuals suffering this problem have been found to have lost most or all of the otolithic organ and/or the receptor epithlium necessary to detect its movement under the pull of gravity.[171]

Vestibular ataxia is a staggering gait controlled largely by visual, not vestibular cues. Schuknecht[10] has suggested that the symptoms imply loss of vestibular control of the lower limbs and that the lesion is likely in the CNS, either at the level of the vestibular nerve or deeper, lying in the brain stem or spinal cord.

While the visual and auditory systems have received intensive study, the remaining sensory systems have been rather inadequately studied with regard to age effects. Thus, outside of vision and audition there are few mechanisms that have been documented to aid in understanding how some of the changes take place. The changes with age, when they occur, are generally those of a loss of function. However, the changes that can take place are of a wide variety and have a wide variance in their probability of occurrence. In the face of lack of evidence, many of the changes cannot yet be assessed as pathological or normal. As the number of older persons increases, the study of the sensory functions of older persons will certainly receive the increased interest they deserve.

REFERENCES

1. Botwinck, J. *Aging and Behavior.* New York: Springer, 1973.
2. Fozard, J. L., Wolf, E., Bell, B., McFarland, R. A. and Podolsky, S. Visual perception and communication. In J. E. Birren and K. W. Schaie (eds.) *Handbook of the Psychology of Aging.* New York: Van Nostrand Rheinhold Co., pp. 497–534, 1977.
3. Leighton, D. A. Special senses: Aging of the eye. In J. C. Brocklehurst (ed.) *Textbook of Geriatric Medicine and Gerontology.* Edinburgh, Great Britain: Churchill Livingston, pp. 254–64, 1973.
4. Panck, P. E., Barrett, G. V., Sterns, H. L. and Alexander, R. A. A review of age changes in perceptual information processing ability with regard to driving. *Exp. Aging Res.* 3: 387–449 (1977).
5. Corso, J. F. Sensory processes and age effects in normal adults. *J. Gerontol.* 26: 90–105, 197.
6. Corso, J. F. Sensory processes in man during maturity and senescence. In J. M. Ordy and K. R. Brizzee (eds.) *Neurobiology of Aging.* New York: Plenum Press, pp. 119–43, 1975.
7. Corso, J. F. Auditory perception and communication. In J. E. Birren and K. W. Schaie (eds.) *Handbook of the Psychology of Aging.* New York: Van Nostrand Rheinhold Co., pp. 535–53, 1977.
8. Fisch, L. Special senses: The aging auditory system. In J. C. Brocklehurst (ed.) *Textbook of Geriatric Medicine and Gerontology.* Edinburgh, Great Britain: Churchill Livingston, pp. 265–79, 1973.
9. Engen, T. Taste and smell. In J. E. Birren and K. W. Schaie (eds.) *Handbook of the Psychology of Aging.* New York: Van Nostrand Rheinhold Co., pp. 554–61, 1977.
10. Schuknecht, H. F. *Pathology of the Ear.* Cambridge, Mass.: Harvard University Press, 1974.
11. Schmidt, P. H. Presbycusis: The present status. *Internat. Audiol.* 6, suppl. 1: 1–36 (1967).
12. Meyerson, M. D. The effects of aging on communication. *J. Gerontol.* 31: 29–38 (1976).
13. Chamberlain, W. Restriction in upward gaze with advancing age. *Trans. Am. Opthalmol. Soc.* 68: 235–44 (1970).
14. Lopping, B. and Weale, R. A. Changes in corneal surface during occular convergence. *Vision Res.* 5: 207–15 (1965).
15. Burch, P. R. J., Murray, J. J. and Jackson, D. The age-prevalence of arcus senilis, greying of hair, and baldness. Etiological considerations. *J. Gerontol.* 26: 364–72 (1971).
16. McFarland, R. A. The sensory and perceptual processes in aging. In K. W. Schaie (ed.) *Theory and Methods of Research on Aging.* Morgantown, West Virginia: West Virginia University Press, pp. 3–52, 1968.
17. Leopold, I. H. The eye. In J. T. Freeman (ed.) *Clinical Features of the Older Patient.* Springfield, Ill.: Charles C Thomas, pp. 420–27, 1965.
18. Weale, R. A. On the eye. In A. T. Welford and J. E. Birren (eds.) *Aging, Behavior and the Nervous System.* Springfield, Ill.: Charles C Thomas, pp. 307–25, 1965.
19. Said, F. S. and Weale, R. A. The variation with age of the spectral transmissivity of the living human crystalline lens. *Gerontologia* 3: 213–31 (1959).
20. van Heyningen, R. The lens: Metabolism and cataract. In H. Davson (ed.) *The Eye, vol. 1.* (2nd edition) New York: Academic Press, pp. 381–488, 1969.
21. van Heyningen, R. What happens to the human lens in cataract. *Sci. Amer.* 233(6): 70–81 (1975).
22. Birren, J. E., Casperson, R. C. and Botwinick, J. Age changes in pupil size. *J. Gerontol.* 5: 267–71 (1950).
23. Weale, R. A. *The Aging Eye.* New York: Harper & Row, 1963.
24. Gordon, D. M. Eye problems of the aged. *J. Amer. Geriat. Soc.* 13: 398–417 (1965).
25. Bruchner, R. Longitudinal research on the eye. *Gerontol. Clin.* 9: 87–95 (1967).
26. Weale, R. A. Senile changes in visual acuity. *Trans. ophthal. Soc. U. K.* 95: 36–38 (1975).
27. Fisher, R. F. Presbyopia and the changes with age in the human crystalline lens. *J. Physiol., (London)* 228: 765–79 (1973).
28. Birren, J. E. and Shock, N. W. Age changes in rate and level of dark adaptation. *J. Appl. Physiol.* 26: 407–11 (1950).
29. McFarland, R. A., Domey, R. G., Warren, A. B. and Ward, D. C. Dark adaptation as a function of age: I. A statistical analysis. *J. Gerontol.* 15: 149–54 (1960).
30. Gregory, R. L. "Neurological noise" as a factor in aging. *Proceedings of the Fourth Congress of the International Association of Gerontology.* Merano, Italy: International Association of Gerontology, pp. 314–24, 1957.

31. McCarter, A. and Atkeson, B. M. Simultaneous brightness contrast in young and old adults. *Exp. Aging Res.* **3:** 215–24 (1977).

32. Burg, A. Light sensitivity as related to age and sex. *Percept. Mot. Skills* **24:** 1279–88 (1967).

33. Shinar, D. Driver visual limitations and treatment. Indiana University Institute for Research in Public Safety, Contract DOT–HS–5–1275, Department of Transportation, 1977.

34. Wolf, E. Glare and age. *Arch. Ophthalmol.* **64:** 502–14 (1960).

35. Wolf, E. and Gardiner, J. S. Studies on the scatter of light in the dioptric media of the eye as a basis of visual glare. *Arch. Ophthalmol.* **74:** 338–45 (1965).

36. Burg, A. Lateral visual field as related to age and sex. *J. Appl. Psych.* **52:** 10–15 (1968).

37. Wolf, E. Studies on the shrinkage of the visual field with age. *Highway Res. Rec.* **167:** 1–7 (1967).

38. Harrison, R. and Wolf, E. Ocular studies with special reference to glaucoma in a group of 107 elderly males. *Am. J. Ophthalmol.* **57:** 235–41 (1964).

39. Baker, C. H. and Steedman, W. C. Perceived movement in depth as a function of luminance and velocity. *Human Factors* **3:** 166–73 (1961).

40. Ohta, Y. and Kato, H. Color perception changes with age; test results by P-N anomaloscope. *Mod. Probl. Ophthal.* **17:** 345–52 (1976).

41. Gilbert, J. G. Age changes in color matching. *J. Gerontol.* **12:** 210–15 (1957).

42. Lakowski, R. Is the deterioration of colour discrimination with age due to lens or retinal changes? *Farbe* **11:** 69–86 (1962).

43. Janis, S. N. The age factor in stereopsis screening. *Am. J. Optom.* **43:** 653–55 (1966).

44. Bell, B., Wolf, E. and Bernholz, C. D. Depth perception as a function of age. *Aging Human Dev.* **3:** 77–88 (1972).

45. Misiak, H. The decrease of critical flicker frequency with age. *Science* **113:** 551–52 (1951).

46. Wolf, E. and Schraffa, A. M. Relationship between critical flicker frequency and age in flicker perimetry. *Arch. Ophthalmol.* **72:** 832–43 (1964).

47. McFarland, R. A., Warren, A. B. and Karis, C. Alterations in critical flicker frequence, as a function of age and light:dark ratio. *J. exp. Psychol.* **56:** 529–38 (1958).

48. Weekers, R. and Roussel, F. Introduction à l'étude de la fréquence de fusion en clinique. *Ophthalmologica* **117:** 305–19 (1946).

49. Ericksen, C. W., Hamlin, R. M. and Breitmeyer, R. G. Temporal factors in visual perception as related to aging. *Percept. Psychophys.* **7:** 354–56 (1970).

50. Kline, D. W. and Nestor, S. Persistence of complementary afterimages as a function of adult age and exposure duration. *Exp. Aging Res.* **3:** 191–201 (1977).

51. Walsh, D. A. and Thompson, L. W. Age differences in visual sensory memory. *J. Gerontol.* **33:** 383–87 (1978).

52. Kline, D. W. and Baffa, G. Differences in the sequential integration of form. *Exp. Aging Res.* **2:** 333–43 (1976).

53. Kline, D. W. and Birren, J. E. Age differences in backward dichoptic masking. *Exp. Aging Res.* **1:** 17–25 (1975).

54. Walsh, D. A. Age differences in central perceptual processing: A dichoptic backward masking investigation. *J. Gerontol.* **31:** 178–85 (1976).

55. Green, M. F. Incidence of deafness from wax. Paper presented at the annual meeting of the Brit. Geriatric Soc., 1970. As quoted in Fisch, L. Special senses: The aging auditory system. In J. C. Brocklehurst (ed.) *Textbook of Geriatric Medicine and Gerontology.* Edinburgh, Great Britain: Churchill Livingston, pp. 265–79, 1973.

56. Nixon, J. C., Glorig, A. and High, W. S. Changes in air and bone conduction threshold as a function of age. *J. Laryng. Otol.* **76:** 288–98 (1962).

57. Davis, H. and Fowler, E. P. Hearing and deafness. In H. Davis and S. R. Silverman (eds.) *Hearing and Deafness.* New York: Holt, Rhinehart, and Winston, pp. 80–124, 1960.

58. Belal, A. and Stewart, T. Pathological changes in the middle ear joints. *Ann. Otol. Rhinol. Laryng.* **83:** 159 (1974).

59. Etholm, B. and Belal, A., Jr. Senile changes in the middle ear joints. *Ann. Otol. Rhinol. Laryngol.* **83:** 49–54 (1974).

60. Glorig, A. and Davis, H. Age, noise and hearing loss. *Ann. Otol. Rhinol. Laryng.* **70:** 556–71 (1961).

61. Goetzinger, C. P., Proud, G. O., Dirks, D. and Embrey, A. J. A study of hearing in advanced age. *Arch. Otolarygn.* **73:** 662–74 (1961).

62. Sataloff, J., Vassalo, L. and Menduke, M. Presbycusis air and bone conduction thresholds. *Laryng.* **75:** 889–901 (1965).

63. Miller, M. M. and Ort, R. G. Hearing problems in a home for the aged. *Acta Otolarygn.* **59:** 33–44 (1965).

64. Dayal, V. and Nussbaum, M. Patterns of puretone loss in presbycusis: A sequential study. *Acta Otolaryng.* **71:** 382–84 (1971).

65. Sercer, A. and Krmpotic, J. Über die ursacher der progressiven altersschwerhörigkeit (Presbyacusis) *Acta Otolarygn.* Suppl. 143 (1958).

66. Kirikae, I., Sato, T. and Skitara, T. Auditory function in advanced age with reference to histological changes in the central auditory system. *Laryng.* **74:** 205–20 (1964).

67. Hansen, C. C. and Reske-Nielsen, E. Pathological studies in presbycusis. *Arch. Otolaryng.* **82:** 115–32 (1965).

68. Hansen, C. C. and Reske-Nielsen, E. Cochlear and cerebral pathology in aged patients. *Internat. Audiol.* **7:** 450–52 (1968).

69. Spoor, A. Presbycusis values in relation to noise

induced hearing loss. *Internat. Audiol.* **6:** 48–57 (1967).

70. Lebo, C. P. and Reddell, R. C. The presbycusis component in occupational hearing loss. *Laryngoscope* **82:** 1399–1409 (1972).

71. Mathog, R. H., Paparella, M. M., Huff, L., Siegel, L., Lassmen, F. and Bozarth, M. Common hearing disorders, methods of diagnosis and treatment. *Geriatrics* **29:** 49–88 (1974).

72. Konig, J. Pitch discrimination and age. *Acta Otolaryng.* **48:** 473–89 (1957).

73. Nordlund, B. Directional audiometry. *Internat. Audiol.* **3:** 186–92 (1964).

74. Herman, G. E., Warren, L. R. and Wagener, J. W. Auditory lateralization: Age differences in sensitivity to dichotic time and amplitude cues. *J. Gerontol.* **32:** 187–91 (1977).

75. Matzker, J. and Springborn, E. Richtungshören und lebensalter. *Zeitschr. Laryng.* **37:** 739–45 (1958).

76. Matzker, J. M. and Springborn, E. Die Fehlerbreite bei der Schallokalisation in verschiedenen Altersklassen. *Acta Otolargyn.* **50:** 463–68 (1959).

77. Potash, M. and Jones, B. Aging and decision criteria for the detection of tones in noise. *J. Gerontol.* **32:** 436–40 (1977).

78. U.S. Dept. Health, Education and Welfare Reports. Hearing status and ear examinations (1960–1962). *Nat. Cent. Health Stat., Ser. 11, No. 32* (1968).

79. Pestalozza, G. and Shore, I. Clinical evaluation of presbycusis on the basis of different tests of auditory function. *Laryng.* **65:** 1136–63 (1955).

80. Eby, L. G. and Williams, H. I. Recruitment of loudness in the differential diagnosis of end-organ and nerve fibre deafness. *Laryng.* **61:** 400–14 (1951).

81. Bergman, M. Changes in hearing with age. *Gerontologist* **11:** 148–51 (1971).

82. Bergman, M. Hearing and aging: implications of recent research findings. *Audiology* **10:** 164–71. (1971).

83. Calearo, C. and Lazzaroni, A. Speech intelligibility in relation to the speed of the message. *Laryng.* **67:** 410–19 (1957).

84. Hirsh, I. J. *The Measurement of Hearing.* New York: McGraw-Hill, 1952.

85. Corso, J. F. Conformation of the normal threshold for speech on C. I. D. Auditory Test W-2. *J. Acoust. Soc. Am.* **29:** 368–70 (1957).

86. Melrose, J., Welsh, O. L. and Luterman, D. M. Auditory responses in selected elderly men. *J. Gerontol.* **18:** 267–70 (1963).

87. Punch, J. L. and McConnell, F. The speech discrimination function for elderly adults. *J. Aud. Res.* **9:** 159–66 (1969).

88. Carhart, R. Problems in the measurement of speech discrimination. *Arch. Otolaryngol.* **82:** 253–60 (1965).

89. Bergman, M., Blumenfeld, V. G., Cascardo, D.,

Dash, B., Levitt, H. and Margulies, M. K. Age-related decrement in hearing for speech: sampling and longitudinal studies. *J. Gerontol.* **31:** 533–38 (1976).

90. Clark, L. E. and Knowles, J. B. Age differences in dichotic listening performance. *J. Gerontol.* **28:** 173–78 (1973).

91. Obusek, C. J. and Warren, R. M. A comparison of speech perception in senile and well-preserved aged by means of the verbal transformation effect. *J. Gerontol.* **28:** 184–88 (1973).

92. Warren, R. M. and Warren, R. P. Some age differences in auditory perception. *Bull. N. Y. Acad. Med.* **47:** 1365–77 (1971).

93. Rosen, S. and Olin, P. Hearing loss and coronary heart disease. *Arch. Otolaryng.* **82:** 236–43 (1965).

94. Rosen, S. Dietary prevention of hearing loss—long-term experiment. *IX Int. Cong. Oto. Rhino. Laryng. Exerpta Med.* **189:** 134–35 (1969).

95. Rosen, S., Bergman, M., Plester, D., El-Mofty, A. and Satti, M. H. Presbycusis study of a relatively noise-free population in the Sudan. *Ann. Otol.* **71:** 727–43 (1962).

96. Rosen, S., Plester, D., El-Mofty, A. and Rosen, H. V. High frequency audiometry in presbycusis: A comparative study of the Mabaan tribe in the Sudan with urban populations. *Arch. Otolaryng.* **79:** 18–32 (1964).

97. Rosen, S., Plester, D., El-Mofty, A. and Rosen, H. V. Relation of hearing loss to cardiovascular disease. *Trans. Amer. Acad. Ophthal. Otol.* **68:** 433–44 (1964).

98. Hinchcliffe, R. The threshold of hearing as a function of age. *Acoustica* **9:** 303–8 (1959).

99. Hinchcliffe, R. The threshold of hearing of a random sample rural population. *Acta Otolaryng.* **50:** 411–22 (1959).

100. Hinchcliffe, R. Correction of pure tone audiograms for advancing age. *J. Laryng. Otol.* **73:** 830–32 (1959).

101. Hinchcliffe, R. Aging and sensory thresholds. *J. Gerontol.* **17:** 45–50 (1962).

102. Hinchcliffe, R. Neuro-otolaryngology in West Africa. In W. Taylor (ed.) *Disorders of Auditory Function.* New York: Academic Press. pp. 237–48, 1973.

103. Macrae, J. H. Noise-induced hearing loss and presbycusis. *Audiol.* **10:** 323–33 (1971).

104. Arey, I. B., Tremaine, M. J. and Monzingo, F. L. The numerical and topographical relations of taste buds to human circumvallate papillae throughout the life span. *Anat. Rec.* **64:** Suppl. 1 (1936).

105. Allara, E. Ricerche sull'organo del gusto dell'unomo. I. La struttura delle papille gustative nella varie eta della vita. *Arch. ital. Anat. Embriol.* **42:** 506–64 (1939).

106. El-Baradi, A. F. and Bourne, G. H. Theory of tastes and odors. *Science* **113:** 660–61 (1951).

107. Harris, W. Fifth and seventh cranial nerves in

relation to the nervous mechanism of taste sensation: A new approach. *Brit. Med. J.* **1:** 831–36 (1952).

108. Cooper, R. M., Bilash, M. A. and Zubek, J. P. The effect of age on taste sensitivity. *J. Gerontol.* **14:** 56–58 (1958).

109. Byrd, E. and Gertman, S. Taste sensitivity in aging persons. *Geriatrics* **14:** 381–4 (1959).

110. Balogh, K. and Lelkes, K. The tongue in old age. *Gerontol. Clin.* **3**(Suppl.): 38–54 (1961).

111. Bourliere, F., Cendron, H. and Rapaport, A. Modification avec l'âge des sénils gustatifs de perception et de reconnaissance aux saveurs salée et sucrée chez l'homme. *Gerontologia* **2:** 104–12 (1958).

112. Richter, C. P. and Campbell, K. H. Sucrose taste thresholds of rats and humans. *Am. J. Physiol.* **128:** 291–97 (1940).

113. Glanville, E. V., Kaplan, A. R. and Fischer, R. Age, sex, and taste sensitivity. *J. Gerontol.* **19:** 474–78 (1964).

114. Cohen, T. and Gitman, L. Oral complaints and taste perception in the aged. *J. Gerontol.* **14:** 294–98 (1959).

115. Schiffman, S. Food recognition by the elderly. *J. Gerontol.* **32:** 586–92 (1977).

116. Langan, M. J. and Yearick, E. S. The effects of improved oral hygiene on taste perception and nutrition of the elderly. *J. Gerontol.* **31:** 413–18 (1976).

117. Hughs, G. Changes in taste sensitivity with advancing age. *Gerontol. Clin.* **11:** 224–30 (1969).

118. Pangborn, R. M., Trabue, I. M. and Barylko-Pikielna, N. Taste, odor, and tactile discrimination before and after smoking. *Percept. Psychophy.* **2:** 529–32 (1967).

119. Kaplan, A. R., Glanville, E. V. and Fischer, R. Cumulative effect of age and smoking on taste sensitivity in males and females. *J. Gerontol.* **20:** 334–37 (1965).

120. Vaschille, N. L'état de la sensibilité olfactive dans la vieillesse. *Bull. Laryng.* **7:** 323–33 (1904).

121. Kimbrell, G. McA. and Furchgott, E. The effect of aging on olfactory threshold. *J. Gerontol.* **18:** 334–37 (1965).

122. Chalke, H. D., Dewhurst, J. B. and Ward, C. W. Loss of sense of smell in old people. *Public Health (London)* **72**(6): 223–30 (1958).

123. Rovee, C. K., Cohen, R. Y. and Shlapack, W. Life span stability in olfactory sensitivity. *Devel. Psychol.* **11:** 311–18 (1975).

124. Engen, T. Taste and smell. In J. E. Birren and K. W. Schaie, (eds.) *Handbook of the Psychology of Aging.* New York: Van Nostrand Rheinhold, pp. 554–61, 1977.

125. Moncrieff, R. W. *Odour Preferences.* New York: John Wiley, 1966.

126. Moncrieff, R. W. Changes in olfactory preferences with age. *Rev. Laryng. Otol. Rhin.* **86:** 895–904 (1966).

127. Liss, L. and Gomez, F. The nature of senile changes of the olfactory bulb and tract. *Arch. Otolarygn.* **67:** 167–71 (1958).

128. Smith, C. S. Age incidence of atrophy of olfactory nerves in man. *J. Comp. Neurol.* **77:** 589–95 (1942).

129. Cauna, N. The effects of aging on the receptor organs of the human dermis. In W. Montagna (ed.) *Advances in Biology of Skin, Vol. VI: Aging.* New York: Pergamon Press, pp. 63–96, 1965.

130. Bolton, C. F., Winklemann, R. K. and Dyck, P. J. A quantitative study of Meissner's corpuscles in man. *Neurol.* **16:** 1–9 (1966).

131. Hunter, R., Ridley, A. and Malleson, A. Meissner corpuscles in skin biopsies of patients with Presenile Dementia: A quantitative study. *Brit. J. Psychiat.* **115:** 347–49 (1969).

132. Pearce, R. H. and Grimmer, B. J. Age and the chemical constitution of normal human dermis. *J. Invest. Dermatol.* **58:** 347–61 (1972).

133. Ma, C. K. and Cowdry, E. V. Aging of elastic tissue in human skin. *J. Gerontol.* **5:** 203–10 (1950).

134. Jackson, R. Solar and senile skin: Changes caused by aging and habitual exposure to the sun. *Geriatrics* **27:** 106–12 (1972).

135. Montagna, W. Morphology of the aging skin: The cutaneous appendages. In W. Montagna (ed.) *Advances in Biology of Skin, Vol. VI: Aging.* New York: Pergamon Press, pp. 1–16, 1965.

136. Whitton, J. T. New values for epidermal thickness and their importance. *Health Phys.* **24:** 1–8 (1973).

137. Ronge, H. Altersveranderungen des beruhrungs sinnes. I. Druchpunktschwellen und bruckpunktfrequenz. *Acta Physiol. Scand.* **6:** 343–52 (1943).

138. Zobel, H. Die sensibilität der kornhaut in den verschledenen lebensaltern. *Albrecht Graefes Arch. Ophthal.* **139:** 668–76 (1938).

139. Jalavisto, E., Orma, E. and Tawast, M. Aging and relation between stimulus intensity and duration in corneal sensibility. *Acta Physiol. Scand.* **23:** 224–33 (1951).

140. Corbin, K. B. and Gardner, E. D. Decrease in number of myelinated fibers in human spinal roots with age. *Anat. Rec.* **68:** 63–74 (1937).

141. Gardner, E. Decrease in human neurones with age. *Anat. Rec.* **77:** 529–36 (1940).

142. Bender, M. B., Fink, M. and Green, M. Patterns in perception on simultaneous tests of the face and hand. *Arch. Neurol. Psychiat.* **66:** 355–62 (1952).

143. Bender, M. B. and Green, M. A. Alterations in perception in the aged. *J. Gerontol.* **7:** 473 (1952).

144. Fot, K., Richard, J., Tissot, R. and DeAjuriaguerra, J. Le phénoméne de l'extinction dans la double stimulation tactile de la face et de la main chez les dements degeneratifs du grand age. *Neuropsychologia* **8:** 493–500 (1970).

145. Goldstein, G. and Shelly, C. H. Similarities and

differences between psychological deficit in aging and brain damage. *J. Gerontol.* **30:** 448–55 (1975).

146. Clark, W. C. and Mehl, L. Thermal pain: A sensory decision analysis of the effect of age and sex on d′, various response criteria, and 50 percent pain threshold. *J. Abnorm. Psychol.* **78:** 202–12 (1971).

147. Kenshalo, D. R. Psychophysical studies of temperature sensitivity. In W. D. Neff (ed.). *Contributions to Sensory Physiology.* New York: Academic Press, pp. 19–74, 1970.

148. Rohles, R. H. Preference for the thermal environment by the elderly. *Human Factors* **11:** 37–41 (1969).

149. Krag, C. L. and Kountz, W. B. Stability of body functions in the aged. I. Effect of exposure of the body to cold. *J. Gerontol.* **5:** 227–35 (1950).

150. Verrillo, R. T. A duplex mechanism of mechanoreception. In D. R. Kenshalo (ed.) *The Skin Senses.* Springfield, Ill.: Charles C Thomas, pp. 139–59, 1968.

151. Kokmen, E., Bossemeyer, R. W., Barney, J. and Williams, W. J. Neurological manifestations of aging. *J. Gerontol.* **32:** 411–19 (1977).

152. Goff, G. B., Rosner, B. S., Detre, T. and Kennard, D. Vibration perception in normal man and medical patients. *J. Neurol. Neurosurg. Psychiat.* **28:** 503–9 (1965).

153. Perret, E. and Regli, F. Age and the perceptual thresholds for vibratory stimuli. *Eur. Neurol.* **4:** 65–76 (1970).

154. Magladery, J. W. Neurophysiology of aging. In J. E. Birren (ed.) *Handbook of Aging and the Individual.* Chicago: University of Chicago Press, pp. 173–86, 1959.

155. Lascelles, R. G. and Thomas, P. K. Changes due to age in internodal length in the sural nerve in man. *J. Neurol. Neurosurg. Psychiat.* **29:** 40–44 (1966).

156. Horwitt, M. K., Liebert, E., Kriesler, O. and Wittman, P. Studies of vitamin deficiency. *Science* **104:** 407–8 (1946).

157. Howell, T. H. Senile deterioration of the central nervous system. *Brit. Med. J.* **1:** 56–68 (1949).

158. Laidlaw, R. W. and Hamilton, M. A. A study of thresholds in appreciation of passive movement among normal control subjects. *Bull. Neurol. Inst.* **6:** 268–73 (1937).

159. Landahl, H. D. and Birren, J. E. Effects of age on the discrimination of lifted weights. *J. Gerontol.* **14:** 48–55 (1959).

160. Benjamin, F. B. Effect of aspirin on suprathreshold pain in man. *Science* **128:** 303–4 (1958).

161. Birren, J. E., Schapiro, H. and Miller, J. The effect of salicylate upon pain sensitivity. *J. Pharmacol. exp. Therap.* **100:** 67–71 (1950).

162. Hardy, J. D., Wolff, H. G. and Goodell, H. The pain threshold in man. *Amer. J. Psychiat.* **99:** 744–51 (1943).

163. Schludermann, E. and Zubek, J. P. Effect of age on pain sensitivity. *Percept. Mot. Skills* **14:** 295–301 (1962).

164. Sherman, E. D. and Robillard, E. Sensitivity to pain in the aged. *Can. Med. Assoc. J.* **83:** 944–47 (1960).

165. Collins, L. G. and Stone, L. A. Pain sensitivity, age and activity level in chronic schizophrenics and in normals. *Brit. J. Psychiat.* **112:** 33–35 (1966).

166. Woodrow, K. M., Friedman, G. D., Siegelaub, A. B. and Collen, M. F. Pain tolerance: Differences according to age, sex and race. *Psychosomat. Med.* **34:** 548–56 (1972).

167. Melzack, R. *The Puzzle of Pain.* New York: Basic Books, 1973.

168. Lasagna, L., Mosteller, F., von Felsinger, J. M. and Beecher, H. K. A study of the placebo response. *Amer. J. Med.* **16:** 770–79 (1954).

169. Lasagna, L. Influence of age on analgesic pain relief. *J. Amer. Med. Assoc.* **218:** 1831 (1971).

170. Bellville, J. W., Forrest, W. H., Miller, E. and Brown, B. W. Influence of age on pain relief from analgesics. A study of postoperative patients. *J. Amer. Med. Assoc.* **217:** 1835–41 (1971).

171. Harkins, S. W. and Chapman, C. R. Detection and decision factors in pain perception in young and elderly men. *Pain* **2:** 253–64 (1976).

172. Harkins, S. W. and Chapman, C. R. The perception of induced dental pain in young and elderly women. *J. Gerontol.* **32:** 428–35 (1977).

173. Arslan, M. The senescence of the vestibular apparatus. *Pract. Oto. Rhino. Laryng.* **19:** 475–83 (1957).

174. Bruner, A. and Norris, T. Age-related changes in caloric nystagmus. *Acta Otolaryng.* Suppl. 282 (1971).

175. Johnsson, L. Degenerative changes and anomalies of the vestibular system in man. *Laryng.* **81:** 1682–94 (1971).

Chapter 8

The Psychology of Adult Development and Aging[1,2]

Ilene C. Siegler, Ph.D.
Duke University Medical Center

INTRODUCTION

The focus of this chapter is the review of the psychologic changes that occur in adult life and in aging. The psychology of adult development and aging can be considered a part of development psychology—where the goal is to describe, understand and predict the changes that come with age. The orientation of the chapter is that of lifespan developmental psychology.[1-7] In this orientation, the emphasis is on the continuity of developmental processes, and many of the theoretical and methodological issues are in common with child development and focus on developmental processes which attain their saliency in a life span context.[8,9] The interest in adult development and aging is relatively new to psychology; yet the field does have a history,[8,10,11] starting in the 1920s and becoming formalized with the founding of the Gerontological Society and

Division 20: Maturity and Old Age in the American Psychological Association in 1945 (now Adult Development and Aging). The growth of the field has been phenomenal[10,12-14] with a doubling of the literature in the past 15 years.[15]

Developmental psychology is a multidisciplinary field in many ways which cut across the standard areas of psychological study. Psychology covers a broad range of topics. One useful way of organizing psychology is as psychology as a natural science and psychology as a social science. This chapter is organized into three main sections: (1) the introduction including general theoretical orientation of the chapter and methods of research; (2) psychology as a natural science including the following topics: learning, memory, motor performance, intelligence and problem solving; and (3) psychology as a social science in-

[1] Preparation of this chapter was facilitated by grants from the National Institute on Aging, AG00364 and AG00029 to the Center for the Study of Aging and Human Development, Duke University Medical Center.

[2] I would like to give a special thanks to my colleagues who generously supplied me with preprints of their current work, and to my colleagues at the Center for the Study of Aging and Human Development for access to their reprint files, libraries and comments.

cluding: personality, coping and adaptation, and the family and social change. Clinical psychological approaches are covered in another chapter of this volume.

This review must of course be selective. The recently published *Handbook of the Psychology of Aging*[16] contains over 700 pages, this chapter significantly less than that. The emphasis is placed on describing the parameters of normal development in various age ranges. The research reviewed is limited to human studies. While the area of psychology of adult development and aging has relatively few textbooks,[17-22] there are many excellent collections of review papers that will be cited in the appropriate sections of this chapter. The central question asked in each area reviewed is what proportion of the variance of the behavior under study can be attributed to age? This is a deceptively simple question, and one that can only be answered by carefully controlled studies.

Aging research involves many fascinating methodological issues. One of the major contributions of the developmental psychological approach has been methodological[23,24] and has focused around what has been called the developmental model,[25,26] which seeks to separate out the variance in presumably age-related behaviors into those due truly to phenomena intrinsically related to the aging process (or age), to variance due to the effects of the historical time at which the measurement was made (time of measurement), or due to the unique social historical conditions operative in the developmental history of the person under study (cohorts).[27] The cohort effect can also be seen as an age by time of measurement interaction that happened in the past.

Additionally, the cohort perspective is important in understanding that the research literature (as well as our own training) is fixed in a sociohistoric context that will influence the ways that reality is interpreted. In summary, those changes that are truly age-related are those that are observed independent of cohorts studied at the time of measurement. In essence this test requires

special kinds of replication. By combining longitudinal and cross-sectional designs, it is possible to observe combinations of ages and cohorts at different times and make such assessments. The accepted conventions now refer to "age changes" as changes observed longitudinally in the same persons (or random samples from the same cohort) and to "age differences" in reference to cross-sectional studies where people of various ages are measured at the same point in time and the inference made that the younger people "will become like" or perform as the older people studied concurrently.

There are some other special problems in developmental research. Kuhlen[28] discusses stimulus equivalence—will the stimulus mean the same thing to different age groups (e.g., a TAT card with a couple in their sixties may represent peers to older people and grandparents to younger people). Response equivalence, the psychological meaning and interpretation of the response, may also differ. This is a particular problem in that the age grading of society makes age appropriateness a criterion for evaluating behavior, and this is often implicit rather than explicit.[29] The statistical problems in measuring change are of concern to many branches of science, but the problems are particularly acute when studying aging.[30,31]

In addition, as will be seen more clearly in the remaining sections, the selection of an appropriate control group is not always obvious. Should older college graduates be compared to younger college graduates? We know that in the past a much more select group graduated from college. In clinical studies, where older people have known diseases (either medical or psychiatric), should the control group be younger persons with the same disease, older persons who are disease free, or both? Nice discussions and summaries of special problems of aging research can be found in a variety of sources.[15,22,32]

Throughout the chapter, special attention will be focused on longitudinal studies. Longitudinal studies provide uniquely valuable information about the different patterns of aging. A second focus of the chapter will be on characterizing the stages within adult life. Although the research literature is unequally distributed across the adult lifespan, attention will be focused on 4 major periods where feasible: young adulthood (21–34), midlife (35–54), young-old (55–74), and old-old (75 +).[33]

PSYCHOLOGY AS A NATURAL SCIENCE

The research reviewed in this section includes cognitive and intellectual performance and experimental work in learning, memory, and human performance. A major goal of this research has been to understand the brain-behavior relationships and how they change as a function of age. Two major modifiers of cognitive performance are physical health status and the so-called "noncognitive" factors in cognitive performance, such as cautiousness and other motivational and personality constructs. These two topics will be evaluated in separate parts of this section. The emphasis of this section is on basic research findings. This research is particularly important because of the clinical implications for diagnosis, assessment, and the development of treatment programs.

Learning

Botwinick[21] defines learning as the acquisition of information or skills. The processes of learning are of obvious importance throughout the lifecycle. Older people are capable of learning, this is no longer in question. The research questions are now focused on understanding the conditions under which learning is facilitated or hampered as a function of age and on elucidating the mechanisms and their probable locus of operation in the nervous system. Two areas of learning are reviewed: conditioning studies and verbal learning studies in the laboratory. The linkages between learning and memory are strong. In order to assess learning, the material must be remembered long enough to be tested. The area of learning research is becoming a historical curiosity within experimental psychology. The current paradigms in experimental psychology adopt an information processing view of cognitive performance as a system. Learning, then, becomes a part of the input. Thus, most of the research in learning has been more than adequately reviewed in the major texts on the psychology of aging,[17,21,22] in the first *Handbook of Aging and the Individual* published in 1959, in the Handbook chapters by Kay emphasizing theory[34] and Jerome emphasizing empirical findings,[35] and more recently by Arenberg and Robertson-Tchabo.[36] The conclusions of this research will be summarized.

Conditioning Studies. Classical and instrumental conditioning paradigms represent relatively simple forms of learning and one of the few psychological areas where human and animal studies can be compared. However, a current review of the animal learning literature[36] fails to report consistent findings in the conditioning area. There is relatively little human work on conditioning. Botwinick[17,21] reports only four studies, three of which concerned eyelid conditioning of the galvanic skin response. In all four studies, older people were harder to condition, required more trials, and in three of the four studies, extinguished more quickly. These results imply reduced behavioral reactivity in the older nervous system. These results are in agreement with the findings of Cautela and Mansfield[37] who review behavioral therapy techniques used with older people and suggest that older patients required more therapy sessions than younger patients.

Verbal Learning Studies. Verbal learning research is based on associative learning developed from conditioning and behavior theory.[34,38] In these stimulus-response paradigms, words or nonsense syllables form the basic experimental stimuli. Two main paradigms have been employed: paired associate learning (PAL) and serial learning (SL). In PAL, a list of paired stimulus-response items is presented; the subject's task is to learn the list. In the next presentation, only the stimulus is presented and the subject must anticipate the response. The time allowed for the stimulus and response to be shown together is called the inspection interval. These intervals can be manipulated separately. In SL, the words are chained together so that each word is both the response to the previous word and the stimulus for the next word. In both paradigms, various experiments may vary the times for the anticipation and inspection intervals and the difficulty of the task by the number of items in the list and the degree of association between the stimuli and responses. Pairs range from those with high associative value (e.g., dog-bone) to those of low associative value (e.g., TL-RQ). The literature is consistent in reporting that, for both PAL and SL, learning performance declines with advancing age. Early studies by Gilbert[39] reported that PAL was particularly sensitive to the effects of aging. This has been an active area of research. Differences between age groups were accentuated when the material was presented at a fast pace and minimized but not eliminated when the material was presented at a slower pace,[40-47] when the task was self-paced (under control of the subject),[41,43] or when the total time for both stimulus and response intervals was longer.[48,49] Similar findings were reported in SL studies.[50-52]

The major dependent variables in these studies have been either the number of trials required to learn the list to one or more perfect recitations or the number of errors made in a set number of trials. Special attention has also focused on the types of errors made. Older people have been found to make omission errors (not respond at all) while younger people make more commission errors (give a response, but not a correct one).[52]

These findings raised questions as to the causes of the poorer learning performance of older persons. The main questions have been concerned with assessing whether the lowered performance represented a true learning deficit indicative of central nervous system changes, or was due to a set of performance factors that are noncognitive in nature.

The effects of additional time in improving performance are suggestive that at least part of the deficit may be reduced by procedural changes. One potential aid in such learning tasks is the formation of mediators to help remember the relationship between the stimulus and response. A mediator is a link (either a visual image or a word) between the two words of the pair. For example, "babysitter" would be a mediator for the pair baby-chair. Hulicka and Grossman,[53] in a study of PAL, reported that the older subjects did not spontaneously produce mediators while the younger subjects did. They then instructed the subjects to use mediators and the performance of the older people was significantly improved. In a study by Canestrari, the subjects were given mediators by the experimenter. Again, the age differences were reduced but not eliminated.[42] However, the reasons for this difference in strategy are not well understood. The findings are similar in studies where meaningfulness of the pairs is manipulated.[54-56] However, manipulations that made the task more meaningful by increasing the associative strength of the words also made the tasks easier. Thus performance improved both for young and for old, and in general more for the older subjects than for the younger subjects. Wittels[57] attempted to develop stimuli that would be particularly meaningful for older people. This manipulation did not differentially improve performance. Botwinick and Storandt,[58] as part of a large cross-sectional study, investigated performance on three PAL tasks that differed in meaningfulness. They employed a relatively slow pace (5 seconds). The results indicated that with words of high associative strength no age differences were found from the twenties to the seventies. As the tasks increased in difficulty, so did the age differences. Thus, differences in meaningfulness and the ease of the task can reduce or even eliminate age differences. The results, however, point to a real learning deficit.

Eisdorfer and his colleagues' work on a serial learning,[50-52] noting the particularly large number of omission errors, hypothesized that caution, caused by increased arousal, was largely responsible for the poor learning performance. Eisdorfer, Nowlin and Wilkie[59] tested this hypothesis by administering a drug to block autonomic arousal or a placebo to groups of elderly subjects before their participation in a serial learning task. Those subjects who received the drug made fewer errors. Froehling[60] failed to replicate these results. Her work suggests that the overarousal may be reduced by adapting the subjects to the laboratory fully before testing. These findings do not rule out, however, the role that arousal may play.

Okun, Siegler, and George[61] investigated the role of cautiousness in verbal learning performance. Young and old subjects were tested in the SL paradigm using the same stimuli as Eisdorfer, et al.[50] Subjects were also assessed on two measures of cautiousness. There were significant age differences in both learning performance and in cautiousness. Age differences in cautiousness were found to account for the age differences in omission errors, but not for the differences in overall learning performance.

In many of the studies reviewed above, the comparisons were between a young group (college students or young adults in their twenties) and an old group (typically aged in the sixties and seventies). Those studies that covered the full adult age span by decades[46,58] tended to report learning deficits occurring in the forties and fifties for the difficult tasks and generally apparent across all tasks and conditions for those in their seventies. An additional performance factor may be generational differences. The research in intellectual development indicates that parts of the differences in in-

tellectual performance can be shown to be related to differences in early experiences in the education system and to cultural change. There are relatively few longitudinal studies of learning performance. Arenberg[36] presented some unpublished data on both PAL and SL from the Baltimore Longitudinal Study, which is a longitudinal follow-up of work in which the cross-sectional results indicated small age differences before age 60, larger differences after age 60, with the differences accentuated at the faster pace.[62] At the first time of measurement (1960–1964) the subjects were aged 30–76; subjects were retested an average of 6.8 years later. At the time of the second testing, new samples from the same cohorts were taken. Both the longitudinal results and the data from samples of the same cohorts confirmed the original cross-sectional results, indicating a deficit in verbal learning in the later years of life. An inspection of Figs. 1 and 2 in Arenberg and Roberts chapter[36] indicate declines in PAL starting in the forties and accelerating in the sixties while the declines for SL do not appear to be significant until the sixties. However, as no statistical tables are presented, it is hard to interpret which of the differences are large enough to be statistically significant. Nonetheless the pattern is clear.

In summary, the learning literature suggests that there are true learning deficits found in older people and also that performance factors affect learning performance. The reasons for the learning deficits remain largely unexplained by the principles of the learning theories but may well be accounted for by memory factors and other components of information processing to be explored next.[63] The findings of the performance modifiers, while not as useful theoretically, have been of tremendous practical importance. The results of the work on performance factors have led to the development of teaching methods in applied work settings based on known characteristics of older learners. The bulk of this work has been done in Great Britain and has been reviewed by Belbin and Belbin[64] and by

Welford.[65] The techniques developed have emphasized generous time limits, meaningful training materials, the avoidance of errors during early learning, and procedures which tend to reduce anxiety.

Memory

Studies of memory performance are a major focus of current work in experimental aging research. The associative learning model that guided the learning studies has been replaced by an information processing model. This model presents a system for handling information and is organized into sequentially related components. The first component is called sensory memory, which receives information from the visual and auditory systems. It is thought to be extremely time limited (¼ to 2 seconds). Information is coded into the next part of the memory system or it decays. Attentional processes are seen as critical in controlling the flow of information at this point of the system. Cognitive performance of older persons has been shown to be particularly sensitive to tasks which required divided attention. Failures at this early stage of the memory process may be related to deficits in recall because the information was never fully registered. Age differences in situations which do not require divided attention have been minimal whereas age differences in situations which required divided attention have been found to be large.[8]

Information received from sensory memory is transferred to primary memory. Primary memory is seen as the main working memory where information is coded, organized, and then passed to secondary memory for storage. Primary memory is seen as extremely limited in capacity, and information still in mind is assumed to come from primary memory. Primary memory is thought to be the conscious control system for memory—the "ego" of the information processing system. A typical measure of primary memory is digit span, which averages about seven digits, and is relatively stable over the life span. Few age differences

have been reported on tasks which require the retrieval of the most recent information presented. Thus there are thought to be few age differences in primary memory *per se*.[38,66] However the speed with which items can be retrieved from primary memory has been shown to increase with age.[67] These differences in speed of the operations of primary memory may be particularly important in tasks which require the rapid processing or encoding of information into secondary memory.

Secondary memory, or long-term memory, is the major storage system. It is seen to be highly organized, presumably by the semantic characteristics of verbal information. Secondary memory contains what is commonly meant by memory and is the major locus of reported age decrements. Information that is no longer in mind must be retrieved from secondary memory. Deficits in secondary memory are generally attributed to failures in acquisition or original learning or to failures in retrieval. Failures in retrieval are presumed to result from the ways the material is organized or encoded, much in the same way an inefficient filing system can lend to problems in retrieval. The multistage model described is representative of most of the work in memory. However, Craik and Lockhart[68] have suggested that viewing memory as a continuum might be more useful. They argue that memory is a function of the durability of the memory trace. The durability of the trace is determined by the level of processing of the material during acquisition. Material that is coded semantically, or more elaborately, is described as being deeper. And, it is suggested, the material which is entered into the system with the most optimal set of mental operations will be most likely to be remembered. Thus, encoding and retrieval are seen to be complementary and interdependent processes.[66]

Due to the theoretical developments within experimental psychology, research on age differences in memory has become sophisticated and has produced an interesting set of results where various types of memory have been shown to be well pre-served at least until the middle of the seventh decade for relatively healthy, community-dwelling older persons.

Age differences seem to be accentuated when the material to be learned and therefore remembered, is unfamiliar[67,69] or consists of nonverbal or spatial figural stimuli.[58,70] Age differences are found to be minimal or nonexistent in tasks with semantic content (sentences) and semantic encoding mechanisms,[71,72] particularly when only recognition is required,[66] and age differences have been shown to be large in conditions of experiments which require shallow processing but eliminated in the conditions of experiments which require deep processing.[73,74] In agreement with some of the learning studies reviewed earlier,[42,53] older persons were found to be able to generate mediators, but not to use them spontaneously, or as efficiently as younger persons,[75] suggesting the older people show a production deficiency.[76]

Three recent studies provided nice summaries of the "state of the art" in memory research. Waugh, Fozard and Thomas[77] investigated retrieval time from primary and secondary memory and included a measure of retrieval time to index the amount of time required to perceive the stimulus and generate the response not related to memory. The subjects ranged in age from 31–79 years old. The results indicated that the perceptual motor component remained relatively constant across the life span until about age 70; the time required to retrieve information from primary memory increased with age and was most marked in the sixties; the time required to retrieve information from secondary memory had the largest increase and was shown the earliest, in the fifties. These findings suggest that the reason why older persons are hampered on learning tasks[36] is because they do not have time to perform the required operations necessary for good memory performance.

Robertson-Tchabo and Arenberg[78] factor-analyzed a large battery of memory measures in a sample of men ranging in age

from 20–80. They extracted four factors, which were then correlated with age. The factors and their correlations with age were: attention (−.40), information processing speed (−.35), secondary memory (−.30), and primary memory (−.15), essentially replicating the levels of age deficits found in the memory literature.[66]

Perlmutter[76] did an excellent study investigating various aspects of memory, including individuals' experiences with memory in real world situations. She tested four groups of subjects: two groups of young people aged 20–25—one group had a high school education only and a second group were doctoral level students. The two older groups were aged 60–65, high school only vs. completed Ph.D.'s. Thus it was possible to evaluate the effects of age and of education independently. All subjects provided basic background information including reported mental and physical health symptoms and ratings. Subjects were given a 60-item memory questionnaire about memory problems in everyday life, any perceived changes in memory, and any memory strategies that they used. Subjects were then tested on a series of memory tasks including some traditional, experimental, word-memory tasks, and a task about memory for facts about general information. The results present an interesting set of similarities and differences: older subjects reported more memory problems, academicians reported more memory demands, older subjects and those with less education reported that their memories were more likely to get worse, and all subjects reported using memory strategies and exhibited a good general knowledge about factors which influence memory.

Age differences were found in the traditional memory tasks; age differences were largest in recall and reduced in recognition. Age differences in recall were found for the conditions of the task that required both deep and shallow processing; in recognition there were no differences in the deeper processing task. Overall, performance was significantly worse for the older subjects and for those with less education. Intercorrelations of the variables indicated a low relationship between the traditional word-memory tasks and fact-memory (r = .16) tasks. Other task factors, preparation time and memory monitoring, were shown to be related to good memory performance independent of age.

For the traditional experimental task, good performance was predicted by preparation time (18%), age (18%), physical health ratings (6%), and education (5%). Fact memory was predicted by education (15%) and age (9%).

The results of the set of studies reviewed suggest that at least until very old age, memory performance for middle-aged and older persons is sensitive to the particular requirements imposed by the experimental paradigm. Thus, in evaluating memory in older persons, particular types of memory can be compared to the expected patterns of maintenance of ability and decline. This literature is starting to be incorporated into clinical memory testing. This is certainly a promising new direction for the field.[79,80]

Motor Performance and Speed of Behavior

In studies of age-related behavioral change, the observed slowing of behavior is the most consistent finding: across wide ranges of behavior, from simple motor movements to complex cognitive process, and from the earliest studies starting with Galton in the 1880s up to the current research findings. Birren[81] argues convincingly that the speed of behavior is an intrinsic property of behavior and one of the most logical ways to relate behavior to the functioning of the central nervous system (CNS). Birren goes on to suggest that, with increased age, the speed with which the particular behavior can be performed becomes critical in determining the efficiency and quality of the response.

The role of the speed of various processes in aging has been studied in a variety of contexts including measures of CNS functions as assessed by psychophysiology,[82] motor performance,[83] and decision making.[85]

There is almost a political nature to the set of arguments as to the meaning of this finding. On one side, declines in speed of behavior represent an index of CNS function and the ultimate measure of competence of the older person. On the other side speed is seen as extrinsic to behavior, representing a performance factor that demeans older persons' capacities unfairly. Birren's position is essentially correct, but the counter arguments have generated a set of studies aimed at manipulating variables that can reduce age differences and thus improve performance within the limits of capacity.

Welford,[83] in a masterly review, has summarized the literature on human motor performance with the goal of specifying the location of the changes observed with age and the reasons underlying those changes. While there are known changes in the capacities of the sensory systems with age (see Marsh, Chapter 7) and in the responses of effector muscles, by and large the data indicate that the rates of changes of the peripheral components of these systems are not large enough to account for the observed age differences. In addition, studies that partition the changes in reaction time (RT) into movement time and decision time consistently report that the decision time components are the primary locus of the age deficit.

Changes with age in simple motor times or simple RT studies generally report a time increase of about 26% from age 20 to age 60. Studies of complex reaction time, in which decisions must be made, indicate significantly larger changes.[83] Research by Fozard and his colleagues,[67,69,77,86-88] however, is beginning to suggest that, in RT studies where the material is familiar (which reduces the difficulty of the decision), perceptual motor time, which increases slightly with age, is sufficient to account for the age differences. In addition, aside from the reported increases in average RT, an increase is seen in the variance of RT with age. This increase in variance is particularly important. On certain trials of the RT task, the older person is performing as fast or faster than younger persons. However, this more optimal behavior cannot be sustained. This may be related to motivational factors. Welford[89] points out that the maintenance of performance under speeded conditions requires considerable effort. Older people who may well be performing closer to the limits of their capacity may choose not to expend the effort.

Salthouse[90,91] investigated the meaning of the declines in speeded tasks by reanalyzing data from a variety of tasks ranging from simple RT tasks to age records in track and field events. All of the tasks were selected to be those with minimal cognitive demands. Performance of each age group was calculated as a percentage of the time obtained at maximal performance. He reported steeper declines of up to 40% more time at age 60 than at age 20 for the running events. Choice RT tasks required about 15% to 20% more time at age 60, and simple RT tasks only about 5% more time. Performance for all of the nonrunning tasks declined between the forties and the fifties and for running performance about a decade earlier. Thus the "universal slowing with age" was found, but it varied in magnitude and age of onset as a function of task characteristics.

Modifiers of Speeded Behavior. In choice RT experiments the subject is required to perform under instructions that demand both speed and accuracy. Welford[83] suggests older persons adopt a cautious strategy as a way to compensate for the loss of speed of their behavior while maintaining accuracy.

Signal detection theory presents a paradigm for studying the role of caution in decision making. In the typical signal detection experiment, the individual must scan for the appearance of a particular signal and respond only to that (monitoring a radar screen for enemy aircraft is an example of a typical task). There are two correct responses (hit—reporting the signal is there when it is, and correction rejection—not responding when the signal is not there) and two types of errors (false alarm—reporting the signal is present when it is not, and

miss—failing to report that a signal has occurred). Two parameters are calculated by comparing the numbers of these 2 types of correct and incorrect responses: d' which is a measure of perceptual acuity and Beta which is a measure of response bias and also an index of cautiousness.

Salthouse[91] suggested another approach to this problem. He designed a study in order to compare the performance of young and old with instructions to perform at different levels of accuracy by varying the payoff for fast responses vs. accurate responses. The performance characteristics of the task determine what the optimal speed-accuracy ratio should be to achieve the best performance. He evaluated whether the age differences suggested that older persons were operating on the same curve of optimal performance but at different rates, implying differences in strategy, or whether older people, due to capacity limitations, were operating on a different curve. In the first study, the young were faster than the old only at the extremes (100% accuracy and 40% accuracy). This suggested no capacity differences, only a strategy difference, as the performance was equal at 50% accuracy. As this result was unexpected, he replicated the study with new groups of young and old subjects. This time the results were the reverse: the young were faster than the old at all levels of accuracy, suggesting a strategy difference. However, comparing the performance of all four groups, the main difference was in the performance of the young subjects. The young subjects in the second study were an average of 200 milliseconds faster in all conditions than the young subjects in study one. Salthouse concluded that the results overall indicated strategy differences were most important and capacity differences could not be addressed. This study has been reviewed in some detail because it points up the critical nature of the young "control" group, making inferences about age differences. The young subjects in the second study were college students; in the first study (run during the summer) the subjects were recruited from an employment office. The older subjects were unspecified "community volunteers." Thus, particularly in studies where cognitive behaviors are studied, it is important that subjects of different ages be matched so that they are similar in educational achievement, and, if possible, on measures of other cognitive functions which can be used as a covariate to test for the effects of any age-related sample differences.

Findings of increased cautiousness have been shown to be characteristic of older people across a wide variety of situations.[17,93] Various tasks which attempt to manipulate cautiousness have been done, indicating that cautiousness can be manipulated by proper changes in the payoff matrix,[94] by changes in instructions with monetary incentives for performance,[95] and by training.[83] It is clear that older persons' cautious behavior can be successfully manipulated; whether these manipulations are sufficient, however, to account for age differences in performance remains unclear.[17,61]

Other factors that have been shown to modify reaction time performance include biofeedback,[96] practice,[83,87,89] fitness,[97-100] and health status (particularly changes in cardiovascular function).[101-104] Practice has been shown to reduce age differences but rarely eliminate them. Studies of subjects with cardiovascular disease indicate that slower performance times are more closely related to disease than to age.

The performance differences among people of different ages in the experimental psychology laboratory can be summarized as follows: (1) Most changes appear to become noticeable in midlife (35–54) and accelerate slowly through the young-old years (55–74). Relatively little is known about the performance of the old-old (75 and over) as they are rarely tested. In the few studies that included very old persons, deficits were significantly greater than for the young-old group. (2) The age at which decrements are reported varies as a function of the task employed. To the extent that speed is an important parameter in the measurement, the age differences are likely to be reported earlier, during midlife; to the extent that the tasks are related to semantic content and not speed, performance tends to be maintained through the sixties. (3) There are relatively few longitudinal or sequential studies in this area. However, the few that have been done tend to suggest maintenance of performance through midlife, with increasing deficit in old age. (4) It is rare for interventions, either in the form of specifically designed experimental treatment conditions, or specifically designed programs, to eliminate age differences entirely. However, it is also rare that these manipulations fail to significantly reduce the magnitude of the age differences.

The findings in learning, memory, and human performance studies have generally been concerned with the isolation of particular cognitive processes at a molecular, or specific and basic, level of analysis. These processes are the components of cognitive and intellectual functioning. The role of physical health has only been mentioned briefly, as most of the data relating health to behavior has been in terms of intellectual performance. Thus, the role of physical health factors will be reviewed after the findings in intelligence.

Cognitive and Intellectual Development

Intelligence represents the sum of the cognitive abilities, generally assessed in omnibus tests which have been shown to be dependent upon and related to learning, memory, problem solving, reasoning, thinking, and the abilities required to deal with both verbal and nonverbal (or spatial-pictorial) information. There are two major traditions in the study of intelligence. The first is represented by the mental test movement and includes most tests of intelligence currently in use; the second is more directly concerned with the processes of reasoning and problem solving. The second is more experimental in nature, and is represented by current work in the Piagetian framework and earlier work in problem solving.

Intelligence. Intelligence is typically measured by fairly extensive test batteries. While there are no intelligence tests that have been developed exclusively for work with older people, there is a set of tests developed for the broad category of adults. Two excellent source books provide descriptions of psychological tests, Anastasi's text on psychological testing,[105] and Buros' *Mental Measurements Yearbook.*[106]

The study of age differences in adult intelligence, started in the 1920s, has one of the longest traditions in aging research. These early studies reported that the peak level of intellectual performance was reached at the end of adolescence[19,20] and declined after that.[107,108] Research done in the 1940s[109] indicated that the peak was reached around age 25, and had a gradual fall-off up to age 65. Research in the 1950s[109] indicated that the peak was reached around age 30 and declined gradually towards age 75. Note that in the approximately 25 years covered by this set of cross-sectional studies (1932–1955) the cross-sectional curve indicated that the peak intelligence increased by almost 10 years. In the 1950s the results of the first longitudinal studies of adult intelligence became available.[110-112] While the oldest subjects in these studies were middle-aged (up to about age 50), the results indicated that intellectual performance was maintained at least for verbal abilities well into the forties and for nonverbal abilities through the mid thirties. This discrepancy between longitudinal and cross-sectional findings in intelligence had a major impact on the field.[113] Three major foci of the intelligence and aging literature can be related to this discrepancy: (1) a concern with factors, aside from age, that could explain the results, particularly cultural change,[114,115] and the development of a set of methodological strategies that would provide a new way of considering developmental data;[25] (2) the development of tests of more specialized measures of intellectual functioning that would be predicted to have differential age trends;[116-119] and, (3) particularly as the ages of subjects studied expanded to include large groups of subjects in the seventies and older, a concern with physical health and terminal changes in intelligence that might be death-related.[120-122] Botwinick,[123] reviewing the literature on intellectual abilities and age including the work from the three traditions noted above, suggests that the differences between longitudinal and cross-sectional studies of intelligence are more apparent than real. He argues, convincingly, that both types of data indicate a maintenance of intellectual abilities through late middle age (up to the fifties and sixties in most cases), with declines increasing in frequency through old age; that verbal abilities are maintained significantly longer than nonverbal abilities (by almost a two-decade difference); that abilities which require speed for optimal performance are intrinsically related to the aging process and show the earliest and most consistent declines (thirties to forties in some cases); and that there are individual differences in the level of intellectual performance that are maintained well into old age. His conclusions are basically correct. However, it is instructive to review here some of the work in the past 20 years that has produced a remarkably consistent set of findings within the aging literature. The findings in intelligence provide some of the best normative data about the course of the aging process and, as such, are most helpful for the clinician in attempting to disentangle the effects of aging from the effects of disease.

Cultural Change and the Developmental Model. Kuhlen,[114] in an article reviewing the evidence about the discrepancy between longitudinal and cross-sectional studies, suggested that both research strategies might be biased by cultural or environmental change. In the work in intelligence, environmental effects have been assumed to be positive, with each generation benefiting from a more sophisticated cultural milieu. Thus, cross-sectional studies overestimated the age decrement because younger subjects, on the average, have been exposed to a more positive cultural milieu and in general to more formal education, which is reflected in indices of intelligence. Longitudinal studies tend to underestimate the age decrement, because all subjects tend to share the same cultural milieu as they age, and, if this effect is positive, they will also improve as they age, not due to any effect of aging but due rather to a reflection of the cultural changes. Cultural change need not always be positive however. Current speculations about the decline in SAT scores and the role of TV may suggest a negative bias in future studies. A more serious problem leading to the underestimation of age decrements in longitudinal studies is the effect of sample attrition. It has been well established that individuals who continue to participate in research studies do not represent a random sample of the original participants.[124,125] This is true across broad age ranges[125,126] and accelerates in seriousness with the number of repeated observations.[127] Additionally, if exactly the same tests are used, gains can be due to practice.

Schaie[25] proposed a set of strategies for the analysis of developmental data that combine longitudinal and cross-sectional designs. These strategies are called sequential designs and involve taking measures of two or more cohorts at two or more times of measurement over the age range of interest. By comparing various groups of subjects who differ in age (but not cohort or time of measurement) or who differ in cohort (but not age or time of measurement) or in time of measurement (but not age), it is possible to estimate the three parameters by analyzing various parts of the data set. These three parameters are important in understanding development at all phases of the lifecycle,[128] but these strategies have been applied more often in studies of aging where the age ranges are larger. Schaie suggests taking random samples from the same cohort as a way to control for attrition, and obviate practice effects, and thus composite longitudinal gradients can be constructed. While many parts of Schaie's formulation have caused controversy, his work has produced a methodological "revolution" of a sort. Some of the theoretical development of these constructs can be found in papers by Baltes[129] with a reformulation by Schaie,[130] with the best summary to be found in Schaie.[26] The data collected is analyzed by a statistical procedure called analysis of variance (ANOVA), which is the most common analytic technique in experimental psychology. Schaie's formulations have been criticized on statistical terms [131,132] and alternative statistical procedures have been suggested where random samples are taken from the same cohorts.[133,134] Nonetheless, the impact of the developmental model has been substantial. Researchers in all areas of psychology of aging, not just intelligence, have been made aware of competing explanations for their findings.

Measures of Intelligence. A set of tests provide most of the data on adult intelligence. The Wechsler Adult Intelligence Scale (WAIS), introduced in 1955,[109,135,136] (a revised version of the Wechsler-Bellevue[137] which was in use before 1955) is the main, individually administered intelligence test. The test is given by a trained examiner and generally takes 1½ to 2 hours to complete. The WAIS is composed of 11 subtests which represent aspects of intellectual abilities and are organized into two major components: verbal and performance intelligence. Six scales are summed to get an assessment of verbal intelligence: information, comprehension, arithmetic, similarities, digit span, and vocabulary. Five scales are summed to get an estimate of performance intelligence: digit-symbol substitution, blocking design, picture arrangement, picture completion, and object assembly. These scaled scores are summed to get an estimate of total intelligence. Intelligence as defined by the Wechsler scales is an age-linked measure, as scaled scores are converted to intelligence quotients (IQ's) so that IQ is defined as the individual's standing relative to his/her age peers. Adult intelligence tests originated from the tests developed for children by Binet. IQ was defined as the ratio of a child's mental age (determined by passing a certain number of items that were passed by most children of that age) to the child's chronological age. When this same principle was transferred to adult intelligence, norms were developed that set the expected number of items correct for the average of each age range. The test is designed so that average intelligence, independent of age, is always 100. The test has a standard deviation of 15 points. The sum of the scaled scores is converted to IQ by means of a set of tables provided with the test manual.[135] Verbal, Performance, and Total scaled scores, which are not age corrected, provide the basic data for much of the aging research. The norms were developed on the basis of a large cross-sectional study of adults aged 16–64[109,135] and an additional cross-sectional study of older persons aged 60–80+.[138] On the basis of the findings from these studies, peak performance was found in the 20–34 year age range where 110 full-scale points are required for an IQ = 100, while for those 75 and older only 68–69 points are required for IQ = 100. Verbal intelligence tends to increase until the sixties and then to fall off gradually, while performance intelligence increases until the forties with a gradual decline until the sixties and a sharper decline after that. Botwinick calls this the "classic age pattern."

Due to the time required for a full WAIS, research investigations often use only some of the subtests or other intelligence tests that can be given to groups of subjects. The work of Schaie and his group[139-143] has used Thurstone's Primary Mental Abilities test (PMA).[144] The PMA has 5 subtests: verbal meaning, space, reasoning, number and word fluency. Two additional indices, intellectual ability and educational aptitude, can be calculated from the 5 subtests as well as an overall composite score. Schaie's studies also included measures of three types of rigidity: motor-cognitive, personality-perceptual, and psychomotor speed,[145] as flexibility of thought has long been seen as an important correlate of intellectual perfor-

mance.[146] Schaie's group has been primarily concerned with attributing the variance observed in age differences to age, cohort, or time of measurement effects. They report that cohort differences account for most of the differences up through the decade of the sixties for all subtests except for word fluency, which is highly speeded and shows age changes relatively early in life, with age changes in general not becoming important until the seventies or potentially later. Botwinick[123] reanalyzed Schaie's data concentrating on the composite score and concluded that the methods of analysis point to a lesser role for cohort than Schaie has concluded.

Another approach to the assessment of adult intelligence is represented by testing a large number of abilities with separate tests and factor-analyzing the results. This set of studies have developed from Cattell's theory of fluid and crystallized intelligence and are summarized in a set of papers by Horn.[116-119] Horn and Cattell suggest that different factors of intelligence have different age patterns. They propose two general factors: crystallized intelligence (G_c) which is the result of learning and acculturation is presumed to increase with age over the life span, unless some degenerative disease process is apparent; and fluid intelligence (G_f) which involves the manipulation of new information, complex problem-solving capacity and speed, which is seen to decline linearly with age from a peak in the early twenties. Overall intelligence is seen to be relatively stable over the life span. This work was based on data from subjects aged approximately 15-60 years old and appears to be a good description of the age patterns. The findings from other measures of intelligence will then behave more like G_f or G_c depending on the particular types of abilities measured by the test.

Two other tests, developed in Britain,[147] have also been used: the Mill-Hill Vocabulary test and the Raven Progressive Matrices test. The fluid/crystallized distinction is a useful one. WAIS verbal intelligence, other vocabulary tests, and the verbal meaning, space and reasoning subtests of the PMA appear to be primarily crystallized measures; the WAIS performance, PMA word fluency and Raven appear to be primarily measures of fluid intelligence.

Organization of Abilities. Most of the findings reviewed so far have been in terms of differences in level of functioning as related to age. Implied by the G_f/G_c notions of intelligence are potential age differences in the structure of the abilities that make up intelligence. Cunningham and his colleagues have investigated structural changes in intelligence with age.[148-150] (As a test of G_f/G_c notions.) Cunningham[148] reasoned that measures of fluid and crystallized intelligence should be more highly correlated in the young than in the old. He reported a correlation of .672 between WAIS vocabulary and Raven matrices for the young while the same correlation was .386 for the old, supporting the prediction of the theory that G_f and G_c should be more highly related during early adult life than in old age.

In a more direct test, data from Owen's longitudinal study[112] was factor-analyzed in order to compare the organization of abilities at age 19, 50, and 60, as measured by the Army Alpha,[151] a group test developed to test inductees in World War I. The factor structure did not change between age 19 and age 50, but the factor structure at age 60 was different suggesting that speed had become an important component which was represented on its own factor.[149] A reanalysis of this data with more sophisticated forms of factor analysis replicated the initial findings.[150]

A number of factor analyses have been done with the WAIS and are reviewed by Matarazzo.[136] The studies generally find the factorial nature of the WAIS to be stable with age. However, very few of the studies have included significantly large numbers of individuals over age 70 or have been based on longitudinal data. Some preliminary work in our own laboratory[152,153] on the Duke Longitudinal subjects suggests that the WAIS in old age becomes unifactorial and

that its correlation with other tests of more highly speeded functions (RT) is reduced, thus replicating Cunninghams's finding of a speeded factor emerging in old age. Arenberg,[154] using data from the Baltimore Longitudinal Study, reported with sequential analysis techniques that WAIS vocabulary was well maintained over a 6-year period, with only slight decrements into the eighties, but that memory for designs as indexed by the Benton Visual Retention Test declined significantly in the seventies and eighties. This finding is consistent with increased age deficits in intellectual functions that involve spatial relationships and increased memory loads and are thus closer to G_f.

Modifiers of Intellectual Performance. Two important factors implied in the G_f/G_c distinction are the role of formal education and the role of speeded tasks. As intelligence tests were originally developed to predict school achievement, it is perhaps not surprising that intelligence is so closely related to education. G_c attributes are defined partially as those types of abilities that can be learned and represent the accumulated knowledge of a culture, as they are most closely defined by measures of vocabulary. In some early research on the WAIS standardization sample, Birren and Morrison in 1961[155] reported higher correlations of the subtest scores with educational achievement than with age (ranging from .40–.66) and correlations of total scores have been reported to as high as .70.[136] These correlations imply that anywhere from 16% to 35% of the variance in intelligence as measured by the WAIS can be accounted for by differences in amount of formal education. However, this still leaves the majority of the variance unexplained. Education is seen as one of the major cohort effects and has also been given as an explanation for the differences in cross-sectional versus longitudinal results.[156] Theoretically it is still not fully understood, as a correlation only describes a relationship, not the causality. Thus, whether brighter people are those who attain more formal education, or whether formal education makes people brighter (probably both are true to some extent), this very consistent finding suggests that assessments of intellectual functioning cannot be correctly interpreted unless the educational background of the person is known. Additionally, while levels of formal education are definitely related to the level of intellectual achievement, particularly in tasks which are highly loaded with G_c, this is less true in tests highly loaded with G_f. However, there is data to suggest that the patterns of growth and decline of verbal abilities with age share a similar pattern within high and low education groups.[157] As with education, there have been fairly consistent reports of sex difference in intelligence. Typically, women do better on verbal tasks and men on spatial tasks; however, in a recent investigation of the structure of intellectual abilities in old age, Cohen, Schaie and Gribben[158] reported that organization of the abilities was the same.

As in the areas of learning, memory and human performance, the question of the role of speeded tasks in the measurement and assessment of intelligence has been of concern since at least 1936 when Lorge[159] pointed out that older people were hampered by speeded tasks. Doplett and Wallace[138] evaluated the role that speed played in the various subtests of the WAIS where speed is a factor. When testing the older subjects for the standardization, they allowed extra time and calculated the scores both in the standard fashion and without time as a factor. The correlations for the two types of scoring ranged from .88 for block design to between .93-.95 for the other speeded subtests. They concluded that speed did not therefore account for the age differences in performance. Recent studies have criticized the Doplett and Wallace work because they did not provide a young control group to test the effects of extra time.[160,161] Other similar studies have investigated the role of memory,[162] fatigue,[163] practice,[164] and training on component

skills.[165] In general, the results of this set of studies suggest that increased time significantly improves scores on arithmetic, picture completion, block design, picture arrangement, and object assembly[160] but this is true only for older people with high verbal ability,[161] that manipulations that reduce the memory load are equally successful for young and old,[162] that fatigue does not appear to be a particular problem for older people (aged 57-91),[163] and that practice and training on the component abilities are translated into improved scores.[163,164] Thus, intelligence as measured by current instruments is not a fixed, immutable quality, and older people's performance on intelligence tests can be improved by manipulations that would be expected to do so. These manipulations should lessen the gap between observed performance and presumed underlying ability. There have been many arguments in the literature about whether intelligence declines in old age.[166-169] The answer to the question depends to a large extent on the prior beliefs of the questioner. Compared to earlier research findings and the general "popular wisdom," intellectual functions are remarkably well preserved with age; compared to the maximal level that an individual can achieve, except in extremely rare instances, declines can almost always be found, at least in some of the important components of intellectual functioning. Nonetheless, one of the most interesting and consistent findings about adult intelligence is the relationship between intellectual performance and survival.

Intelligence and Survival. Level of intellectual performance has been shown to be positively related to survival across the life span at age 22,[170] age 30,[171] age 44,[111] age 50,[172] and beyond.[120-122,173] Siegler[122] reviewed the relevant set of longitudinal studies in aging that relate intellectual performance to survival, to distance from death, and to the terminal drop hypothesis.[120] Ten research programs are represented in Table 8-1 which contains an update of that report.

Table 8-1a. Descriptive Studies of Survival, Distance from Death and Terminal Drop.

STUDY	INITIAL AGE	AVERAGE[b] IQ	YEARS TESTED	HEALTH[c]	ANALYTIC "CROSS"	STRATEGY[d] "LONG"	PROVIDES EVIDENCE FOR: SURVIVAL	DISTANCE DEATH	TERMINAL DROP
Moosehaven[120,174]	65–79	94–104	1949–61	below	no	yes	NA	NA	+
NYS Twins[175,176,177,178,179]	69–76	100–106	1947–67	average	yes	yes	+	NA	+
Bath, VA[180,181,182,183,184]	50–84	100	1950–65	below	yes	yes	-	-	+
Chicago[185,186]	65–91	?	1962–65	below	yes	yes	-	+/-	+
Hamburg[121,124]	55–75+	100–104	1956–71	average	yes	yes	+	+	+
NIH[187,188]	65–91	108–120	1956–67	above	yes	no	+	NA	NA
Newcastle[189]	60–75+	100	1963–71	average impaired	yes	no	+	+/-	NA
Duke[153,190,191,192,193]	60–94	100–104	1955–75	average	yes	yes	+	-/+	+/-
Bonn[194,195]	60–65	100	1965–73	average	yes	no	+	NA	NA
Washington U.[196]	60–89	100	1973–74	average	yes	yes	+	NA	-

[a] Adapted from Table 1 of Siegler (1975).[122]

[b] Not all of the authors presented their data the same way. IQ's when not reported were estimated from the sub-tests reported and Wtd. scores were converted according to Wechsler for the Wechsler-Bellevue and Wechsler (n.) for the WAIS.

[c] Health status was rated as average unless exceptional health was reported or the subjects were institutionalized.

[d] "Cross" = cross sectional analysis of longitudinal date; "Long" = longitudinal analysis.

Studies of survival and the relationship of performance to death are hampered by special methodological problems. Research subjects do not often die at the appropriate time vis à vis the measurement interval. Thus, two common techniques of data analysis have been used. In the "cross-sectional" analysis of longitudinal data, data is analyzed typically from the first measurement point when all subjects were alive, on the basis of how long the subjects survived after that measurement point. In the "longitudinal" analysis of longitudinal data, rates of change in intellectual functioning, typically on a per year basis, are calculated for groups of subjects differing in survival; the pattern of change over time is evaluated. Three related, yet conceptually distinct, questions are addressed by this research: (1) the level of intellectual performance and its relationship to survival; (2) the relationship between intellectual performance and the distance from death of the individual at the time the measurement was made; and (3) the terminal drop hypothesis which postulates that cognitive performance is stable during adult life but declines rapidly as death approaches. The terminal drop hypothesis suggests that there will be an accelerated rate of change in cognitive performance, typically within five years before death. All of these studies share the practical problem that data cannot be fully analyzed until sufficient members of the subject population have died. This set of studies raises two major issues. The first is a measurement issue. That is, findings of cognitive change in old age may be biased because of the results of those subjects about to die. Such findings are not accurate representations of normal aging because such results overestimate the true age differences and thus constitute a sampling problem,[123] as subjects who differ in age also differ in their probability of dying. The second issue is an important theoretical issue: death is rarely a random event. Whatever processes are related to death might also be the same processes underlying cognitive decline, and, thus, issues of physical health become critical variables in understanding terminal changes in cognitive functioning.

As can be seen in Table 8-1, the studies are listed primarily by the place where they were done. The superscript numbers refer to the major papers about each of the studies. The age range at the start of the study, years of data collection, average IQ for the sample, and general health status of the subjects are included as descriptors of the studies. The results and analytic strategies employed are presented in the right-hand side of the table.

Higher intellectual performance at the start of the study was significantly related to survival in 7 of the 10 studies. In the three studies where this was not true, all of the subjects were in institutional settings and thus in relatively poor health. Blum and Jarvik[179] investigated the role of initial ability and educational achievement on survival in a reanalysis of data from the NYS Twin Study[175-179] and included in their discussion a review of other studies on the same issue. They concluded that, whether initial ability is indexed by level of intellectual performance or by educational attainment, and whether the subsequent rate of change is measured by a comparison of mean scores, by an index of percentage decline, or by rate of change, those with higher initial ability exhibited patterns of lower decline and increased survival. While intelligence is not the only correlate of survival, it appears to be a significant one.[198]

The evidence relating to distance from death is clear. All of the studies that find a relationship between initial level of performance and survival imply that distance from death should be a factor; however, the requirements for a direct test of this notion are more severe. All subjects must have a known date of death in order to do an analysis. Five of the ten studies addressed distance from death, and the results are equivocal. One reason for the lack of agreement is that the distance from death varied greatly between studies. For example, in the Hamburg study,[121-124] Riegel and Riegel found a linear relationship for subjects originally aged 55-64, with those 10 years from death the highest, those 5 years from death intermediate; however, in the age range 65-74, there was no difference between those 5 and 10 years from death. Berkowitz[183,184] and Eisdorfer and Wilkie[191] both reported nonsignificant correlation coefficients between initial peformance and distance from death. Eisdorfer and Wilkie compared the third measurement point after 10 years of testing on groups of nonsurvivors who survived up to an additional 3 years. When the mean differences were tested by ANOVA, there were no significant differences in this group of 37 nonsurvivors. However, Siegler[192] using the same longitudinal population after eight examinations and therefore a total distance from death from the first measurement point of up to 19 years, reported a significant relationship for verbal, performance and total intellectual performance for the 192 subjects who had died. Thus, it would appear that when the distance from death is at least 7-10 years, and the age range of the subjects is large, significant effects are found.

Terminal drop implies an accelerated rate of change before death. In order to study terminal drop, the investigator must have two or more data points. The rate of change on a per year basis can be calculated with only two data points, but three or more data points are required to evaluate whether the rate changes as death approaches. Four of the studies provided evidence favoring the terminal drop hypothesis, two of the studies reported ambiguous findings, and one study found negative evidence. Kleemeier's[120] original report on terminal drop included data from only 13 subjects; all 13 had 4 measurement points, 9 survived and 4 died shortly after the fourth examination. An inspection of the curves and the average rates of decline indicated that terminal drop was a good description of the data. Kleemeier then tested this hypothesis by comparing the data from 37 subjects who were alive and 33 who had died who had at least 2 measurement points. The group were both aged 79 years at the last testing. He found an accelerated rate of decline for the deceased subjects, but only for the performance score of the WB. In the NYS Twin studies,[175-179,197] an index of critical loss was developed. This index included any change in vocabulary, an annual decline of at least 10% on the similarities subtest, and a 2% decline on digit symbol substitution. Death was related to critical loss on any two of the three indices of loss. These data, which are particularly impressive for critical loss also predicted the earlier death within twin pairs. Lieberman[185] reported that declines in performance discriminated between death within 3 months versus survival of at least a year. Wilkie and Eisdorfer[191] reported that an increased rate of decline was related to death but that the major decline occurred within 7-10 years prior to death. Siegler et al.,[193] in her analyses from the same population, found evidence for terminal drop. However, when initial age and age at death were controlled for, the relationship was no longer apparent. This finding is in agreement with the negative finding of the Washington University study in which the subjects were carefully matched.[196]

The Duke Longitudinal Study stopped data collection in 1976. On the basis of the full scale WAIS score only, predictions were made for 61 of the remaining 71 survivors (10 subjects had moved, or refused testing, and thus did not have sufficient information). Deaths in the sample are monitored. Since the predictions were made, 32 of these subjects have died and 39 are currently alive (10/78). Of those with stable IQ patterns, 61% have survived and 39% died; of those with terminal drop patterns 39% have survived and 61% have died. Of those subjects currently alive, 11 have patterns which indicate drop, and 20 have stable patterns. The mean age of the survivors is approximately 84 years old. Some of the mispredictions between 1974-76 occurred when an individual was ill when tested or missed an exam due to illness. When they recovered from the illness, their WAIS score recovered as well. Analyses are underway to explore this further. Thus, the terminal drop hypothesis remains a hypothesis. However, the results do point to the significant role that physical health status plays in the assessment of cognitive functioning late in life. An additional important implication from the terminal drop literature is that sudden, large drops in cognitive performance in older people are unexpected and not "normal" aging. Any large change in the cognitive capacity of an older person should be treated with suspicion—it may be a terminal sign, or it may indicate a potentially treatable illness.

Intelligence and Health. In addition to the other modifying factors in intellectual performance, poor health, particularly changes in the cardiovascular system, has been shown to be related to poorer cognitive performance,[101-104,174,187-189,198,199] while fitness[87,99] has been related to increased performance. Intelligence has been used in a number of studies which indicate a direct relationship between intellectual performance and blood pressure,[200,201] cerebral blood flow and EEG,[174,202] the performance of the immune system,[203-204] and reduced stress.[205-206] This is seen most clearly in the NIH study[187,188] where 47 men were intensively studied. During the physical examination about half of the group was found to be suffering from asymptomatic disease (the healthy group). Botwinick and Birren[207] compared the performance of the healthy and the suprahealthy (those without evidence of disease even after extensive medical screening) men on 23 tests of cognitive and intellectual performance. They found the suprahealthy group better on 21/23 measures including the WAIS subtests and the Raven progressive matrices test; however, the patterns of differences typically found in aging studies (verbal higher than performance and better performance on nonspeeded versus speeded tasks) were maintained within each health group. Thus, in studies of intellectual and cognitive functioning, controls for health are critical.

Functional Age. Functional age is a construct that combines concerns about performance and health that has been primarily employed in work-related contexts. Implied in all of the performance literature so far reviewed is the notion that individuals age at different rates and thus age by itself is a relatively poor predictor of function. The construct was first introduced by McFarland[208] to emphasize the skills that older workers have. Functional age studies typically measure a large number of cognitive and physiological functions. One of the best examples of this type work was done by Heron and Chown[147] who established that variance in performance increases with age, meaning that the performance of the best older person may be better than the best younger person, although, as a group, younger people may score better than older people. Their results stressed individual differences within the various aspects of a persons's behavior, and suggest that specific measures of cognitive performance or health are better predictors of an individual's ability than is age. The functional age literature has recently been reviewed by Edelman and Siegler[209] and by Costa and McCrae[210] and argues against age-based criteria for retirement, suggesting instead specific testing situations where performance and health criteria replace age. The original goal of the functional age research was to come up with a factor that would indicate how old the person was behaviorally and physiologically. Thus a particular 65-year-old might have the functional age of someone aged 40 or aged 80. While the research has not been particularly successful in finding a single index of function to replace age, it has been particularly useful in establishing the specific relationships between health, physiological and behavioral functioning and age.

Problem Solving

The abilities presented in this section on cognition and problem solving are both the processes that underlie intelligence (e.g., reasoning and concept formation) and the "products" of intelligence (lifelong achievement and creativity). Three separate literatures are reviewed in this section: the first includes traditional studies of problem solving capacities and their changes with age; the second deals with productive achievement throughout the lifecycle; and the third, a relatively recent approach to cognitive functioning across the life span derived from the theoretical formulations of Jean Piaget.

Traditional Studies. Problem-solving tasks are generally abstract and difficult. They are similar in content to many measures of G_f but are more often tested in experiments under various conditions which manipulate attributes of the task. Rabbitt[211] sees the task for problem-solving research as discovering why older persons are not able to solve complex problems as well as they were presumed to in their youth, or when they are compared to younger persons. In problem-solving studies it is important to equate the young and old groups of subjects for intelligence. Arenberg[212,213] reported that studies that matched subjects on measures of performance (or fluid) intelligence tend not to find age differences in problem solving as the same abilities are measured. In a recent study,[214] a correlation of .72 was reported between problem-solving ability and a measure of performance intelligence based on the block design and picture completion subtests of the WAIS. Matching for verbal intelligence, however, does not reduce age differences. Older subjects also appear to have particular difficulty when concepts are tested with abstract stimuli rather than concrete stimuli.[212] Arenberg found that he could not get his older subjects to understand the directions for the problem-solving task when the stimuli were shapes of various colors and sizes; but when the problem was converted into one with names of foods, that were either poisoned or not, the subjects could understand the practice problem and proceed to do the task. With subjects matched for verbal ability (about average in both age groups), significant differences were found in favor of the younger subjects, even with the concrete stimuli. Arenberg[213] also studied problem

solving longitudinally with participants from the Baltimore Longitudinal Study. The subjects ranged in age from 24–87 at the first measurement, were matched for verbal intelligence, and were all above average in intelligence. The task involved manipulating a series of switches in the proper combinations in order to turn on a light. The cross-sectional results indicated little change up to age 60 but significant decrements after age 60. In the longitudinal follow-up, 6 years later, all groups improved their performance significantly except for those subjects initially over 70 years of age. Problem-solving ability at the first examination was also related to survival over the 6-year period. In a concept learning task, statistically significant declines in performance were observed by age 35 but did not become large until age 50. The performance decrement was related to the encoding of memory components of the task.[215] In a study of perceptual problem solving, Lee and Pollack[216] reported a major shift in performance at age 50, in both the time required to solve the problems and in the number of problems correctly solved. Subjects were matched for verbal intelligence and there were no age differences in the abstractness of the solutions picked, the cognitive style of the individuals, or their personalities. Studies of categorization[217-219] which ask subjects to sort items and then evaluate the dimensions of the sorting report that older people are less likely to use abstract dimensions as the basis for their sorts. Their responses tend to be more relational, which is typical of the sorting behavior of young children. However, studies that employed a modeling,[218,219] or specific training,[220] paradigm reported that older subjects were able to switch to the more abstract strategies with little difficulty. The results were interpreted as suggesting that older persons have the capacity but do not use it; a simpler explanation is that they did not fully understand the instructions and chose to categorize the items in what they might have perceived to be a more complex way (by relationship) rather than by the more abstract notions of color and form.

Kogan[221] did a similar study with young and older subjects of high educational achievement and verbal ability. He reported more thematic and less analytic strategies but interpreted the differences as being stylistic rather than indicating a decline in problem-solving ability.

In sum, the results of the problem-solving studies are consistent with the findings in intelligence. Age differences are reduced when the subjects have high verbal ability; and when the task is primarily a measure of nonverbal or performance intelligence, matching subjects on such measures removes age differences entirely. While some deficits are reported earlier, deficits do not appear consistently until the fifties or later, with longitudinal findings suggesting no real decrement until the seventies. Hultsch and Hickey[222] raise the question of external validity. That is, how well do results in the laboratory generalize to other situations?

Achievement Across the Lifecycle. Lehman,[223,224] in a set of now classic studies, investigated the relationship of creative artistic and scientific contributions and age, using the careers of eminent persons whose full history is known. He reported consistent age-related peaks in major contributions, with the contributions in the physical sciences and mathematics made, on the average, earlier (twenties to thirties), while in fields such as philosophy, history and literature, the major contributions were made later (forties to fifties). Dennis[225] criticized some of the work on methodological grounds and studied productivity with controls for length of life and reported the major productivity during the thirties and forties for most fields with artistic productivity dropping off the earliest. Alpaugh and Birren[226] investigated the reasons for such reported differences in creative production. Individuals ranging in age from 20–87, of high verbal ability, were tested with a set of tests which measure divergent thinking and preference for complexity as indices of the abilities that underlie creativity. They found that age differences on the tests of divergent thinking were apparent by the thirties, with a slight decline through the forties and another larger decline after age 50. Preference for complexity was maintained through the forties. While both were related to age in a similar way, the two components were independent when the variance due to age was removed. Kogan,[227] in reviewing the literature on creativity and cognitive styles in adulthood and old age, suggests that more than just particular abilities may be involved. As individuals age and follow the progressions of their careers, there are often fewer opportunities for creative production. In addition, individuals who early in their career made a major discovery, and then continued the same work in that area, would no longer be seen as creative, although the quality of the work might be maintained. The motivational components of achievement and creativity are probably involved, and they will be explored in the section of this chapter on personality and adjustment. Rabbitt[211] concluded his review of the problem solving literature with a question: given the measured deficits of older persons on many laboratory measures, the real problem is to account for the continued problem-solving abilities that are manifested by most middle-aged and many older persons and to specify the adaptive strategies that are used to cope with some real declines in measured performance.

Piagetian Approach to Cognitive Development. There are two implicit models of development employed in most developmental studies: the mechanistic/-quantitative and the structuralist/-qualitative.[222,228] Most of the research discussed so far has been of the first type: the same developmental processes are assumed to underly behavior at all ages, with the age differences seen primarily in the amount, precision, or speed of the behavior. Piaget's work is clearly in the structuralist/ qualitative model. In such models, age differences are the results of different structural organizations of behavior, and the differences are in level of organization. A structuralist approach is more obvious when one considers the massive changes in the cognitive capacities of the organism between birth and even early childhood, or for the first 15 years of life. Piaget's work has been exclusively with children and adolescents and his theoretical formulations and experimental procedures are best described in a volume by Flavell.[229] Piaget's view of cognitive development is exceedingly complex. Developed and organized into a set of four main stages, these stages are highly organized internally, and sequentially ordered. Behavior at any stage (or substage) is indexed by an evaluation of the way the subject responds to the task, rather than just a correct or incorrect answer. The four stages with the approximate ages at which the stages are primarily observed are: sensorimotor (birth—2 years), preoperational or representational (2, or with the development of language, to 7–8 years), concrete operations (7–8 to 11–12 years), and formal operations (from 11–12 years until ?). The work in adult development has been focusd on the two operational stages. Concrete operations involve the child's interaction with the physical real world and include such constructs as the development of the understanding of number, length, width, volume, seriation, and the classification of objects. Formal operations are concerned with abstract thought and are best represented by the calculus of formal logic. They represent the set of abilities that not only deal with abstractions such as reversibility, identity, and casuality, but also the capacity to think about thought.[230] Most of the current work on the problem-solving abilities of adults and older people has been done within a piagetian perspective.[14] Two reviews of the literature[14,231] report consistent problems for adults and older people on tasks of both formal and concrete operations. However, age differences do not appear to be substantial until the sixties in most cases; and are accentuated when the

older subjects are drawn from institutional settings, or have known chronic brain syndrome, and are mitigated when the older subjects are well educated and are known to have high verbal ability. Thus, the results of the studies that employ Piagetian tasks are not all that surprising. By far, the more interesting contributions from the Piagetian perspective have been theoretical. Piaget's theory suggests that cognitive growth is a reciprocal, interactive process between the developing capacities of the organism and the environmental inputs, and only by resolving discrepancies caused by mismatches between cognitive structure and the requirements of the environment does growth occur. Piaget's descriptions of the mental worlds of children are charming—and his theory is best illustrated with descriptions of children's thought and behavior. For example, a young child will not search for a missing object until the child has a concept of the object.

In discussing the application of Piagetian constructs to adult development, Flavell[232] highlighted the major difference between child and adult development. Cognitive development for children can be described as inevitable (barring some neurological deficit), massive, cumulative and positive in direction, and essentially permanent and irreversible. In addition, the sequencing of the stages of development are invariant across children. On the other hand, changes in adult cognition appear to be primarily quantitative, at least until some dementing process is observed, primarily small, and less characteristic of adults in general. Flavell suggests that the obvious difference in the rate of biological change between children and adults implies that whatever cognitive change is seen in adult life must, therefore, be found in the domain of experience. It may well be that the structural changes in adult cognition are found not in cognitive abilities but in personality. Inhelder and Piaget[230] see one of the main tasks of adulthood as the development of the personality which can now be accomplished because the adolescent has the capacity to think about such abstract concepts as the self.

Research on formal operations in adults and the elderly[231-234] indicates that most adults are not particularly comfortable when asked to solve tasks which present formal operational problems in the laboratory. Piaget[234] discussed the implications of his theory of cognitive development for adults and presented three possible interpretations of the differences in adult cognition: (1) There may be differences in the speed of development as a function of the quality and amount of intellectual stimulation received; therefore formal operations could fail to develop under certain conditions or be delayed until the conditions needed to support its emergence are met. (2) Aptitudes may diversify with age; thus, formal operations might not be a universal stage but rather a structured advancement in particular areas of specialization. This, however, seems unlikely, as Piaget notes. It would seem foolish to assume a different cognitive structure for members of various professions. (3) All normal individuals reach formal operations; however, they are expressed most appropriately within the domain of professional specialization or aptitude. The third proposition would appear to fit the data best. Sinnot[233] found that age differences in the ability to solve formal operational problems were reduced when the materials were familiar rather than abstract, and when the subjects had college degrees.

Kuhn, Langer, Kohlberg and Haan[235] investigated the development of formal operations over the age range of 10 to 50 in a set of studies which employed two measures of formal operations that were scored qualitatively as to the level within formal operations achieved by the subjects, and compared levels of logical reasoning with the development of levels of moral reasoning. Although none of the subjects had fully achieved formal operational reasoning, there was an increase with age, up to the age 21–30 group, in the level of formal reasoning achieved, with a slight but not significant proportion of the oldest group (45–50) at a somewhat lower level. The age relationship for levels of principled moral reasoning was similar. Comparing the patterns of logical and moral reasoning, intelligence was measured and level of intellectual performance was related to level of achievement of principled levels of moral development. Most of the analyses in this excellent monograph focus on the relationships among stages of logical and moral development, thus the age relationships were not highlighted. Yet the results suggest acceptable levels of formal thought and moral reasoning through age 50.

Not all researchers see the Piagetian approach as the best way to explore cognitive development in the adult years. Arlin[236] postulated a fifth stage of cognitive development, drawing on the work in creativity, which suggest that increases in divergent thinking abilities and more long-term patterns of dealing with ideas would better represent the contents of this stage. She developed a measure of problem finding as an index of divergent thinking abilities[222-225] and, with a group of college seniors, reported evidence supporting her hypothesis. In a replication of her study with a broader age range (18–35), no evidence for such a stage of cognitive development was found. However, there was not enough information about the subjects to evaluate the reason for this lack of replication. Riegel[238] has developed a dialectic view of human development. He argues that Piagetian theory is an inappropriate framework for understanding cognitive development, particularly in adults. Riegel suggests that it is improbable that adults use formal operational strategies except in exceptional circumstances, and that they would rarely calculate all possible outcomes in a situation before making a decision, although the individual would have the capacity to do so. Riegel proposes that dialectical operations are characteristic of mature thought and that the acceptance of contradiction and the ability to operate at all of Piaget's levels of thought as the situation demands are indeed the hallmarks of adult cognition. Dialectic paradigms emphasize the situational determinants of behavior and thus should provide important data about cognitive development in adult life. As the major part of the literature from the dialectical perspective has been theoretical,[239] it is still too soon to evaluate the empirical usefulness of the paradigm in studies of adult development and aging.

PSYCHOLOGY AS A SOCIAL SCIENCE

In this section psychological studies of personality, adjustment, and the interaction of the individual in complex social environments (the family, society) are reviewed. In contrast to the natural science aspects of psychology, the research and theory reported here tend to come from organismic/qualitative models of development rather than mechanistic/quantitative models. In this literature, age plays a less important role, with the emphasis more often on stage of life. There are broad-gauged descriptions of the psychological reality of midlife and old age. The current work on midlife is somewhat reminiscent of earlier work in adolescence, postulating an internally caused crisis exacerbated by escalating external demands. The "midlife crisis" is a will-o'-the-wisp, often reported in studies which focus intensively on the lives of their respondents but are not, in general, confirmed by studies which include large numbers of middle-aged persons. In old age, the focus is less often on internal feelings, and the image of crisis is replaced by a concern with the individual's capacity to adapt to an increasingly hostile world. The imagery of old age is that of loss. As in the intelligence data, the findings are significantly more optimistic than common stereotypes.

This literature has its own set of methodological problems. Experimental paradigms are of limited usefulness. Most studies report careful observations and descriptions of behavior assessed by inter-

viewers according to a particular rating system, or by so-called "objective" measures of personality which are primarily self-report indices. In addition, the appropriate frame of reference for the time scale of the development of various aspects of personality is not agreed upon. Nonetheless, at least at the descriptive level, this literature has been successful in elucidating a set of patterns of adult development and of aging. An excellent review of the issues in current life span personality research is given by Livson.[240]

Personality

Major theorists in personality have been primarily concerned with achievement of adult status, and not personality development during adult life and old age. There are three notable exceptions: Bühler,[241,242] Jung,[243,244] and Erikson.[245,246] The contributions of their work are discussed in three excellent review papers by Havighurst[247] and Neugarten.[248,249] Bühler studied the life cycle by charting the importance of motives and goals at different phases of development by the use of published biographies and clinical material. Bühler's framework formed the basis for Kuhlen's work.[1,28,250,251] Kuhlen suggested that the first half of life was organized by motives for growth and expansion, while the second half of life was organized by motives related to conservation and constriction as a way of dealing with increased threats. There has not been very much other developmental work on motivation across the life cycle; however, White's work on the development of competence motivation[252,253] would appear to have substantial implications across the life cycle,[254] but, as yet, this has not been well worked out or translated into researchable terms in adult life and aging. In similar fashion, Jung's theoretical formulations suggest the necessity for the reorganization of personality at midlife, but research which makes use of these insights is still rare.[255] Erikson's psychosocial, developmental formulations, which divide the life cycle into eight stages, give the tasks of intimacy versus isolation to young adulthood, generativity versus stagnation to midlife, and ego-integrity versus despair to old age. His ideas have been instrumental in perspectives which seek to define specific developmental tasks for each age period[247] and in perspectives which define psychological maturity and adjustment within the requirements of each stage of the lifecycle.[256] The research literature is reviewed in four overlapping sections: antecedents of adult personality, developmental changes within the adult years, coping and adaptation, and personality and coping in old age.

Antecedents of Adult Personality. The research reported in this section comes from three of the longest ongoing developmental studies, the Fels Study (birth through mid-twenties);[257,258] Terman's study of intellectually gifted children (from childhood through the sixties);[110,111,171,172,259-261] and the Institute of Human Development Studies at Berkeley (infancy and childhood through the fifties).[262-274]

In the Fels Study, the data, including psychological tests, behavioral observations, and interview materials, were rated for four periods during childhood (0-3, 3-6, 6-10, 10-14) and one adult follow-up session (age 19-29, average age, 24) for 71 children who had data at all of the ages of interest. Rating scales were developed for a set of behaviors of interest. The results indicated a fairly high degree of stability of behavior based on the correlations of the ratings of different time periods, and significant sex differences. Behaviors that exhibited stability for both sexes were: indices of achievement and mastery, anxiety in social interaction, and introspection. Behaviors that were stable for men but not for women were: aggression, sexual activity and anxiety, and physical harm anxiety. Behaviors that were stable for women but not for men were dependency and fear of failure. Ratings of compulsivity were unstable for both sexes, and ratings of nurturance had a complex pattern.[257] In an adult assessment at ages (18-26) of an additional 74 children, intellectual achievement was predictable for both sexes but opposite characteristics predicted academic achievement for males and females.[258] The results of the Fels studies are important in exploring the role that socialization plays in personality development. Their findings are consistent with sex-role socialization practices in the decades studied (1929-39; 1957-59).

Terman's study of gifted children started in 1921 and included 1,528 children in the superior IQ range. Most of the children were from the 1910 cohort and were aged about 11 at the start of the study. The subjects were retested in 1927, 1940, and 1950 and followed-up by mail in 1936, 1945, 1955, 1960, 1972, and 1977. The overall purpose of the study was to investigate the consequences of superior intellectual endowment. There were relatively few measures of personality *per se*, but the subjects were regularly evaluated for mental and physical health and for achievements and interests in work, family, and community participation. The sample as a whole maintained excellent physical and mental health; and while there were a few suicides and mental breakdowns, the level of mental illness was generally less (3%) than reported for the general population.[111] Personality was assessed by ratings made by the subjects, by their spouses, and by their parents and was used primarily to explore the differences in achievement between the 150 most successful and 150 least successful men in the study population. As the groups were equal in intelligence, the four personality factors that best discriminated the groups were: persistence in accomplishment of end, integration towards goals, self-confidence, and freedom from inferiority feelings.[111,172] In general, these superior children became superior adults. R. R. Sears[259] investigated sources of life satisfaction and predictors of coping style in the gifted men at age 62. The results indicated a high degree of consistency in affective feelings and constructs pertaining to the self. P. H. Sears and Barbee[260] investigated sources of life satisfaction and career choices in the Terman women at age 62. Measures of satisfaction were more complex for the women, as there were various patterns of childbearing and work histories for the group. Marriage was generally positive, and the findings for having children vary with the particular combination of work and career paths of the women. Three types of satisfaction were studied: general, work pattern, and joy in living. Early ratings of self-confidence and attachments to their own parents were particularly important contributors to these women's sense of satisfaction 30 years after the measurements were made. Data from the most recent follow-up[261] has not yet been reported. However, this extraordinary study has the potential to tell us much about the life styles, choices, and patterns of aging.

The Berkeley studies [262-274] have also made extraordinary contributions to our understanding of human development. A bibliography of publications from the Berkeley studies and reprints of 63 of the publications through 1970 are found in a volume edited by Jones, Bayley, Macfarlane, and Honzig.[262] The Berkeley studies contain three major studies: the Guidance Study, which started in 1928, and included regular assessments between the ages of 21 months to 18 years, with adult follow-ups at approximately ages 30 and 40; the Berkeley Growth Study, started in 1928, with frequent assessments between 4 days old to 15 months, every 3 months until 3 years of age, every 6 months to age 18, with follow-ups at ages 21, 26, and 36; and the Oakland Growth Study, started in 1932, with periodic assessments from the ages of 11 through 45. Findings from the Berkeley Growth Study have primarily concerned the growth of intelligence.[275] In addition the parents of the children have been studied, once at age 30 and again at age 70.[272] Most of the adult personality data comes from adult assessments of the Guidance and Oakland Growth Study children.

The major assessment of personality has been with the Q-sort. The Q-sort[263,264] is a complex rating system where descriptors of personality traits or characteristics are sorted into a forced distribution (e.g., for 100 items, the distribution would be 5, 8, 12, 16, 18, 16, 12, 8, 5) with equal numbers of statements rated most and least characteristic on a 9-point scale. These ratings derived from the Q-sort form the basic set of data that can then be analyzed by a variety of techniques. The Q-sorts can be performed on the basis of an interview with the subjects, or, as was more often the case, by reading the full case records for each subject for a specific time period. An index of psychological adjustment was constructed by having trained clinicians do a Q-sort for a hypothetical, maximally adjusted person. The correlation of the observed Q scores with this ideal Q-sort is thus taken as an index of adjustment. This set of methods provides extremely rich personality descriptions which can then be combined in various typologies. The reader is referred to the original sources for the specifics of the findings; general patterns of results are described below.

Block and Haan[263,265] developed Q descriptions of personality for three age ranges from the Oakland Growth and Guidance studies: junior high school, senior high school, and adulthood (30 or 37). Seven patterns of sameness and change were evaluated for the 100 characteristics over the three time periods. The men were more stable than the women, particularly in terms of cognitive orientations, dependability, and impulsivity. Indices of productivity converged for the men with increased age, and measures relating to interpersonal skills diverged. None of the traits for the women met the criteria for sameness. Persistence in personal style was seen (traditional feminine versus rebellious) as well as the distribution of cognitive-intuitive orientation. For both sexes there were trends for increases in conventional femininity and psychological mindedness, convergence for measures of responsibility and self-control, and divergence for measures of self-resiliency and bodily concern. The results of this set of analyses were compared to the findings from the Fels Study[257] on variables that had been defined in similar ways. While the overall findings of sex differences were confirmed, the results did not replicate on a construct by construct basis. Typologies were then developed by factor-analyzing the data at junior high school and adulthood as a single set of measures for men and women separately, in order to develop patterns of personality development which included both characteristics at both points in time and the observed transformations. The men were classified into five types, the women into six types, with a residual category for each sex, classifying about 75% of each sex into the various types. The 11 types developed represent a large number of styles. In general, there were two adaptive styles for the men and two for the women. In the first types for each sex (Ego Resilient men; Female Prototype women), the pattern of development was progressive with increasingly adapted scores and characteristics at each phase studied. The second adjusted types (Belated Adjusters (men) and Cognitive Copers (women)) indicated patterns of recovery from less than ideal descriptions in junior or senior high school profiles. Other correlates of the types and full descriptions are presented in Block.[263] Haan[265] provides a succinct review of the findings discussed,[263] noting that there were no universal patterns observed and that patterns of both continuity and discontinuity were related to good adjustment as adults, and points out that the average correlation between Q-types at senior high school and adulthood was about .50, and that the developmental patterns observed were sex-typed.

Peskin and Livson[260] looked at personality development in 31 men and 33 women from the guidance study using Q-sort data from ages 5–7, 8–10, 11–13, 14–16, and age 30, with the ideal Q-sort at age 30 as the criterion for psychological health. They reported that the data from 11–13 appeared to be the most predictive and that the data from ages 14–16 tended to be in the opposite direction from both the earlier and the adult data. They suggest that their results imply that an adolescent crisis is predictive of adult mental health.

Haan and Day[267] added the findings at the second adult follow-up (ages 40–44 and 47–51) for the subjects in the earlier studies.[263,265] Criteria were developed in order to assess the patterns of changes in the 100 Q-traits across 4 times of measurement for 4 samples (the men and women in each of the 2 studies). The Q-traits were organized into four groups: information processing skills, interpersonal reactions, responses to socialization, and presentation of self. Statistical criteria were developed in order to differentiate unaltered sameness, where both the rank order of the trait were the same; transposition, where the order of the subjects was maintained but the level of the trait changed in importance; and systematic changes that did not preserve individual differences, which was called experimental change. Block[268] pointed out that some of the coefficients had been incorrectly calculated, and thus the data were reanalyzed and presented in Haan.[269] Traits related to presentation of self were the most stable, with responses to socialization primarily stable. Interpersonal reaction traits were found in all three categories of change, as were information processing skills. However, the information processing traits were the most likely to be in the experimental change category.

Livson[270] focused her analysis on personality change in women during midlife. She studied 24 women from the Oakland Growth Study at ages 11, 18, 40, and 50. At age 50, against the criterion of the ideal Q-sort, there were two very different groups of women, 17 called traditionalists who had maintained a highly adjusted Q-picture in the decade from 40 to 50 compared to a group of 7 women called independents whose adjustment at 40 had been minimal, but who by age 50 were as equally adjusted as the first group. She found that the traditionalists had fairly well completed Erikson's tasks and, given that their personality style was consistent with cultural demands, had displayed a relatively continuous pattern of development. The independents had a rougher time, with low points both in early adolescence and at age 40. She suggests that these women displayed a midlife crisis of sorts, yet they were able to reorganize and restructure their lives by age 50 as Jung would predict. Honzig and Macfarlane[271] investigated the personality correlates of intellectual growth in the Guidance Study of men and women from childhood through age 40. Overall IQ was quite stable with correlations between age 18 and 40 equal to .74 and .75 and between age 6 and 40 equal to .60. They used Q-sort personality descriptions of the first 18 years of life, at 30, and at 40 to investigate differences between the 7 men and 3 women who had gained at least 8 full-scale IQ points by the age of 40. As children, these individuals had been rated as less gregarious and less sex role stereotyped; at age 30 they were more likely to be satisfied with the appearance and to be turned to for advice. In a second analysis, they evaluated the relationship between personality factors and intellectual achievement at age 40. For women, more of the childhood variables were predictive, whereas for men, more of the variables at age 30 were predictive. They reported the particular characteristics at each age for each sex. However, their most interesting finding was that measures of social intelligence did not appear to be related to measures of intellectual performance. One further study is mentioned briefly here, but will be reported in more detail in the section on coping and adaptation. Maas and Kuypers[272] studied the parents of the children who were first interviewed when they were about 30 years of age and again when they were 70 years of age. They used Q-sort personality descriptions and measures of ego defenses[273] as well as measures of the current lifestyles of the participants. In general, the men were more consistent than the women, and there were no direct relationships between personality patterns and life style clusters in old age.

Clausen[274] developed occupational, family, and marriage histories for these subjects and reported that continuity, rather than crisis at midlife, appeared to best describe the subjects as a whole.

The findings from the Berkeley studies are complex, and it is difficult to evaluate the various particular findings from the variety of analyses done. However, in general these studies suggest that (1) continuity of personality is more often reported than discontinuity; (2) there appear to be 4–6 reliably different patterns of development for both men and women; (3) at least in the developmental history of the men and women studied, sex differences are significant in determining those patterns; (4) personality changes cannot be understood without reference to the socio-historical conditions operating at the time; and (5) continuity of personality does not mean complete identity of personality characteristics over time. Thus, even if future research fails to replicate all of the specific findings of the Berkeley studies, their major finding will stand. Naïve views of personality development during adulthood are surely wrong. The precise specification of the "laws" of such development remain a challenge for the future.

Developmental Changes in the Adult Years. Midlife appears to be the new developmental stage. Keniston[276] notes that childhood and adolescence are relatively modern concepts whose emergence was tied to particular social and economic conditions. He argues for the emergence of a new optional stage, called youth (between adolescence and adulthood), as a result of the particular conditions of the 1960s. The characterizations of this youth stage are similar to current conceptions of midlife with a state of tension between self and society, a major issue of movement versus stasis, fear of death, and ideological conflict as some of the major descriptors. One can hypothesize that the current conceptualizations of midlife crisis are reactions of an earlier generation who were too old to be in the stage of youth but nonetheless faced the same issues. Cox[277] studied a group of college student leaders of the classes 1946–1952 and found reasonable progress towards adult status during the first 10 years following graduation. Two recent books have focused on midlife: Vaillant's report of the Grant Study Subjects, a prospective longitudinal study between the ages of 18–50,[278,279] and Levinson and his colleagues' report of their investigation of the adult lives of 40 men aged 35–45.[280–282]

The Grant Study men were selected from the 1939–41 and 1942–44 classes at Harvard on the basis of their independence, academic performance and overall psychological soundness. They were intensively studied as undergraduates and followed regularly by mail after graduation. The original group included 268 men. A random selection of 95 men from the classes of 1942–44 were interviewed around the time of their 25th college reunion. Vaillant's major analyses are aimed at exploring the components of adaptation and mental health in this sample, and he develops a typology of defensive styles which he suggests mature during adulthood. He further divides the sample into the best and worst outcomes and looks at predictors of success, defined by traditional criteria within this group of elite and relatively successful men. Thus his findings are not organized in a fashion to speak to patterns of psychological development during the adult years. He reports that intimacy, career consolidation and generativity are the major tasks of the decades of the twenties, thirties and forties, and that, when a midlife crisis occurs, it generally implies a reorganization that leads to increased adjustment. One of the most important aspects of this study is that retrospective data (the subjects' statements when interviewed in midlife about their college years) could be checked with the archival materials in the files. Vaillant reports that often the past had been transformed to give a better fit with the individuals' current life situation.[278] Thus, when the data consists of biographical material, it is important to remember that,

aside from any potential effects of memory, the data are a reconstruction of the past which is influenced by the outcome of events, and may or may not be a "true" reflection of past. However, even longitudinal data do not always provide the optimal information: it is the rare study that is able to anticipate all of the questions that should be asked early in the study so that, 20–25 years later, the data will reflect the current concerns of the investigators.

Levinson's work[280–282] is primarily concerned with building a theory of adult development, which started with its focus on midlife. The theory developed from an intensive study of 40 men aged 35–45. The men were members of four occupational groups: hourly workers, executives, academic biologists, and novelists; were born between 1923–34; and were primarily interviewed in 1969. The data consisted of life history interviews supplemented by some psychological testing. The main finding of the study is the theory of adult development that emerged from the interviews, with the relatively narrow age ranges attached to the stages of adult development. The theory and findings are summarized in a recent book.[282] Adult life is organized into eras: 0–22, 17–45, 40–65, 60–80?, 80?–?. These eras are further subdivided into periods of stability and transition, with the transitional stages providing linkages between the eras. The major task of adult development is to build a life structure. This life structure is composed of the choices made by the individual and the consequences of those choices. The stages are described as sequential and age-linked but not hierarchical. Thus, in contrast to the cognitive stage theories, the same level of operations occurs at each stage; it is the content of the stage that is different. Each stage has its own set of tasks that are important to building the life structure at that phase of the lifecycle. In the transitional stages between the stable periods, evaluations of the life structure are made, and things are reorganized. The names of the life stages are descriptive and the modal age ranges are: 22–28—Entering the Adult

World; 28–33—Age 30 Transition; 33–40—Settling Down; 40–45—Midlife Transition; 45–50—Entering Middle Adulthood; 50–55—Age 50 Transition; 55–60—Culmination of Middle Adulthood; 60–65—Late Adult Transition. Transitional stages are reported as such by 60–80% of the respondents. The tasks given for each period of the lifecycle are not surprising and involve building a career, a family, and a self. Levinson and his colleagues place special importance on the building of a dream as an important component of the life structure, on the provisional nature of choices made until the midthirties, and on the emotional and psychic components of the midlife transition. The system of adult development builds on the theoretical work of Erickson, Jung, Bühler and Frenkel-Brunswick[283] and is particularly concerned with the role of individuation during the midlife transition and the confrontation with death and issues of mortality.[284] The book is a fine summary not only of the work of Levinson and his group but also of most of the major writings on midlife.

There are other excellent discussions of the character of midlife.[285-288] Neugarten and Datan[285] emphasize the social matrix surrounding midlife and the special concerns that revolved around power, responsibility and control. For men, they suggest midlife concerns are more often played out in the work place, and for women within the family. Levinson's study included no women, but findings reviewed in the book suggest that the same structure will probably hold.[282] Neugarten and Datan also review the epidemiological literature suggests to that patterns of mental health and illness at midlife do not support the view of a generalized crisis at this time of life; rather, they point to the timing of events as one predictor of crisis. Brim[286] reviewed the evidence for a male midlife crisis, and, while generally supportive of the transitional nature of midlife, did not conclude that such a crisis was generally to be predicted. Rosenberg and Ferrell[287] review the imagery of midlife and find themes similar to those

of Levinson; additionally, their reading of the epidemiological literature suggests to them that crisis in midlife is fairly widespread. Bardwick[288] defines the crisis as one of self-awareness and self-definition, with an existential flavoring. She reports that the mid-life concerns of professional women are more likely to be similar to men. Thus, while there is a wide acceptance of the components of midlife and of the nature of the transitions that must be made, there is little agreement as to whether this should be considered a crisis. Research paradigms that rate the level of emotional involvement tend to support the notion of crisis: paradigms that focus on adaptation or adjustment do not tend to support the notion of crisis. However, as both sets of paradigms may be talking about different parts of the same process, this gap may not be as wide as it seems from a reading of the literature.

Costa and McCrae[289] report one of the few studies designed to test the notion of a male midlife crisis. A 36-item scale was developed that focused on midlife concerns and symptoms. The items were based on Gould's[290] analysis of midlife, which is similar in content to the work discussed above.[282] The midlife crisis scale was administered to a group of 315 men aged 33–79. There were no differences between midlife and post-midlife groups. The scores approached statistical significance only for the contrast of 45–50 versus 50–55. The total scores on the scales were correlated with other personality measures, and the scale correlated .51 with neuroticism and .15 with extroversion. As these traits were measured approximately 10 years before the midlife measure, Costa and McCrae conclude that midlife crisis represents longstanding psychological problems. Most men in the study did not experience a midlife crisis, and for those who reported problems with similar content, there was no particular age range that emerged. This research area has become a "hot" one. Thus, when the results of studies currently in progress are available, a clearer picture of adult development during the midlife crisis period (40–45) should become available. Most of the work on personality and adjustment has not been focused on the intrapsychic aspects of personality. Rather, there has been a concern with the psychological components of personality as they interact with changes in the social structure and responses to particular events characteristic of various phases of the lifecycle (retirement, empty nest). Emphasis is given to studies which focus on the psychological components of personality and adjustment as social factors are reviewed in Chapter 9.

In her recent review on personality and aging, Neugarten[249] is pessimistic about the state of the art. Other reviews of the personality literature[289,291] are not quite as pessimistic but agree that, while there is evidence for both stability and change of personality during middle and later life, it is difficult to fully document either position, particularly for specific personality traits. Neugarten,[249] after reviewing the literature on a large set of traits, found consistent evidence only for increased introversion. Personality research shares the same measurement problems as the intelligence literature. However, there are fewer agreed-upon personality measures that are used consistently across studies. Often the failure to replicate a particular finding can be as easily explained by the use of a different scale to measure the construct as by anything else about the respondents. Changes in physical health have been shown to have only a small effect on personality[292] but a somewhat larger role in studies of personality change.[293] Methods of measuring personality are not, in general, as reliable as measures of learning, memory, or intelligence. The unreliability of the measures makes the assessment of stability or change much more difficult[30,31] and may also account for part of the lack of convergence in this literature.

For many years, personality research was concerned with arguments about disengagement theory.[249,291,294] Briefly, disengagement theory (introduced in 1960–61) postulated a mutual withdrawal of both the older individual and society that met the needs of all concerned. The critical index of disengagement theory was the relationship between degree of activity or social engagement and its relationship to life satisfaction, psychological well-being, or morale. The research that followed[295-300] found various personality types within the older population (4–6 types were common) that had multiple relationships to activity level and satisfaction and indicated that disengagement was an appropriate prediction for only a small subsample of older persons. Yet this controversy provided a major stimulus for research in personality[247,301] and for research on lifestyle patterns during middle and late life.[302]

As in the cognitive literature, dialectical perspectives, which relate inner biological and psychological changes to outer historical and social events, have produced an excellent set of thoughtful essays[303-306] which are particularly relevant to studies of dynamic relationships within the family. Relatively few studies have been concerned with the inner dynamics of personality change. Gruen[307] and Peck and Berkowitz[308] evaluated the Eriksonian adult stages by use of interviews and projective tests data. Both studies used individuals aged 40–65 and neither study reported any consistent age relationships among the Eriksonian stages. However age differences have been reported in dream content,[309] daydreams,[310] and themes assessed by projective tests.[311] Neugarten and Gutmann,[311] in a now classic study, investigated the responses of subjects aged 45–70 to a specially designed TAT (Thematic Apperception Test) card which was called the adult family scene. The card had four figures, two men, two women, who were either relatively young or relatively old. The card was consistently seen as a two generation family. The subjects were asked to tell a story about the card and to give an age and a description to each of the characters. The results indicated that, as the respondents aged, the roles of the characters changed. For the younger subjects, the older man was seen as dominant, the older woman nurturant; but, for the older subjects, (split at 55) the reverse was true. The evidence for the interaction of age and sex changes is strong and consistent in the patterns of changes seen with age. This finding has been supported by studies which used paper and pencil measures of personality or personality inventories.

Studies of personality measured with objective tests used primarily for research purposes have been concerned with the assessment of stability and change in personality during the adult years and, where the design makes it possible, with the attribution of any age changes to maturational process or to cohort effects. Reliable age differences have been reported with a number of instruments: the Edwards Personal Preference Schedule,[312,313] Cattell's Sixteen Personality Factor Questionnaire (16PF).[58,289,314-317] The Guilford-Zimmerman Temperment Survey,[318] the interpersonal check list,[293,318] and the California Test of Personality.[320] In studies which have included both men and women,[313,316-320] there tend to be more sex differences than age differences and, in general, the sex differences are stable across time.[316,317] In studies with longitudinal data,[289,315-318,320] more of the factors measured are stable than show any reliable change with age. This is true of the cross-sectional studies as well,[312-314] where fewer age differences are reported than sex differences and the general picture is one of trait stability. Studies that evaluate the contribution of age and cohort in accounting for the observed age changes generally report more cohort differences,[316,320] or an equal number,[318] or in all cases more change attributed to age/cohort where it can be separated than to the time over which the subjects have been studied (generally 7–10 years).[315-318] Thus, at the trait level of personality measurement, the results indicate stability of the majority of traits, with little agreement about which of the few traits that change with age change across studies and instruments, and stability of sex differences in measures of personality. There are also no clear findings on the role of changes in personality and changes in ability.[312,321]

A large number of other social psychological indices which are related to personality have been studied, e.g., social responsibility,[322] self-concept,[323] locus of control,[324-337] openness to experience,[289,314,315] person perception,[338-341] as well as a number of constructs that relate to both personality and cognitive styles,[227,343] egocentrism,[342] cognitive tempo (reflexive versus impulsive),[344] coronary prone personality (Type A),[345] field independence versus field dependence,[346] and cautiousness or rigidity.[17,61,93-95,121,145,146,291,247] No age differences have been reported for social responsibility, cognitive tempo, or Type A behavior (ages 50–90).[322,344,345] Consistent age differences have been reported, with older people more field dependent,[216,346] cautious and rigid.[17,61,93-95,121,145,146,291,347] There are complex relationships between rigidity or cautiousness and intellectual functioning. Differences in cautiousness sometimes disappear when the subjects are matched for intelligence, and differences in cognitive performance are reduced when the subjects are matched for cautiousness; however, the full nature of the relationship is not completely understood. There is evidence both for and against age differences in egocentrism[342,343] and openness to experience.[289,314,315]

The findings for person perception, self-concept and locus of control are more complex. Studies of person perception have age groups rate themselves (or their age peers) and persons of another age group on measures of personality or self-concept. These studies indicate a high degree of misperception across age groups. There is not, however, consistency about the characteristics that tend to be misperceived.

In a study of self-concept over the life cycle (ages 9–98), Monge[323] indicated that the same general factors of self-concept could be identified across the lifecycle achievement/leadership, congeniality/ sociability, adjustment, and masculinity/ femininity. There were age and sex differences in each of the components of self-concept and age by sex interactions for achievement and masculinity/femininity.

Sex differences on these two components of self-concept were large in young adulthood but tended to converge for the older subjects. Unpublished data from the Duke Adaptation Study indicated that the self-concept is stable over a 6-year period.[348] Studies of age relationships and changes in self-concept are important in understanding adult personality. This should be an important area for future research.

Locus of control[337] is a construct that describes a belief system about the relationship between individual action and responsibility and outcomes. Internal locus of control is the belief that reinforcements are related to behavior, or that your own behavior is causal in determining what happens, and implies responsibility for one's own actions. External locus of control is a belief in fate, chance, or powerful others having primary control or responsibility for what happens. A variety of scales which force a choice between two alternatives (one internal, one external), comprise the major locus of control scales. Special instruments have been developed to measure locus of control in institutional settings.[333] Locus of control is a construct that is related to perception of responsibility and control rather than actual responsibility and control. Locus of control, in the general social psychological literature,[349,350] has been related to numerous characteristics. The development of internal control is seen as a relevant therapeutic outcome, and internal control has been related to measures of achievement, success, adaptation and adjustment. Aging studies have been concerned with the level of internality/externality observed across the lifespan and with locus of control as a measure of adjustment or adaptation in the elderly. In a set of cross-sectional studies,[325-328,330] older people have been found to be as internal as college students, or more internal, through age 60. After age 60, either the same level of internality is maintained, or the subjects become more external.[331,333,335] Externality is more likely to be reported when the older subjects are institutionalized. Internal control has also been related to increased levels of ad-

justment and indices of success in middle-aged and community-dwelling older persons;[329-332,334-336] however, externality was related to adaptation in institutionalized subjects.[331,333] Three questions remain: (1) the level of locus of control in old age; (2) whether internality or externality is more adaptive for older persons; and (3) the longitudinal stability of locus of control. Differences in locus of control scales and dimensions within locus of control suggest that some components of locus of control should be stable and not change with age, while other components are expected to vary as a function of experience, suggesting that both linear increases in internality and a curvilinear shift to externality may be a true representation of the cross-sectional data.[351] The adaptive nature of locus of control is most likely related to the environmental situation of the person. Longitudinal work with locus of control suggests that for about 70% of middle-aged and older people locus of control is stable; however, about 15% of the sample changed from internal to external or vice-versa over a 6-year period. The meaning of the patterns is being explored.[352]

Coping and Adaptation

Coping and adaptation, from a life span perspective, have been studied primarily by focusing on significant life events and the responses to those events. One view considers life events as normative life crises.[7] The events are mainly events that are part of the family lifecycle. In a superb chapter, Hultsch and Plemons[353] reviewed the literature on life events. They suggest that two models (mechanistic or traditional versus organismic or lifecycle) are seen in this literature. Traditional models of stress and adaptation see events as potentially stressful stimuli that require adaptation. This tradition is best represented by the work of Meyer,[354] Selye,[355] and Holmes and Rahe.[356] The most common index of maladaptation in this context, is physical illness. In general, this research has not been concerned with special problems of aging, but has instead focused on specifying various models of adaptation and measurement of the characteristics associated with events, represented most prominently by the work of the Dohrenwends.[357] Recent findings from Duke's second longitudinal study on stress and adaptation[358-360] illustrate the application of this paradigm to middle-aged and older persons. The study included 375 individuals aged 45–70 who were followed over a 6-year period (1969–1975). Five common life events were selected for study: subject's retirement, spouses' retirement, widowhood, last child leaving home, and a major physical illness which required hospitalization. Of the study population, 36.5% (137 individuals) experienced none of the five events over the six year study period. All subjects were at risk for experiencing a major medical event, whereas the likelihood of experiencing the other events varied (e.g., one must have a job to retire from, a spouse to be widowed or experience the retirement of a working spouse). In this study population, 61.6% were eligible for retirement, 45% for spouses' retirement, 54.8% for widowhood, and 29.8% for having the last child leave home. The percentages of elligible individuals actually experiencing the event were: 33.7% retired, 46.15% had a spouse retire, 7.86% were widowed, 50.89% had the last child leave home, and 63.56% experienced a major medical event. The incidence of the events is presented in some detail to illustrate a major problem with research in this area: if one wishes to look at adaptation to typical events during the life course of middle-aged and older persons, one can only hope to have a sufficiently large sample that enough events happen to permit conclusions to be drawn. A different approach is to pick individuals who are specifically likely to be at risk for such events; but, as the data presented above indicate, this varies event by event. A simple model of adaptation was developed that evaluated the adaptation to the events. In this model, the individual's resources were considered to moderate the event, both in potentially determining whether an event would happen and in

determining the response to the event. Three groups of resources measured at the start of the study were considered: health, as measured by level of physical functioning; psychological resources, a combination of intelligence and adaptive capacity as measured by the Cattell 16PF factor Q_{II}; and social resources, measured as a combination of income, education and the density of the social network. The results indicated that, when subjects who experienced events were compared to a control group (those eligible for the event who did not experience it), only level of psychological resources was related to experiencing events: that is, those with low psychological resources were more likely to experience events. The events were then looked at separately. Those with lower health resources were more likely to retire and to experience a major medical event during the study, those with lower social resources were more likely to become widowed, and those with low psychological resources were more likely to have a major medical event. Thus, these resource variables, measured before any of the events that were included in the study occurred, were differentially related to the experiencing of events.[358] Resources also played a role in the adaptation to the events, when adaptation was indexed by a series of health indices[359] or by measures of self-esteem, activity, and life satisfaction.[360] An analysis of the response to the events indicated a homeostatic pattern of response: an initial disorganization tended to return to pre-event levels of functioning for the health indicators[359] and for social-psychological indices, some positive effects were associated with the last child leaving home, no effects were determined for spouses' retirement, essentially no effects for medical events, small declines were observed in life satisfaction, and some increases in activity were reported after retirement and widowhood. Thus, when adaptation to potentially disorganizing events is studied over time, the level of adaptation tends to be higher than one would expect. If the individual's response had been studied immediately after the event, the negative effects most likely would have been stronger.

A different approach to this same area is the work done by Marjorie Fiske Lowenthal and her colleagues.[361,366] This research is more in the organismic tradition and focuses on groups of individuals dealing with a particular event. Thus groups of individuals are sampled because they are going through major transitional periods of the lifecycle (high school seniors, newlyweds, middle-aged persons whose youngest child is a high school senior, and individuals who are planning to retire). The study of these four groups of individuals was designed as a longitudinal study to measure the individuals before the event and then five years later. The findings from the initial evaluation are presented in an interesting volume by Lowenthal, Thurner and Chiriboga.[363] Their findings about friendship patterns, lifestyles, self-concept, well-being, time perspective and value orientations will not be reviewed here; rather, the concentration will be on their model of adaptation, stress, and adaptation to stress.

The study included 261 subjects with approximately equal numbers of males and females at each stage of life. The approximate mean ages of the groups were 17, 24, 50 and 60 years old; the subjects were primarily working and middle class and lived in San Francisco neighborhoods. The data included an intensive interview of social and psychological characteristics, some psychological testing, the TAT and two WAIS subtests (vocabulary and block design), and personality ratings derived from the items from Block's Q-sort.[264] A model of adaptation was developed that included measures of psychological resources (intelligence and ratings for accommodation, growth, hope, and mutuality) and psychological deficits (reported emotional problems, symptoms, and assessments of anxiety and hostility from the responses to the projective tests). Overall, about 25% of the sample reported emotional problems, with most reported by the newlyweds. The two younger groups were more accommo-

dating, more growth-oriented, and more hopeful. There were no age differences in mutuality. Respondents were then classified into a typology where psychological resources and deficits were considered jointly. This resulted in two major types of persons: the complex who were high on both, and the simple who were low on both. Relatively complex younger people and relatively simple older people were reported to be the best adjusted.

An interesting stress typology was also developed by cross-classifying people on the basis of high or low presumed stress and whether or not the stress was perceived by raters as thematic in the interview material. This resulted in four groups: of those with frequent or severe stress—the challenged (those for whom the material was not thematic) and the overwhelmed (those who indicated high stress in the interview) and for those with infrequent or midstress: self-defeating (those in whom stress was thematic) and the lucky (those in whom it was not thematic). Interestingly enough, while the older groups had experienced more stress (as much as a function of time as of age), the biggest shift was between the high school seniors and the newlyweds; and there were few age differences in the way that the two younger and two older groups were distributed among the four cells of the stress typology. For those with presumed heavy stress, the percentages of overwhelmed and challenged were nearly identical, 32% and 30.5% for the overwhelmed and 18.5% and 18% for the challenged in the two age groups. There were very slight age differences in the two light-stress groups, with about 4% more of the young overwhelmed (19 versus 23) and 4% of the old lucky (26 versus 31). Sex differences were larger than age differences, with more women reporting stress. Overall, the sex differences in the study were more striking than the age differences. This was particularly true for their middle-aged women (age 50). No age range was given for this group, who were defined by having their last child as a high school senior. It would appear that this group is about 10 years older than Levinson's midlife males but one cannot conclude that the men have completed their midlife crisis and are thus better adjusted than the women, who may be having their crisis ten years later. Even though these subjects were selected particularly because they were undergoing transitions, there was little evidence of planning. The results of their five year follow-up should be fascinating.

Personality and Coping in Old Age

There are relatively few studies of personality development and coping from a psychological perspective in the very old (seventies, eighties, and nineties). Many of the studies of personality in the elderly were in response to disengagement theory and developed from various personality patterns that were found among the elderly;[295-298] however, in general these types were not age-related within the elderly range, nor were they studied longitudinally with an emphasis on personality changes within the elderly years. A second approach in this literature has been the use of personality tests as diagnostic instruments rather than as descriptors of normal personality.[367-369] This will be reviewed in another chapter of this volume. As there has been a renewed interest in the clinical psychology of aging,[370-372] this literature can be expected to grow in the future. Four sets of studies are reported here: findings from the NIH Human Aging Study; [187,188,292,374,375] the Newcastle studies;[189,376] Maas and Kuypers study of the Berkeley parents;[272] and work done at the University of Chicago by Lieberman and by Tobin and their colleagues. [15,186,377,378]

Singer[292] evaluated the performance of the 47 suprahealthy men in the NIH study on a variety of psychological tests used to assess personality and subtle aspects of cognitive functioning. The mean age of the group was 71 with a range from 65–91 years of age. The performance was not markedly different from what would be expected in the general adult population and there were no significant differences between the groups when evaluated for symptomatic disease; however, the performance of those with a symptomatic disease was in the direction of poorer performance. This indicated a smaller role for physical health than had been found for the cognitive and intellectual measures. However, for the 11 subjects who had been rated by psychiatrists to display "senile qualities"[373] poorer performance on these tests was noted. Analysis of the MMPI profiles of this group indicated only an elevated D (depression) scale.[374] At the 11-year follow-up the tests were treated cognitively, as personality factors were taken from the psychiatric exam, but were found to be related positively to survival.[375]

The Newcastle studies[376] included six different samples of older persons drawn from the community and from various institutional settings between 1964–1973. Personality was evaluated in normal and psychiatrically diagnosed groups of elderly. Most of the subjects were over 70 years of age and for the two community samples had mean ages of 74.8 years and 79.6 years. Different personality instruments were given to different samples, but the data set as a whole contains information on the MMPI, the Maudsley Personality Inventory, and Cattell's 16PF. The results indicated many more changes on the MMPI than had been previously reported when the scale scores were compared to adult norms; these differences were accentuated in the older subjects who had a psychiatric diagnosis of a functional illness and were not in general related to the age of the subjects between 70–90+ years of age. Neither extroversion nor neuroticism were found to be related to age within the samples, and, while many of the 16 factors assessed by Cattell's 16PF showed differences from the standardization sample, there were no age differences (but consistent sex differences) within the older population. A series of factor analyses were performed which indicated four personality patterns descriptive of these older persons. These patterns were also not age-related, suggesting considerable stability of personality patterns even in extreme old age. As these samples are so different from the typical young standardization samples to which they were compared, and a complete literature on these instruments with other samples is sparse in this age range, the particular cross-sectional age differences reported cannot as yet be fully evaluated.

Maas and Kuypers[272] studied 97 mothers and 47 fathers of the Berkeley children who were aged 60–82 at the time of their second testing. They developed 10 life style and 7 personality clusters for this group of parents and evaluated the antecedents of each of the clusters. As in other studies that developed personality typologies, a full range of styles were reported for each sex. The various personality types were reasonably well-distributed across the life-style clusters, and personality change was shown not to be related to significant life cycle transitions (e.g., retirement and widowhood) in this sample. Changes in physical health, however, were important in discriminating among the personality types. In general, there was greater continuity of personality among the mothers than the fathers, especially for the personality styles which included the fewest adaptive traits. There was greater continuity of life style patterns for the fathers.

These studies as a group suggest that, in old age, the view of personality is relatively consistent with the patterns identified in young adulthood and midlife. There is a large variability with no single personality pattern identified as characteristic of "the aged." Various personality trait measures have tended to find more stable sex differences than age differences. To the extent that personality change can be estimated from cross-sectional studies within old age, there appears to be a high degree of stability between adjacent age groups. There is insufficient longitudinal or sequential data to fully evaluate the stability of various traits in the later years.

The work of Lieberman and his colleagues[185,186,377,378] used measures of personality as a way of studying coping and adaptation in the very old. Coping and adaptation were studied in response to a particular stress often characteristic of old age: relocation into institutional settings. Lieberman[377] developed a model of adaptive processes in late life on the basis of a series of studies of various groups of older persons undergoing the stress of relocation. Approximately 870 older persons were studied who moved from the community into various homes for the aged, or were transferred between institutional facilities, or were elderly psychiatric patients being transferred between institutional facilities. The studies are particularly useful, as careful attention was paid to the assessment of appropriately selected and well-matched control populations. The measures included various cognitive, personality, and coping indices developed from interviews and projective tests. A model was developed which included measures of resources, current functioning (with measures of amount of stress and social support system as modifiers of current functioning), crisis management skills, and personality traits related to dealing with threats and losses and adaptive outcomes. The results of this set of studies indicated that coping and adaptation for the very old were different than the findings that had been reported for younger persons. The major defining element of the crisis for this population was seen to be related to the amount of change required of the persons, rather than to the perceptions of the crisis in terms of meaning of the event or the amount of loss entailed. The processes that were related to coping with loss were not the same processes that were related to coping with stress. Cognitive and physical resources were reported to act as a threshold: those with poor resources were unable to adapt, but good resources did not guarantee adaptive outcomes. Most interesting was a personality constellation that was related to survival and to adaptation to the crisis which included the traits of being aggressive, irritating, narcissistic and demanding. These results support a comment of Len Gottesman, "It's not that older people become crabby; but rather that crabby people live longer." Lieberman thus suggests that a special view of the components of mental health is required when working with the very old. Along with the aggressive personality constellation, the ability to maintain the self system and levels of hope, and the ability to introspect were found to be important parameters of adaptation.

Tobin and Lieberman[378] present the findings from an in depth study of the parameters involved in the processes of institutionalization in older persons. A few of the statistics they quote are important in order to put this work in perspective. The average age of the older person in a long-term care facility is 82 years old, with about 20% of the population residing in institutions over the age of 90. The figure that only 5% of the elderly reside in institutions of all types is well-known. However, when this figure is broken down by age, less than 2% of those 65–75 are in institutions, 7% of those 75–85, and 16% of those 85 and older. Thus, while institutionalization is a major fear of older people and their families, and a major social problem, the majority of even the very old do not reside in institutions.

The major population under study[378] included 100 older persons who were on waiting lists for three homes for the aged. Those with severe mental and physical illness are excluded from such facilities and were thus excluded from the study population. These individuals were interviewed and tested between 1964–1966. A one year follow-up after approximately 2 months and 1 year in the institution was completed in 1968. About 75% of the sample was foreign born, averaged 8 years of formal education, was aged about 78 (61–91), and about 70% of the respondents were female. There were two control groups: a sample of 37 residents from within those institutions who had lived there between 1–3 years and who were matched for level of self-care and mental functioning to the group on the waiting list, and a community sample of 40 individuals who did not apply for admission to institutional facilities. A large number of psychological variables were assessed which

are fully explained in the appendix of the book. Their findings were fascinating, as they present a very different picture than one would expect. Their results suggest that (1) many of the "effects of institutionalization" were found in the waiting list sample and thus psychological changes that have been associated with institutionalization start prior to the actual residence within the institution (these findings relate primarily to the older person's attempt to deal with feelings of loss and abandonment); (2) no common personality type distinguished persons who became residents of institutions; (3) adjustment to the institution during the first 2 months indicated a remarkable stability of functioning (To the extent that functioning was low, this was in general, due to declines in function before entry); (4) the individual's self-system was maintained by effective uses of defense mechanisms; and (5) after admission, children tended to be "mythicized."

Of the 85 subjects who entered institutions, five levels of change were noted after the first year: 6% had enhanced functioning, 16% had no essential changes, 30% had some negative changes, 33% deteriorated, and 15% died. Thus, the majority of the sample experienced significant and severe negative outcomes. The main psychological variable that was related to death and severe decline was passivity. For those who survived the first year, preadmission characteristics were related to the level of adaptation, with stability of functioning the norm.

It is difficult to characterize the world of the very old from this set of studies. In many respects, the literature on the "normal" older person in the community suggests a persistence of personality patterns from adult life, significant sex differences, and a wide range of adaptive styles. However, the divergence from this general pattern is large when radical changes in lifestyle are required due to changes in physical or mental health. The severely impaired elderly are forced to cope with massive changes at a time when their resources to do so are often severely limited. Nonetheless, the research findings indicate that the adaptive capacities of even the very old are significant. In an essay on personality and psychopathology among the elderly, Robert Kastenbaum[379] suggests that perhaps the emphasis on age, in understanding and treatment of the elderly, is somewhat counter-productive. He suggests, instead, a focus on the types of problems often seen in an older population (bereavement and its consequences, depression, family problems, role loss, psychosomatic complaints) as a way to develop therapeutic approaches and research paradigms that will then lead back to a full psychology of old age.

The Family and Social Change.

Many of the topics in this final section have not been the exclusive focus of psychological research and are thus discussed elsewhere in this volume. Yet a few comments about the family and social change as they relate to psychological changes and age are in order.

Rosow[380] argues that one of the major problems of old age is that people are not socialized for old age. Other views of socialization across the lifecycle[381,382] do not adopt as extreme a position, but Rosow is correct in saying that there are·fewer guidelines for appropriate behavior in old age. This could be seen as a liberating rather than a problematical situation. However, old age appears to be a time of liberation only for the highly creative who have always defined life, at whatever stage, pretty much on their own terms. The length of time between learning about old age as a child and being able to practice what you have learned as an old person is great and is further complicated by the effects of social change.

The family is seen as the primary socialization force and evidence suggests that the family itself has changed. In considering historical trends in the family, Rosow[383] argues that our notions of the close-knit, multigenerational family in the past ignore the fact that this interdependence may well have been based more on a relative lack of affluence than on any increase in sentiment. He suggests that one of the consequences of an expanding economy with the concomitant growth in affluence is

that the generations are able to live independently. With social mobility comes geographic mobility, and increasingly, social distance, such that children are different from their parents not only in age or generation but, potentially more importantly, in terms of social class as well. Nonetheless, families are quite involved with their older members. Laurie[384] estimates that family members provide about 50% of the services received by older persons and up to 70% of the services received by very impaired older persons. Children, grandchildren, and siblings all play a role in older persons' lives. Brody[385] reports that the multigenerational family is common. For those 65 and older, 70% have grandchildren, and 40% have great-grandchildren, while Cicerelli[386] notes that 38% of people 65 and older have a spouse, 61% have children and 93% have living siblings. Many families have 2 generations of older persons. Brody[385] reported that 5% of people over 65 live with their own aged parent, 25% share a household with an adult child, and 84% of those with children live within an hour of at least one child. In reviewing the therapeutic approaches used with families that contain older persons, Brody is optimistic that the family "crises" that come with aging are both predictable and treatable. She defines two normative crises. The first is the attainment of filial maturity of the adult children. The task for the adult child is to see the parents as individuals who both give and receive support, and for the older person, to be able to accept the maturity of the children and establish a new relationship. For many, a second crisis is the task of dealing with institutional arrangements for a parent with failing health. This can produce a crisis for the adult child which is characterized by intense anxiety about one's own aging, a denial of the older parent's problems, projection of guilt onto the institution, and avoidance of the older parent once separation has occurred. Attention to these issues has been primarily by social workers who deal with the problems on a day-to-day basis, and helpful books with practical advice for family members have started to appear.[387,388] Research which explores the processes of institutionalization such as that by Tobin and Lieberman[378] and research which explores ethnic variations in family experiences[389] still leave many of the questions in this important area unanswered. Good psychological studies and multidisciplinary approaches to understanding the importance of family have started to appear.[390] This will probably be one of the most important areas of aging research in the future.

Most of the work concerned with the family and the effects of social change has been focused earlier in the life cycle and been concerned with the changing role of women,[391-396] and transitions to parenthood,[397-402] with some interest in the marital relationship during the postparental stage.[363,403-405] The family is seen as a major source of satisfaction across the life cycle[406] and in old age.[259] However, the relationship between family, children, career, and satisfaction is more complex for older women.[260] The meanings of parenthood and family relationships for men have yet to receive full attention, particularly in the aging literature. Parenthood is seen as the phase of the life cycle that requires the maximal sex-role differentiation between husband and wife, in order for effective parenting to occur. The literature suggests that before parenthood, and after the children have left the home, sex-role differences are smaller and there is increased androgeny. However, although culturally sex roles appear to be becoming more androgenous, whether this will remain the model pattern remains to be seen. Data from persons currently old tend to be extremely sex stereotyped. Thus the effects of changes in sex roles have yet to show up in the "aging" literature *per se*. The real meaning of the observed sex differences which are consistent and omnipresent have yet to be fully understood.

Research in psychology of aging is now firmly established. While there are few studies that cover the entire lifecycle, the literature in most areas of psychology can speak to most phases of the lifecycle. There are, however, important gaps to be filled. Relatively little is known about cognitive development in the middle years and in very old age. Personality has been well explored in the middle years but not as fully in later life.

Work in the applied psychology of aging is just beginning. Fozard and Popkin[407] define applied psychology of aging to include all areas of psychology, not just the traditional clinical and counseling areas. The baselines have been established and the future should contain good clinical research with special attention to applying the findings of experimental psychology to the assessment and treatment of memory problems, as well as the development of better diagnositc and therapeutic methods based on the findings from developmental studies. The literature has developed methodological sophistication, and a large variety of instruments and paradigms are of proven usefulness across the lifespan. The real task ahead lies in replication of the findings—convergence in personality measurement has yet to be achieved—and in the building of theoretical models of aging.

REFERENCES

1. Pressey, Sidney L., and Kuhlen, Raymond G. *Psychological Development Through the Lifespan.* New York: Harper & Row, 1957.
2. Baltes, P. B. (ed.) Lifespan models of psychological aging: A white elephant? *The Gerontologist,* **13:** 457–512 (1973).
3. Schaie, K. Warner (ed.) *Theory and Methods of Research on Aging.* Morgantown: West Virginia University Press, 1968.
4. Goulet, L. R. and Baltes, Paul B. *Lifespan Development Psychology: Research and Theory.* New York: Academic Press, 1970.
5. Nesselroade, John R. and Reese, Hayne W. (eds.) *Lifespan Developmental Psychology: Methodological Issues.* New York: Academic Press, 1973.
6. Baltes, Paul B. and Schaie, K. Warner. *Lifespan Development Psychology: Personality and Socialization.* New York: Academic Press, 1973.
7. Datan, Nancy and Ginsberg, Leon. *Lifespan Development Psychology: Normative Life Crisis.* New York: Academic Press, 1975.
8. Baltes, Paul B. *Lifespan Developmental Psychology: Some Observations on History and Theory.* Presidential Address, Division 20,

American Psychological Association, San Francisco, August 1977.

9. Bayley, N. The lifespan as a frame of reference in psychological research. *Vita Humana,* **6:** 125–139 (1963).

10. Riegel, Klaus F. History of psychosocial gerontology. In J. E. Birren and K. W. Schaie (eds.) *Handbook of the Psychology of Aging.* New York: Van Nostrand Reinhold Co., pp. 70–102, 1977.

11. Riegel, Klause F. On the history of psychosocial gerontology. In C. Eisdorfer and M. P. Lawton (eds.) *The Psychology of Adult Development and Aging.* Washington, D.C. American Psychological Association, pp. 37–68, 1973.

12. Edwards, Willie M., and Flynn, Frances. *Gerontology: A Core List of Significant Works.* Ann Arbor, Michigan: Institute of Gerontology, 1978.

13. Botwinick, Jack. Geropsychology. In P. H. Mussen and M. R. Rosenzweig (eds.) *Annual Review of Psychology.* Palo Alto: Annual Reviews Inc., v. 21, pp. 239–272, 1970.

14. Schaie, K. Warner and Gribbin, Kathy. Adult development and aging. In M. R. Rosenzwig and L. W. Porter (eds.) *Annual Review of Psychology,* Palo Alto: Annual Reviews Inc., v. 26, pp. 65–95, 1975.

15. Birren, James E. and V. Jayne Renner. Research on the psychology of aging. In J. E. Birren and K. W. Schaie (eds.) *Handbook of the Psychology of Aging.* New York: Van Nostrand Reinhold, 1977.

16. Birren, James E. and Schaie, K. Warner. *Handbook of the Psychology of Aging.* New York: Van Nostrand Reinhold Co. pp. 3–38, 1977.

17. Botwinick, Jack. *Aging and Behavior.* New York: Springer, 1973.

18. Kimmel, Douglas C. *Adulthood and Aging: An Interdisciplinary View.* New York: John Wiley & Sons, 1974.

19. Bromley, Dennis B. *The Psychology of Human Aging.* Baltimore: Penguin, 1974.

20. Birren, James E. *The Psychology of Aging.* Englewood Cliffs, New Jersey: Prentice Hall, 1964.

21. Botwinick, Jack *Cognitive Processes in Maturity and Old Age.* New York: Springer, 1967.

22. Elias, Merrill F., Elias, Penelope K. and Elias, Jeffery W. *Adult Developmental Psychology.* St. Louis: C. V. Mosby, 1977.

23. Baltes, Paul B., Reese, Hayne W., and Nesselroade, John R. *Lifespan Developmental Psychology: Introduction to research methods.* Monterey, California: Brooks/Cole, 1977.

24. Wohlwill, Jochaim F. *The study of behavioral development.* New York: Academic Press. 1973.

25. Schaie, K. W. A general model for the study of developmental problems. *Psychol. Bull.* **64:** 92–107. (1965).

26. Schaie, K. Warner Quasi-experimental designs in the psychology of aging. In J. E. Birren and K. W. Schaie (eds.) *Handbook of the Psychology of Aging* New York: Van Nostrand Reinhold, pp. 39–58, 1977.

27. Rosow, I. What is a cohort and why? *Human Development* **21:** 65–75 (1978).

28. Kuhlen, Raymond G. Aging and life adjustment. In J. E. Birren (ed.) *Handbook of Aging and the Individual.* Chicago: University of Chicago Press, pp. 852–897, 1959.

29. Neugarten, Bernice L. and Datan, Nancy. Sociological perspectives in the life cycle. In P. B. Baltes and K. W. Schaie. *Lifespan Developmental Psychology: Personality and Socialization.* New York: Academic Press, pp. 53–69, 1973.

30. Nesselroade, John R. Issues in studying developmental change in adults from a multivariate perspective. In J. E. Birren and K. W. Schaie (eds.) *Handbook of the Psychology of Aging.* New York: Van Nostrand Reinhold Co., pp. 59–69, 1977.

31. Harris, Chester W. (ed.) *Problems in Measuring Change.* Madison: University of Wisconsin Press, 1963.

32. Birren, James E. Principles of research on aging. In J. E. Birren (ed.) *Handbook of Aging and the Individual.* Chicago: University of Chicago Press, pp. 3–42, 1959.

33. Neugarten, Bernice L. The future and the young old. *The Gerontologist.* **15,** Part II: 4–9, (1975).

34. Kay, Harry Theories of learning and aging. In J. E. Birren (ed.) *Handbook of Aging and the Individual.* Chicago: University of Chicago Press, pp. 614–654, 1959.

35. Jerome, Edward A. Age and learning—Experimental studies. In J. E. Birren (ed.) *Handbook of Aging and the Individual.* Chicago: University of Chicago Press, pp. 655–699, 1959.

36. Arenberg, David and Robertson-Tchabo, Elizabeth A. Learning and aging. In J. E. Birren and K. W. Schaie (eds.) *Handbook of the Psychology of Aging.* New York: Van Nostrand Reinhold, pp. 421–449, 1977.

37. Cautella, Joseph R. and Mansfield, Linda A. Behavioral Approach to Geriatrics. In W. Doyle Gentry (ed.) *Geropsychology: A Model of Training and Clinical Service.* Cambridge, Mass.: Ballinger Press, pp. 21–42, 1977.

38. Walsh, David A. Age differences in learning and memory. In D. S. Woodruff and J. E. Birren (eds.) *Aging: Scientific Perspectives and Social Issues.* New York: Van Nostrand Reinhold Co., pp. 125–151, 1975.

39. Gilbert, J. G. Memory loss in senescence. *J. Abnormal Soc. Psychol.* **36:** 73–86 (1941).

40. Korchin, S. J. and Basowitz, H. Age differences in verbal learning. *J. Abnorm. Soc. Psychol.* **54:** 64–69 (1957).

41. Canestrari, R. E. Paced and self-paced learning in young and elderly adults. *J. Gerontol.* **18:** 165–168 (1963).

42. Canestrari, Robert E. Age changes in acquisition.

In G. A. Talland (ed.) *Human Aging and Behavior*. New York: Academic Press, pp. 169–188, 1968.

43. Arenberg, D. Anticipation interval and age differences in verbal learning, *J. Abnorm. Soc. Psychol.* **70:** 419–425 (1965).

44. Taub, H. A. Paired associates learning as a function of age, rate and instructions. *J. Genetic Psychol.* **111:** 41–46 (1967).

45. Arenberg, D. Verbal learning and retention. *Gerontologist.* **7:** 10–13 (1967).

46. Monge, R. H. and Hultsch, D. F. Paired-associate learning as a function of adult age, and length of the anticipation and the inspection intervals. *J. Gerontol.* **26:** 157–162 (1971).

47. Witte, K. L. Paired associate learning in young and elderly adults as related to presentation rate. *Psychol. Bull.* **82:** 975–985 (1975).

48. Kinsbourne, M. and Berryhill, J. L. The nature of the interaction between pacing and the age decrement in learning. *J. Gerontol.* **27:** 471–77 (1972).

49. Winn, F. J., Jr. and Elias, J. W. Age, rate and instructional conditions: Empirical support against the pacing variable. *Exp. Aging Res.* **3:** 305–324 (1977).

50. Eisdorfer, C., Axelrod, S. and Wilkie, F. L. Stimulus exposure time as a factor in serial learning in an aged sample. *J. Abnorm. Soc. Psychol.* **67:** 594–600 (1963).

51. Eisdorfer, C. Verbal learning response time in the aged. *J. Genetic Psychol.* **107:** 15–22 (1965).

52. Eisdorfer, Carl. Arousal and performance: Experiments in verbal learning and a tentative theory. In G. A. Talland (ed.) *Human Aging and Behavior*. New York: Academic Press, pp. 189–216, 1968.

53. Hulicka, I. M. and Grossman, J. L. Age-group comparisons for the use of mediators in paired-associate learning. *J. Gerontol.* **22:** 46–51 (1967).

54. Canestrari, R. E. The effects of commonality on paired associate learning in two age groups. *J. Genetic Psychol.* **108:** 3–7 (1966).

55. Kausler, D. H. and Lair, C. V. Associative strength and paired associate learning in elderly subjects. *J. Gerontol.* **21:** 278–280 (1966).

56. Zaretsky, H. H. and Halberstam, J. L. Age differences in paired-associate learning. *J. Gerontol.* **23:** 165–168 (1968)

57. Wittels, I. Age and stimulus meaningfulness in paired associate learning. *J. Gerontol.* **27:** 372–375 (1972).

58. Botwinick, Jack and Storandt, Martha. *Memory-Related Functions and Age*. Springfield, Ill.: Charles C Thomas, 1974.

59. Eisdorfer, C., Nowlin, J. B. and Wilkie, F. L. Improvement of learning in the aged by modification of autonomic nervous system activity. *Science,* **170:** 1327–1329 (1970).

60. Froehling, Susan. Effects of propranolol on behavioral and physiological measures in elderly males. Unpublished Doctoral Dissertation, University of Miami, Florida, 1974.

61. Okun, M. A., Siegler, I. C. and George, L. K. Cautiousness and verbal learning in adulthood. *J. Gerontol.* **33:** 94–97 (1978).

62. Arenberg, D. Age differences in retroaction. *J. Gerontol.* **22:** 88–91 (1967).

63. Hultsch, D. F., Nesselroade, J. R. and Plemons, J. K. Learning-ability relations in adulthood. *Hum. Dev.* **19:** 234–247 (1976).

64. Belbin, E. and Belbin, R. *Problems in Adult Training*. London: Heinemann 1972.

65. Welford, A. T. Thirty years of psychological research on age and work. *J. Occup. Psychol.* **49:** 129–138, (1976).

66. Craik, Fergus I. M. Age differences in human memory. In J. E. Birren and K. W. Schaie (eds.) *Handbook of the Psychology of Aging*. New York: Van Nostrand Reinhold Co., pp. 384–420, 1977.

67. Thomas, J. C., Waugh, N. C. and Fozard, J. L. Age and familiarity in memory scanning. *J. Gerontol.* **33:** 528–533, (1978).

68. Craik, F. I. M. and Lockhart, R. S. Levels of processing: A framework for memory research. *J. Verb. Learn. Verb. Behav.* **11:** 671–684 (1972).

69. Poon, L. W. and Fozard, J. L. Speed of retrieval from long term memory in relation to age, familiarity and datedness of information. *J. Gerontol.* **33:** 711–717, (1978).

70. Smith, A. D. and Winograd, E. Adult age differences in remembering faces. *Dev. Psychol.* **14:** 443–444, (1978).

71. Walsh, D. A. and Baldwin, M. Age differences in integrated semantic memory. *Dev. Psychol.* **13:** 509–514 (1977).

72. Mistler-Lachman, J. L. Spontaneous shift in encoding dimensions among elderly subjects. *J. Gerontol.* **32:** 68–72, (1977).

73. Smith, A. D. Adult age differences in cued recall. *Dev. Psychol.* **13:** 326–331, (1977).

74. Zelinski, E. M., Walsh, D. A. and Thompson, L. W. Orienting task effects on EDR and free recall in three age groups. *J. Gerontol.* **33:** 239–245 (1978).

75. Marshall, P. H., Elias, J. W., Weber, S. M., Gist, B. A., Winn, F. J., King, P. and Moore, S. A. Age differences in verbal mediation: A structural and functional analysis. *Exp. Aging Res.* **4:** 175–193, (1978).

76. Perlmutter, M. What is memory aging the aging of? *Dev. Psychol.* **14:** 330–345, (1978).

77. Waugh, N. C., Thomas, J. C. and Fozard, J. L. Retrieval time from different memory stores. *J. Gerontol.* **33:** 718–724, (1978).

78. Robertson-Tchabo, E. A. and Arenberg, D. Age difference in cognition in healthy educated men: A factor analysis of experimental measures. *Ex. Aging Res.* **2:** 75–79, (1976).

79. Poon, L. W. A systems approach for the assess-

ment and treatment of memory problems. In J. Ferguson and C. B. Taylor (eds.) *Advances in Behavioral Medicine.* New York: Spectrum Press, (in press).

80. Poon, L. W. (ed.). Toward Comprehensive Intervention Programs for Memory Problems Among the Aged. Veterans Administration Outpatient Clinic, Boston, MA. Technical Report 77-01 (1977).

81. Birren, J. E. Translation in gerontology—from lab to life: Psychophysiology and speed of response. *Am. Psychol.* **29**: 808-815, (1974).

82. Marsh, Gail R. and Thompson, Larry W. Psychophysiology of aging. In J. E. Birren and K. W. Schaie (eds.) *Handbook of the Psychology of Aging.* New York: Van Nostrand Reinhold Co., pp. 219-248, 1977.

83. Welford, Alan T. Motor performance. In J. E. Birren and K. W. Schaie (eds.) *Handbook of the Psychology of Aging.* New York: Van Nostrand Reinhold Co., pp. 450-596, 1977.

84. Welford, Alan T. and Birren, James E. *Behavior, Aging and the Nervous System.* Springfield: Charles C Thomas, 1965.

85. Poon, Leonard W. and Fozard, James L. (eds.) *Design Conference on Decision Making and Aging.* Boston V.A. Geriatric Education and Clinical Center, Technical Report 76-01 (1976).

86. Fozard, J. L., Thomas, J. C. and Waugh, N. C. Effects of age and frequency of stimulus repetitions on two-choice reaction time. *J. Gerontol.* **31**: 556-563, (1976).

87. Poon, Leonard W., Fozard, James L., Vierck, Beby, Darbey, Brian F., Carella, John and Zeller, Pamela. The effects of practise and information feedback on age-related differences in performance speed, variability and error rates in a two-choice decision task. Boston V.A. Geriatric Education and Clinical Center, Technical Report 76-01 pp. 65-81, (1976).

88. Fozard, James L. and Poon, Leonard W. Research, Educational and Clinical Activities in the Psychological Aspects of Aging. Boston Geriatric Education and Clinical Center Technical Report 78-02. (1978).

89. Welford, A. T. Motivation, capacity, learning and age. *International J. Aging and Hum. Dev.* **7**: 189-199, (1976).

90. Salthouse, T. A. Speed and age: multiple rates of decline. *Exp. Aging Res.* **2**: 349-359, (1976).

91. Salthouse, Timothy A. Does speed of performance change with increased age? In L. W. Poon and J. L. Fozard (eds.) *Design Conference on Decision Making and Aging.* Boston V.A. Geriatric Education and Clinical Center Technical Report 76-01 pp. 104-117, (1976).

92. Davies, D. K. and Tune, G. S. *Human Vigilance Performance.* New York: American Elsevier, 1969, American Edition (London: Staples Press, 1970)

93. Okun, M. A. Adult age and cautiousness in decision: A review of the literature. *Hum. Dev.* **19**: 220-233, (1976).

94. Okun, M. A. and Elias, C. S. Cautiousness in adulthood as a function of age and payoff structure. *J. Gerontol.* **32**: 451-455, (1977).

95. Birkhill, W. R. and Schaie, K. W. The effect of differential reinforcement of cautiousness in intellectual performance among the elderly. *J. Gerontol.* **3**: 578-583, (1975).

96. Woodruff, D. S. Relationship between EEG, alpha frequency, reaction time, and age: A biofeedback study. *Psychophysiol.* **12**: 673-681, (1975).

97. Rahe, Richard H. Stress tolerance and the rise and fall of bodily energy. In D. K. Heyman (ed.) *Proceedings of Seminars 1970-1976,* Duke University Council on Aging and Human Development: Durham, North Carolina, pp. 31-47, 1978.

98. Botwinick, J. and Thompson, L. W. Age differences in reaction time: An artifact? *Gerontologist.* **8**: 25-28, (1968).

99. Spirduso, W. W. and Clifford, P. Replication of age and physical activity effects on reaction and movement time. *J. Gerontol.* **33**: 26-30, (1978).

100. Woodruff, Diana S. A physiological perspective of the psychology of aging. In D. S. Woodruff and J. E. Birren (eds.) *Aging: Scientific Perspectives and Social Issues.* New York: D. Van Nostrand, pp. 179-198, 1975.

101. Abrahams, J. P. and Birren, J. E. Reaction time as a function of age and behavioral predisposition to coronary heart disease. *J. Gerontol.* **28**: 471-478, (1973).

102. Botwinick, J. and Storandt, M. Cardiovascular status, depressive effect, and other factors in reaction time. *J. Gerontol.* **29**: 543-548, (1974).

103. Light, K. C. Effects of mild cardiovascular and cerebrovascular disease in serial RT performances. *Exp. Aging Res.* **4**: 3-22, (1978).

104. Speith, Walter. Slowness of task performance and cardiovascular diseases. In A. T. Welford and J. E. Birren (eds.) *Behavior, Aging and The Nervous System.* Springfield, Ill.: Charles C Thomas, pp. 366-400, 1965.

105. Anastasi, Ann. *Psychological Testing.* New York: MacMillan, 1976.

106. Buros, Oscar, K. (ed.) *Mental Measurements Yearbook.* Hiland Park, New Jersey: Gryphon Press, 1972.

107. Miles, C. C. and Miles, W. R. The correlation of intelligence scores and chronological age from early to late maturity. *Am. J. Psychol.* **44**: 44-78, (1932).

108. Jones, H. C. and Conrad, H. S. The growth and decline of intelligence: A study of homogeneous groups between the ages of ten and sixty. *Genetic Psychol. Monographs.* **13**: 223-298, (1933).

109. Wechsler, David *The Measurement and Appraisal of Adult Intelligence.* Baltimore: Williams and Wilkins Co., 1958.

110. Bayley, N. and Oden, M. H. The maintenance of intellectual ability in gifted adults. *J. Gerontol.* **10:** 91-107, (1955).

111. Terman, Lewis M. and Oden, Melita H. *The Gifted Group at Midlife.* Stanford, California: Stanford University Press, 1959.

112. Owens, W. A. Jr. Age and mental abilities: A longitudinal Study. *Genetic Psychol. Monographs.* **48:** 3-54, (1953).

113. Siegler, Ilene C. Lifespan developmental psychology and clinical geropsychology. In W. D. Gentry (ed.) *Geropsychology: A Model of Training and Clinical Service.* Cambridge: Ballinger Press, pp. 87-109, 1977.

114. Kuhlen, R. G. Age and intelligence: The significance of cultural change in longitudinal versus cross-sectional findings. *Vita Humana.* **6:** 113-124, (1963).

115. Owens, W. A. Jr. Age and mental abilities: A second adult follow-up. *J. of Educ. Psychol.* **54:** 311-325, (1966).

116. Horn, J. L. and Cattell, R. B. Age differences in primary mental ability factors. *J. Gerontol.* **21:** 210-220, (1966).

117. Horn, J. L. Intergration of structural and developmental concepts in the theory of fluid and crystallized intelligence. In R. B. Cattell (ed.) *Handbook of Multivariate Experimental Psychology.* Chicago: Rand McNally, pp. 553-562, 1966.

118. Horn, J. L. Organization of abilities and the development of intelligence. *Psychol. Rev.* **75:** 242-259, (1968).

119. Horn, J. L. Organization of data on life-span development of human abilities. In L. R. Goulet and P. B. Baltes (eds.) *Life-Span Developmental Psychology: Research and Theory.* New York: Academic Press, pp. 423-466, 1970.

120. Kleemeier, R. W. Intellectual changes in the senium. *Proceedings of the American Statistical Association.* **1:** 290-295, (1962).

121. Riegel, K. F. and Riegel, R. M. Development, drop, death. *Dev. Psychol.* **6:** 309-316, (1972).

122. Siegler, I. C. The terminal drop hypothesis: Fact or artifact? *Exp. Aging Res.* **1:** 169-185, (1975).

123. Botwinick, Jack Intellectual abilities. In J. E. Birren and K. W. Schaie (eds.) *Handbook of the Psychology of Aging.* New York: Van Nostrand Reinhold Co., pp. 580-605, 1977.

124. Riegel, K. F., Riegel, R. M. and Meyer, G. The prediction of retest resisters in longitudinal research on aging. *J. Gerontol.* **23:** 370-374, (1968).

125. Baltes, P. B., Schaie, K. W. and Nardi, H. Age and experimental mortality in a seven year longitudinal study of cognitive behavior. *Dev. Psychol.* **5:** 18-26, (1971).

126. Rosenthal, R. and Rosnow, R. L. *The Volunteer Subjects.* New York: Wiley, 1975.

127. Siegler, I. C. and Botwinick, J. A long-term longitudinal study of intellectual ability of older adults: The matter of selective subject attrition. *J. Gerontol.* **34:** 242-245 (1979).

128. Kessen, W. Research design in the study of developmental problems. In P. H. Messen (ed.) *Handbook of Research Methods in Child Development.* New York: Wiley, pp. 36-70, 1960.

129. Baltes, P. B. Longitudinal and cross-sectional sequences in the study of age and generation effects. *Hum. Dev.* **11:** 145-171, (1968).

130. Schaie, K. W. Methodological problems in descriptive developmental research on adulthood and aging. In J. R. Nesselroade and H. W. Reese (eds.) *Life-Span Developmental Psychology: Methodological Issues.* New York: Academic Press, pp. 253-280, 1973.

131. Botwinick, J. and Arenberg, D. Disparate time spans in sequential studies of aging. *Exp. Aging Res.* **2:** 55-61, (1976).

132. Adam, J. Statistical bias in cross-sequential studies of aging. *Exp. Aging Res.* **3:** 325-333, (1977.)

133. Mason, K. O., Mason, W. M., Winsborough, H. H. and Poole, W. K. Some methodological issues in cohort analysis of archival data. *Am. Sociol. Rev.* **38:** 242-258, (1973).

134. George, L. K., Siegler, I. C., and Okun, M. A. Analyzing developmental data: An empirical comparison of ANOVA and a multiple regression in age-period-cohort analysis. Manuscript submitted for publication, 1979.

135. Wechsler, David *Wechsler Adult Intelligence Scale Manual.* Psychological Corporation., New York, 1955.

136. Matarazzo, Joseph D. *Wechsler's Measurement and Appraisal of Adult Intelligence.* Baltimore: Williams & Wilkins, 1972. (5th edition).

137. Wechsler, David. *Wechsler Bellevue Intelligence Scale, Form II.* Psychological Corporation, New York, 1946.

138. Dopplet, J. and Wallace, W. L. Standardization of the WAIS for older persons. *J. Abnorm. Soc. Psychol.* **51:** 312-330, (1955).

139. Schaie, K. W. and Strother, C. R. A cross-sequential study of age changes in cognitive behavior. *Psychol. Bull.* **70:** 671-680, (1968).

140. Schaie, K. W. and Strother, C. R. The effects of time and cohort differences on the interpretation of age changes in cognitive behavior. *Multivariate Behavioral Research.* **3:** 259-294, (1968).

141. Schaie, K. W., Labouvie, G. V. and Buech, B. U. Generational and cohort specific differences in adult cognitive functioning: A fourteen-year study of independent samples. *Dev. Psychol.* **9:** 151-166, (1973).

142. Schaie, K. W. and Labouvie-Vief, G. Generational versus ontogenetic components of change in adult cognitive behavior: A fourteen-year cross-sequential study. *Dev. Psychol.* **10:** 305-320, (1974).

143. Schaie, K. W. and Parham, I. A. Cohort-sequential analyses of adult intellectual development. *Dev. Psychol.* **13**: 649-653, (1977).

144. Thurstone, L. L. and Thurstone, T. G. *SRA primary mental abilities test.* Chicago: Science Research Associates. 1949.

145. Schaie, K. W. Rigidity—flexibility and intelligence: A cross-sectional study of the adult lifespan. *Psychol. Monographs.* **72** (Whole No. 462) (1958).

146. Chown, S. M. Age and the rigidities. *J. Gerontol.* **16**: 353-362. (1961).

147. Heron, Alister and Chown, Shelia *Age and Function.* London: S. A. Churchill, 1967.

148. Cunningham, W. R., Clayton, V. and Overton, W. Fluid and crystallized intelligence in young adulthood and old age. *J. Gerontol.* **30**: 53-55, (1975).

149. Cunningham, Walter R. Factorial Invariance of Intellectual Abilities in Adulthood and Old Age, Paper presented at the meetings of the American Psychological Association, New Orleans, September, 1974.

150. Cunningham, Walter R. and Birren, James E. Age changes in factor structure of intellectual abilities in adulthood and old age. *Educational Psychol. Measurements,* in press.

151. Yerkes, R. M. (ed.) Psychological examing in the United States Army. *Memoirs of the National Academy of Sciences,* **15**: 1-890, (1921).

152. Siegler, Ilene C. Structural change in intellectual functioning: An example of Markov Network Analysis. In R. Campbell (Chair), *Research Methods,* Symposium presented at meeting of Gerontological Society, Louisville, KY, October, 1975.

153. Woodbury, M. A., Manton, K. G. and Siegler, I. C. Evaluation of intellectual functioning overtime in the Duke Longitudinal Studies: An application of covariance structures. Paper presented at the conference on Longitudinal Statistical Analysis, Boston, June, 1975.

154. Arenberg, D. Differences and changes with age in the Benton Visual Retention Test. *J. Gerontol.* **33**: 534-540, (1978).

155. Birren, J. E. and Morrison, D. F. Analysis of WAIS subtests in relation to age and education. *J. Gerontol.* **16**: 363-369, (1961).

156. Green, R. F. Age-intelligence relationships between ages sixteen and sixty-four. *Dev. Psychol.* **1**: 618-627, (1969).

157. Gardner, E. F. and Monge, R. H. Adult age differences in cognitive abilities and educational background. *Exp. Aging Res.* **3**: 337-383, (1977).

158. Cohen, D., Schaie, K. W. and Gribbin, K. The organization of spatial abilities in older men and women. *J. Gerontol.* **32**: 578-585, (1977).

159. Lorge, I. The influence of the test upon the nature of mental decline as a functional age. *J. of Educational Psychol.* **27**: 100-110, (1936).

160. Storandt, M. Age, ability level, and method of administering and scoring the WAIS, *J. Gerontol.* **32**: 175-178, (1977).

161. Koldin, V. M. The relationship of scoring treatment and age in perceptual integrational performance. *Exp. Aging Res.* **2**: 303-313, (1976).

162. Salthouse, T. A. The role of memory in the age decline in digit-symbol substitution performance. *J. Gerontol.* **33**: 232-238, (1978).

163. Cunningham, W. R., Sepkoski, C. M. and Opel, M. R. Fatigue effects on intelligence test performance in the elderly. *J. Gerontol.* **33**: 541-545, (1978).

164. Grant, E. A., Storandt, M. and Botwinick, J. Incentive and practice in the psychomotor performance of the elderly. *J. Gerontol.* **33**: 413-415, (1978).

165. Plemons, J. K., Willis, S. L. and Baltes, P. B. Modifiability of fluid intelligence in aging: A short-term longitudinal training approach. *J. Gerontol.* **33**: 224-231, (1978).

166. Schaie, K. W. Translations in gerontology: From lab to life: Intellectual functioning. *Am. Psychol.* **29**: 802-807, (1974).

167. Horn, J. L. and Donaldson, G. On the myth of intellectual decline in adulthood. *Am. Psychol.* **31**: 701-719, (1976).

168. Baltes, P. B. and Schaie, K. W. On the plasticity of intelligence in adulthood and old age: Where Horn and Donaldson Fail. *Am. Psychol.* **31**: 720-725, (1976).

169. Horn, J. L. and Donaldson, G. Faith is not enough: A response to the Baltes-Schaie claim that intelligence does not wane. *Am. Psychol.* **32**: 369-373, (1977).

170. Thorndike, E. L., Begman, E. O., Lorge, I., Metcalfe, Z. F., Robinson, E. E. and Woodyard, E. *Prediction of Vocational Success.* Commonwealth, Fund, 1934.

171. Terman, Lewis and Oden, Melita, H. *The Gifted Child Grows Up.* Stanford California: Stanford University Press, 1947.

172. Oden, Melita H. The fulfillment of promise: 40-year follow-up of the Terman Gifted group. *Genetic Psychol. Monographs.* **73**: 3-93, (1968).

173. Granick, Samual Cognitive aspects of longevity. In E. Palmore and F. Jeffers (eds.) *Prediction of Lifespan.* Lexington, Mass: D.C. Heath, pp. 109-122, 1971.

174. Obrist, W. D., Busse, E. W., Eisdorfer, C. and Kleemeier, R. W. Relation of the EEG to intellectual function in senescense. *J. Gerontol.* **17**: 197-206, (1962).

175. Blum, J. E., Clark, E. T., and Jarvik, L. F. The N.Y.S. Psychiatric Institute Study of aging twins. In L. F. Jarvik, C. Eisdorfer, and J. E. Blum (eds.) *Intellectual Functioning in Adults.* New York: Springer, 1973.

176. Jarvik, L. F. and Blum, J. E. Cognitive decline as predictor of mortality in twin pairs. A twenty-year

long study of aging. In E. Palmore and F. C. Jeffers (eds.) *Prediction of Life-span.* Lexington, Mass.: D.C. Heath & Co., 1971.

177. Jarvik, L. F., Kallman, F. L. and Falek, A. Intellectual changes in aged twins. *J. of Gerontol.* 17: 289–294, (1962).

178. Jarvik, Lissy F., Kallman, Franz J., Lorge, Irving and Falek, Arthur Longitudinal study of intellectual changes in senescent twins. In C. Tibitts and W. Donahue (eds.) *Social and Psychological Aspects of Aging.* New York: Columbia University Press, 1962.

179. Kallmann, Franz J. and Jarvik, Lissy F. Individual differences in constitution and genetic background. In J. E. Birren (ed.) *Handbook of Aging and the Individual.* Chicago: University of Chicago Press, 1959.

180. Berkowitz, B. The Wechsler-Bellevue performance of white males past 50. *J. Gerontol.* 8: 76–80, (1953).

181. Berkowitz, B. Changes in intellect with age. IV. Changes in achievement and survival in older people. *J. Genetic Psychol.* 107: 3–14, (1965).

182. Berkowitz, B. and Green, R. F. Changes in intellect with age. I. Longitudinal study of Wechsler-Bellevue scores. *J. Genetic Psychol.* 103: 3–21, (1963).

183. Berkowitz, B. and Green, R. F. Changes in intellect with age. V. Differential change as functions of time interval and original score. *J. Genetic Psychol.* 197: 179–192, (1965).

184. Remains, G. and Green R. F. Imminence of death and intellectual functioning in the aged. *Dev. Psychol.* 5: 270–272, (1971).

185. Lieberman, M. A. Psychological correlates of impending death: Some preliminary observations. *J. Gerontol.* 20: 181–190, (1965).

186. Lieberman, M. A. and Coplan, A. S. Distance from death as a variable in the study of aging. *Dev. Psychol.* 2: 71–84, (1970).

187. Birren, J. E., Butler, R. N., Greenhouse, S. W., Sokoloff, L. and Yarrow, M. *Human Aging.* Washington, D.C.: Government Printing Office, Public Health Service Document #986, 1963.

188. Granick, S. and Patterson, R. D. (eds.) *Human Aging II. An Eleven-Year Follow-Up: Biomedical and Behavioral Study.* Washington, D.C.: Government Printing Office. DHEW Publication #(HSM) 71-9037, 1971.

189. Savage, R. D., Britton, P. G., Bolton, N. and Hall, E. H., *Intellectual Function in the Aged.* London: Methuen, 1973.

190. Eisdorfer, Carl and Wilkie, Frances Intellectual change with advancing age. In L. F. Jarvik, C., C. Eisdorfer, and J. E. Blum (eds.) *Intellectual Functioning in Adults.* New York: Springer, 1973.

191. Wilkie, Frances and Eisdorfer, Carl Terminal changes in intelligence, In E. Palmore (ed.) *Normal Aging II,* Durham, N.C.: Duke University Press, 1974.

192. Siegler, I. C., Harkins, S. W. and Thompson, L. W. Stability and change in intellectual performance: An examination of the terminal drop hypothesis in the later years of life. Paper presented at the meeting of the Gerontological Society, Portland, Oregon, 1974.

193. Siegler, I. C., Rosenman, J. and Harkins, S. W. Complexities in the terminal drop hypothesis. Paper presented at the meeting of the 10th International Congress of Gerontology, Jerusalem, Israel, June 1975.

194. Thomae, Hans (ed.) Patterns of aging. Findings from the Bonn Longitudinal Studies. *Contributions of Human Development* vol. 3. Basel: Karger 1976.

195. Lehr, U. and Schmitz-Scherzer, R. Survivors and non-survivors—two fundamental patterns of aging. In H. Thomae (ed.) *Patterns of Aging: Contributions to Human Development.* vol. 3. Basel:Karger 1976.

196. Botwinick, J., West, R. and Storandt, M. Predicting death from behavioral test performance. *J. Gerontol.* 33: 755–762, (1978).

197. Blum, J. E. and Jarvik, L. F. Intellectual performance of octogenarians as a function of education and initial ability. *Human Dev.* 17: 364–375, (1974).

198. Palmore, Erdman and Jeffers, Frances C. *Prediction of Lifespan: Recent Findings.* Lexington, Mass.: D.C. Heath, 1971.

199. Thompson, L. W. Psychological changes in later life. In E. W. Busse and E. Pfeiffer (eds.) *Mental Illness in Later Life.* Washington, D.C.: American Psychiatric Association, 1973.

200. Wilkie, Frances L. and Eisdorfer, Carl. Systemic disease and behavioral correlates. In L. F. Jarvik, C. Eisdorfer, and J. E. Blum (eds.) *Intellectual Functioning in Adults.* New York: Springer pp. 83–93, 1973.

201. Wilkie, F. and Eisdorfer, C. Intelligence and blood pressure in the aged. *Science.* 172: 959–962, (1971).

202. Wang, H. Shan. Cerebral correlates on intellectual function in senescence. In L. F. Jarvik, C. Eisdorfer, J. E. Blum (eds.) *Intellectual Functioning in Adults,* New York: Springer, pp. 95–106, 1973.

203. Roseman, J. M. and Buckley, C. E. Inverse relationship between serum IgG correlations and measures of intelligence in elderly persons, *Nature,* 254: 55–56, (1975).

204. Cohen, D., Matsuyama, S. S. and Jarvik, L. F. Immunoglobulin levels and intellectual functioning in the aged. *Exp. Aging Res.* 2: 345–348, (1976).

205. Eisdorfer, Carl Stress, disease and cognitive change in the aged. In C. Eisdorfer and R. D. Friedel (eds.) *Cognitive and Emotional Disturbance in the Elderly.* Chicago: Year Book Medical Publishers, p. 27–44, 1977.

206. Eisdorfer, Carl and Wilkie, Frances. Stress, disease, aging and behavior In J. E. Birren and

K. W. Schaie (eds.) *Handbook of the Psychology of Aging*. New York: Van Nostrand Reinhold, pp. 251–275, 1977.

207. Botwinick, Jack and Birren, James E. Mental abilities and psychomotor responses in healthy aged men. In J. E. Birren, R. N. Butler, S. W. Greenhouse, L. Sokloff, and M. R. Yarrow (eds.) *Human Aging I: A Biological and Behavioral Study*. Washington, D.C.: Government Printing Office, pp. 97–108, 1963.

208. McFarland, Ross A. The need for functional age measurements. *Industrial Gerontol.* **19:** 1–19, (1973).

209. Edelman, Charles D. and Siegler, Ilene C. *Federal Age Discrimination in Employment Law: Slowing Down the Gold Watch*. Charlottesville, Virginia: The Michie Co., pp. 11–36, 1978.

210. Costa, Paul T. and McCrae, Robert. Functional Age: A conceptual and empirical critique. In *Epidemiology of Aging II*. Washington D.C.: Department of Health, Education and Welfare, Government Printing Office in press.

211. Rabbit Patrick. Changes in problem solving ability in old age. In J. E. Birren, and K. W. Schaie (eds.) *Handbook of the Psychology of Aging*. New York: Van Nostrand Reinhold, pp. 606–625, 1977.

212. Arenberg, D. Concept problem solving in young and old adults. *J. Gerontol.* **23:** 279–282, (1968).

213. Arenberg, D. A longitudinal study of problem solving in adults. *J. Gerontol.* **29:** 650–658, (1974).

214. Kesler, M. S., Denney, N. W. and Whitely, S. E. Factors influencing problem-solving in middle-aged and elderly adults. *Hum. Dev.* **19:** 310–320, (1976).

215. Brinley, J. F., Jarvik, T. J. and McLaughlin, L. M. Age, reasoning and memory in adults. *J. Gerontol.* **29:** 182–189, (1974).

216. Lee, J. A. and Pollack, R. H. The effects of age on perceptual problem strategies. *Exp. Aging Res.,* **4:** 37–54, (1978).

217. Cicirelli, V. G. Categorization behavior in aging subjects. *J. Gerontol.* **31:** 676–680, (1976).

218. Denney, N. W. and Denney, D. R. Modeling effects on the questioning strategies of the elderly. *Dev. Psychol.* **10:** 458, (1974).

219. Denney, N. W. Classification abilities in elderly. *J. Gerontol.* **29:** 309–314, (1974).

220. Labouvie-Vief, G. and Gonada, J. N. Cognitive strategy training and intellectual performance in the elderly. *J. Gerontol.* **33:** 327–332, (1976).

221. Kogan, N. Categorizing and conceptualizing styles in younger and older adults. *Hum. Dev.* **17:** 218–230, (1974).

222. Hultsch, D. F. and Hickey, T. External validity in the study of human development: Theoretical and methodological issues. *Hum. Dev.,* **21:** 76–91, (1978).

223. Lehman, H. *Age and Achievement*. Princeton, New Jersey: Princeton University Press, 1953.

224. Lehman, H. C. The creative production rates of present versus past generation of scientists. *J. Gerontol.* **17:** 99–105, (1968).

225. Dennis, W. Creative productivity between ages 20 and 80 years (1966), in nev. (1968) pp. 106–114 *J. Gerontol.* **21:** 106–114.

226. Alpaugh, P. K. and Birren, J. E. Variables affecting creative contributions across the adult life span. *Hum. Dev.* **20:** 240–248, (1977).

227. Kogan, N. Creativity and Cognitive style In P. B. Baltes and K. W. Schaie (eds.) *Lifespan Developmental Psychology: Personality and Socialization*. New York: Academic Press, pp. 145–178, 1975.

228. Baltes, Paul B. and Willis, Sherry L. Toward psychological theories of aging and development. In J. E. Birren and K. W. Schaie (eds.) *Handbook of the Psychology of Aging*. New York: Van Nostrand Reinhold, pp. 128–154, 1977.

229. Flavell, John H. *The Developmental Psychology of Jean Piaget*. Princeton: New Jersey: Van Nostrand, 1963.

230. Inhelder, Barbel and Piaget, Jean. *The Growth of Logical Thinking from Childhood to Adolescence*. New York: Basic Books, 1958.

231. Papalia, D. E. and Bielby, D. D. V. Cognitive functioning in middle and old age adults: A review of research based on Piaget's theory. *Hum. Dev.* **17:** 424–443, (1974).

232. Flavell, J. H. Cognitive changes in adulthood. In L. R. Goulet and P. B. Baltes (eds.) *Lifespan Developmental Psychology: Research and Theory*. New York: Academic Press, pp. 247–253, 1970.

233. Sinnot, J. D. Everyday thinking and piagetian operativity in adults. *Hum. Dev.* **18:** 430–443, (1975).

234. Piaget, J. Intellectual evolution from adolescence to adulthood. *Hum. Dev.* **15:** 1–12, (1972).

235. Kuhn, D., Langer, J., Kolberg, L. and Haan, N. S. The development of formal operation in logical and moral judgement. *Genetic Psychol. Monographs.* **95:** 97–188, (1977).

236. Arlin, P. K. Cognitive development in adulthood: A fifth stage? *Dev. Psychol.* **11:** 602–606, (1975).

237. Cropper, D. A., Meck, D. S. and Ash, M. J. The relation between formal operations and a possible fifth stage of cognitive development. *Dev. Psychol.* **13:** 517–518, (1977).

238. Riegel, Klaus F. (ed.) The development of dialectical operations. *Hum. Dev.* **18:** 1–238, (1975).

239. Riegel, K. F. Dialectic operations: The final period of cognitive development. *Hum. Dev.* **16:** 346–370, (1973).

240. Livson, Norman. Developmental Dimensions of Personality: A Lifespan Formulation. In P. B. Baltes and K. W. Schaie (eds.) *Lifespan Developmental Psychology: Personality and Socialization*. New York: Academic Press, pp. 97–122, 1973.

241. Bühler, C. The curve of life as studies in

biographies. *J. Applied Psychol.* **19:** 405–409 (1935).

242. Bühler, Charlotte and Massarick, Fred. *The Course of Human Life.* New York: Springer, 1968.

243. Jung, Carl G. *Modern Man in Search of a Soul.* New York: Harcourt, Brace & World, 1933.

244. Jung, Carl G. The Stages of Life (Translated by R. F. C. Hull). In J. Campbell (ed.). *The Portable Jung.* New York: Viking (1971).

245. Erikson, Erik H. *Childhood and Society.* New York: Norton, 1950, 1963.

246. Erikson, E. H. Identity and the lifecycle. *Psychological Issues,* 1959 (Whole No. 1).

247. Havighurst, Robert J. History of developmental psychology: Socialization and personality development through the lifespan. In P. B. Baltes and K. W. Schaie (eds.) *Lifespan Developmental Psychology: Personality and Socialization.* New York: Academic Press, pp. 3–24, 1973.

248. Neugarten, B. L. Personality change in late life: A developmental perspective. In C. Eisdorfer and M. P. Lawton (eds.) *The Psychology of Adult Development and Aging.* Washington, D.C.: American Psychological Association, pp. 311–321, 1973.

249. Neugarten, Bernice L. Personality and aging. In J. E. Birren and K. W. Schaie (eds.) *Handbook of the Psychology of Aging,* New York: Van Nostrand Reinhold, pp. 70–102, 1977.

250. Kuhlen, R. G. Personality changes with age. In P. Worchel and D. Byrne (eds.) *Personality Change.* New York: John Wiley, pp. 524–555, 1964.

251. Kuhlen, R. G. Developmental changes with maturity during the adult years. In J. E. Birren (ed.) *Relations in Developmental Aging.* Springfield, Ill.: C. C. Thomas, pp. 209–246, 1964.

252. White, R. W. Competence in the psychosexual stages of development. In M. R. James (ed.). *Nebraska Symposium on Maturation.* Lincoln: University of Nebraska Press, pp. 97–143, 1970.

253. White, R. W. Ego and reality in psychoanalytic theory. *Psychological Issues* **3:** 1–210 (1963).

254. Harter, S. Effectance motivation reconsidered: Toward a developmental model. *Hum. Dev.* **21:** 34–64 (1978).

255. Shows, W. Derek. A psychological theory of the later years: C. G. Jung. In W. D. Gentry (ed.) *Geropsychology: A Model of Training and Clinical Service.* Cambridge, Mass.: Ballinger Press, pp. 79–86, 1977.

256. Cox, Rachel Dunaway. The Concept of Psychological Maturity. In S. Areti (ed.) *American Handbook of Psychiatry.* New York: Basic Books, Vol. 1, pp. 214–238, 1974.

257. Kagan, Jerome and Moss, Howard A. *Birth to Maturity.* New York: Wiley, 1962.

258. Crandall, V. C. The Fels Study: Some contribution to personality development and achievement in childhood and adulthood. *Seminars in Psychiatry* **4:** 383–397 (1972).

259. Sears, R. R. Sources of life satisfaction of the Terman gifted men. *Am. Psychol.* **32:** 119–128 (1977).

260. Sears, Pauline S. and Barbee, Ann H. Career and life satisfactions among Terman's gifted women. In J. C. Stanley, W. C. George and C. H. Solano (eds.) *The Gifted and the Creative: A Fifty Year Perspective.* Baltimore: Johns Hopkins University Press, pp. 28–65, 1977.

261. Sears, P. S. and Sears, R. R. From childhood to middle age to later maturity: Longitudinal study. Paper presented at American Psychological Association Meeting, Toronto, 1978.

262. Jones, Mary C, Bayley, Nancy, Macfarlane, Jean W. and Honzik, Marjorie P. (eds.) *The Course of Human Development.* Waltham, Mass: Xerox College Publishing, 1971.

263. Block, Jack. *Lives through Time.* Berkeley, Ca.: Bancroft Books, 1971.

264. Block, Jack. *The Q-sort Method in Personality Assessment and Psychiatric Research.* Springfield, Ill.: Charles C Thomas, 1961.

265. Haan, Norma. Personality development from adolescence to adulthood in the Oakland Growth and Guidance Studies. *Seminars in Psychiatry* **4:** 399–414 (1972).

266. Peskin, H. and Livson, N. Pre- and postpubertal personality and adult psychologic functioning. *Seminars in Psychiatry* **4:** 343–353 (1972).

267. Haan, N. and Day, D. A longitudinal study of change and sameness in personality development: Adolescence to later adulthood. *Int. J. Ag & Hum. Dev.* **5:** 11–39 (1974).

268. Block, J. Changes and sameness in personality development: Unwarranted conclusions. *Int. J. Ag. and Hum. Dev.* **6:** 277–281 (1975).

269. Haan, N. Change and sameness reconsidered. *Int. J. Ag. & Hum. Dev.* **7:** 59–65 (1976).

270. Livson, F. B. Patterns of personality development in middle-aged women: A longitudinal study. *Int. J. Ag. & Hum. Dev.* **7:** 107–115 (1976).

271. Honzik, Mary P. and Macfarlane, Jean W. Personality Development and Intellectual Functioning from 21 Months to 40 Years. In L. F. Jarvik, C. Eisdorfer & J. E. Blum (eds.) *Intellectual Functioning in Adults.* New York: Springer, pp. 45–58, 1973.

272. Maas, Henry S. and Kuypers, Joseph A. *From Thirty to Seventy.* San Francisco: Jossey Bass, 1974.

273. Haan, N. Proposed model of ego functioning: Coping and defense mechanisms in relation to IQ change. *Psychol. Monographs,* **77:** 1–23 (1963).

274. Clausen, J. A. Glimpses into the social world of middle age. *Int. J. Ag. & Hum. Dev.* **7(2):** 99–106 (1976).

275. Bayley, Nancy. Cognition and aging. In K. W. Schaie (ed.) *Theory and Methods of Research on Aging.* Morgantown: West Virginia University Press, pp. 97–119, 1968.

276. Keniston, K. Youth and its Idealogy. In S. Areti

(ed.) *American Handbook of Psychiatry*. New York: Basic Books, Vol. 1, pp. 399-429, 1974.

277. Cox, Rachel D. *Youth into Maturity*. New York: Mental Health Materials Center, 1970.

278. Vaillant, George E. and McArthur, Charles C. Natural history of male psychologic health. 1. The adult life cycle from 18—50. *Seminars in Psychiatry* **4**: 415-427 (1972).

279. Vaillant, George E. *Adaptation to Life*. Boston: Little Brown, 1977.

280. Levinson, Daniel J., Darrow, Charlotte M., Klein, Edward B., Levinson, Maria H. and McKee, Braxton. The Psychosocial Development of Men in Early Adulthood and the Midlife Transition. In D. F. Ricks, A. Thomas, and M. F. Roff (eds.) *Life History Research in Psychopathology*. Minneapolis: University of Minnesota Press, pp. 243-258, 1974.

281. Levinson, D. J. The midlife transition: A period in adult psychosocial development. *Psychiatry* **40**: 99-112 (1977).

282. Levinson, Daniel J. with Charlotte N. Darrow, Edward B. Klein, Maria H. Levinson and Braxton McKee. *The Seasons of a Man's Life*. New York: Knopf, 1978.

283. Frenkel-Brunswick, Else. Adjustments and Reorientation in the Course of the Lifespan. In B. L. Neugarten (ed.) *Middle Age and Aging*. Chicago: University of Chicago Press, pp. 77-84, 1968.

284. Jaques, E. Death and midlife crisis. *Int. J. Psychoanalysis* **46**: 502-514 (1965). Reprinted in L. R. Allman and O. T. Jaffe, (eds.) Readings in Adult Psychology: Contemporary Perspectives. New York: Harper & Row, Ch. 32, 1978.

285. Neugarten, Bernice L. and Datan, Nancy. The Middle Years. In S. Areti (ed.) *American Handbook of Psychiatry*, Vol. 1. New York: Basic Books, pp. 592-608, 1974 (2nd Edition).

286. Brim, O. G. Jr. Theories of the male midlife crisis. The *Counseling Psychologist,* **6**: 2-9, (1976).

287. Rosenberg, S. D. and Farrell, M. P. Identity and crisis in middle aged men. *Int. J. Ag. & Hum. Dev.* **7**: 153-170, (1976).

288. Bardwick, J. M. Middle age and a sense of the future. *LSA The University of Michigan* **1**, Fall 1977.

289. Costa, Paul T. Jr. and McCrae, Robert R. Objective personality assessment. In M. Storandt, I. C. Siegler, and M. F. Elias (eds.) *The Clinical Psychology of Aging*. New York: Plenum Press, pp. 119-43, 1978.

290. Gould, R. L. The phases of adult life: A study in developmental psychology. *Am. J. Psychiatry* **29**: 521-531 (1972).

291. Chown, S. M. Personality and Aging. In. K. W. Schaie (ed.) *Theory and Methods of Research in Aging*. Morgantown: West Virginia Univ. Press, pp. 134-157, 1968.

292. Singer, Margaret T. Personality measurements in the aged. In J. E. Birren, R. N. Butler, S. W. Greenhouse, L. Sokoloff, and M. Yarrow (eds.) *Human Aging*. Washington, D.C.: Government Printing Office, Public Health Service Document #986, 1963.

293. Angleitner, A. Health, SES, and self perception in the elderly: An application of the interpersonal checklist. *Int. J. Ag. & Hum. Dev.* **8**: 293-299, (1977-78.)

294. Cumming, Elaine and Henry, William E. *Growing Old*. New York: Basic Books, 1961.

295. Reichard, Suzanne, Livson, Florine and Peterson, Paul G. *Aging and Personality*. New York: Wiley, 1962.

296. Havighurst, R. J., Neugarten, Bernice L. and Tobin, S. S. Disengagement and patterns of aging. In B. L. Neugarten (ed.) *Middle Age and Aging*. Chicago: University of Chicago Press, pp. 161-172, 1968 (1963).

297. Neugarten, Bernice L., Crotty, W. J. and Tobin, S. S. Personality types in an aged population. In B. L. Neugarten and Associates. *Personality in Middle and Late Life: Empirical Studies*. New York: Atherton, pp. 158-187, 1968.

298. Neugarten, Bernice L., Havighurst, Robert J. and Tobin, Sheldon S. Personality and Patterns of Aging. In B. L. Neugarten (ed.) *Middle Age and Aging*. Chicago: University of Chicago Press, pp. 173-177, (1968).

299. Maddox, George L. Fact and artifact: Evidence bearing on disengagement theory from the Duke Geriatric Project. *Hum. Dev.* **8**: 117-130 (1965).

300. George, L. K. Predictors of activity and morale patterns in late life. *J. Geront.* in press.

301. Neugarten, Bernice L. and Associates. *Personality in Middle and Late Life: Empirical Studies*. New York: Atherton, 1964.

302. Williams, Richard H. and Wirths, Claudine G. *Lives through the Years*. New York: Atherton Press, 1965.

303. Riegel, K. F. Toward a dialectical theory of development. *Hum. Dev.* **18**: 50-64 (1975).

304. Riegel, Klaus F. Adult life crisis: A dialectic interpretation of development. In N. Datan and L. Ginsberg (eds.) *Lifespan Developmental Psychology: Normative Life Crisis*. New York: Academic Press, pp. 99-128, 1975.

305. Riegel, K. F. The dialectics of human development. *Am. Psychol.* **31**: 689-700 (1976).

306. Datan, N. The life cycle, aging and death: Dialectical perspectives. *Hum. Dev.* **20**: 185-216 (1977).

307. Gruen, Walter. Adult Personality: An Empirical Study of Erikson's Theory of Ego Development. In B. Neugarten and Associates, *Personality in Middle and Late Life: Empirical Studies*. New York: Atherton Press, pp. 1-14, 1964.

308. Peck, Robert and Berkowitz, F. Howard. Personality and adjustment in middle age. In B. L. Neugarten *et al. Personality in Middle and Late Life*. New York: Atherton Press, pp. 15-43, 1964.

309. Brennis, C. B. Developmental aspects of aging in

women: A comparative study of dreams. *Arch. Gen. Psychiatry,* **32:** 429–435, (1975).

310. Giambra, L. M. A factor-analytic study of daydreaming—Imaginal process, and temperament. A replication of an adult male lifespan sample. *J. Gerontol.* **32:** 675–680 (1977).

311. Neugarten, B. L. and Gutmann, D. L. Age-sex roles in personality in middle age: A TAT study. In B. L. Neugarten, *et al. Personality in Middle and Late Life.* New York: Atherton Press, pp. 44–89, 1964.

312. Edwards, A. E. and Wine, D. B. Personality change with age: Their dependency on concommitant intellectual decline. *J. Gerontol.* **18:** 182–184 (1963).

313. Schaie, K. Warner and Strother, Charles R. Cognitive and Personality Variables in College Graduates of Advanced Age. In G. A. Talland (ed.) *Human Aging and Behavior.* New York: Academic Press, pp. 281–308 (1968).

314. Costa, P. T. Jr. and McCrae, R. R. Age differences in personaltiy structure: A cluster analytic approach. *J. Gerontol.* **31:** 564–570 (1976).

315. Costa, P. T. Jr. and McCrae, R. R. Age differences in personality structure revisited: Studies in validity, stability and change. *Int. J. Ag. & Hum. Dev.,* **8:** 261–276, (1977–78).

316. Schaie, K. W. and Parham, I. A. Stability of adult personality traits: Fact or fable? *J. Pers. and Soc. Psychol.* **34:** 146–158 (1976).

317. Siegler, I. C., George, L. K. and Okun, M. A. A cross-sequential analysis of adult personality. *Developmental Psychology,* **15:** 350–351 (1979).

318. Douglas, K. and Arenberg, D. Age changes, cohort differences and cultural change on the Guilford-Zimmerman Temperament Survey. *J. Gerontol.* **33:** 737–747, (1978).

319. Fitzgerald, J. M. Actual and perceived sex and generational differences in interpersonal style: structural and quantitative issues. *J. Gerontol.* **33:** 394–401, (1978).

320. Woodruff, D. S. and Birren, J. E. Age changes and cohort differences in personality. *Dev. Psychol.* **6:** 252–259, (1972).

321. Costa, P. T., Fozard, J. L., McCrae, R. R. and Bosse, R. Relations of age and personality dimensions to cognitive ability factors. *J. Gerontol.* **31:** 663–669, (1976).

322. Schaie, K. W. and Parham, I. A. Social responsibility in adulthood: Ontogenetic and socialculture change. *J. Pers. and Social Psychol.* **30:** 483–492, (1974).

323. Monge, R. H. Studies of the self concept from adolescence thru old age. *Exp. Aging Res.* **1:** 281–291, (1975).

324. Brim, O. G. The sense of personal control over one's life. Invited Address American Psychological Association, New Orleans, September 1974.

325. Duke, M. P., Shaheen J. and Nowicki, S. The determination of locus of control in a geriatric population and a subsequent test of the social learning model for interpersonal distances. *J. Psychol.* **86:** 277–285 (1974).

326. Ryckman, R. M. and Malikioski, M. X. Relationship between locus of control and chronological age. *Psychological Reports.* **36:** 655–658, (1975).

327. Lao, R. The developmental trend of locus of control. *Proceedings of the Division of Personality and Social Psychol.* **1:** 348–350, (1974).

328. Staats, S. Internal versus External locus of control for three age groups. *International J. in Aging and Hum. Dev.* **5:** 7–10, (1974).

329. Palmore, E. and Luikart, C. Health and social factors related to life-satisfaction. *J. Health and Soc. Behav.* **13:** 68–80, (1972).

330. Wolk, S. and Kurtz, J. Positive adjustment and involvement during aging and expectancy for internal control. *J. Consulting and Clinical Psychol.* **45:** 173–178, (1975).

331. Wolk, S. Situational constraint as a moderator of the locus of control adjustment relationship. *J. Consulting and Clinical Psychol.* **44:** 420–427, (1976).

332. Kuypers, J. A. Internal-external locus of control. *Gerontologist.* **12:** Part 1: 168–173, (1972).

333. Felton, B. and Kahana, E. Adjustment and situationally-bound locus of control among institutionalized aged. *J. Gerontol.* **29:** 295–301, (1974).

334. Andrsani, P. J. and Nestel, G. Internal-external control as a contributor to and of work experience. *J. of Applied Psychol.* **61:** 156–165, (1976).

335. Bradley, R. H. and Webb, R. Age-related differences in locus of control orientation in three behavior domains. *Hum. Dev.* **19:** 49–55, (1976).

336. Reid, D. W., Haas, G. and Hawkings, D. Locus of desired control and positive self-concept of the elderly. *J. Gerontol.* **32:** No. 4: 441–450, (1977).

337. Rotter, J. B. Generalized expectancies for internal versus external control of reinforcement. *Psychological Monographs.* **80,** (Whole No. 609), (1966).

338. Lewis, Mary Ann. Psychological well-being and self-concept: Objective and perceived age differences in self-concept for Catholic Sisters. Unpublished doctoral dissertation, Syracuse University, 1972.

339. Nardi, A. H. Person perception research and the perception of lifespan development. In P. B. Baltes and K. W. Schair (eds.) *Lifespan Developmental Psychology: Personality and Socialization.* New York: Academic Press, pp. 285–301, 1973.

340. Labouvie-Vief, G. and Baltes, P. B. Reduction of adolescent misperceptions of the aged. *J. Gerontol.* **31:** 68–71, (1976).

341. Fitzgerald, J. M. Actual perceived sex and genera-

tional differences in interpersonal style: Structural and quantative issues. *J. Gerontol.* **33**: 394–401, (1978).

342. Looft, W. R. Egocentrism and social interaction across the lifespan. *Psychol. Bull.* **78**: 73–92, (1972).

343. Schultz, N. R. and Hoyer, W. J. Feedback effects on spatial egocentrism in old age. *J. Gerontol.* **31**: 72–75, (1976).

344. Coyne, A. C., Whitbourne, S. K. and Glenwick, D. S. Adult age differences in reflection-impulsivity. *J. Gerontol.* **33**: 402–407, (1978).

345. Cohen, D. Sex differences in overt personality patterns in older men and women. *J. Gerontol.* **23**: 262–266, (1977).

346. Panek, P. E., Barrett, G. V., Sterns, H. L. and Alexander, R. A. A review of age changes in perceptual information processing ability with regard to driving. *Exp. Aging Res.* **3**: 387–449, (1977).

347. Chown, S. M. The effect of flexibility-rigidity and age on adaptability in job performance. *Indus. Gerontol.* **13**: 105–121, (1972).

348. George, Linda K. Personal Communication, October 12, 1978.

349. Lefcourt, Herbert M. *Locus of Control.* New York: John Wiley, 1976.

350. Phares, E. Jerry *Locus of Control in Personality.* Morristown, New Jersey: General Learning Press, 1976.

351. Siegler, I. C. and Gatz, M. J. The meaning of age differences in locus of control. Manuscript submitted for publication, 1979.

352. Siegler, I. C. Longitudinal patterns in locus of control. Unpublished manuscript, Duke University, 1978.

353. Hultsch, David F. and Plemons, Judy K. Life and lifespan development. In P. B. Baltes and O. G. Brim Jr. (eds.) *Lifespan Development and Behavior,* Vol. 2, New York: Academic Press, 1979. (in press)

354. Meyer, A. The life chart and the obligation of specifying positive data in psychopathological diagnosis. In E. E. Winters (ed.) *The Collected papers of Adolf Meyer, Vol. III: Medical Teaching.* Baltimore: Johns Hopkins Press, 1951.

355. Selye, Hans. *The Stress of Life.* New York: McGraw-Hill, 1956.

356. Holmes, T. H. and Rahe, R. H. The social readjustment rating scale. *J. of Psychosom. Res.* **11**: 213–218, (1967).

357. Dohrenwend, B. S. and Dohrenwend, B. P. (eds.) *Stressful Life Events: Their Nature and Effects.* New York: Wiley, 1974a.

358. Siegler, I. C. *Stress and Adaptation In Later Life: Strategies, Resources and Events.* In G. Maddox (Chair) Stress and adaptation in later life. Symposium presented at the meetings of the gerontological society. San Francisco, CA., 1977.

359. Nowlin, J. B. *Stress and Adaptation in Later Life:*
Biomedical Response. In G. Maddox (Chair) Stress and adaptation in later life. Symposium presented at the meetings of the gerontological Society. San Francisco, CA., 1977.

360. Palmore, E., Cleveland, W. P., Palmore E., Cleveland, W. P., Nowlin, J. B., Ramm, D. G. Siegler, I. C. *Stress and Adaptation in later life: Social and Psychological aspects. J. Gerontol.,* in press.

361. Lowenthal, M. F. Intentionality: Toward a framework for the study of adaptation in adulthood. *Aging and Hum. Dev.* **2**: 79–95, (1971).

362. Lowenthal, M. F. and Chiriboga, D. Social stress and adaptation: Toward a life course perspective. In C. Eisdorfer and M. P. Lawton (eds.) *The Psychology of Adult Development and Aging.* Washington, D.C., American Psychological Association, 1973.

363. Lowenthal, Marjorie F., Thurner, Majda, and Chiriboga, David *Four Stages of Life.* San Francisco: Jossey Bass, 1975.

364. Lowenthal, Marjorie F. Toward a socio-psychological theory of change in adulthood. In J. E. Birren and K. W. Schaie (eds.) *Handbook of the Psychology of Aging.* New York: Van Nostrand Reinhold, pp. 116–127, 1977.

365. Fiske, Marjorie L. The reality of psychological change. In L. F. Jarvik (ed.) *Aging in the Twenty-first Century: Middle Agers Today.* New York: Gardner Press, 1978.

366. Thurner, Majda. Adaptability of life history interviews to the study of adult development. In L. F. Jarvick, C. Eisdorfer, and J. E. Blum (eds.) *Intellectual Functioning in Adults.* New York: Springer, pp. 137–142, 1973.

367. Bernal, Guillermo A. A., Brannon, Linda J., Belar, Cynthia, Lavigne, John and Cameron, Roy. Psychodiagnostics of the elderly. In W. D. Gentry (ed.) *Geropsychology: A Model of Training and Clinical Service.* Cambridge, Mass.: Ballinger Press, pp. 43–77, 1977.

368. Kahana, Boaz. The use of projective techniques in personality assessment of the aged. In M. Storandt, I. C. Siegler and M. F. Elias (eds.) *The Clinical Psychology of Aging.* New York: Plenum Press, pp. 145–180, 1978.

369. Lawton, M. Powell, Whelihan, William M., and Belsky, Janet K. Personality tests and their uses with older adults. In J. E. Birren (ed.). *Handbook of Mental Health and Aging.* New York: Prentice Hall, in press.

370. Gentry, W. Doyle (ed). *Geropsychology: A Model of Training and Clinical Service.* Cambridge, Mass.: Ballinger Press, 1977.

371. Krasner, J. D. (ed.) Special Issue: Psychotherapy with the elder and dying persons. *Psychotherapy: Theory, Research and Practice.* **14**: 309–415, (1977).

372. Storandt, Martha, Siegler, Ilene C. and Elias,

Merrill F. *The Clinical Psychology of Aging.* New York: Plenum Press, 1978.

373. Pearlin, Seymour and Butler, Robert N. Psychiatric aspects of adaptation to the aging experience. In J. E. Birren, R. N. Butler, S. W. Greenhouse, L. Sokoloff and M. Yarrow (eds.) *Human Aging.* Washington, D.C.: Government Printing Office, Public Health Service Document #986, Chapter 11, pp. 159–213, 1963.

374. Kortensky, Conan. Minnesota multiphasic personality inventory: Results obtained from a population of aged men, In J. E. Birren, R. N. Butler, S. W. Greenhouse, L. Sokoloff and M. Yarrow (eds.) *Human Aging.* Washington, D.C.: Government Printing Office Public Health Service, Chapter 11, pp. 253–?

375. Granick, Samuel. Summary and conclusions. In S. Granick and R. D. Patterson, (eds.) *Human Aging II.* An Eleven-Year Follow-up Biomedical and Behavioral Study. Washington, D.C.: Government Printing Office, DHEW Publication # (HSM) 71-9037, pp. 129–138, 1971.

376. Savage, R. D., Gaber, L. B., Bolten, N. and Cooper, A. *Personality and Adjustment in the Aged.* New York: Academic Press, 1977.

377. Lieberman, Morton A. Adaptive processes in late life. In N. Datan and L. Ginsberg (eds.) *Lifespan Developmental Psychology: Normative Life Crisis.* New York: Academic Press, pp. 135–139, 1975.

378. Tobin, Sheldon and Lieberman, Morton A. *Last Home for the Aged.* San Francisco: Jossey Bass, 1976.

379. Kastenbaum, Robert. Personality theory: Therapeutic approaches and the elderly client. In M. Storandt, I. C. Siegler and M. Elias (eds.) *The Clinical Psychology of Aging.* New York: Plenum Press, pp. 199–224, 1978.

380. Rosow, Irving *Socialization to Old Age.* Berkeley, California: University of California Press, 1974.

381. Brim, O. G. Adult socialization. In J. Clausen (ed.) *Socialization and Society.* Boston: Little Brown, pp. 182–226, 1968.

382. Looft, W. R. Socialization in a lifespan perspective. In P. B. Baltes (ed.) Lifespan models of psychological aging: A White elephant? *The Gerontologist,* 13: 457–512, (1973).

383. Rosow, Irving. Affluence, reciprocity and social bonds. In K. F. Riegel and I. A. Meadiam (eds.) *The Developing Individual Index in a Changing World Vol. II* Chicago: Aldine, pp. 640–652, 1976.

384. Laurie, W. F. Employing the Duke OARS methodology in cost comparisons: Home services and institutionalizational advances in research 2, No. 2: 1–4, (1978).

385. Brody, Elaine M. Aging and family personality: A developmental view. In L. R. Allman and D. T. Jaffee (eds.) *Readings in Adult Psychology: Con-*temporary *Perspectives.* New York: Harper & Row, pp. 355–360, 1978.

386. Cicirelli, Victor. Relationship of siblings to the elderly persons feelings and concerns. *J. Gerontol.* 32: 317–322, (1977).

387. Brody, Elaine M. *Longterm Care of Old People: A Practical Guide.* New York: Human Science Press, 1977.

388. Silverstone, Barbara and Hyman, Helen. *Understanding Your Aging Parent.* New York: Pantheon, 1976.

389. Krause, Corrine A. *Grandmothers, Mothers and Daughters.* New York: Institute on Pluralism Group Identity of the American Jewish Community, June 1978.

390. Maddox, G. L., Blazer, D. G. and Siegler, I. C. The Family Book and older persons. Policy, research and practice. Durham, North Carolina, Center for Aging and Human Development, in press.

391. Henning, Margaret and Jardim, Anne. *The Managerial Woman.* New York: Pocket Books, 1977.

392. Shains, Natalie. The effect of changing cultural patterns upon women. In S. Areti (ed.) *American Handbook in Psychiatry.* New York: Basic Books, Vol. 1, pp. 467–481, 1974.

393. Hoffman, L. W. Effects of maternal employment on Children *Dev. Psychol.* 10: 204–228, (1974).

394. Hoffman, L. W. Changes in family roles socialization and sex differences. *Am. Psychol.* 32: 644–657, (1977).

395. Pearlin, Leonard I. Sex roles and depression. In N. Datan and L. Ginsberg (eds.) *Lifespan Developmental Psychology: Normative Life Crisis.* New York: Academic Press, pp. 191–207, (1977).

396. Block, J. H. Conceptions of sex role: Some crosscultural and longitudinal perspectives. *Am. Psychol.* 28: 512–526, (1973).

397. Russi, Alice S. Transition to parenthood. In L. R. Allman and D. T. Jaffe (eds.) *Readings in Adult Psychology: Contemporary Perspectives.* New York: Harper & Row, Ch. 32 pp. 229–241, 1978.

398. Gutmann, David. Parenthood: A key to the comparative study of the life cycle. In N. Datan and L. Ginsberg (eds.) *Lifespan Developmental Psychology: Normative Life Crisis.* New York: Academic Press, pp. 167–184, 1975.

399. Leifer, Myra. Psychological changes accompanying pregnancy and motherhood. *Genetic psychol Monographs.* 95: 55–96, (1977).

400. Abrahams, B, Feldman, S. S. and Nash, S. C. Sex role self-concept and sex role attitudes: Enduring personality characteristics or adaptations to changing life situations? *Dev. Psychol.* 14, No. 4: 393–400, (1978).

401. Heath, D. H. Competent fathers: Their personalities and marriages. *Hum. Dev.* 19: 26–39, (1976).

402. Bendek, Therese The psychobiology of parenthood. In S. Areti (ed.) *American Handbook of Psychiatry*. New York: Basic Books, Vol. 1, pp. 482–496, 1974.

403. Pineo, P. C. Disenchantment in the later years of marriage. In B. L. Neugarten (ed.) *Middle Age and Aging*. Chicago: University of Chicago Press, pp. 258–262, 1968.

404. Lowenthal, M. F. and Chiriboga D. Transition to empty nest: Crisis, challenge or relief? *Arch. Gen. Psychiatr*. **26**: 8–14, (1972).

405. Thurner, M. Midlife marriage: Sex differences in evaluation and perspectives. *Int. J. Ag. and Hum. Dev*. **7**: 129–135, (1976).

406. Flanagan, John C. A research approach to improving our quality of life. *Amer. Psychol*. **33**: 138–147, (1978).

407. Fozard, J. L. and Popkin, S. J. Optimizing adult development: Ends and means of an applied psychology of aging. *Amer. Psychol*. **33**: 975–989 (1978).

Chapter 9
The Social Factors in Aging

Erdman Palmore, Ph.D.

Duke University Medical Center

INTRODUCTION

Previous chapters have emphasized the important biological and neurological factors in aging. Physical deterioration, intellectual slowing, and perceptual declines among the aged are often so obvious that health professionals overlook the central role that culture and society play in determining individual and group differences in the aging process. Even when some group differences are noted, it may be mistakenly assumed that these differences are caused by biological differences. For example, the fact that a majority of Japanese men past age 65 continue to be in the labor force, while less than a third of those in the United States do so, is explained by cultural, not by biological differences.[1] Similarly, the fact that in the United States almost three times as high a proportion of men as compared with women continue to work past age 65 is less related to any biological differences than it is to our traditional expectations that a man's primary role is to work outside the home, while a woman's primary role is to work inside the home.

Many people believe that the aged inevitably suffer a steady deterioration in physical and mental abilities and therefore should withdraw from the central arenas of our society. We often forget that in other cultures the aged are the most powerful, the most engaged, and the most respected members of the society. When some aged persons show depression, hopelessness, feelings of inferiority, and paranoia, we may forget that these symptoms may have been caused by deprivation of basic satisfactions, reduction to an inferior status, and discrimination against those with 65 or more birthdays, rather than by any biological process.

Indeed, the noted biologist and gerontologist Alex Comfort estimates that only 25% of aged-related changes are accounted for by physical aging. The other 75% is accounted for by "sociogenic aging, the role which our folk-lore, our prejudices, and our misconceptions about age still impose on the old."[2]

In order to clarify the social factors in aging, this chapter will discuss cross-cultural differences in aging, group differences within in the United States, ageism, social stress on elders, social support, government programs for elders, implications for health practitioners, and aging in the future.

CROSS-CULTURAL DIFFERENCES

Modernization and the Aged*

When we compare the status of the aged in different cultures around the world and in different societies throughout history, we may first be impressed by the bewildering variety of situations. In some cultures the aged are revered and considered closest to the gods. In others they are considered outcasts and ostracized. In some societies they are the most powerful and important members, while in others they have almost no role and are often considered worse than useless.

Yet when we examine the types of societies in which these contrasts occur, a pattern begins to emerge. This pattern could be represented by a curvilinear graph of the rise and fall in status of the aged in the following general form. The baseline or zero point would be represented by animal groups in which there seem to be no instincts or inborn propensities to sustain aged parents or grandparents. The usual pattern among animals is to abandon the aged of the species as soon as their ability to function has seriously declined.[4] It is only through the development of human culture that the aged have been able to achieve any security. Beginning with primitive hunting, fishing, and collecting societies, the status and security of the aged rises until it reaches its peak in highly developed agricultural societies. Simmons and others have argued that the graph would show substantial decline as it moves to our modern industrial societies.[5]

The reasons for the rise in status of the aged from the primitive to the stable rural

* Some of this material is adapted from Palmore and Maddox, 1977.[3]

societies involve six factors that may be summarized as follows:

1. Stable agricultural societies were able to develop greater surpluses of food and shelter to share with the aged. As long as the next day's or the next week's meals were uncertain, as long as food storage was inadequate, and as long as families had to migrate from one area to another when the local supply of food was exhausted, the aged and infirm were likely to suffer and to be left behind. It is true that, in order to counter this tendency, the aged in many primitive societies developed food taboos or food preferences that gave them some advantage over the younger tribe members in the competition for scarce food. But when food became more plentiful and more assured with the development of grain storage and animal husbandry, the security of the aged increased markedly.

2. Stable agricultural societies developed more capital and more personal property, which increasingly came under the control of the aged. Through their ability to dictate who had access to the property, who would inherit it, and so on, the aged were able to exert a strong influence on the society as a whole and thereby maintained their position of power.

3. The growing importance of extended family relations could also be manipulated by the aged to support their status and power. The aged members of the extended family usually were able to influence marriage and birth rates and the economic and social roles that various members of the family assumed, thus assuring the well-being of the clan and of their own position in it.

4. In agricultural societies there are generally more opportunities for auxiliary but useful tasks for the aged than in the more primitive ones. As societies shifted to cultivation of the soil and animal husbandry, the aged could move more easily to lighter tasks, so that they seldom suffered from abrupt retirement and usually found useful functions until near the end of life. Simmons[4] states, "Self-employment or ancillary services in agrarian systems probably

have provided the most secure and continuous occupational status that society at large has yet afforded for the majority of its aged."

5. Stable agrarian societies accumulated more and more knowledge and technical skills for adapting to the environment and meeting the needs of its members. The aged tended to be the best authorities on this accumulated knowledge and often the most skilled practitioners of the growing arts and crafts. When most of what was known had to be retained by memory, the aged were the best source of information and were usually in the best position to make the best judgments. This semimonopoly on knowledge, wisdom, and skills reinforced the high status of the aged.

6. Similarly, because of their greater experience and knowledge, the aged were usually able to become the main leaders in the growing political, civil, judicial, and religious institutions in the agrarian society. These roles were even more rewarding than their auxiliary tasks. Simmons found that most of the tribes he surveyed had old men as chiefs, councilmen, and advisors. He pointed out that the term *elder* had commonly implied leader, head man, or councilman.[4] Also, as magic and religion were associated with complex ceremonies and institutions among the sedentary societies, the aged were usually able to control the most important roles in these structures.

Two qualifications of this general picture of the high status of the aged in agricultural societies should be kept in mind. First, the aged in some foraging, hunting, and fishing societies had relatively high status, and the aged in some agricultural societies had relatively low status.[6] Second, among all societies, the extremely old and helpless person is viewed as a living liability.[4] This discussion does not generally consider the very frail elderly.

There seems to be little question that the status of the aged in most stable agricultural societies tended to be higher than in most primitive societies. However, the assumption that the status and satisfactions of the aged have declined markedly as a result of industrialization is more debatable. Shanas et al.,[7] Friedmann,[6] and others have challenged the view that today's aged are less socially integrated and are worse off than the aged were a century ago.

Several distinctions need to be made in resolving this issue. First, the different types of status or satisfaction need to be specified, (e.g., health, economic, family, political, prestige). For example, there is evidence that the health, education, and income status of the aged as a group are improving as younger and healthier cohorts move into the aged category and as health care improves.[8] Also, the actual standard of living of the aged has probably improved over the past century just as it has for the average younger person. On the other hand, the proportion of the aged living with children or other relatives has declined,[9] although the extended kinship network remains strong.[7]

The status of the aged relative to younger people has declined substantially in several industrial societies, although this decline may be leveling off or even reversing itself in the most advanced nations, such as the United States and Canada.[10]

Finally, trends in the status of the aged vary substantially by race, sex, and socioeconomic status. Therefore it is neither useful nor accurate to make such a broad generalization as "the status of the aged declines as a result of industrialization." Accurate resolution of the issue requires specification of the country, the kind of status meant, how status is measured, and which type of aged person is being referred to.

Oriental Societies*

The status of the aged in Asian societies appears to have suffered much less decline than in Western societies. For example, aging in Japan is almost the opposite of aging in the United States. Despite high levels of industrialization and urbanization, the Japanese have maintained a high level of respect for their elders and a high level of in-

* Some of this material is adapted from Palmore, 1975.[1]

tegration of their elders in the family, work force, and community. While there is considerable prejudice and discrimination against the aged in America, old age is recognized by most Japanese as a source of prestige and honor. The most common word for the aged in Japanese, *Otoshiyori,* literally means "the honorable elders." Respect for the elders is shown in the honorific language used in speaking to or about the elders; rules of etiquette which give precedence to the elders in seating arrangements, serving order, bathing order, and going through doors; bowing to the elders; the national holiday called Respect for Elders Day; giving seats on crowded public vehicles to the elders; and the authority of the elders over many family and household matters.

The high level of their integration into Japanese society is demonstrated by the following facts. Over 75% of all Japanese aged 65 and older live with their childen, in contrast to 25% in the United States. The majority of Japanese men over 65 continue to be in the labor force, compared to 29% of men in the United States over 65. Most of the Japanese elders who are not actually employed continue to be useful in housekeeping, child-care, shopping, and gardening, often freeing their daughters or daughters-in-law for employment outside the home. The vast majority of Japanese elders also remain active in their communities through Senior Citizens Clubs, religious organizations, and informal neighborhood groups. Most surprising of all, there appears to have been little decline in these high levels of integration during the past 20 or 30 years.

Observers in the Peoples Republic of China and in Taiwan also report relatively high status for the aged there.[5] Thus, Asian societies prove that the aged in industrial societies need not suffer from the ageism they experience in our society.

Communist Societies

Reports on the situation of the aged in communist countries, such as the U.S.S.R., the German Democratic Republic, and Hungary, may be somewhat idealized, but one thing seems to be clear: there is little or no mandatory retirement based on age alone.[11] On the contrary, there are special incentives for older persons to keep working. These countries claim that, because of their communist system, they can and do provide useful employment for all aged who wish to keep working, even though their abilities may have declined. This is in sharp contrast to our common practice of forcing all workers to retire at age 65, regardless of their wishes and abilities.

Federal legislation will prohibit such mandatory retirement, until age 70, but the effectiveness of such legislation remains to be seen. Considerable age discrimination in employment will probably continue for many years despite such changes in the law.

Furthermore, the reports from communist countries claim that all age discrimination is prohibited and that the aged are guaranteed adequate income, housing, medical care, transportation, recreation, and all the other things necessary for a good and long life. They also claim that the aged are respected and honored for their years of contribution to the society. If true, these reports provide another dramatic contrast to the situation of many aged in our country.

Dependency Ratios

It is generally known that the number of aged in the United States has and will continue to increase rapidly. In 1950 there were only about 12 million persons age 65 and over; now the number has almost doubled to 23 million persons and the number is expected to increase to about 32 million by the end of this century.[12] Many people view this rapid increase with alarm. They wonder if our society can provide adequate medical care, housing, and other necessities to such a large and growing number of dependent persons.

However, these numbers become much less alarming when they are viewed in the context of other factors. (1) The proportion of our population 65 or over is substantially less than in many European countries. In 1975, 10% of our population was 65 or over, while at least 13 European countries had higher proportions, including Norway with 14%, Austria with 15% and the German Democratic Republic with 16%. These countries with much higher proportions of the aged have managed to provide for their aged without unusual difficulty. (2) Despite the large increase in absolute numbers, the proportion over 65 is not expected to increase by more than two percentage points by the year 2000.[12] In other words, while the number of aged is increasing rapidly, the number of persons under 65 is increasing almost as rapidly. (3) The *aged dependency ratio* (number of persons over 65 divided by the number age 20–64) is presently about .19 and is expected to increase to .21 by the year 2000. Thus the burden of older persons on "working age" persons will be slightly greater. However, this will be more than offset by the current and expected lower fertility. The *total dependency ratio,* which includes dependent children (number of persons over 65 and under 20 divided by the number 20 to 64) will go down from the current .75 to about .72 in the year 2000. In other words, the increase in dependent aged will be more than made up for by the decrease in dependent children. Thus, we need not fear an inability to support the increasing numbers of aged. The problem will be how to transfer the savings from decreased numbers of children to support for the increased number of aged.

DIFFERENCES WITHIN THE UNITED STATES*

One of the most common misconceptions about the aged is that most are pretty much alike. There is a common tendency to talk about "the aged" as if they were a homogeneous group. On the contrary, persons over 65 are at least as heterogeneous as any other age category spanning 35 or more years. The major social differences among the aged are age, sex, marital status, class,

* Some of this material was adapted from Palmore and Maddox, 1977.[3]

race and residence. Furthermore, longitudinal studies have found that variability in most characteristics generally tends to increase among the aged as they grow older.[13] Age and sex grading are probably the most pervasive bases of differentiation in all societies, since they are permanent differences.

A basic difference between the sexes is that women live longer than men: in our society, women live eight years longer than men. One consequence of this is that, while two-thirds of the aged men are still married, only one-third of the women are still married.[14]

When women become widowed, they are more likely to live with their children or other relatives. Widowed men are more likely to live alone or end up in an institution. In general, men have fewer contacts with their families: they live farther away from their families, they see their children less often, and they exchange services less with their families.[7] These differences may be related to the general cultural expectation that women should remain closer to their families, and men should be more independent and more interested in things outside their families.

Aged men also claim to be healthier than aged women: they less often say they are housebound, report fewer incapacities and fewer illnesses within the past year, and see a physician less often.[7] It is difficult to tell whether this is due to actual better health among men or to the cultural expectation that men should be "tough" and should not admit illness as readily as women. Since women actually outlive men, it seems likely that the cultural expectation is the major explanation of these differences in reported health.

A clear and fundamental difference between the sexes is that aged men are more often employed than aged women, just as they were in their younger years. Of men over age 65, 38% continue some employment, compared with 14% of the women.[15] Among those who are retired, more of the men were forced to retire because of compulsive retirement policies, poor health, and the like, while women more often report that they retired voluntarily. These differences are explained by the cultural expectation that man's primary role should be gainful employment, while the married woman's primary role is usually thought to be in the home. Men also are able to earn substantially more than women on the average, even when the number of hours and weeks is controlled.[16] Partly as a result of this difference in earning power, there are about twice as many aged women living in poverty as there are aged men.[17]

Differences between age groups also persist among persons over 65. In general, the older aged (those over 75) are in poorer health, are hospitalized more often, are more often widowed and more often live alone, are isolated and lonely, are rarely employed, and have less income than those between ages 65 and 75.[7,18]

Socioeconomic differences also persist among the aged, although there is some evidence that these differences become somewhat attenuated in comparison with younger groups. For example, income differences become smaller because the income of those on the upper economic level is reduced with retirement, and those in the lower economic groups are supported by Social Security and welfare payments.[14] However, the general stratification patterns remain among the aged: those with less income have less education and come from the blue collar or manual occupations. They have less adequate diets and poorer housing, see doctors less often, and, as a result, their health is poorer. They are more incapacitated, have a higher death rate, are more likely to double up and live with their children and have more serious unmet needs.[7,14,19] The lower strata are also less likely than the more affluent to belong to organizations, be church members, travel, and read newspapers. On the other hand, they are more likely to hold fundamentalist views, such as a belief in the existence of the devil, and they are more often anomic, depressed, and unhappy.[20]

There is less known about the differences between aged whites, blacks, and other minority groups. We do know that aged members of minority groups tend to be in lower socioeconomic positions substantially more often than white aged. But it should also be remembered that aged minority members are not homogeneous groups either. There are substantial numbers of wealthy and well-educated aged among minority groups.

In addition, there is some scattered evidence that aged blacks have some relative advantage compared with aged whites (e.g., aged blacks do not usually suffer as great a reduction in income as do aged whites.)[21] There is also some evidence that aged blacks, as compared with aged whites, feel generally more accepted by their children and receive more assistance from their children.[22] It appears that, relative to their previous status and insecurity during youth and middle age, many of the black aged enjoy somewhat higher status and security because of a more stable income; because surviving to old age is an achievement in itself; because intergenerational family ties are strong; and because some progress toward racial equality has been made.

AGEISM AND OTHER PREJUDICES

Just as racial groups suffer from racism and women suffer from sexism, the aged in our society suffer from ageism. Ageism may be defined simply as prejudice and discrimination against the aged. Because ageism is a relatively new concept[23] and is so much a part of our "way of life," much of it tends to be unrecognized and unconscious. It is none the less real and damaging to the health and happiness of our elders. It probably accounts for a major part, if not the majority, of the "problems of aging."

Health professionals, because of their education and training, should know better than most people that prejudices against the aged have little basis in fact.* Yet health professionals are particularly subject to a biased view of elders because of the type of elderly person they most often come into

* Some of this material is adapted from Palmore, 1976.[8]

contact with. Health professionals primarily see the one-fourth of the elderly who are sick, senile, disabled, institutionalized, or have other major problems. They rarely see the three-fourths who are healthy, capable of living in their own homes, taking care of themselves, and carrying out their manual activities. As a result health professionals tend to overestimate the prevalence of illness, senility, and other problems among elders. More seriously, this bias may lead to the belief that illness and senility are "natural and inevitable" among the aged and that nothing can be done about it, (or that the little that can be done is hardly worth doing). It is therefore particularly important that health professionals examine the facts and avoid these prejudices in order to maximize the effectiveness of their treatment.

Illness

One of the most common prejudices against elders is that most are ill or disabled. From one-fifth to two-thirds of various groups agree with the following statements: Older people "spend much time in bed because of illness;" "have many accidents in the home;" "have poor coordination;" "feel tired most of the time;" and "develop infection easily".[24] Other common stereotypes are that large proportions of the aged are living in hospitals, nursing homes, homes for the aged, or other such institutions, and that the health and abilities of the aged show a steady decline with each passing year.[25]

The fact is that these stereotypes do not apply to the vast majority of elders. For instance, it comes as a great surprise to those unfamiliar with study findings that only 5% of persons aged 65 and over live in homes for the aged, nursing homes, hospitals, or other institutions.[12] In an ordinary group of uninformed persons the estimates of the proportion of the aged who live in institutions usually range from 20% to over 50%.

As for the idea that the aged spend much time in bed due to illness, it is true that they spend almost twice as many days in bed per year as younger persons, but this is still only 3% of the total days in the year (10 days for men, 13 days for women).[26] Also, most aged persons are able to perform their major activity most of the time. Only 16% of the aged outside institutions say that they are unable to perform their major activity. The average number of restricted activity days is only 38 per year.

In reference to the stereotype that the aged develop infections easily and have many accidents, there are actually fewer acute conditions among the old than among the young (1.1 per person per year for the aged compared to 2.3 for persons under age 65). It is true that the elderly have more chronic conditions (81%), but this is only one and one half times more than those aged 17 to 64 (54%), and including such minor conditions as needing glasses, mild hearing loss, and allergies.

Regarding the belief that the health and physical ability of most aged decline steadily, the Duke Longitudinal Study of Aging found that from 44% to 58% of survivors who returned for examinations had no decline in physical functioning or actually had some improvement over time, depending on the time interval (3 to 13 years).[27] The aged actually show great variability in patterns of change. A few decline precipitously and quickly become totally disabled. For the majority of aged, health and abilities seem to remain fairly level or fluctuate slightly when illnesses are contracted, accidents occur, and recoveries are made; 51% of the aged rate their health as good, 33% as fair, and only 16% as poor.[14] Some aged pride themselves on remaining extremely healthy and capable. There are frequent reports of aged persons who run marathons, climb mountains, swim great distances, and carry out other feats demonstrating their high level of physical functioning. A recent study reports that a 1-year program of exercise for men 70 and over so improved their health and fitness that their body reactions became similar to those of men 30 years younger.[28] Such evidence suggests that much of the decline in abilities that does occur among the aged may be due more to declining exercise and activity than to any inevitable aging process itself.

Impotency

A related prejudice against the aged is the belief that most no longer have any sexual activity or even sexual desire and that those few who do are morally perverse or at least abnormal. Evidence from all the surveys show these beliefs to be false. The Duke Longitudinal Study of Aging indicates that large proportions of the elderly continue to be sexually active, with even larger proportions reporting continuing interest in sexual activity. For example, 70% of the men who were relatively healthy reported that they were still sexually active, and 80% reported continuing sexual interest.[29] Sexual activity and interest did tend to decline with advancing age, but the majority of men continued to be sexually active up through their seventies. This bias against sexual activity among the aged often causes resistance to remarriage and other normal sexual interests. Clinicians should be aware that frustration of sexual desire among the aged, as at any age, may cause depression and other psychiatric symptoms.

Mental Decline

Another common belief is that mental abilities begin to decline steadily from age 20 onward, especially the abilities to learn and remember, so that "you can't teach an old dog new tricks," and the aged are generally mentally incompetent. It is true that reaction time tends to slow somewhat with advancing age, but among healthy aged this slowing is only about two-tenths of a second on the average and has little practical significance for most tasks and functioning.[30] Furthermore, there is great variability in reaction times and many older persons have faster reaction times than the average young person. It is also true that older persons often require somewhat longer to learn new

material, but, given extra time, they can learn as well as younger persons.

As for general intelligence, longitudinal studies have found little or no overall decline with age among the healthy aged until a few years before death. Tests of vocabulary and information also show less decline than performance tests involving speed response. Similarly there tends to be a decline in speed of response but not in accuracy. Seven different studies have found that subjects with advanced education and superior ability, working without time pressure, show little or no deterioration with age.[31] There is considerable evidence that many aged continue to be creative in later life.[32] Some have concluded that the potential peak performance for abstraction and philosophy occurs between the ages of 45 and 83.[33] Dennis found that creativity remained high among inventors and scholars in the humanities, mathematics, and botany during their 70s, although it decreased sharply among biologists, chemists, geologists, and artists.[34]

Mental Illness

A similar prejudice is that many or most aged are "senile" and that mental illness is common, inevitable, and untreatable among most aged. This belief is particularly vicious because it can become a "self-fulfilling prophecy" in which the belief that mental illness is inevitable and untreatable leads to lack of prevention and treatment, which in turn tends to confirm the original belief.

The facts clearly contradict such beliefs. Less than 1% of persons over 65 are patients in mental hospitals. An additional 1% or 2% have significant psychiatric disturbances and reside in other institutions.[35] As for those living outside institutions, a series of eight community surveys found the prevalence of psychosis to vary from 4% to 8%.[36] All the studies agree that severe mental illness is not inevitable for the majority of older persons, even with the current levels of social and psychological stress in our society. The prevalence of milder forms of mental illness becomes largely a matter of arbitrary definition, and the estimates of psychoneurosis range from 7%[37] to over 50%.[38]

It is more difficult to determine what proportion of mental illness among the aged is reversible or responsive to some form of treatment. Much of this book is devoted to discussing the usefulness of various methods of diagnosis and treatment. It is sufficient to point out here that many or most of these methods have not been applied on a large scale because of limited personnel and funds. We cannot determine the large scale effectiveness of these methods until they are tried. A defeatist attitude that little can be done tends to assure that in fact little is done.

It is a central thesis of this chapter that much of mental illness among the aged, as at other ages, is at least partly caused by social and psychological stress and therefore can be reduced or ameliorated by the reduction of stress and by proper treatment.

Uselessness

Because of the above-mentioned beliefs that the majority of the aged are disabled by physical or mental illness, many people conclude that the elderly are unable to continue working and that those few who do continue to work are unproductive. It is true that, in this country, the majority of the aged are retired, but evidence indicates that this is due less to disability than to discrimination in employment, (such as compulsory retirement) and other pressures for the aged to withdraw from the labor force.[39] In some countries, such as Japan, older workers are highly valued and the majority continue to work past age 65.[1] Even in this country, most persons over 65 either continue to be employed (12%), continue to work as housewives (17%), do volunteer work (another 19%), or are retired but would like to be employed or do volunteer work (30%). Thus, a total of 78% are working (including housework and volunteer work) or would like to have some kind of work to do.[40]

Isolation

The idea that most aged are lonely and isolated from their families and normal social relations is clearly false About 80% of the aged in the United States live with someone else, 75% say they are not often alone, and 86% say they have seen one or more relatives during the previous week.[7] Two studies also found that there is even more social interaction and less isolation among aged who live in neighborhoods with a high proportion of aged like themselves.[41,42] About two-thirds say they are never or hardly ever lonely,[43] or say that loneliness is not a serious problem.[40] Most older persons have close relatives within easy visiting distance and contacts are relatively frequent.[44] About one-half of the aged say they "spend a lot of time" socializing with friends.[40] Three-fourths are members of a church or synagogue,[45] and about half attend services at least three times per month.[46] Over half belong to other voluntary organizations.[47] Thus, between visits with relatives and friends and participation in church and other voluntary organizations, the majority of old people are far from socially isolated. However, when isolation and loneliness do occur, it may contribute to mental illness, especially depression and cognitive disorientation.

Thus it is not "normal," either statistically or clinically, for older persons to be isolated. Good clinicians will do what they can do to help their patients avoid becoming isolated.

Poverty

Views about the economic status of the aged range from those who think that most of the aged are in poverty, to those who think that a large proportion of the aged are rich with substantial assets. Neither of these extreme views is correct. It is true that the average income of older persons is approximately cut in half after retirement and about 15% of persons over 65 have incomes below the poverty level according to the official government definitions.[48]

Economic decline is a major problem for many of the aged. There are very few with substantial financial assets other than their equity in their home.[14] Most aged are primarily dependent on social security and pensions or what little they can continue to earn. But poverty among the aged is concentrated primarily among the single or widowed. Later we will discuss how the multiple stresses of loss of role, reduced income, and widowhood may combine to produce or exacerbate mental illness.

But the point here is that poverty also is "abnormal" among the aged, and clinicians must not neglect economic difficulties in the evaluation and treatment of patients.

Depression

A final set of stereotypes about the aged is that they are "grouchy," "feel sorry for themselves," "touchy," and "cranky." The evidence on this stereotype is somewhat mixed. Many studies have found more depression, neuroticism, and unhappiness among aged persons, although these studies do not show large differences by age.[36] On the other hand, a detailed item analysis of the Minnesota Multiphasic Personality Inventory found greater amounts of satisfaction and happiness indicated in the young and older ages as compared to the middle ages.[49] A review concluded that "the typical older person is not only as likely as a younger person to have a sense of adequacy and self-worth but also as likely to seem content with his occupational and familial roles."[36] The Duke Longitudinal Studies of Aging found little or no significant decline in happiness or life satisfaction, nor increase in depression.[50] A recent national survey found that less than a fourth of persons 65 and over reported that "This is the dreariest time of my life," while a majority said "I am just as happy as when I was younger."[40] The discrepancies in the conclusions of these various studies are probably due to the differences in groups studied, aspects of happiness or depression measured, and methods used. However, none of the studies would support the stereotype that the majority of

aged are extremely depressed or unhappy. Thus depression among the aged is also "abnormal" and should be treated as such rather than ignored.

The main danger of such prejudices against the aged is that they will encourage or excuse discriminatory behaviors which are the direct causes of, or at least contributory factors, in the problems of the aged.

Employment

Perhaps the most obvious and serious form of discrimination is in the area of employment: from hiring and promotions to firing and compulsory retirement. Despite the existence of the Age Discrimination in Employment Act since 1967, which is designed to protect workers aged 40–65 from discrimination, there was considerable evidence that widespread discrimination against older workers persists, especially against workers over age 65 who have no legal protection.[44] Compulsory retirement based on age is by definition discrimination against an age category. Compulsory retirement is a policy which prevents employment of older persons regardless of their personal merit, abilities, or qualifications. Various sources of data indicate that about half of all male workers retiring at age 65 or beyond are affected by compulsory retirement policies.[39]

Contrary to the prejudices against older workers, the facts indicate that most older workers can work at least as effectively as younger workers. Despite declines in perception and reaction speed under laboratory conditions among the general aged population, studies of older workers under actual working conditions generally show that they perform as well as young workers, if not better on most measures. When speed of reaction is important, older workers sometimes produce at lower rates, but they are at least as accurate and steady in their work as younger workers. Consistency of output tends to increase with age, as older workers perform at steadier rates from week to week than younger workers do. In addition, older workers have less job turnover, less accidents, and less absenteeism than younger workers.[36]

The evidence does not justify age discrimination on most jobs. The main detrimental effects often resulting from such discrimination are loss of income, loss of role and status, isolation, depression, and declining health and vigor because of inactivity.

Segregation

A sizable and growing proportion of the aged are concentrated in certain states and counties, in certain sections of cities, and in special residences for the aged.[9] Surveys show that only about one-fourth of the aged live with their adult children.[7] This is a decline from 1952, when one-third of the aged lived in a household with two or more generations.[51] The concentration of the aged in certain counties is dramatically shown in the special Census Bureau map of the United States that color-codes each county in terms of the proportion of aged. The urban aged are concentrated in the central sections of the city, and the rural aged are concentrated in Villages.[52]

The growing segregation of the aged has been described by Breen[52] as follows:

Homes for the aged, public housing projects, medical institutions, recreation centers, and communities which are devoted to the exclusive use of the retired have been increasing in number and size in recent years. Retirement "villages" have been sponsored by philanthropic organizations, unions, church groups, and others. Even established communities which are now known as "retirement centers" have become inundated by older migrants seeking identification and spatial contiguity with "the clan."

The question that cannot be answered at present is how much of this segregation is voluntary or self-segregation, and how much of it is subtly or overtly forced on the aged by the younger majority. In all probability, voluntary segregation is more likely to occur among the aged than among other minority groups. There is some evidence that most elders living in age-segregated communities prefer such living arrangements to age-integrated ones. They are at least as satisfied with their communities and their life as are other elders. Regardless of the causes of the segregation, the consequences to the aged and to the rest of society may well be similar to the familiar consequences of segregation of other minority groups. For example, Friedmann[6] warns that the duplication of community facilities and services for segregated aged communities may prove to be as economically unfeasible as attempts to provide "separate but equal" facilities for other groups in our society. He also points out other indirect losses, such as the loss of needed skills in the industrial system and the loss of the potential contribution of this new leisure class in performing nonpaid functions essential in the conduct of political and civil affairs.

Inadequate Medical Care

It is difficult to assess the adequacy of medical care for elders. On the one hand, elders are the only age group covered by national health insurance (Medicare), and they certainly consume a larger proportion of health services than any other group. On the other hand, there are several indications that they still receive less adequate care than other age groups. First, the widespread belief (often shared by the aged themselves) that most of the illnesses and health conditions of older persons are "normal" and irreversible, prevents the adequate treatment of many illnesses that are in fact reversible. This is another example of "self-fulfilling prophecy", the belief that something is untreatable leads to neglect which may eventually make the condition untreatable. Second, there is extensive evidence that most health professionals tend to give low priority to treating the aged and prefer to treat children and young adults.[25] Third, despite

Medicare, there are still formidable barriers to adequate care including financial and transportation barriers, as well as ignorance and denial among elders.[53] Fourth, despite the fact that elders consume more health services, these moderately higher rates of consumption are still lower than might be expected based on the much higher rates of illness and health concerns among elders.[53] It is probable that many elders do not get as adequate medical care as they would if they were younger.

Other Discrimination

There are many other areas where subtle and sometimes not-so-subtle discrimination against elders is practiced. The aged sometimes have more difficulty getting a loan or mortgage, even though their actuarial life expectancy would cover the period of payments on the loan. They are usually not given the educational opportunities younger persons have. Civic and community organizations often drop them out of active leadership roles. Commercials and advertisements depicting older persons usually show them as suffering from arthritis, constipation, insomnia, or some other ailment. Slang epithets for older persons are widely used: dirty old man; old geezer; old codger; old maid; old biddy; old bag; hag; senile; and decrepit. Most jokes and sayings about the aged tend to reinforce prejudice against them.[54,55,56] Even supposed compliments such as "You don't look that old" and "You haven't changed a bit" imply that to look old or older is to look ugly or infirmed.

As a result of these prejudices and discriminations most older persons tend to deny their age and suffer from lowered self-esteem when they have to admit their age. Some stop having birthdays, other give their age as "39" for the rest of their lives. One of the most common types of joke about the aged involves denial of age. In normal conversation with elders it is considered rude and embarrassing to ask about or discuss the elder's age. If the elder's age is revealed, he or she is usually reassured that "You don't look that old." Billions of dollars are spent each year in attempts to hide signs of aging including hair dyes, toupes, hair growers, wrinkle removers, face lifts, etc. The elderly should not be criticized for these attempts to look handsome or beautiful, yet these attempts are a demonstration of our basic assumption that youth is beautiful and desirable while old age is ugly and undesirable.

In contrast, many cultures in less industrialized countries and in Asia still admire and venerate old age. Gray hair, baldness, and wrinkles tend to be respected as badges of maturity, experience, wisdom, and service. In Japan, for example, it is generally considered respectful to ask an elder's age and then to congratulate the elder on his or her advanced age and venerability.[1] The effects of age denial or self-hatred on the mental and physical health of the aged are manifold and include depression, neurosis, alcoholism, drug abuse, psychosomatic illness, withdrawal, isolation, inactivity, and high rates of suicide.

SOCIAL STRESS

While ageism is probably the most pervasive stress that elders in our society have to endure, there are several other forms of stress that may contribute to mental and physical illnesses.

Income Loss

While the majority of the aged do not live in poverty, 15% are in poverty, and another 10% are among the "near poor." These proportions are about one-third higher than among the nonaged.[48] Furthermore, the average elder usually faces a substantial loss of income upon retirement. The median income of persons over 65 is less than half that of younger persons. Regardless of whether the older person is reduced to poverty, any substantial loss of income may produce many kinds of stress such as reductions in nutrition, clothing, shelter, recreation, and other social activities.

Loss of Role and Status

Old age has been called the "roleless role." This is an exaggeration because most elders have the normal roles of citizen, community member, neighbor, friend, and family member, regardless of what other roles they may have. Each of these roles has a complex set of rights and responsibilities which the elder is expected to fulfill, as would any other person. But it is true that retirement (especially involuntary retirement), loss of parental role as children leave home, and reductions in other roles often produce a sense of uselessness, isolation, and loneliness among the aged.

A loss of status, prestige, and respect often accompanies these role losses. Unless elders find some alternate source of status and self-esteem they may suffer from feelings of worthlessness and depression as a result. The antidote is to remain active or become active in some meaningful and satisfying role(s) which will maintain self-esteem and status.

Bereavement

Death of spouse has been rated as *the* most serious life change in the Holmes and Rahe Schedule of Life Changes.[57] Death of other relatives and friends are also considered serious potential stressors. Yet there is some evidence from the Duke Longitudinal Studies that in middle and old age, death of spouse does not usually result in significant long-term negative consequences.[31,58] Apparently, most normal older persons are able to adjust to widowhood within a period of a few years.

Nevertheless, widowhood is probably one of the most traumatic events that most persons are likely to experience. Loss of spouse is, at least, a temporary stress requiring adaptive mechanisms.

Furthermore, it appears that when widowhood is compounded with other stresses, such as income loss, loss of role and status, illness, etc., it is more likely to result in deterioration of mental health and, occasionally in overt mental illness. The health practitioner should be aware of the special problems that may be caused by widowhood, especially when it occurs in combination with other stressors.

Isolation through Disability

Earlier in this chapter it has been pointed out that the vast majority of elders are not seriously isolated. Nevertheless, isolation often results from various forms of physical and mental disability. It is well known that the aged suffer from more physical disabilities and chronic conditions. Disability and illness are obviously stressful and are associated with higher rates of mental illness,[59] but, in addition to the obvious physical stress of illness and disability, various kinds of social and psychological stress can be caused by disability. Isolation from normal social interaction and psychological support is probably one of the most important. For example, failing eyesight or hearing often interfere with normal communication. There is evidence that loss of hearing is associated with impaired cognitive functioning.[60] Thus, isolation from disability (or from other causes) is a frequent stressor in old age.

Involuntary isolation, which begins in old age, must be distinguished from voluntary preference for being alone over a life time. There is evidence that it is mainly the involuntary isolation beginning in old age which causes stress. Life-long "loners" apparently prefer little interaction and might find increased interaction stressful.

Loss of Cognitive Functioning

Although many older persons show no loss of cognitive functioning, most studies conclude that "the general trend in cognitive functioning is downhill."[30] Such loss, whether it be slowing of response speed, loss of intellectual ability, learning ability, memory, or integrative functions, can produce severe stress in adapting to the problems of old age. If such stress becomes severe enough it can result in mental illness.

Community Disintegration

The neighborhood one lives in may be an additional source of stress, especially for older persons. Dr. Alexander Leighton and colleagues have carried out a series of community studies which indicate that social disintegration is a major factor in producing mental illness. He describes the symptoms of a disintegrated community as "defective communication among the members of the group; lack of leadership and followership; inability to arrive at group decisions; defective child rearing, training, and education; deficiencies in work and productivity; lack of recreation; and weak control of hostile impulses".[61] The main cause of such community disintegration appears to be rapid social change which creates widespread poverty, relative deprivation or even sudden affluence.[62] In his study of a Nova Scotia community over a 10-year period, Leighton found that an increase in community integration resulted in a decrease in mental illness.[38] A partial explanation for the higher rates of mental illness among the aged is the fact that many of the aged are left behind in disintegrating rural communities and central city areas. Since older persons tend to be less mobile and less able to get out of their neighborhood, they are likely to be more intensely affected by the condition of their neighborhood than others. Thus, the health professional should be aware of an older person's neighborhood as a stressor which may cause mental and physical illness.

In summary, there is considerable evidence that the multiple stresses associated with old age, such as loss of income, loss of social role, bereavement, isolation, loss of cognitive functioning, and community disintegration often combine to produce the higher rates of severe mental illness found among the aged in our society.

SOCIAL SUPPORT

Family

Despite alarms about the "disintegration of the family" and family neglect of elders, families remain the single most important and frequent source of aid and support for elders in our society. Families typically provide at least three main types of support. First, they provide financial and material aid when needed, usually on an emergency basis, but sometimes on a continuing basis. Second, they provide care and nursing when illness and disability strike, either on a temporary or continuing basis. Third, and perhaps most important, they are usually the primary source of affection, esteem, and emotional gratification for most elders.

However, the United States could learn from such countries as Japan about how to better integrate elders in their families. In Japan, about three-fourths of the aged live with their children and most of the rest live near their children. Most of the Japanese elders have important roles to perform in the homes of their families, ranging from advice and counsel to housework, shopping, household repair and care of grandchildren. Usually the elders in Japan have a "special friend" relationship with their grandchildren in which they help them with their studying, chores, and even in their play. These roles free the father and mother for employment outside the home. Thus, the elders are usually considered important and respected members of the family. Health professionals should do what they can to encourage the family as a most important source of meaningful roles, aid, and support. For those few elders without immediate family to provide such support, support from other sources becomes most important.

Community

Community support can be of great importance for those elders without immediate family, but can also be of major support even for those with families. Both formal and informal support exists in communities. Formal support can be provided by churches (most elders belong to a church), unions, fraternal and civic organizations, and various community programs for elders. In addition, the informal network of neighbors and friends may be even more pervasive and provide more support than the formal organizations. Community support is one of the main reasons that remaining socially active is so important for the aged. Social activity keeps one involved in a social network which provides, or can provide, crucial support in time of need.

Religious Institutions

Churches and synagogues deserve special consideration because they are the single most pervasive community institution to which elders belong. All the other community institutions considered together, including senior citizen centers, clubs for elders, unions, etc., do not involve as many elders as churches and synagogues. Elders belong and are active in religious organizations at a higher rate than any other age group. This is not because elders have become more religious as they aged, but rather because they were raised in a more religious era and have remained religious throughout their lives.[63]

Because most elders belong to a religious organization, the church has a special opportunity to provide more support than other organizations. This support can take many forms: emergency financial and material aid; visitation and care during illness; personal counseling; referral to other organizations for aid; special recreational, educational, and devotional programs for elders; and meaningful roles for the elders through their work in the church organization. Many elders are willing to turn to the church for aid in time of need because of the elders' years of contributions to the church, and because aid from the church does not have the stigma of "welfare" associated with aid from public institutions. Similarly,

personal counseling from ministers and church members does not have the stigma of "mental illness" often attached to counseling and therapy from psychiatrists, social workers, and public agencies. Various studies have shown that few aged go to mental health clinics or psychiatrists as outpatients, but prefer to go to ministers or other private counselors with their emotional and personal problems.[35]

Thus, the health professional who sees an elderly patient with less difficult emotional problems in need of counseling (e.g., adjustment reactions, mild depressive symptoms, etc.) may be more successful in referring the elder to a minister skilled in counseling than to a psychiatrist or mental health clinic. Of course, there are some problems of mental illness so serious that a psychiatric or mental health clinic is needed (e.g., severe depression).

Employment

While the majority of elders are retired, a substantial minority continue to be employed on a full or part-time basis. At any given point in time, about 17% of men over 65, and 9% of women over 65, are employed.[40] Employment rates are about double these percentages among those aged 65–69, and are higher among those in the higher socio-economic occupations such as professionals and managers as well as among farmers. In fact earnings constitute a major source of income for elders, about 30% of their total income.[14]

While there has been a long-term trend toward less employment among elders, recent events may reverse that trend. A major factor will be the new federal law prohibiting mandatory retirement based on age for all federal employees and for most nonfederal employees prior to age 70. Many expect that after problems in administering this initial law have been worked out, the law will be extended to cover all workers regardless of age. Thus, most elders who wish to keep working and are capable of working will be able to do so. In addition, discrimination against older workers is increasingly being recognized and reduced by new laws, enforcement policies, and growing public recognition that age discrimination may be as unjust as racial or sexual discrimination. Various federal and local programs are also growing to increase job opportunities for elders.

Employment provides many benefits which can contribute to better mental health. First, it provides additional income which reduces the stress of poverty or sharp income reductions. Second, it tends to provide physical exercise which contributes to better physical health, which in turn helps mental health. Third, it tends to provide cognitive stimulation which is important for maintenance of cognitive function. Fourth, it tends to provide meaning in life and a feeling of usefulness and high self-esteem. Finally, it tends to integrate the elder in a wider social network which provides emotional support on a daily basis and is a source of help and support in emergencies.

Thus, some kind of at least part-time employment may be the best "medicine" that can be prescribed for many elders suffering from boredom, loneliness, meaninglessness, mild or depressive symptoms.

Leisure Activities

Satisfying leisure activities provide important social support for both employed and retired elders, but they are especially important for the retired. A major problem with the leisure activities of many elders is their limited nature and scope. For maximum benefit, elders need to develop and learn to enjoy a wide variety of leisure activities to meet various needs and various conditions.

The major dimensions by which leisure activities vary are locomotor vs. sedentary (or physical vs. mental), social vs. solitary, and indoor vs. outdoor. Combining these three dimensions result in eight basic types of leisure activities: locomotor-social-indoor (square dancing), locomotor-social-outdoor (shuffle-board), locomotor-solitary-indoor (woodworking), locomotor-solitary-outdoor (walking), sedentary-social-indoor (card games), sedentary-social-outdoor (picnicking), sedentary-solitary-indoor (reading), and sedentary-solitary-outdoor (sunbathing alone). Elders who enjoy at least one activity in each of these types are likely to derive maximum benefit and rarely have "nothing to do."

GOVERNMENT PROGRAMS FOR ELDERS

Social Security

Social Security is the single most important government program for elders. In 1977 it provided 78 billion dollars in benefits to over 33 million retired or disabled persons.[64] In addition to the regular Social Security benefits that retired persons receive, the new Supplementary Security Income (SSI) program guarantees a minimum income to all persons over age 65. Some aged are eligible for SSI but do not apply, either through ignorance of their eligibility or reluctance to apply for "welfare" benefits.

One general misconception about Social Security is that it "prevents" retirees from working at all, or from earning more than a few hundred dollars a year. This misconception is based on the "earnings test" provision which specifies that if a retiree earns more than a certain amount (in 1978 it was $4,000, but this will increase to $6,000 by 1982) he will lose $1 in benefits for every $2 of earnings over that amount. Thus, it is possible for a person with large benefits (say, $4,000 a year) to earn up to $12,000 a year and still be drawing some Social Security benefits. The purpose of this provision is to restrict Social Security benefits to those who need them because they do not have large earnings. However, income other than earnings, such as pensions and income from investments are not included in this earnings test. Thus, some retirees with high pension and investment income also draw full Social Security benefits.

One of the best things about Social Security benefits is that they now contain an automatic cost-of-living adjustment, so beneficiaries need not worry about their benefits being eroded by inflation.

A number of recent media presentations about the Social Security system have given the impression that the system is going bankrupt. There was a need to raise Social Security taxes in 1978 and some subsequent years to compensate for the effects of unemployment and inflation. Yet Social Security benefits continue to be one of the most secure sources of income available to elders.

Medicare

Another important program administered by the Social Security Administration is Medicare, which has two parts. Part A covers hospitalization and is free to elders. Part B covers physician and certain other services and is optional to elders willing to pay a monthly premium ($7.70 in 1978). This is an excellent bargain in health insurance and all elders should be encouraged to take advantage of it.

However, Medicare pays only about half the total medical expenses of elders because it does not cover out-patient drugs, dental services, optical services, and certain other medical expenses. Furthermore it contains deductible provisions which require the elder to pay the first portion of most medical bills, as well as co-insurance provisions which require the elder to pay a percentage of many of the medical bills. Therefore, it is advisable to secure private supplementary health insurance specifically designed to cover these gaps in Medicare.

Employment

In the previous section we pointed out how valuable employment is for those elders willing and able to work. The federal and state governments have recognized this and have provided several programs to encourage more employment opportunities for elders. The Senior Community Service Employment Program (title IX of the Older Americans Act) pays for part-time community service jobs for low-income persons 55-years-old and older. In 1976 about 20,000 individuals participated at a cost of 85 million dollars.[64] The Senior Opportunities and Services program funds projects which serve or employ older persons. In 1976 about one million persons were served at a cost of 10 million dollars. The Department of Labor also provides special job placement services for older workers. There is also a federal law prohibiting discrimination against workers aged 40 to 65. Finally, many local agencies provide special employment opportunities for elders such as Home Help Aides, Green Thumb (landscaping and park beautification projects), Foster Grandparents, Mr. Fixit (home repairs, sheltered workshops, and various training programs to increase work skills).

Despite continuing discrimination against elders in employment, such government programs are expanding employment opportunities for elders.

Retired Senior Volunteers Program (RSVP)

RSVP is a program for those who do not want (or cannot find) gainful employment, and yet want to do something useful in the community. It develops community volunteer service opportunities for elders. In 1977 about 250,000 older volunteers served in this program and about 19 million dollars was devoted to it. While the program does not pay its volunteers, it does provide lunch and transportation money to facilitate the work of those who give their services.

Senior Centers

Many of the programs mentioned above are administered or coordinated by local Senior Centers. Senior Centers often provide or coordinate a wide range of services including employment and training programs, nutrition programs, recreation programs, information and referral, transportation, telephone contact (for persons living alone), lectures, and physical fitness programs. In

1977 the Federal Government devoted $20 million to Senior Centers (Title V).

Some programs that Senior Centers administer or coordinate are funded through the Model Projects on Aging Program (Title III of the Older Americans Act). In 1977 $12 million were devoted to these projects.

Activities of the Senior Centers and other agencies for elders are coordinated on the regional level by Area Agencies on Aging, and at the state level by state administrations on aging. In 1977 over $150 million were appropriated for over 500 area and state agencies on aging.

Nutrition

A recent addition to federal programs for elders is the Nutrition Program for the Elderly (Title VII of the Older Americans Act). This program includes the delivery of meals to the homes of elders ("Meals on Wheels") who have difficulty shopping and cooking for themselves, as well as providing nutritious meals at congregate dining sites (such as senior centers or churches) for a nominal charge. The purpose of these congregate dining projects is to improve both nutrition and socialization among the elders. Elders who initially come to senior centers for the low-cost meals, often stay to participate in other programs of the center. In 1977 this program served about 435,000 meals at about 8,500 sites for a cost of $225 million. This is a particularly valuable program for the frail elderly whom health professionals are more likely to serve.

Day Care or Geriatric Day-Hospitals

In an attempt to reduce unnecessary institutionalization, day care centers and geriatric day-hospitals have been set up in some areas to care for elders who need care during the day, but who can take care of themselves, or be taken care of, at night in their own homes. Such centers usually provide a full range of medical, nutrition, psychiatric, rehabilitative and recreational services. It has been estimated that such centers, combined with home help and other support services, can reduce the number of institutionalized elders by about one-third.

Other Social Services

Other governmentally financed social services for elders include legal services, respite services (to relieve primary caretakers, such as adult children, from their continuing responsibilities over weekends and vacations), protective services (for mentally impaired elders), visiting nurses, and social work. Needy elders, along with all other needy citizens, are also eligible for services such as food stamps, public welfare, vocational rehabilitation, education, etc.

IMPLICATIONS FOR MENTAL HEALTH PROFESSIONALS*

Social Policy

As an influential citizen and a specialist in treating the elderly, the geriatric mental health professional has a special opportunity to improve various social policies in order to reduce the stresses that cause mental illness among the aged. He/she can influence social policy through speaking engagements with civic and religious groups, by writing articles for professional and popular journals and newspapers, appearing on television and radio talk shows, and in informal discussions with friends and colleagues.

What policies need to be improved or instituted? On a most general level, the status and integration of the aged in our society should be improved. For specific policy recommendations, the clinician can consult the proceedings of the 1971 White House Conference on Aging. Most of these recommendations have not yet been implemented. For example, the section on physical and mental health policy includes recommendations for special health care of the aged, coordinated health service delivery systems, expanding Medicare into a comprehensive

* Some of this material is adapted from Palmore, 1976.[8]

national health insurance system, health education, training of manpower for health care of the aged, funding for research, service, and education, and protection of individual rights during treatment for mental illness. Other important recommendations cover employment and retirement, housing, income, nutrition, transportation and spiritual well-being for the aged.

Nutrition

Obviously, adequate nutrition is a prerequisite for both physical and mental health. The elderly are particularly vulnerable to poor nutrition of several kinds. Many elders have such a small income that they cannot afford to maintain an adequate balanced diet. Even those with sufficient income may have many barriers between them and an adequate diet, such as lack of transportation, disabilities which prevent them from shopping and preparing meals or even ignorance about adequate nutrition. The aged also may need special vitamin or mineral supplements because of problems in their digestion, metabolism, or other assimilative functions. At the same time, the aged need to be protected against food quackery and unfounded nutritional claims. Another problem is obesity, which is frequent among the aged because of lack of exercise and lack of other gratifications that may cause overeating. It has been estimated by the 1973 White House Conference on Aging that one-half to one-third of the health problems of the elderly are related to nutrition. Thus, it is of primary importance that clinicians become aware of nutritional inadequacies in their patients and do whatever is necessary to correct them. This may require referral to welfare agencies to provide adequate income, arrangement of transportation for shopping, provision of a home help service to aid in preparation of some meals, or referral to the local food stamp agency, the local "meals on wheels" program, or a "hot lunch" program. More generally, it may require information about what is a balanced diet and how it may be

obtained. This information and advice on nutrition is of special importance for older patients because they are less likely to have knowledege of and interest in good nutrition.

Exercise

If poor nutrition accounts for up to one-half of the health problems of the elderly, lack of exercise and activity probably accounts for much of the loss of physical function. It is clear that most older people get less exercise than the young. We have already mentioned how exercise programs can improve health and fitness so that the bodies of older persons can respond as well as those of middle-aged persons. For example, older people who have kept in training are able to compete in various vigorous sports, and training can preserve the physical abilities of many elders at a far higher level than those who allow their bodies to atrophy through inactivity. Such fitness also contributes to mental health.[65]

Obesity is a common problem among the aged which is directly related to lack of exercise. It is well known that obesity is a serious health hazard, primarily because of the extra strain obesity places on the heart, bones, and other organs. Less recognized is the probability that obesity often has various indirect detrimental effects on mental health and adjustment. Despite the fact that many people in our society are obese, obesity is often viewed as a weakness, if not a moral failing. Societal views may lower a person's self-esteem which may lead to even greater food intake and various forms of neurosis, such as depression.

Therefore, the sedentary life of the majority of older persons may be one of the most dangerous threats to their longevity and adjustment. Clinicians can perform an important service for their sedentary or obese patients by giving them information about the benefits of regular exercise and by prescribing a program of suitable exercise. It should be understood that suitable exercise will vary, depending on a person's interests and abilities. Too strenuous or sudden exercise may be just as dangerous as lack of exercise. The simple act of walking is one of the safest forms of exercise and it is universally available. The amount and speed of walking can be easily graduated to fit the needs and abilities of a wide variety of patients.

Medical Care

Any competent clinician will be concerned with providing adequate medical care. Good comprehensive medical care is important to both physical and mental health, and second to discuss the obstacles to good medical care for the aged. Studies have shown that health is the single most important factor related to life satisfaction in the later years.[66] Low life satisfaction in turn leads to depression and other forms of mental illness.

There is evidence that, despite Medicare and Medicaid, the elderly's share of medical care is not commensurate with their proportion of illness.[39] There are at least four major obstacles to adequate medical care for the aged—finances, transportation, attitudes of the aged, and attitudes of medical personnel.

Financial Obstacles. Financial considerations appear to have been more important before the passage of Medicare, but it is difficult to assess Medicare's actual impact. The relatively low income of the aged and the relatively high cost of their medical care are well known and were the major justifications of Medicare legislation. However, Medicare clearly has not eliminated all financial obstacles, particularly among the aged poor. It has been estimated that the voluntary part of Medicare does not even cover some 15% of the aged poor, presumably because they cannot afford, or believe they cannot afford, the premiums.[67]

Even for those who are covered by Medicare there are various deductibles, limitations, restrictions, and coinsurance provisions that limit the amount of medical services for which Medicare pays. Medicare pays less than half of the total medical charges incurred by the aged.[68] Of course, Medicare does not cover charges for dental care, drugs, and optometrist's services. Medicare, Medicaid, and all other public sources combined still pay only two-thirds of the total expenditures for medical care of the aged.

Therefore, clinicians should not assume that Medicare has dissolved all financial obstacles between them and their older patients. They should be aware that the aged sick may avoid treatment because of limited income.

Transportation Difficulties. Combined circumstances make transportation difficulties particularly formidable to older persons. As the young tend to move from rural areas toward the city and from the inner city to the suburbs, the aged are likely to be left behind and become concentrated in rural areas and older sections of cities. Unfortunately, these are the very areas in which physicians and medical facilities usually are scarce. Thus, the aged must travel great distances to reach medical service, yet they are the least mobile and have the greatest difficulty with transportation. For example, the Project FIND survey determined that about one-third of the aged poor had transportation difficulties.[67] Thus, clinicians may need to make special transportation arrangements for their aged patients or arrange to visit them more often in their homes.

Attitudes of the Aged. The characteristics and attitudes of the aged themselves constitute major obstacles to more adequate medical care. The aged have substantially less education on the average than younger people, and this education was acquired in an earlier era when less was known about health and medicine. Thus, many aged are ignorant about many physical symptoms that a more informed person recognizes as serious enough to require a medical examination, if not treatment. The elderly may simply dismiss these symptoms as signs of aging that do not warrant any medical treatment. For example, in the Duke Longitudinal Study of Aging, over half of those in poor health according to the physician's evaluation rated their own health as good or excellent.[69]

Even when the aged recognize that a symptom indicates the need for some treatment, they are less likely to seek professional help. They are more likely to listen to lay advice, quacks, old wives' tales, or to use patent medicines or nostrums. This may result from ignorance about the value of professional treatment, fear of doctors and the uncomfortable and expensive regimen they may prescribe, fear of hospitals (ie. a place to die) or greater gullibility in believing the claims of quacks and patent medicine advertisments. Therefore, the physician should be particularly sensitive to such fears, denials, and lack of understanding of the many principles of health and medicine that he may mistakenly assume everyone knows. He may need patience and extra effort to educate and inform his aged patients.

Attitudes of Medical Personnel. Many medical personnel are less interested in treating the aged than in treating younger people, and may even avoid the aged because their care seems to be less rewarding psychologically and financially. Lasagna noted "the disinclination of many doctors to be interested in the patient with a chronic illness not likely to yield dramatically—or at all—to therapeutic maneuvers."[70]

Many doctors, as well as the rest of our society, view most of the symptoms of the aged as hopeless. They tend to confuse aging with illness and assume that most symptoms among the aged are inevitable, untreatable concomitants of normal aging. Fortunately, many physicians now question these older assumptions and consider many of these symptoms to be reversible or at least manageable by proper treatment. Arteriosclerosis and senility are two examples of disorders once considered irreversible effects of aging itself, but now more widely attributed to environmental factors such as diet, stress, drug intoxication, and social losses, which can be manipulated to reverse or control the disorders.

Institutionalization of the aged may be necessary for adequate medical care of those unable to care for themselves, yet many factors combine to prevent the delivery of adequate geriatric care even in institutions. One overall problem is the lack of coordination of the many types of institutions, such as general hospitals, chronic disease hospitals, rehabilitative facilities, nursing homes, and home care programs. Since older patients usually have multiple, recurrent problems and their hospital experiences usually are not for isolated or self-limited illnesses, there is need for a "smoothly geared mechanism for rapidly admitting chronically ill persons to a hospital for acute medical care as well as for quickly facilitating transfer to the home, or a rehabilitative facility, or long-term custodial care as the needs change".[70] This requires a much closer liaison than now generally exists among these various institutions.

Another general problem is the severe limitations of both short-stay and long-stay hospitals in their ability to care adequately for the chronically ill, aged patient. As the name implies, the short-stay general hospital is usually better equipped to handle acute rather than chronic illnesses. For example, bedsores or limb contractures may develop rapidly in a stroke patient in a short-stay general hopsital because the physicians and nurses have had little experience with the needs of such patients. On the other hand, long-stay hospitals "are all too often third-rate custodial facilities with staffs that are badly deficient in numbers, quality, or both; where patients become pathetic vegetables waiting to die, as remote from imaginative attention as they are from the outside world."[70]

Most nursing homes have even lower standards for medical care. The inadequacies of many nursing homes have become common knowledge with the recent proliferation of various exposés, such as the Ralph Nader group report,[71] the 1971 Senate Special

Committee on Aging hearings, and the 1971 conference on nursing homes sponsored by the American Association of Retired Persons and the Duke Center for the Study of Aging and Human Development.

Various investigations of nursing homes have produced charges that some are filthy, fetid, unsafe, overcrowded, and understaffed and that patients are often ill-kept, neglected, undernourished, forbidden to leave their rooms, kept in bed needlessly, and given excess sedatives and tranquilizers to reduce their complaints.[72] It is difficult to determine how widepread and serious these practices are, for many nursing homes provide excellent care for their patients.

Because of such inadequacies, many persons argue that institutionalization should be a last resort and have urged various alternatives. Clearly, the aged themselves and, to a lesser degree their families, hold a generally negative view of living in an institution. For example, only 3% of the aged say they would most like to live in a home for the aged, whereas 61% say they would like this plan least of all.[73] Even when the question refers only to the aged who can no longer care for themselves, only a minority (38%) think that a nursing home is the best living arrangement.[74]

Mortality is higher among those who are institutionalized than among those who are not, even controlling for factors of age. Does institutionalization contribute to earlier death or are persons who are sicker more likely to be institutionalized? There is some evidence that any kind of transfer or change in living arrangements may have seriously deleterious effects on the health and longevity of the aged, particularly the more frail and infirm.[75]

The following alternatives to institutionalization are being used successfully.

1. Day care services at centers outside the home for those ambulatory aged needing medical or nursing care during the day.
2. Organized home care with visiting nurses, physical therapy, rehabilitation services, "meals on wheels," homemaker services, and social casework for homebound geriatric patients.
3. Special housing for the aged designed to meet the needs of the infirm, with elevators, specially designed kitchens and bathrooms, centrally located dining rooms, and transportation.
4. Foster home care in which the aged person lives in the home of foster children who are paid to care for their foster parents.
5. Sheltered workshops that provide meaningful and rehabilitative activities and some income for the aged.
6. Information and referral centers to facilitate delivery of these and other types of services.

Brecher and Brecher[72] estimated that the effective combination of all these services could take 40% of the residents out of nursing homes.

The physician obviously has a crucial role in the delivery of more adequate care for the aged. In treating elderly patients, physicians must follow a narrow path between the twin pitfalls of too little and too much treatment. On the one hand, they must avoid the trap of placing the elderly patient into a single most obvious disease classification, and treating only that one disease. Elderly patients are more likely to have multiple problems, many of which may have subtle beginnings overshadowed by earlier chronic conditions. Complications are more likely to develop during hospitalization in the aged than in younger people, and physicians should be alert to prevent or treat them. Such complications develop in as many as three-fourths of hospitalized geriatric patients and are often fatal. On the other hand, physicians need to avoid overtreating elderly patients. For example, a rapid-fire series of diagnostic tests and x-rays involving restrictions on food and drink, cleansing enemas, etc., may produce only discomfort in a healthy young person but may push the debilitated older patient into a crisis.

Effective medical care balances the probable benefits of treatment against the cost in discomfort, as well as in money and time. If an aged patient is rapidly deteriorating and has only a few more months or years to live, ideally the physician should weigh the advantages against the disadvantages before depriving the patient of favorite foods, or habits such as tobacco and alcohol that may give substantial comfort and support.

Mental and Social Stimulation

Erroneous beliefs exist that most elderly people are mentally ill or senile, that they have no sexual interests or needs, that they are unable to be productive, and that they are socially isolated. In addition the multiple stresses of loss of social role, bereavement, isolation, and loss of cognitive functioning often combine to produce mental illness among the aged. These stresses may also combine to reduce longevity. For example, we found that one of the strongest predictors of longevity in our longitudinal study of aging was the amount of work satisfaction a person had.[31] Work satisfaction was interpreted broadly to include either paid employment or work around the house, hobbies, or community service. Thus the older person with some meaningful social role from which he derived considerable satisfaction lived substantially longer than the person who had no such role. Presumably this meaningful social role operated at three levels to increase his longevity. At the physical level the activity provided exercise and a healthy routine. At the mental level it provided the necessary stimulation and exercise of cognitive abilities, and at the social level it provided a route to integration into a helpful social network, gave life social meaning, and maintained self-esteem.

In their therapeutic role with patients, clinicians have a unique opportunity and obligation to encourage the maintenance of such meaningful social roles. They can encourage patients to continue or develop some full- or part-time work, community service, or productive hobbies. They can encourage patients to remain or become active in the many community organizations, churches, and clubs that can provide valuable mental and social stimulation. They can counsel against hasty divorce or advise remarriage for the sexual and emotional gratification and security it provides. They can encourage the maintenance or development of family and friendship ties to provide mental and social stimulation and security. They can prescribe various prostheses to compensate for those physical disabilities which interfere with communication and interaction, especially losses of hearing, sight, and mobility which are so common in advanced old age.

Adequate Income

Next to adequate health, adequate income is probably the most important ingredient in a successful, happy adjustment to old age. Persons of any age without adequate income for the essentials of a good life obviously suffer from stresses that undermine mental health. This is a special problem for the aged because of their reduced income.

It may appear that concern with adequate income and providing mental and social stimulation are far removed from the traditional clinician's role. However, they come within the concept of treating the whole patient rather than treating an isolated symptom. Furthermore, they can be thought of as a part of preventive medicine. Without this holistic and preventive approach, treatment of symptoms will be palliative and at best only temporarily successful.

It may be that the physician will help in this area more through referral and information than through direct personal intervention. Yet clinicians *can* help patients get a more adequate income by urging them to apply for Social Security, veteran's benefits, and welfare benefits to which they may be entitled. The clinician could investigate the possibilities of financial help from relatives or one of the many charitable organizations that aid needy older persons, or find part-time employment to supplement the elderly patient's income.

One reason for the unique opportunity of

physicians to help older persons reduce these stresses is that older persons tend to consult physicians more frequently than younger persons. In fact, physicians (together with clergymen) are the primary sources of aid to whom older persons go when seeking help for personal problems.[76] The mentally ill aged are even more likely to consult a physician.[77] Thus physicians probably have more opportunity to reduce stress among older persons than any other group in the community.

AGING IN FUTURE SOCIETIES

Predicting the future has always been a hazardous undertaking. Nevertheless, just as some planning is usually better than no planning, tentative predictions are usually more useful than no predictions at all. Thus, I will venture to make three predictions relevant to the mental health of elders in the future.

First, we can be fairly sure that, barring some major catastrophe or precipitous drop in the birth rate, the proportion of the population over age 65 in the United States will only increase slightly during the rest of this century (to about 12% in the year 2000) and reach its peak around the year 2030 of about 15%.[12] Furthermore, as pointed out earlier, the total dependency ratio (numbers of aged and children divided by number aged 21–64) will actually *decline* because the increase in proportion aged will be more than offset by the decrease in the proportion of children. Thus, our society should have adequate resources and enough "productive age" adults to care for the mental health needs of its elders in the future. Fears that our society will be overrun by unmanageable numbers of aged in the future are unwarranted. On the other hand, we will need substantially more mental health professionals to adequately care for the increasing numbers of elders needing such care.

My second prediction is that the unnecessary suffering produced by the prolongation of dying among terminally ill patients will be reduced. This prediction is based on the growing interest in and acceptance by both professionals and laymen of the idea that prolonging death by the use of costly machines and personnel when a patient has a hopeless and terminal illness and is suffering from intense and increasing pain or is in an irreversible coma is often a wasteful and inhumane practice.

I believe the following trends will tend to decrease the prolongation of dying:

1. The increasing number of persons who reach very old age when prolonged but terminal illness becomes the typical cause of death.
2. The trend toward more rational allocation of scarce and expensive medical equipment (e.g., kidney machines) and personnel to those who can benefit from them the most.
3. The growing belief in the right of all persons to do what they want with their own bodies, so long as it does not harm others, as reflected in the growing acceptance of contraceptives, abortion, masturbation, premarital intercourse, and cremation. The right to die under certain circumstances may become another generally accepted civil right.

Several states, such as California and North Carolina, have now legalized the right of terminally ill patients to request the withdrawal of artificial means of prolonging their life, and the right of physicians to carry out these requests. This trend should reduce the fear of many persons, old and young, who do not fear death as much as they fear a prolonged and painful process of dying.

Finally, I predict that the relative status of elders in terms of health, education, occupation, and income will continue to rise for the foreseeable future. There is a widespread belief that the lot of elders is getting worse in our society and that the gaps between their health, income, and other measures of the good life and that of the rest of society are increasing. Indeed, there was some evidence that this was true until around 1967. However, since that time various indices show that these gaps are narrowing, and careful projections through the year 2000 show that they probably will continue to narrow. Data from the National Health Interview Survey show that four out of five indicators of health reveal improvements in the health status of the aged relative to that of the rest of the population, and the fifth indicator has remained fairly level.[78] Similarly, U.S. Census data on mean incomes show increasing ratios of aged to nonaged incomes since 1967. Also, the proportion of aged in poverty has declined at a faster rate than in the general population. Projections of both occupational and educational status of the aged relative to the middle aged also show increases at least through 1990.

All these indicators of rising status for the aged may also indicate less mental illness because higher status persons generally appear to suffer from less mental illness than lower status persons.

SUMMARY

While this chapter has reviewed many serious problems in our society which contribute to mental illness among our elders, such as ageism with its prejudice and discrimination against elders, and the many sources of social stress, it has also reviewed many sources of social support and government programs which can contribute toward mental health of elders. Mental health professionals can make important contributions toward better physical and mental health of the elderly. Finally, the outlook for the mental health of future aged is relatively bright, if the progress made in recent decades continues.

REFERENCES

1. Palmore, E. *The Honorable Elders*. Durhan, N.C.: Duke University Press, 1975.
2. Comfort, A. *Proceedings: Governor's Conference on the Quality of Life for our Senior Citizens*. Raleigh, N.C.: N.C. Department of Human Resources, 1977.
3. Palmore, E. and Maddox, G. Sociological aspects of aging. In E. Busse and E. Pfeiffer, (eds.) *Behavior and Adaptation in Late Life* (Second Edition). Boston: Little Brown, 1977.
4. Simmons, L. Aging in preindustrial societies, In C. Tibbets (ed.) *Handbook of Social Gerontology*. Chicago: University of Chicago Press, 1960.
5. Cowgill, D. and Holmes, L. *Aging and Modernization*. New York: Appleton-Century-Crofts, 1972.
6. Friedmann, D. The impact of aging on the social structure. In C. Tibbets (ed.) *Handbook of Social Gerontology*. Chicago: University of Chicago Press, 1960.
7. Shanas, E. *et al. Old People in Three Industrial Societies*. New York: Atherton Press, 1968.
8. Palmore, E. Social and economic aspects of aging. In L. Bellak, and T. Karasu, (eds.) *Geriatric Psychiatry*. New York: Grune and Stratton, 1976.
9. Golant, S. Residential concentrations of the future elderly. *Gerontologist*, **15:** 1, 16 (1975).
10. Palmore, E. and Manton, K. Modernization and status of the aged. *Journal of Gerontology*, **29:** 2, 205 (1974).
11. Palmore, E. *International Handbook on Aging*. Westport, Conn: Greenwood Press in press.
12. Bureau of Census. *Projections of the Population of the U.S. 1977 to 2050*. Current Population Reports, Series P-25, No. 704. Washington: USGPO, 1977.
13. Maddox, G. and Douglas, E. Aging and individual differences. *Journal of Gerontology*, **29.** 5: 555 (1974).
14. Epstein, L. *The Aged Population of the U.S.* Washington: USGPO, 1967.
15. Palmore, E. Differences in the retirement patterns of men and women. *Gerontologist*, **5:** 4, (1965).
16. Palmore, E. Employment and retirement. In Epstein, L. (ed.), *The Aged Population of the United States*. Washington: USGPO, 1967.
17. Orshansky, M. Living in retirement. *Social Security Bulletin*, **31:** 3 (1968).
18. Neugarten, B. Age groups in American society and the rise of the young-old. *The Annals*, September, 1974.
19. Palmore, E. The elderly poor in America. In J. Ossofsky (ed.) *The Golden Years: A Tarnished Myth*. Washington: National Council on the Aging, 1970.
20. Broom, L. and Selznick, P. *Sociology*. New York: Harper and Row, 1968.
21. Orshansky, M. The aged Negro and his income. *Social Security Bulletin*, **27:** 3 (1964).
22. Roberts, R. Ethnic and Racial Differences in the Characteristics and Attitudes of the Aged in Selected Areas of Rural Louisiana. M. A. Thesis. Baton Rouge: Louisiana State University, 1964.
23. Butler, R. Ageism: another form of bigotry. *Gerontologist*, **9:** 243 (1969).
24. Tuckman, J. and Lorge, I. The projection of personal symptoms into stereotypes about aging. *Journal of Gerontology*, **13:** 70 (1958).

25. Palmore, E. Facts on Aging: a short quiz. *Gerontologist*, **17**: 4, 315 (1977).

26. National Center for Health Statistics. *National Health Survey*, Series 10. Washington: USGPO, 1977.

27. Dovenmuehle, R. H., Busse, E. W. and Newman, G. Physical problems of older people. *Journal of the American Geriatrics Society*, **9**: 208 (1961).

28. Devries, H. *Report on Jogging and Exercise for Older Adults*. Washington: Administration on Aging, 1968.

29. Pfeiffer, E., Verwoerdt, A. and Wang, H. S. The natural history of sexual behavior in a biologically advantaged group of aged individuals. *Journal of Gerontology*, **24**: 193 (1969).

30. Botwinick, J. and Thompson, L. W. Components of reaction time in relation to age and sex. *Journal of Genetic Psychology*, **108**: 175 (1966).

31. Palmore, E. *Normal Aging II*. Durham, N.C.: Duke University Press, 1974.

32. Butler, R. The destiny of creativity in later life, in B. Levin, and R. Kahana, (eds.) *Psychodynamic Studies on Aging*. New York: International Universities Press, 1967.

33. Soddy, K. *Men in Middle Life*. Philadelphia: Lippincott, 1967.

34. Dennis, W. Creative productivity between twenty and eighty years. *Journal of Gerontology*, **21**: 1 (1966).

35. Redick, R. W., Kramer, M. and Taube, C. A. Epidemiology of mental illness and utilization of psychiatric facilities among older persons. In E. W. Busse and E. Pfeiffer (eds.) *Mental Illness in Later Life*. Washington: American Psychiatric Association, p. 199, 1973.

36. Riley, M. and Foner, A. *Aging and Society I*. New York: Russell Sage Foundation, 1968.

37. Pasamanick, B. A survey of mental disease in an urban population. *Mental Hygiene*, **46**: 567 (1962).

38. Leighton, A. Poverty and social change. *Scientific American*, **212**: 21 (1965).

39. Palmore, E. Compulsory vs. flexible retirement. *Gerontologist*, **12**: 343 (1972).

40. Harris, L. *The Myth and Reality of Aging in America*. Washington: National Council on the Aging, 1975.

41. Rosenberg, G. Age, poverty, and isolation from friends in the urban working class. *Journal of Gerontology*, **23**: 533 (1968).

42. Rosow, I. *Social Integration of the Aged*. New York: Free Press, 1967.

43. Dean, L. Aging and decline of affect. *Journal of Gerontology*, **17**: 440 (1962).

44. Binstock, R. and Shanas, E. *Handbook of Aging and the Social Sciences*. New York: Van Nostrand Reinhold, 1976.

45. Erskine, H. The polls. *Public Opinion Quarterly*, **28**: 679 (1964).

46. Catholic Digest. Survey of religions in the U.S. **7**: 27 (1966).

47. Hausknecht, M. *The Joiners*. New York: Bedminster Press, 1962.

48. Fowles, D. *Income and Poverty Among the Elderly*. Washington: Administration on Aging, 1977.

49. Pearson, J. Age and sex differences related to MMPI response. *American Journal of Psychiatry*, **121**: 988 (1965).

50. Palmore, E. *Normal Aging*. Durham, North Carolina: Duke University Press, 1970.

51. Steiner, P. and Dorfman, R. *The Economic Status of the Aged*. Berkeley: University of California Press, 1957.

52. Tibbets, C. *Handbook of Social Gerontology*. Chicago: University of Chicago Press, 1970.

53. Palmore, E. Medical care needs of the aged. *Postgraduate Medicine*, May and June, 1972.

54. Palmore, E. Attitudes toward aging as shown by humor. *Gerontologist*, **11**: 3, 181 (1971).

55. Richman, J. The foolishness and wisdom of age. *Gerontologist*, **17**: 3, 210 (1977).

56. Davies, L. Attitudes toward old age and aging as shown by humor. *Gerontologist*, **17**: 3, 220 (1977).

57. Holmes, T. and Rahe, R. The social readjustment rating scale. *Journal of Psychosomatic Research*, **11**: 213 (1967).

58. Palmore, E. *et al*. Stress and adaptation in later life. *Journal of Gerontology* (in press).

59. Blazer, D. G. The OARS-Durham survey, In *Multidimensional Functional Assessment: The OARS Methodology* (Second Edition). Durham, N.C.: Duke University Center for the Study of Aging, 1978.

60. Eisdorfer, C. Developmental level and sensory impairment in the aged. *Journal Protective Techniques and Personality Assessment*, **24**: 129 (1960).

61. Leighton, A. Is social environment a cause of psychiatric disorder? in Monroe (ed.) *Psychiatric Epidemiology and Mental Health Planning*. Washington: American Psychiatric Association, 1967.

62. Leighton, A. and Smith, R. A comparative study of social and cultural change. *Proceedings of the American Philosophical Society*, **99**: 2 (1955).

63. Blazer, D. and Palmore, E. Religion and aging in a longitudinal panel. *Gerontologist*, **16**: 82 (1976).

64. Office of Management and Budget. *Catalogue of Federal Domestic Assistance*. Washington: USGPO, 1977.

65. Harris, R. Physical activity and mental health in the aged, In U. Simki (ed.) *Physical Exercise and Activity for the Aging: Proceedings of an International Seminar*. Jerusalem: Wingate Institute, 1975.

66. Palmore, E., Luikant, C. Health and social factors related to life satisfaction. *Journal Health and Social Behavior*, **13**: 68 (1972).

67. Ossofsky, J. *The Golden Years: A Tarnished Myth*. Washington: National Council on the Aging, 1970.

68. Cooper, S. and Piro, P. Age differences in medical

care spending. *Social Security Bulletin,* **17:** 3 (1974).

69. Maddox, G. L. Self-assessment of health status. *Journal Chronic Diseases,* **17:** 449 (1964).

70. Lasagna, L. Aging and the field of medicine, In M. Riley, J. Riley and M. Johnson (eds.) *Aging and Society II.* New York: Russell Sage Foundation, 1969.

71. Townsend, C. *Old Age: The Last Segregation.* New York: Grossman, 1971.

72. Brecher, R. and Brecher, E. Nursing homes. *Consumer Reports,* **29:** 30 (1964).

73. Shanas, E. *The Health of Older Persons.* Cambridge: Harvard University Press, 1962.

74. Beyer, G. and Woods, M. *Living and Activity patterns of the Aged.* Ithaca: Center for Housing and Environmental Studies, Cornell University, 1963.

75. Palmore, E. and Jeffers, F. *Prediction of Life Span.* Lexington, Mass.: Raytheon, Health, 1971.

76. Gurin, G. *Americans View Their Mental Health.* New York: Basic Books, 1960.

77. Kay, D. Old age mental disorders in Newcastle-upon-Tyne. *British Journal of Psychiatry,* **110:** 668 (1964).

78. Palmore, E. The future status of the aged. *Gerontologist,* **16,** 4: 297 (1976).

Chapter 10
The Epidemiology of Mental Illness In Late Life

Dan Blazer, M.D.

Duke University Medical Center

INTRODUCTION

The epidemiology of mental illness in late life is a study of both the distribution of mental illness among the elderly and the factors that influence this distribution.[1] The rationale for such studies is apparent when one considers the increasing percentages of older people in developed countries. There were approximately 22,405,000 individuals 65 and over in the United States in 1975 but the number is expected to increase to 45,102,000 by 2020.[2] This increase results from decreased birth rates and greater life expectancy. The "baby boom" of the late 1940s has produced a bulge of individuals who are presently in their late twentys and early thirtys. As these individuals age, society must necessarily attend to their needs. Moreover, the average life expectancy in developed countries (such as the United States, England and Wales, Sweden and Japan) is approximately 70 years for males and approximately 76 years for females. Yet

at the age of 65, the life expectancy for males is approximately 13 years and for females is 17 years.[2] The elderly will therefore receive increasing attention in the future because of their mere numbers alone. (See Table 10-1).

Epidemiologic methods of study are valuable to clinicians and health care planners for the elderly. Primarily they focus on:[3] (1) the *identification* of cases, e.g., can the symptom patterns of schizophrenia be reliably identified across cultures in the elderly?; (2) the *distribution* of mental illness in the population, e.g., what is the prevalence and/or incidence of the neuroses among the elderly?; (3) The *historical trends* of mental illness among the elderly, e.g., have the rates of organic mental disease among the elderly?; (3) the *historical trends* over the past 75 years?; (4) the *etiology* of mental illness in late life, e.g., what factors contribute to the occurrence of depression in late life?; (5) the present *utilization* of mental health facilities by the elderly, what types of mental health services are most [or least] used by the elderly?; (6) the planning for

Supported by Grant #5 K01 MH00115-02 from the National Institute of Mental Health.

Table 10-1.   Life Expectancy at Birth and at Age 65 in Certain
Developed Countries.[2]

		MALE	FEMALE
Life expectancy at birth:	United States	68.7	76.5
	England and Wales	69.2	75.6
	Sweden	72.1	77.9
	Japan	71.8	77.0
Life expectancy at age 65:	United States	13.7	18.0
	England and Wales	12.3	16.3
	Sweden	14.0	17.3
	Japan	13.8	16.6

new mental health services, e.g., what new services will be needed and what will be the level of utilization?; (7) *intervention and outcome,* e.g., what types of mental health services are most effective in treating the elderly mentally ill?

This chapter describes each of these factors in detail. First the methods of study will be described with emphasis placed on those methodologic problems that might bias past, present and future studies. Then the results of previous epidemiologic studies will be reviewed together with their implications for clinicians.

THE IDENTIFICATION OF CASES

When a group of individuals with a mental health impairment is chosen for study, primary consideration must be given to the diagnostic criteria for the particular impairment. This criteria, which determines inclusion (or exclusion) of individuals in the group, should be clearly defined, specific, and reproducible. A number of approaches to case identification have been used beneficially in psychiatric epidemiological studies. Each can be valuable but can also present unique problems with the elderly. These will be discussed here.

The most commonly used method of case identification has been that of *chart review* or the *establishment of case registeries.*[4,5,6] Chart review assesses the distribution of categorical cases diagnosed within a certain hospital or specific case load. Case registration is a continued report to health

authorities of diseases deemed important enough to the public health to ask or require their occurrence to be reported. The diagnosis of a particular condition (e.g., schizophrenia, manic depressive illness, anxiety neurosis, etc.) is based on the clinician's evaluation of the patient. These studies, therefore, have inherent biases based on variability of patients' socioeconomic status, the clinician's diagnostic criteria,[7] and determinations of age-related illness. The latter especially affects the elderly. Where the diagnostic and statistical manual has created age specific diagnostic categories for children,[8] no such categories have been included for psychiatric illness in late life. This omission reflects our ignorance of the unique symptom presentations in late life (e.g., depression among the elderly may be associated with many symptoms of cognitive impairment). This in turn effects mental health care for the elderly.

Another approach to case identification is the use of self-administered symptom scales and personality inventories. Examples of these instruments include the Goldfarb Mental Status Questionnaire,[9] the MMPI, the Cattel 16 Personality Factors test,[10] the Zung Self-Rating Depression,[11] and so on. Although such scales avoid the problem of subjectively assigning patients to a diagnostic category, they suffer from a lack of age-specific criteria. For example, what degree of anxiety (as might be reported on a self-rated anxiety scale) would be considered normal and what degree would be considered abnormal in late life? What is the retest reliability of such instruments? Self-administered scales do not take advantage of interviewer assessment and frequently do not consider the factor of time. The studies to date concerning the usefulness of such instruments is debatable.

Some of the better known epidemiologic studies have used the technique of asking clinicians to rate the probability that a psychiatric disorder is present on the basis of either interviews or survey questionnaires.[12] For example, psychiatrists may be asked to make an estimate of the chances that intensive diagnostic study would reveal an individual to be (or have been) a psychiatric case. This approach tends to maximize the clinical judgment of the clinician in a forced response framework. The method suffers from not distinguishing between the different types of psychiatric impairment and therefore possibly being less valuable in the planning of services. For the elderly especially, the identification of the presence of psychiatric impairment does not imply a mobilization of professional services.

Another frequently used method of case identification is that of functional status.[13,14] Functional status basically measures the level of well-being or impairment of an individual. Status can be measured in a number of areas of functioning, such as social resources, economic resources, physical health, mental health and self-care capacity. The presence of definite psychiatric symptoms and/or moderate intellectual impairment would usually incapacitate an individual's ability to handle at least the major problems of life. Such an individual would suffer from an impairment in mental health functioning. Functional impairment in mental health is definitely correlated with the need for professional intervention, yet the method suffers from not specifying the type of problem (and therefore the type of intervention) necessary.

The most comprehensive method of objective psychiatric evaluation is the use of structural interviews. The Present State Examination[15] is an example of a structured interview that can be computerized. It assesses the mental state of adult subjects during the month preceding the interview. Such an examination should provide reliable and fairly precise data while at the same time take advantage of the clinician's judgment in data collection. Subjects may be placed in various diagnostic categories, following examination, according to the presence or absence of different symptom patterns. This instrument has not been used extensively with the elderly but does provide a framework for the development of more systematic diagnostic categories in future epidemiologic studies. A similar approach has been described by Feighner, et al.[16] The presence or absence of objective symptoms provide a clinical basis for diagnostic inclusion or exclusion in categorical groups.

Case identification continues to be a major obstacle to the development of psychiatric epidemiology, especially in late life. Studies often cannot be compared because the definition of a case is not comparable. The advent of more precise interview techniques and the use of parameters other than the typical diagnostic category, such as mental health impairment, should make the studies more complete in the future.

THE DISTRIBUTION OF MENTAL ILLNESS

Descriptive epidemiologic studies provide evidence of the patterns of disease occurrence in human population. Such studies may begin as general observations concerning the relationship of mental illness to such basic characteristics as age, sex, race, occupation and social class. Once basic trends of mental illness have been established, such as the increased occurrence of mental illness among the elderly, then studies identifying the specific rate of occurrence of mental illness in a given population can be determined through more vigorous experimental conditions. The frequency of a mental illness, such as depression, or an impairment in mental health, would usually be presented in terms of a *rate,* or the frequency of a disease or characteristic expressed per unit of size of the population or group in which it is observed. Three pieces of information are necessary for a rate to be useful to the epidemiologist: (1) The numerator of the fraction (the number of cases or persons affected); (2) The denominator (the population among whom the affected persons are observed); and (3) Some specification of time.[1] Most of the studies presented below are cross-sectional studies, in that they report the rate of the cases at one point in time.

Table 10-2 shows the rate (percentage) of psychiatric impairment among the elderly in three populations from a number of cross-sectional studies. Though selection of cases varied considerably in each of these studies, the degree of impairment in the community is remarkably similar. The rate of significant (definite) or severe psychiatric impairment among the community based elderly is approximately 5% to 10%. Mild to moderate impairment is seen in an additional 10-40% of the population, yet 50-80% are considered to be without impairment. If one looks at a second population, namely those individuals attending a medical outpatient clinic (as demonstrated in Moore's data)[17] one can see that the rates of psychiatric impairment are very similar to those of the community rates, but do show an increase in the number of individuals with mild to moderate impairments. This might indicate that some individuals with mild but definite psychiatric difficulties may be using the medical outpatient clinic as a point of entry to deal with a difficulty. This has been confirmed by a number of studies that show that the primary complaint of individuals attending medical outpatient clinics for all ages is often an emotional one.[18,19]

The rate of psychiatric impairment in long-term care facilities is definitely increased. As demonstrated in the OARS data,[20] 47% of the individuals in long-term care facilities have significant psychiatric impairment and 39% have mild to moderate psychiatric impairment. Teeter,[21]

found that 32% of institutionalized elderly have significant psychiatric impairment.

As can be seen in Table 10-3, the rates of psychiatric disorders according to diagnostic categories among the elderly in the community vary considerably from study to study. This variation in rates emphasizes the need of more persistent and reproducible methods of measuring psychiatric syndromes among the elderly, such as a criterion for distinguishing the dysphoric symptoms of late life from true depressive illness. However, this data does enable us to identify certain trends in the distribution of psychiatric illness across diagnostic categories. For example, it can been seen that the rate of schizophrenia and paranoid psychosis is remarkably consistent from study to study (1-3.5%). The rate of affective psychosis also is quite consistent (1-2%). The rate of organic mental syndromes is generally quite high for this population (even in the community) and the rates vary from 2.5% to 12%. The lower values appear to be secondary to the restrictions placed on the diagnosis of organic mental syndromes by these particular studies. For example, Bremer[22] and Eaton and Weil[23] looked for the psychotic manifestations of organic mental syndrome rather than just the presence of cognitive impairment.

Neurotic symptoms are quite common among the elderly (as demonstrated by Leighton).[12] However, the actual prevalence of psychoneurosis is much less, according to other studies, and ranges between 10% and 25%. The rate of psychiatric syndromes according to the various diagnostic categories in institutions also shows considerable variation (see Table 10-4). For example, the rate of organic mental disease varies between 15% and 60% in mental hospitals and between 35% to 70% in long-term care facilities. The lower levels of organic mental syndromes probably relates to the more restrictive diagnostic categories in addition to the cross-cultural differences in admission policies to mental hospitals. The rate of organic mental disease in mental hospitals

Table 10-2. Rate (%) of Psychiatric Impairment Among the Elderly in Three Populations.

	SETTING									
	COMMUNITY			MEDICAL OUTPATIENT			LONG-TERM CARE			
NORMAL	MILD TO MOD.	SIG. OR SEVERE	NORMAL	MILD TO MOD.	SIG. OR SEVERE	NORMAL	MILD TO MOD.	SIG. OR SEVERE	(AGE RANGE)	AUTHOR
64	32	4	—	—	—	14	39	47	(≥65)	Blazer[17] (OARS Data)
—	—	—	52	43	5	—	—	—	(≥60)	Moore[18] (OARS Data)
82	11	7	—	—	—	—	—	—	(≥65)	Sheldon[19]
55	40	5	—	—	—	—	—	—	(≥60)	Leighton[12]
60	30	10	—	—	—	—	—	—	(≥60)	Lowenthal[20]
74	←—26—→		—	—	—	—	—	—	(≥65)	Kay and Roth[21]
—	—	—	—	—	—	—	—	32		Teeter[22]
←—82.2—→		17.8	—	—	—	—	—	—	(≥60)	Essen-Moller[23]
←—93.3—→		6.7	—	—	—	—	—	—	(≥60)	Bremer[24]
←—96—→		4	—	—	—	—	—	—	(≥60)	Primrose[25]
—	—	—	61	17	22	—	—	—	(≥65)	Harwin[37]

Table 10-3. Rates (%) According to Diagnostic Categories Among the Elderly in the Community.

AUTHOR	RANGE	SCHIZOPHRENIA AND PARANOID PSYCHOSES	AFFECTIVE PSYCHOSES	PERSONALITY DISORDER	NEUROSES	ORGANIC MENTAL DISEASE	PSYCHOPHYSIO-LOGICAL SYMPTOMS
Leighton[12] (1963)	60-69	1	—	6	61*	2.5**	81*
	≥70	2.5	—	7	51*	12**	85*
Sheldon[26] (1948)	≥65	←3.9→		3.2	9.4	11.3	—
Primrose[32] (1962)	≥60	←1.4→		2.2	10.4	11	—
Bremer[22] (1951)	≥60	←4.2→		12.6	5	2.5**	6.7
Essen-Moller[27] (1956)	≥60	1	2	10.6	11.4	5	7
Kay & Roth[28] (1964)	≥65	2	1.3	3.6	8.9	10	
Eaton-Weil[23] (1955)	≥65					4	

* Leighton's rates are quite high because he records the presence of symptoms, not actual diagnosis.
** Records only psychotic manifestations of OMS.

Table 10-4. Rates (%) According to Diagnostic Categories Among the Elderly in Institutions (Public Facilities) Rates (%) (Differentiated by sex when available).

AUTHOR	SCHIZOPHRENIA AND PARANOID PSYCHOSES	AFFECTIVE PSYCHOSES	PERSONALITY DISORDERS	NEUROSES	ORGANIC MENTAL DISORDERS
Reddick[67] (Mental Hospital) (LTCF)	35		.5	1.4*	44* 35
Teeter[21] (LTCF)	11	5	3	17	70
Stromgren[48] (Mental Hospital)	62.2(M) 57.1(F)	6.7(M) 9.6(F)		12.1(M) 14.9(F)	16.4(M) 14.7(F)
Lowenthal[29] (Mental Hospital)					60
Juel-Nielsen[48] (Mental Hospital)					23

* Calculated by Blazer

255

and long-term care facilities probably approaches 50%. The diagnosis of schizophrenia and paranoid psychosis appears to be quite high in mental hospitals varying between 35% and 60%. Many of these patients are individuals who were admitted to state and county mental hospitals earlier in life and have not been discharged.

Table 10-5 presents the percent distributions of admissions to psychiatric outpatient facilities of persons 65 and over by diagnostic category. The figures of Reddick, which take into account census data during 1969 throughout the country, indicate that the most common conditions to be seen in psychiatric outpatient facilities are organic mental syndromes and psychoneuroses. The comparison of this data with data from a new type of facility, the OARS Clinic at Duke University, demonstrates some interesting findings. The OARS Clinic was developed to specifically reach community based elderly with general problems of adaptation. The staff was made up of individuals with specific training in mental health. It became known to most professionals as a mental health facility, but it was not labeled as such for the community at large. Therefore, the rate of psychoneurosis and adjustment reactions is considerably higher than the usual rates in community mental health centers and outpatient psychiatric facilities

and the rate of drug problems and schizophrenia is lower. These findings provide evidence that the orientation of the treatment facility will be associated with the type of patient attracted to that facility.

Another approach to considering the distribution of mental health disorders is to study the distribution of certain symptom complexes (not diagnostic categories). Two recent studies at Duke demonstrate the use of such methods. First, a scale was developed for detecting the presence of dysphoric symptoms and the symptoms that are the criteria for the diagnosis of depressive illness,[16] and it was administered to a stratified random sample (n = 992) of individuals 65 years and older living in Durham County. The point prevalence of dysphoric symptoms was 14.7%. Four subgroups of subjects with dysphoria were identified: (1) those with symptoms of primary dysphoria (4.5%); (2) those with symptoms of primary depression (1.8%); (3) those with symptoms of secondary depression (1.9%) and; (4) those with symptoms of dysphoria associated with physical health impairment (6.5%).[24] In a separate study, using the same sample, the perception of poor health in healthy older adults (i.e., a possible indication of hypochondriasis) was seen in 14%.[25] The use of symptom scales and checklists can be of value in com-

Table 10-5. Percent Distribution of Admissions to Outpatient Facilities of Persons 65 Years and Over by Diagnostic Category.

	REDICH[29]		BLAZER[20]
	OUTPATIENT PSYCHIATRIC FACILITY	CMHC	OARS CLINIC
Alcoholism	3.4	5.6	0
Drug Dependence	.8	.5	0
Organic Mental Syndromes	23.9	31.8	24
Schizophrenia	10.6	7.5	5
Other Psychoses	10.3	13.8	6
Psychoneuroses	16.8	16.3	27
Personality Disorders	6.0	4.0	2
Other (Total)			
Adjustment	28.2	20.5	32
Reactions			22
No Disorder			10

munity diagnosis. Yet the investigator must take care in distinguishing symptomatology from actual mental illness. A rate of 15% for dysphoric symptoms does *not* imply that 15% of the population should be treated for depressive illness.

Descriptive epidemiology studies may also take into account the basic demographic and social characteristics of persons. Among these characteristics age, sex, race or ethnic groups and social class are the most frequent and appropriate to consider in the elderly. Age can be considered from at least two viewpoints. First, there is a differential rate of psychiatric illness in individuals 65 and older when compared to those under the age of 65. In many studies, the prevalence of neurosis declines with age.[12,26,27] Four studies, however, show the rate of overall psychiatric impairment to be increased with age.[4,22,27,28] Two studies show a general ascending order of psychiatric impairment with advancing age among women but not among men.[19,29] It appears that the prevalence of schizophrenia declines with age but the prevalence of psychosomatic complaints and especially organic brain syndrome increases with age.[12] The overall findings are therefore equivocal. Some studies have considered only the elderly (e.g., the Newcastle[28] and the OARS surveys[20]) whereas others have only considered the young and middle aged groups (e.g., the Mid-Manhattan Study[13]). Of even greater importance, however, is the lack of adequate definitions of what constitutes mental health impairment and/or psychiatric illness at various stages of the life cycle.

Second, old age is not a static position of the life cycle. It may be useful to distinguish between the young-old (the 65 to 74) and the old-old (75 and above). As one enters the old-old age group the probability of developing organic mental disease increases markedly, whereas many of the other conditions (schizophrenia in particular) decline considerably. The average age of onset of the Alzheimer's senile dementia is 74 years.[30] When all psychoses are considered together, there is an associated increase in the average annual incidence rate with increase in age. The rate for the 75 and older is almost doubled for the 65 to 74 age group.[31]

Sex differences must also be taken into account in epidemiologic studies. Six studies show a higher prevalence of psychiatric impairment among women.[12,22,26,28,29,32] Constitutional factors may be of etiologic significance, but the researcher must also consider the possible increase in psychosocial stress among women e.g., the increased likelihood of being identified as suffering from psychiatric symptomatology by the usual methods of case identification. It is well known that elderly males are more at risk for committing suicide, whereas elderly males and females are usually equally represented in typical prevalence studies for depressive symptomatology.[24] Though the rate of all psychoses for females 54 and under is greater than for males, this comparison is reversed after the age of 55 and is approximately 1.5 times greater in males in the 75 and over age group.[31]

Data on the distribution of psychiatric symptomatology by race is virtually non-existent, as demonstrated by Jackson.[33] Suicide rates for blacks are known to be low, yet the pattern of increased suicide with advancing age is beginning to appear among black men.[34] Dysphoric symptomatology and perception of poor health in the healthy elderly are not significantly different when white and nonwhite populations are compared.[24,25] Clearly more work must be done in this area.

Studies of the rates of psychiatric illness, impairment or symptomatology in the elderly according to social class are difficult to perform methodologically. How do you measure social class in the elderly? Late life is the great "equalizer" in terms of income, especially when an individual is faced with extensive medical expenses or long-term institutionalization. Most people 65 and older are retired, so occupation is not a good indicator. Previous occupation and/or education may be better measures of social class, but become biased when more immediate factors, such as economic impoverishment or social discrimination secondary to age occur in individuals previously economically secure or from the professional and managerial occupations.

Descriptive studies of the rate and distribution of psychiatric symptoms, syndromes or impairment can be of value in (1) alerting the medical community as to what types of older persons have a greater probability of being affected; (2) assisting in the rational planning of mental health care facilities and; (3) providing initial clues to the etiology of conditions.[35] Such studies are a preliminary step and associates between the outcome variable (i.e., the case) and independent variables do not necessarily reflect etiologic factors intrinsic within an individual.[1] Unfortunately, most studies of psychiatric epidemiology in the elderly have been descriptive studies. They have their uses, but suffer from the deficit described above.

THE HISTORICAL TRENDS IN MENTAL ILLNESS

Historical studies relate the frequency of events among populations to different points in time.[3] The rates of disease in the population increase and decrease over time. There are a number of psychiatric diseases that have decreased over time, such as general paresis, pellagra psychosis and conversion disorders.[36] The decrease in general paresis is particularly relevant to geriatric psychiatry. Clinicians certainly encounter less cases today than 20 years ago. Yet sporadic cases continue to appear and young clinicians may not consider general paresis in the differential diagnosis of organic mental disorders and psychotic reactions in late life.

Because of the increasing numbers of older people in our society and medical advances, it is expected that the absolute numbers of mentally impaired elderly will increase. In particular, senile dementia of the Alzheimer's type has reached such severe proportions that Katzman and Karasu[37] estimate that the senile form of Alzheimer's disease may rank as the fourth or fifth most common cause of death in the United States today. This increase, in part, is due to the increased life expectancy of older persons and the decreased mortality in late life secondary to infectious disease.

Yet there has been very few studies that have looked at the historical trends of mental illness in the elderly, and many problems continue to exist.[38] Changes in diagnostic criteria for certain illnesses have rendered the comparison of data of studies over the last 50 to 75 years much less than optimal. The change in orientation from preoccupation with survival to a preoccupation with the quality of life has brought certain problems, such as depressive symptomatology, to the forefront.[3] In addition, the changing attitudes toward mental disorders in late life and changes in orientation of mental health services toward the mentally impaired elder will have a definite effect upon our perception of historical trends. Dysphoric symptoms that are considered pathological in 1978 were accepted as a normal concomitant of aging in the past.

THE ETIOLOGY OF MENTAL ILLNESS

One of the most important functions of epidemiology in the study of the mental illness of late life is to aid in establishing the etiology of these illnesses. The determination of a biological mechanism through experimentation is the most direct method of finding a causal relationship between a factor and a disease. Epidemiological studies can provide the initial support for such causal relationships and can be most valuable in supporting or rejecting a given hypothesis. Initial studies generally demonstrate a relationship between some suspected causative factor or factors and the disease under investigation at a given point in time (*prevalence studies*). Results are presented in terms of the strength of the association between the factor(s) and the disease with other factors being controlled (such as age, sex, socioeconomic status and physical health status). The next step is to develop an *incidence study*. A group of individuals who are not suffering from the disease under study are selected. The group is then followed over a period of time (usually months or years) for the development of the disease. Some (or all) of the group may be exposed to the suspected causative factor. This study provides the rate of the development of the disease or condition over a period of time and is expressed in terms of the number of new cases per the number of persons in the study population at the beginning of the study. Further evidence of causation can be obtained through: (1) experimental reproduction of the disease in animals or man, such as experimentally induced psychoses in animals with hallucinogenic drugs; (2) elimination of the cause, such as removing a soldier with an acute traumatic neurosis from the battlefield; (3) modification of the subject's response to the cause, such as relaxation training. The total knowledge gained through these activities may never sort out the absolute cause of a given psychiatric illness, symptom or impairment because of the multifactorial etiology of most psychiatric illness. However, accumulated data in each of these areas can be of significant benefit to the geriatric psychiatrist.

In addition to genetic and biochemical abnormalities, at least five psychosocial factors have been considered to be of etiologic importance in the onset of mental illness in late life: psychosocial stress,[12] loss of social support,[28] maladaptive personality development,[28] previous history of mental illness[39] and physical illness.[20] Mental illness in late life provides an excellent example of multidimensional etiology of impairment in health. Unfortunately these factors have typically been studied in isolation. Therefore a comprehensive model of causation has yet to be developed. Following a review of the literature on causation to date, a model will be presented that can be used in developing future epidemiologic studies of mental illness in late life.

The role of psychosocial stress has been given great attention in psychiatric literature as a causative factor in the etiology of mental illness. The early studies of Farris and Dunham[5] and later studies by Hollingshed and Redlich (New Haven Study),[40] Shrole, Langner and Michael (Midtown Manhattan Study),[13] and Leighton (Stirling County Study)[41] demonstrate an increased prevalence of mental illness among the lower socioeconomic groups. These findings generally hold true for the elderly, though some studies (e.g., the Midtown Manhattan Study) do not include the elderly. A more comprehensive review of the role of psychosocial stress has been presented by Leighton[41] in the Stirling County Study. Social disintegration was postulated as being causative in the development of mental illness and Leighton's use of anthropological techniques to classify communities as socially integrated or socially disintegrated provided a mechanism for testing this hypothesis. Leighton demonstrated that social disintegration was indeed associated with an increased prevalence of mental illness.[12] These findings held true for the elderly as with other age groups within the population study.

Holmes and Rahe[42] have taken a step forward in the measurement of stress by developing the Social Readjustment Rating Scale. By identifying the number and types of stressful factors encountered by an individual (i.e., life events), they have shown that social stress is related to mental illness onset. The relationship between changes in life events and mental health has not been extensively studied among the aged. In fact, Heyman and Gianturco[43] found that loss of a loved one was associated with little or no health deterioration in the over 65 years of age. The number of life changes apparently decreases with increasing age.[44,45,46] This could indicate, on the one hand, that, in old age, fewer changes would be required to produce health changes. On the other hand, different life events not typically considered in schedules (e.g., change in attendance at religious assemblies, success or failure of a child in a business venture, etc.) or a rearrangement of numerical weights for other life events (e.g., bereavement, retirement, etc.) may produce more valid studies.

In recent years, the role of the loss of social support in the etiology of illness in general, and mental illness in particular, has been given increased attention. Such considerations should be particularly applicable to the elderly who are uniquely at risk for the loss of social support. Kay and Roth,[47] by gathering historic data from psychotic and nonpsychotic patients, have shown that individuals with psychoses are far more often the youngest members of their families and have fewer surviving relatives. Other individuals with psychoses were shown to be isolated by their illness and by physical symptoms such as deafness. Juel-Nielson and Stromgren[48] have shown an increase in the risk of patients with senile dementia for be hospitalized if they are socially isolated. They also demonstrated that those with decreased social interaction and who live alone are more inclined to develop or to demonstrate impairment. The OARS Survey of Durham County revealed a significant correlation ($r = .42$) between impaired social resources and mental health impairment.[20] Isolation is one measure of loss of social support. Yet the study of isolation in the elderly has produced certain difficulties. For example, Garside, Kay and Roth[49] found that respondents' complaints of loneliness did not correlate well with the number of their daily contacts with other people. Other elderly persons appear to adapt quite well to isolation and usual measures of social interaction do not accurately predict the risk of developing mental impairment.

The role of personality development has also been considered as a causative factor in the development of mental illness in late life. Verwoerdt's[50] clinical experience has lead him to believe that individuals with certain personality styles (e.g., the hysterical personality) may be especially prone to the development of psychiatric symptomatology in late life. Kay, Beamish and Roth,[28] using retrospective case histories, found abnormalities in personality for four to five decades before psychotic breakdowns developed in late life. For example, one-fourth of the female patients with psychotic breakdowns in late life studied in Stockholm had illegitimate children in their twenties. These figures were very different from those with the diagnosis of depression. The association of social isolation and mental disorder is substantiated by the increased prevalence of mental disorders in immigrants, the unmarried urban residents, and certain occupational groups. This association may be a reflection of premorbid abnormalities in personality of these individuals (which in turn are prone to lead to social failure). A number of authors[51,52] have demonstrated that personality traits are usually powerful predictors of adaptation in late life. Vispo found differences between the premorbid personalities among a sample of elderly subjects with functional disorders and those of a group of normal controls.[53]

It is obvious that a previous history of psychiatric disorder may also contribute significantly to the development of psychiatric illness in late life. Stotsky[39] demonstrated that "psychiatric patients" admitted to nursing homes show more intellectual impairment and more evidence of severe psychiatric disturbances than patients placed from general hospitals or the community. The individual with a history of depressive illness would certainly be more inclined to develop depressive episodes in late life. However, one cannot generalize. For example, individuals with schizoid personality styles may feel relatively comfortable with the loneliness of old age.[50]

There is much evidence indicating that physical illness and mental illness are related in late life. Roth and Kay[54] demonstrated a relationship between physical illness and depressive states in the elderly. The loss of sensory perceptual abilities may also lead to the development of certain psychiatric illnesses. Lowenthal,[29] Kay and Roth[55] and Post[56] demonstrated the significant health problems among those who have mental health impairment. A community survey of Durham County showed a correlation of $r = .55$ between physical health and mental health impairment.[20] This positive correlation is related to a number of factors, but the most important predictor may be the reduced capacity for self-care in the physically impaired elderly. Garside, Kay and Roth[49] found reduced mobility and capacity for self-care as the highest distinguishing factors separating organic mental impairment from normality and functional impairment. The OARS Survey reveals a correlation between mental impairment and impairment in activities of daily living of $r = .61$, the highest correlation recorded among the five factors assessed.[20]

Each of the studies presented above are cross-sectional or prevalence studies. They provide good initial evidence of a number of factors that might relate to the development of psychiatric impairment or illness in late life. Yet such studies do not aid the investigator in the development of a model of the sequence of events that lead to the outcome of an identified case. Historical reviews of a subject's past can be of significant help in developing a group of antecedent, precipitant and accompanying factors related to a case. Unfortunately they suffer from the bias of the unique perception of the subject-historian. In the elderly this process may be further complicated by poor memory. Validation of the historical sequence of illness development by family members or friends can make a significant contribution to this process.

Longitudinal studies of the elderly would seem to be the logical source of incidence data. Yet the number of subjects included in such studies is small and the attrition rate, usually by death, is high so only the more common symptom patterns might be followed. Typically such studies have included psychiatric interviews at the initiation of the study but not subsequently.

THE WEB OF CAUSATION

The epidemiologist must organize the complex multifactoral processes that lead to the development of mental illness in late life. One such method is to view disease etiology as a "web of causation."[1] This concept of disease considers all the predisposing factors and the complex relations between these factors and disease outcome. For example, a causal model of the development of depression in late life is demonstrated in Table 10–6. Despite its apparent complexity, even this model is undoubtedly an over simplification and must be modified with further research. Effects are not dependent on single causes. Each causative factor shown is influenced by many other factors not shown and the complexity of the model can easily reach unmanageable proportions. Nevertheless, such a model can provide a concept of disease etiology that might spawn a variety of interventions which in turn might reduce the occurrence of depression in late life. Though it is tempting to search for a "primary cause" of depression, the benefits of such a search may not be as great as one might hope for. In terms of prevention, it may be more practical to attack the cause or web at a point that is relatively remote from the depressive illness itself. For example, increased social stress and decreased social support may be of more importance in the increased prevalence of depression in late life than personality style, and intrapsychic conflicts, or genetic predisposition.

SOCIAL STRESS AND SOCIAL SUPPORT

Two possible etiologic factors deserve special attention in geriatric psychiatry: social stress and social support. Though genetic factors may play a significant causative role in mental illness, they are less likely to be of significance in those illnesses that have their onset in late life. Biological changes in late life certainly contribute to the etiology of certain conditions, but these changes are known to be intimately related to the social environment. Social factors, such as the frequent losses of late life, often precipitate decreased function in individuals who are suffering from biologically determined psychiatric illness (e.g., organic mental disorders). Of more importance, how-

Table 10-6. Some Components in the Etiology of Depression in Late Life.

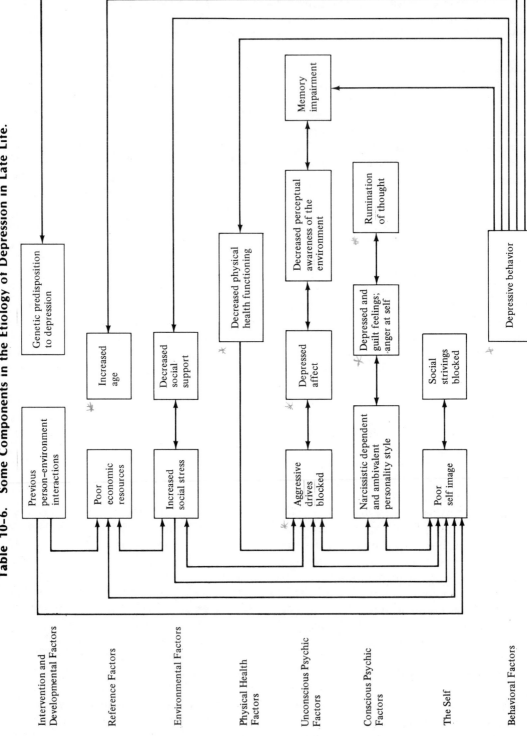

ever, is the role of social factors in the natural history of a late life disorder once it has had its onset. The depressions of late life are frequently recurrent, anxiety is often persistent, and cognitive impairment often is progressive and accompanied by many secondary symptoms. How much of a role do social factors play in the course of late life psychiatric disorders?

In order to understand the effect of social stress and social support on the individual, it is necessary to define these two phenomena as they occur within the environment. Cassel, among others, in looking at the social environment as a factor in the development of disease, has shown that psychosocial processes should no longer be considered unidimensionally.[57] There are factors in the environment which may be stressful to the organism, and other factors that may be protective or beneficial. Social stress is stimuli or feedback from the social environment that blocks goal-directed behavior and/or places demands on the person that interrupts the steady state. In other words social stress impinges on the individual in such a way as to initiate a change in self-perception and accustomed patterns of social relatedness. Stressors in the environment have been typically conceptualized as discrete and definable environmental events with a definite point of origin (e.g., an electric shock, confinement, separation from a significant object).[58] "Life events" research exemplifies this orientation.[42] Yet the environment may also be chronically stressful over a period of time (e.g., the continual high level of noise in a factory or the continued threat of war in an unstable country).

Social support is the provision of meaningful, appropriate and protective feedback from the social environment to the person, enabling the person to negotiate intermittent and/or continual environmental stress. The beneficial effects of social support are less likely to be conceptualized in terms of specific life events and more in terms of the individual's general experience with the en-

vironment over a period of time.[57,59,60,61] Yet the provision of meaningful feedback in a time of crisis can be most protective (e.g., the explanation to the public of the meaning and probable outcome of a political or economic crisis).

Social stress and social support may be harmful or beneficial respectively to the person at the unconscious and even physical level, influencing such phenomena as health outcomes in crisis situations.[62] These effects of the social environment may be mediated through conscious perceptions of the environment. However, certain stressful and supportive stimuli (or components of stimuli) may bypass consciousness and be directly shunted from the sensory organs to other organ systems within the human body, or may provide "parallel" input into consciousness and other bodily systems.[63] For example, Hofer has shown that interruption of nursing in young rat pups at a critical time in their development leads to certain behavioral phenomena within these pups at later stages of development. At the same time, the lack of mother's milk during these same critical periods of development may determine the response of the cardiovascular system to stress at a later point in time.[64]

As mentioned above, the research of "life events" is an example of the measurement and quantification of discrete changes in the environment of the person.[42] To complement this research, the development of a typology of the social system for research in epidemiology would be most valuable in evaluating the continuing effects of social stress and social support. When considering the measurement of the social system from which social stress or social support originates, it is important to remember that this system can be assessed by observation (e.g., an anthropologist observing a community, a therapist observing a family, etc.) or can be assessed indirectly through the perceptions of the individual. Either method may generate potential bias. Perceptions of the social system are influenced by a person's characteristics although the perceptions may actually be more closely associated with mental impairment than the objective nature of the social system.[65]

Regardless of the method chosen to measure the nature of the social system of an individual or group of individuals, certain characteristics of this system should be considered.[66] As previously mentioned, social systems are typically open systems and are therefore influenced by factors outside the system. Systems, like individuals, change over time secondary to internal alterations and interchanges with other systems. To understand and measure the social system, it would be helpful to develop certain criteria of measurement. Table 10-7 presents a typology which may be used in measuring and evaluating the social system. It would be highly unlikely that any one study would consider all of the factors listed, but the relative contributions of whatever factor is studied, should be considered in light of the overall picture. For example, a "stressful life event" such as loss of a spouse, may effect the social system of a subject at many different points. Though the boundaries of the system may be unchanged, one of the roles of the system is unfilled and the density of the system is decreased by one. If the spouse provided a product (or service) to the subject, such as transportation, the survivor may find the remainder of the social system less reachable. Often the loss of a key member of the social system will lead to decreasing linkage between other members of the system. The loss would also decrease the heterogeneity of the system by a factor of one. The durability of the system may also be threatened. As can be seen, the researcher can potentially break up the stressful event of "loss of spouse" into its component effects on the social system.

In summary, the individual negotiates life by a continual series of interchanges with the environment (see Figure 10-1). The genetic characteristics of the individual, the nature of the environment and the nature of the interchanges between the individual and the environment over time determine the individual characteristics of the individual at a given point in time. Most epidemiologic studies focus on the social environment of the person, as described above, but the physical environment (e.g., the provision of an adequate diet, warmth, etc.) is also important. A model for the study of the causative factors of mental illness in late life must encompass each of these elements: (1)

Table 10-7.   A Typology of the Social System.*

A. *Structural Characteristics of the System*
1. *Units, roles and boundaries:* The individuals and groups of individuals within the system, the uniform patterns of behavior expected of persons and the determinants of those included in and excluded from the system.
2. *Density:* The size of the system and the number of persons or groups within physically defined areas.
3. *Reachability:* The extent to which individuals can contact and use other individuals or other groups that are of importance.
4. *Interconnections:* The linkage between members of the system.
5. *Range:* The heterogeneity of the system.

B. *Interactional Characteristics of the System*
1. *Durability:* The stability of the system over time.
2. *Intensity:* The degree of interaction within a system.
3. *Frequency:* The actual number of times interaction within a social system takes place.
4. *Process:* The structure of the interactions of the system.
5. *Flexibility:* The fluidity of the system's roles and procedures.

C. *Value Orientations:* The cognitive, affective and directive elements which give order and guidance to the stream of interactions within the system.

D. *Products:* The output or behavior (both tangible and intangible) of the system.

E. *External Stimuli:* Stimuli from without the system that impinge upon the system.

F. *Orientation of Assessment* (direct or indirect).

* Concepts modified from Weiss[65] and Kaplan.[60]

PHYSICAL ENVIRONMENT

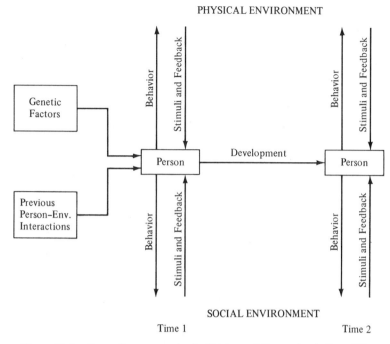

Figure 10–1.   Some Components in the Etiology of Depression in Late Life.

genetic predisposition; (2) previous person-environment interaction; (3) physical environment; (4) social environment; and (5) development. The investigator may concentrate on one or at the most two of these elements, but must always be aware that only a portion of the etiology may be explained by such limitations. Unfortunately, the instruments for valid measurement of each of these areas remain to be developed and the methodology for analyzing their relative importance longitudinally are not available as yet.

UTILIZATION OF MENTAL HEALTH FACILITIES

The development of an effective methodology for the study of the utilization is based on the effectiveness of community diagnosis; namely the prevalence, incidence and distribution of mental disorders among the elderly in the community. Data from psychiatric institutions and outpatient facilities provide information on only those individuals who come in contact with the facilities under study. Such data has value in

that it provides information concerning patient flow, the extent to which the elderly mentally ill use available resources, the characteristics of patients coming under care, etc.[67] Nevertheless, a critical question remains unanswered. Why do certain elderly individuals in the community who are mentally impaired fail to utilize services that would be beneficial to their well-being?

According to the 1970 U.S. Census, 4% of the total population 65 years of age and older were living in institutions. Of the institutionalized elderly, 15% were residents of psychiatric hospitals (approximately 124,000 persons, the majority of which were in state and county mental hospitals).[67] Yet the elderly accounted for only 9% of the total "patient care episodes" in mental health facilities during 1969 (an underutilization of psychiatric services given the rates of mental illness among the elderly compared to other age groups). In contrast, the 65 and over age group tend to utilize inpatient psychiatric facilities to a much greater degree than the entire population.

Resident patients 65 and older in state and county mental hospitals are almost equally divided between those with the diagnosis of organic brain syndromes and those with the diagnosis of psychotic disorders.[67] The latter group is made up of those with the diagnosis of schizophrenia who were often admitted at a younger age. Sixty-five percent of the 65 and older who were admitted to state and county mental hospitals were diagnosed as having organic brain syndrome. Patients 65 and over admitted to private mental hospitals are much more likely to be diagnosed as having psychoneurotic and psychotic processes other than schizophrenia.

Females outnumber males in the utilization of all psychiatric facilities except state and county mental hospitals (where the percentages are approximately equal).[67] This is probably due to the longer life expectancy of females and possibly the greater likelihood of females utilizing psychiatric services.

Outpatient psychiatric services are greatly underutilized by the elderly. In the years 1966 through 1969 the elderly accounted for only 2% of the total outpatient episodes.[67] In 1969, the 65 and older group accounted for only 4% of the total patient care episodes in mental health centers.[67] We might expect to see these percentages increase with a specific mandate for services for persons 65 years of age and older in the extension of the Community Mental Health Centers Act in 1975. Yet the elderly in North Carolina accounted for only 4% of the outpatient services in 1977.[68]

Data from the psychiatric case register in Monroe County, New York indicates that the rate of use of private psychiatrists for the 65 and older group are probably quite small (one-half to one-third the rate for the 35 to 44 age group).[69] Studies by Shepard determined that the psychiatric morbidity rate among persons 65 years of age and over who consulted a general practitioner during a year's period was 11% for males and 15% for females.[70] This indicates that the elderly may tend to utilize other physicians in private practice than psychiatrists for the treatment of psychiatric problems.

The availability of Medicare has probably led to the increased utilization of psychiatric services in general hospitals by the elderly. During the period 1966 through 1969, the 65 and older group accounted for about 12% of the total patient care episodes for these types of hospitals.[67]

Though the utilization patterns for different types of psychiatric facilities has changed over the past 15 years, there is no indication that the need for psychiatric services by the elderly has decreased. For example, though the number of elderly being discharged from state and county mental hospitals has definitely increased, almost 40% have been referred to nursing homes and 15% have been referred to outpatient psychiatric clinics.[71]

Few studies have addressed the critical issue of the untreated in the community. In the OARS Durham Survey,[20] only 1% of the community elderly were receiving some type of counseling or psychotherapy from any source. Twenty percent of the subjects were receiving a tranquilizer or nerve medicine (almost all being prescribed by their primary care physician). Upon systematic questioning, 9.6% of the subjects perceived a need for some type of trained counselling. Thirty-one percent of those with mental health impairment perceived the need for a trained counselor whereas only 8% of the nonimpaired perceived a need for counseling. When a new service for the mentally impaired elderly was developed in Durham County, the planning team anticipated that only 15% of those in need of such services would, in fact, make use of the services. Over the next 5 years, these estimates proved to be quite accurate.[72]

PLANNING FOR NEW MENTAL HEALTH SERVICES

Epidemiologic data can be of value in at least three areas in the planning for services. First, prevalence rates and projections can be of value in predicting the future levels of impairment of mental illness among the elderly in the community (and in institutions) along with future predictions of the use of mental health services by the elderly. If we assume that approximately 10% of the population of 65 and older suffering from significant or severe mental impairment would seek psychiatric services, between 2 and 2.5 million individuals would need services in the year 1980 and that number would continue to increase over the next few decades. If present patterns persist, however, the great majority of these individuals would not receive services in defined psychiatric facilities. In fact, only 20% of those needing services would actually seek out services (between 400,000 and 425,000 individuals). This 20% level of utilization may continue over the next few years. However, a number of factors may change this utilization rate thus decreasing the accuracy of present data in predicting future utilization. Factors that might lead to an increased utilization of psychiatric facilities over present predicted values include: (1) the future elderly, by virtue of their social and cultural background, are more likely to use psychiatric services; (2) psychiatric services may become more available secondary to recent legislation (especially the Community Mental Health Centers Act of 1975); (3) the medical community will become increasingly aware of psychiatric disability among the elderly and its potential for treatment, etc. Factors that might decrease utilization rates include: (1) financial constraints that decrease the availability of public services to an elderly population who may not be able to purchase private services; (2) a greater utilization of nonpsychiatric services (e.g., day care centers, pastoral counsellors, peer counseling, etc.); and (3) changes within the socioeconomic environment that decrease the risk of developing psychiatric illness among the elderly (e.g., changing retirement laws). Therefore past utilization rates alone cannot be expected to provide accurate predictions of future utilization of psychiatric services by the elderly.

Survey data, however, has an additional value in planning for services. For example, the OARS Community Survey provided guidelines for staffing of the OARS Clinic.[73]

Survey data indicated that those older people who seek mental health services tend to have multiple impairments. (Over one-half having two or more functional impairments). A multidisciplinary staff would therefore be required to assess and respond to interacting impairments of social, economic, psychological and biological functioning. The use of survey data coupled with clinical experience provided an estimate of the total amount of staff time required from professionals and supportive staff to assess, process and manage patients referred to the clinic (i.e., the full-time equivalents of a psychiatrist, a physician with experience in internal medicine, family medicine and geriatrics, nurses, social workers, etc. could be determined).

INTERVENTION AND OUTCOME

Psychiatric and other mental health services may be accepted as a norm, but the "norm" is often empirical and not based on objective observation, much less research.[3] The question must be asked, "What good does a service do, or what are the results rather than the intention?" This is the classic question of the evaluation of services. Mental health services contribute to mental health, but other factors, such as the physical and social environment, adaptive qualities of the individual, etc. may be even more important. Social policy usually demands that services created be both utilized and effective. The first issue to be addressed in the development of a program of evaluation is the desired outcome. Previous discussions in this chapter concerning the identification of a case certainly apply, but the outcome of a service might not always be the elimination of a condition, such as organic mental disease. Outcomes appropriate to mental health intervention might include improved mental health functioning, the elimination of certain target symptoms, evidence of greater adaptability, etc. An additional bit of information, however, is needed. What is the outcome of a given psychiatric condition if no intervention is available? In other words, what is the natural history of the condition? The course of an illness may be determined by either retrospective studies, such as obtaining a history from persons suffering from a given condition or prospective studies, such as following an individual at periodic intervals once the illness is diagnosed or the cause identified. A combination of these methods is the normal process of data collection.

Once outcomes have been defined, it is necessary to address the issue of intervention. Definitions of intervention techniques must be discrete and separate from the provider of the intervention if evaluative studies are to be translated from one setting to another. One reason evaluative studies of particular drugs have been more effective and convincing than studies of the outcomes of psychotherapy is that the drug is more easily defined than psychotherapy and its effects are less varied from one service provider to another.

Unfortunately, there is little known about the prognosis of mental impairment in late life. Individuals with Alzheimer's disease show a marked decrease in life expectancy, depending on the age at onset of symptoms. Kay found in a prospective study that the average survival period was 2.6 years for demented males compared to 8.7 years for the age matched nondemented male population, and 2.3 years for demented females compared to an expected survival of 10.9 years.[74] Wang and Whanger in a prospective study found somewhat better rates in that the average of onset for senile dementia was 74.1 years with 5.1 remaining years of life on the average when the life expectancy for aged matched controls of life was 9.6 years.[30] The prognosis for schizophrenia and the paranoid psychosis of late life appears definitely to have improved with the advent of phenothiazine therapy in the early 1950s. There are few studies, however, that document a definite improvement in individuals who initially develop schizophrenic or paranoid symptomatology in late life. The outcome for individuals who develop affective psychosis in late life appears much more

hopeful. Though again definitive studies are sparse, most clinicians recognize a definite clinical improvement in individuals with affective psychoses when appropriate pharmacotherapy is administered.

If one looks at overall mental health functioning, the OARS data indicates that within the community 40% of the 65 and over age group show a definite decline in mental health functioning over a one year period whereas only 19% show improvement during the same time span.[20] Individuals attending a psychiatric outpatient clinic show a greater trend toward improvement but still, overall, 36% of individuals showed a decline whereas only 30% showed improvement over a one year's period in mental health functioning.[20]

There has been a definite trend in recent years to release elderly patients from psychiatric facilities after shorter periods of stay than previously. Data from New York State indicate that during the 4-year period from 1966–1969, the median length of stay of individuals who were 65 years of age and older decreased from 146 to 130 days.[75] This gradual decrease in the number of days hospitalized may be indicative of various state policies which discourage state mental hospitals from continuing to be the caretakers of dysfunctional elderly. As mentioned previously, one cannot assume that intervention techniques have improved, for the percentage of individuals transferred to nursing homes from these state hospitals remains quite high.[71]

Suicide is a frequent outcome variable for studies of mental health. Data from 1966 reveal that 28% of the 21,281 persons committing suicide in the United States were over the age of 60.[76] Among men there is an almost linear increase in suicide rates with advancing age, though these rates level off for middle-age for females. The elderly account for a disproportionately higher number of suicides. While many more young persons attempt suicide than commit suicide,[75] the number of old people attempting suicide is roughly the same as the number actually committing suicide. These data indicate that suicide remains a serious problem among the elderly, and highlights the prominent role of mental health when considering total health care services delivered to the elderly.

There are at least two examples of evaluation in the literature. Sainsbury and Grad de Alarcon[77] compared a community psychogeriatric service with a more traditional hospital based service. The two populations at risk were demographically similar and the only psychiatric facilities available to each were those provided by the respective services. They found that community care was quite successful. The community-based service encourage an increased referral rate of old people and a decrease in suicide rates following its introduction. An additional finding was that the community oriented service, with its greater flexibility and range of facilities is better able to consider the needs of the patient and the family, for the needs of the family are easily recognized. Wertheimer, Gilliand et al.[78] also evaluated the impact of the establishment of a psychogeriatric outpatient center. This institution, serving as an outpost for a psychogeriatric hospital, made it possible to avoid or postpone a substantial number of admissions to the hospital.

The evaluation of services to older persons in the community, albeit quite sparse, points to the need for improved outpatient care for the elderly mentally ill. Not only do such facilities decrease the number of admissions to institutions but they provide substantial intervention for the patient in his or her social environment.

Multidisciplinary assessment of the community and patients referred to such facilities can be of great value in planning for such services and the determination of the success of impact of these services.

REFERENCES

1. MacMahon, B. and Pugh, T. F. *Epidemiology: Principles and Methods.* Boston: Little Brown, 1970.
2. Myers, G. C., Covar, M. G., Matten, K. G., Poss, S. S. and Hogue, C. C. Symposium: Mortality Trends Among the Elderly. Gerontological Society Annual Meeting, 1977.
3. Morris, J. N. *Uses of Epidemiology* (Second Edition). London: E. & F. Livingston, 1970.
4. New York State Department of Mental Hygiene. Mental Health Research Unit: *Mental Health Survey of Older People.* Utica, New York: State Hospital Press, 1960; 1961.
5. Farris, R. E., Dunham, H. W. *Mental Disorders in Urban Areas.* Chicago: University of Chicago Press, 1939.
6. Pasmanick, B., Roberts, D. W. and Lamkau, D. W. *et al.* A survey of mental disease in an urban population: Prevalence rate by race, and income, In B. Pasamanick, (ed.) *Epidemiology of Mental Disorder.* Washington: American Association for the Advancement of Science, 1969.
7. Clausen, J. A. and Cohn, M. L. Relation of schizophrenia to the social structure of a small city, In B. Pasamanick, (ed.) *Epidemiology of Mental Disorder.* Washington: American Association for the Advancement of Sciences, 1959.
8. *Diagnostic and Statistical Manual of Mental Disorders* (Second Edition). Washington, D.C.: American Psychiatric Association, 1968.
9. Goldfarb, A. I. The evaluation of geriatric patients following treatment, In P. H. Hoch, J. Zubin (eds.) *Evaluation of Psychiatric Treatment.* New York: Grune and Stratton, 1964.
10. Cattel, R. B., Eber, H. J. and Tatsuoks, M. *The Sixteen Personality Factor Questionnaire* (Edition 3). Champagne, Ill.: Institute of Personality and Ability Testing, 1970.
11. Zung, W. W. K. A self-rating depression scale. *Archives of General Psychiatry,* **12:** 63, (1965).
12. Leighton, D. C. *et al. The Character of Danger.* New York: Basic Books, 1963.
13. Langner, T. S. and Michael, S. T. *Life Stress and Mental Health.* New York: Free Press, 1963.
14. *Multidimensional Functional Assessment: The OARS Methodology.* Second Edition Durham, N.C.: Center for the Study of Aging and Human Development, 1978.
15. Wing, J. K., Cooper, J. E. and Sartorius, N. *The Measurement and Classification of Psychiatric Symptoms.* Cambridge: Cambridge University Press.
16. Feighner, J. P., Robbins, E. and Guse, S. B., *et al.* Diagnostic criteria for use in psychiatric research. *Archives of General Psychiatry* **26:** 57 (1972).
17. Moore, J. Functional disability of geriatric patients in a family medicine program: implication for education service and research. (Unpublished manuscript), 1977.
18. Burns, B. J., Orso, C., Jacobsen, A., Laet, R. and Goldner, N. Utilization of health and mental health outpatient services in organized medical care settings. *Final Report for National Institute of Mental Health:* Contract #278-76-0027, 1977.

19. Hilkevitch, A. Psychiatric disturbances in outpatients of a general medical outpatient clinic. *International Journal of Neuropsychiatry,* **1:** 371 (1965).

20. Blazer, D. G. The OARS Durham surveys: description and application, in *Multidimensional Functional Assessment: The OARS Methodology* (Second Edition). Durham, N.C.: Center for the Study of Aging and Human Development, 1978.

21. Teeter, R. B., Garetz, S. K., Miller, W. R. and Hailand, W. F. Psychiatric disturbances of aged patients in skilled nursing homes. *American Journal of Psychiatry,* **133:** 1430 (1976).

22. Bremer, J. A. A social investigation of a small community in northern Norway. *Acta Psychiatric et Neurologic Scandinavia Supplement,* **62,** 1951.

23. Eaton, J. W. and Weil, R. J. *Culture and Mental Disorder: A Comparative Study of Hutterites and Other Populations.* New York: Free Press of Glencoe, 1955.

24. Blazer, D. G. and Williams, D. Epidemiology of late life dysphoria and depression. Paper presented at the Annual Meeting of the American Psychiatric Association, May, 1979.)

25. Blazer, D. G. and Houpt, J. Perception of poor health in the healthy older adult. *Journal of the American Geriatrics Society* (in press).

26. Sheldon, J. H. *The Social Medicine of Old Age: Report of an Inquiry in Wolfehampton* London: Oxford University Press, 1948.

27. Essen-Moller, E., Larson, H., Euddenberg, C. E. and White, G. Individual traits and morbidity in a Swedish rural population. *Acta Psychiatric et Neurologic Scandanavia Supplement,* **100,** 1956.

28. Kay, D. W. K., Beamish, P. and Roth, M. Old age mental disorders in Newcastle-upon-Tyne: a study of prevalence. *British Journal of Psychiatry,* **110:** 146–158, 668–682 (1964).

29. Lowenthal, M. F. and Berkman, P. L. *Aging and Mental Disorder in San Francisco.* San Francisco: Jossey-Bass, 1962.

30. Wang, H. S., Whanger, A. Brain impairment and longevity, in E. Palmore and F. C. Jeffers (eds.) *Prediction of the Life Span.* Lexington, Mass.: Heath, 1971.

31. Jaco, E. G. *The Social Epidemiology of Mental Disorders.* New York: Russell Sage Foundation, 1960.

32. Primrose, J. R. *Psychologic Illness: A Community Study.* London: Tavistock, 1962.

33. Jackson, J. J. Epidemiological aspects of mental illness among aged: black women and men. (Unpublished manuscript). Solomon Memorial Lecture, 1978.

34. Model Statistics of the United States, Volume II, Mortality, Part A. Washington, D. C.: U.S. Public Health Service, 1968.

35. Friedman, G. D. *Primer of Epidemiology.* New York: Blakiston, 1974.

36. Group for the Advancement of Psychiatry Committee on Preventive Psychiatry. *Problems of Estimating Changes in Frequency of Mental Disorders.* Report 50. Group for the Advancement of Psychiatry, New York, 1961.

37. Katzman, Karasu, T. B. Differential diagnosis of dementia, In W. Fields (ed.) *Neurologic and Sensory Disorders in the Elderly.* New York: Stratton and Continental Medical Book Corporation, 1975.

38. Gruenberg, E. M. Epidemiology of mental disorders in aging, In *The Neurological and Psychiatric Aspects of Disorders of Aging.* Baltimore: Williams and Wilkins, 1956.

39. Stotsky, B. A. *The Nursing Home and the Aged Psychiatric Patient.* New York: Appleton-Century-Crofts, 1970.

40. Hollingshed, A. D. and Redlich, F. C. *Social Class and Mental Illness: A Community Study.* New York: John Wiley, 1958.

41. Leighton, A. H. *My Name is Legion.* New York: Basic Books, 1959.

42. Holmes, T. H. and Rahe, R. H. The social readjustment rating scale. *Journal of Psychosomatic Research,* **11:** 213 (1967).

43. Heyman, D. K. and Gianturco, D. T. Long-term adaptation of the elderly to bereavement. *Journal of Gerontology,* **28:** 359 (1973).

44. Holmes, T. S. and Holmes, T. H. Short-term intrusion into the life-styles routine. *Journal of Psychosomatic Research,* **14:** 121 (1970).

45. Masuda, M., Holmes, T. H. Life events: Perceptions and frequencies. *Psychosomatic Medicine,* **40:** 236 (1978).

46. Ander, S., Lindstrom, B. and Tibblin, G. Life changes in random samples of middle-aged men, In E. K. E. Gunderson and R. H. Rahe, (eds.) *Life Stress and Illness.* Springfield, Ill.: Charles C Thomas, 1974.

47. Kay, D. W. K. and Roth, M. Environmental and hereditary factors in the schizophrenias of old age (late paraphrenia) and their bearing on the general problems and causation in schizophrenia. *Journal of Mental Sciences,* **107:** 649 (1961).

48. Juel-Nielsen, N., Stromgren, E. Ten years later. A comparison between census studies of patients in psychiatric institutes in Newmark in 1957, 1962 and 1967. *Acta Jutland XLX:* **2** (1969).

49. Garside, R. S., Kay, D. W. K. and Roth, M. Old age and mental disorders in Newcastle-upon-Tyne, Part III. A factorial analysis of medical, psychiatric and social characteristics. *British Journal of Psychiatry,* **111:** 939 (1965).

50. Verwoerdt, A. *Clinical Geropsychiatry.* Baltimore: Williams and Wilkins, 1976.

51. Lowenthal, M. F., Chiribaga, D. Social stress and adaptation: toward a life course perspective, In C. Eisdorfer and M. P. Lawton (eds.) *The Psychology of Adult Development in Aging.* Washington, D.C.: American Psychological Association, 1973.

52. Lieberman, M. A. Adaptive processes in late life,

In N. Datan and L. Ginsberg, (eds.) *Life Span Development Psychology: Normative Life Crises.* New York: Academic Press, 1975.

53. Dispo, R. H. Premorbid personality in the functional psychosis of the cenium. A comparison of ex-patients with healthy controls. *Journal of Mental Sciences.* **108**: 790 (1962).

54. Roth, M. and Kay, D. W. K. Affective disorder arising in the cenium. II. Physical disability at an etiologic factor. *Journal of Mental Sciences,* **102**: 141 (1956).

55. Kay, D. W. K. and Roth, M. Physical accompaniment of mental disorders in old age. *Lancet,* **2**: 740 (1965).

56. Post, F. The relationship of physical health to affective illness in the elderly. Proceedings of the 8th International Congress of Gerontology. Washington, D. C., **1**: 198 (1969).

57. Cassel, J. The contribution of the social environment to host resistance. *American Journal of Epidemiology,* **104**: 107 (1976).

58. Paykel, E. S. Life stress and psychiatric disorder, In B. T. Dohrenwnd and B. S. Dohrenwnd, (eds.) *Stressful Life Events: Their Nature and Effects.* New York: John Wiley, 1974.

59. Caplan, G. *Support Systems and Community Mental Health.* New York: Behavioral Publications, 1974.

60. Cobb, S. Social support as a moderator of life stress. *Psychosomatic Medicine,* **38**: 300 (1976).

61. Kaplan, B. H., Cassel, J. C. and Gore, S. *Social Support in Health and Medical Care,* 1977.

62. Nuckols, K. B., Cassel, J. C. and Kaplan, B. H. Psychological assets, life crisis and prognosis of pregnancy. *American Journal of Epidemiology,* **95**: 431 (1972).

63. Weiner, H. *Psychobiology of Human Disease.* New York: Elsevier, 1977.

64. Hofer, M. A. and Weiner, H. Physiologic mechanisms for cardiac control by nutritional intake after early maternal separation in the young rat. *Psychosomatic Medicine,* **37**: 8, 1975.

65. Dohrenwnd, B. T. and Dohrenwnd, B. S. *Stressful Life Events: Their Nature and Effects.* New York: Wiley, 1974.

66. Blazer, D. Social support: toward a unified theory. Unpublished manuscript.

67. Redick, K. R. W., Kramer, M. and Taube, C. A. Epidemiology of mental illness and utilization of psychiatric facilities among older persons, In E. W. Busse and E. Pfeiffer (eds.) Mental Illness in Later Life. Washington, D.C.: American Psychiatric Association, 1973.

68. Blazer, D. G. Annual Report, Committee on Aging, North Carolina Neuropsychiatric Association, 1978.

69. Bahn, A. K., Gardner, E. A., Alpop, L., Knatterud, D. L. and Solomon, M. Admission and prevalence rates for psychiatric facilities in four register areas. *American Journal of Public Health,* **56**: 2033 (1966).

70. Shephard, M., Cooper, B., Brown, A. C. *et al. Psychiatric Illness in General Practice.* London: Oxford University Press, 1966.

71. National Institute of Mental Health, Biometry Branch: Referral of discontinuations from inpatient services of state and county mental hospitals. United States, 1969, Statistical Note #57. Washington, D. C.: U.S. Government Printing Office, 1971.

72. Blazer, D. G. The use of epidemiologic survey data in planning for geriatric mental health services. Paper presented at the Annual Meeting of the Southern Psychiatric Association, October, 1978.

73. Blazer, D. G. and Maddox, G. L. Developing Geriatric Services in a Community Mental Health Clinic: Case History of a University-Based Affiliate Clinc, Final Report of a contract supported by the Centers for the Study of the Mental Health of the Aging, National Institute of Mental Health (278–76–0012–SM).

74. Kay, D. W. K. Outcome and cause of death in mental disorders of old age: a long-term follow-up of functional and organic psychoses. *Acta Psychiatric Scandanavia,* **38**: 249 (1962).

75. New York State Department of Mental Hygiene: Recent trends of population and admissions to New York State hospitals. Presented at Willard State Hospital Continual Symposium, October, 1969.

76. Model Statistics of the U.S. Volume II, Mortality, Part A. Washington, D. C.: U.S. Public Health Service, 1968.

77. Sainsbury, P., Grad de Alarcon, J. Evaluating a service in Sussex, In J. K. Wing and H. Hafner (eds.) *Roots of Evaluation.* London: Oxford University Press, 1973.

78. Wertheimer, J., Gilliland, T., Bircher, L. and Perier, M. Evaluating a service in Lausanne, In J. K. Wing, H. Hafner (eds.) *Roots of Evaluation.* London: Oxford University Press, 1973.

Part II
The Diagnosis
and
Treatment
of
Psychiatric
Disorders of
Late Life

Chapter 11
The Psychosocial Evaluation of the Elderly Patient

Eric Pfeiffer, M.D.

University of South Florida

Successful treatment of elderly patients with psychiatric disorders depends to a major extent on the adequacy of the initial evaluation of psychological and social functioning. While the *diagnosis* may be based largely on the presence of specific *psychological symptoms,* the *prognosis* will depend heavily on the *social context* in which those psychological symptoms exist. For it is social factors which will affect, favorably or unfavorably, the degree of success of correctly chosen treatment modalities.

In keeping with a life-cycle approach to the psychiatry of aging, this chapter will focus in turn on (a) communicating with the elderly; (b) evaluation of present psychological functioning; (c) evaluation of previous psychological functioning; (d) evaluation of present social functioning; (e) evaluation of past social functioning. This approach is predicated on the assumption that there is a differential significance to present psychosocial malfunctioning where it occurs in persons with good as opposed to poor psychosocial functioning in the past. The chapter will also address (f) issues

related to the nature of informal social support systems in the community; and (g) briefly describe a comprehensive multidimensional functional assessment methodology.

COMMUNICATING WITH THE ELDERLY

Factors Influencing Communication with the Elderly

In every human interaction, each participant makes a contribution that will influence the outcome. Both the patient and the physician must be considered as individuals before interaction can be understood properly. Factors influencing each may be assets or barriers to effective communication.

Patient Factors

Anxiety. Many elderly individuals may function continually at a high level of anxiety. Thus, the increased stress of a new situation may lead to intense arousal, impairing the elderly person's ability to communicate effectively.[1] Every physician realizes that a visit to the doctor is often a stressful experience. Fear, shame, anxiety, and a host of other feelings may play an important role in the communication process in the physician's office.

Sensory Deprivation.[2] Hearing loss is a widespread problem among the elderly. It affects men more than women and occurs in some 30% of all older people. Hearing loss is potentially the most difficult sensory loss for the elderly patient. Although 80% of the elderly have fair to adequate vision, some visual problems may occur. For example, poor orientation, a decreasing ability to read, and an occasional frightening visual impression may complicate communication in the physician's office.

Cautiousness. Older people tend to make few errors of commission but are likely to make errors of omission.[3] When the physician takes a history, he or she must be aware that older people may omit important aspects of their illnesses. Older people also take longer to respond to inquiries. The physician who rushes through the history-taking may overlook valuable information.

Unrealistic Views of the Physician. The elderly patient may develop an unrealistic perception of the physician based on previous experiences (the process that psychiatrists call transference). The elderly person is likely to view the physician as a parent (leading to a marked dependence on the patient's part), or as a child (leading to instruction-giving, or inquiries about the physician's health and behavior). A positive transference can be of benefit in the management of the patient if handled properly. In fact, this country's malpractice crisis probably results more from poor communication between physicians and patients than from incompetent medical care.

Persistent Themes. The elderly patient may concentrate on particular themes in com-municating with the physician. The more common themes include:

Somatic concern. Patients may spend much time complaining of ailments or recounting detailed histories of bodily functions. At a time when friends and loved ones have died and sensory input is decreased, the body, in many ways, keeps the patient company. It is therefore quite usual for the elderly patient to be somatically oriented.[4]

Loss reactions. The elderly patient may spend considerable time discussing the many losses experienced in late life. These include loss of friends and loved ones, loss of physical functioning, loss of employment and previous activities, and loss of self-esteem.

Life review.[5] There is a tendency in the elderly to reflect and reminisce. This is a normal process brought about by disillusion and the realization that death is approaching.

Fear of losing control.[6] Many elderly patients agonize over the loss of physical and mental functions, including physical strength, bowel and bladder control, motor functions, and, especially, the ability to regulate one's thoughts and emotions. One of the greatest fears of late life is the fear of "going crazy."

Death. The elderly are not, as a rule, obsessed with approaching death, but it nevertheless is a frequent topic of conversation. The major fear is of being alone at the end of life. The physician must remember the importance of continued relationships for the elderly person.

Physician Factors

Attitudes Toward the Elderly. It is quite common to find fears of aging and death among members of our youth-oriented society.[7] The recognition of such fears, and of the physician's personal feelings about these issues, is of utmost importance in establishing effective communication with the elderly.

Lack of Understanding. The physician must attempt to separate myths about aging from reality. For example, the labeling and stereotyping of the elderly may be a significant barrier to communication. The elderly are especially sensitive to being labeled "senile," "mentally ill," or "hypochondriac." The physician should try to empathize with the elderly patient. Putting yourself in the other person's shoes is an ability not easily taught by textbooks and can only be learned through personal experiences.

Techniques of Effective Communication

Approach the elderly patient with respect. The physician should knock before entering the examining room and try to approach the patient from the front. Greet the patient by surname (Mr. Smith, Mrs. Ross) rather than by given name (Johnny, Mary), unless he or she wishes to be addressed by a given name.

Position yourself near the older patient. The physician should place himself or herself near enough to be able to reach out and touch the patient if desired. The most comfortable arrangement of chairs for both parties is at a 45-degree angle to each other. If possible, chairs should be of the same height and the physician should not stand or walk during the interview.

Speak clearly and slowly. The elderly patient may have a hearing problem or may not understand a physician's accent. Clarity of speech and the use of simple sentences is most effective in communicating with an elderly patient, especially for those who have hearing loss or organic brain disease.

The staff of the OARS Clinic at the Center for the Study of Aging at Duke University found that telephone interviews with older patients are effective for gathering initial information and for follow-up. The telephone enables the patient to take advantage of preserved bone conduction in mild to moderate hearing loss.

Inquire actively and systematically into the problems presented. The physician should inquire into common physical symptoms of late life (such as visual and auditory defects, falls, and weight loss) and typical psychosocial problems (death of a loved one, change in living arrangements, recent retirement, financial setbacks, feelings of decreased self-esteem, hopelessness, and anxiety).

Pace the interview. The elderly patient must be given enough time to respond to the physician's questions. The elderly are not, as a rule, uncomfortable with silences, which give them an opportunity to formulate answers to questions, and to elaborate on certain points. A slow and relaxed pace in the interview will do much to decrease anxiety.

Pay attention to nonverbal communication. The physician should be alert for changes in facial expressions, gestures, postures, and touch as auxiliary methods of communication in the elderly. These nonverbal signs can provide considerable information about conditions such as depression or anxiety.

Touch may also be an effective way to relax and make contact with the elderly patient. As a rule, the elderly are less inhibited than the young about physical touch. Holding the patient's hand or resting your hand on his arm may be very reassuring.

Be realistic but hopeful. Physicians who work with the elderly often deny the problems of late life. But neither the patient nor the physician believes phrases like "You'll live to be a hundred," or "It's nothing to worry about," and the physician should avoid using them. He/she should never abandon all hope for a particular patient, but should work in the here and now, avoiding unrealistic expectations. Two or three pain-free days may be most rewarding to the patient dying of cancer, a fact too often overlooked by the frustrated physician.

Continue the relationship with the elderly patient. The internist and family physician should avoid, as much as possible, permanent transfer and termination of care of elderly patients. A visit to the physician's office is often a social event in the elderly patient's life. The physician and other health care personnel become important individuals to the elderly. Getting "well" may mean the loss of contact with treasured associates.

Many clinicians working with the elderly have found that regular but infrequent checkups are quite reassuring for elderly patients. Most of them will not abuse an open door policy.

ASSESSMENT OF PRESENT PSYCHOLOGICAL FUNCTIONING

In this presentation we will not discuss formal psychological testing as it might be carried out by a clinical psychologist or a psychometrics technician or laboratory. We will focus instead on evaluations which can be performed during an initial psychiatric interview.

Evaluation of Cognitive Functioning.

Patients in this age group (65 and older) are at high risk for cognitive impairment. For this reason the *presence* and, when present, the *degree* of cognitive deficit must be ascertained. While many methods are available, one of the simplest, most reliable and valid methods is the Short Portable Mental Status Questionnaire developed by the author.[8] It consists of 10 cognitive performance items which test orientation, short-term memory, long-term memory, information necessary for activities of daily living, and capacity for serial mathematical operations. The test questions are reproduced below.

Each question must be scored as correct or incorrect. The total number of errors constitutes the score in the SPMSQ.

The test is sensitive to educational attain-

SHORT PORTABLE MENTAL STATUS QUESTIONNAIRE (SPMSQ)
Eric Pfeiffer, M.D.

Instructions: Ask questions 1–10 in this list and record all answers. Ask question 4A only if patient does not have a telephone. Record total number of errors based on ten questions.

+	−	
		1. What is the date today?_____
		Month Day Year
		2. What day of the week is it?_____
		3. What is the name of this place?_____
		4. What is your telephone number?_____
		4A. What is your street address?_____
		(Ask only if patient does not have a telephone)
		5. How old are you?_____
		6. When were you born?_____
		7. Who is the president of the U.S. now?_____
		8. What was President just before him?_____
		9. What was your mother's maiden name?_____
		10. Subtract 3 from 20 and keep subtracting 3 from each new number, all the way down.

_____   Total Number of Errors

To be Completed by Interviewer

Patient's Name:_____Date_____

Sex: 1. Male   Race: 1. White
2. Female   2. Black
3. Other

Years of Education:_____1. Grade School
2. High School
3. Beyond High School

Interviewer's Name:_____

ment. For persons with 9–12 years of education (high school), the following scoring system applies:

0-2 ERRORS   INTACT INTELLEC-
              TUAL FUNCTIONING
3-4 ERRORS   MILD INTELLECTUAL
              IMPAIRMENT
5-7 ERRORS   MODERATE INTEL-
              LECTUAL IMPAIR-
              MENT
8-10 ERRORS   SEVERE INTELLEC-
              TUAL IMPAIRMENT

For persons with 8 or fewer years of education, one additional error is allowed for each scoring category. For persons with more than 12 years of education, one less error is allowed for each category.

The test is not capable of distinguishing between reversible organic brain deficit (delirium) and irreverisible organic brain deficit (dementia). However, it can be used repeatedly, over days, weeks, months, or years, to quantitatively follow the course of drug-induced delirium or of Alzheimer's type of senile dementia, for example.

There are two sets of practical implications which stem from the results of this test. A finding of "intact intellectual functioning" means that the patient is, from an intellectual standpoint, capable of living independently, capable of understanding instructions and of taking his own medication as prescribed. No further diagnostic studies of intellectual functioning are generally indicated. Evidence of "moderate" or "severe" intellectual impairment should in-

itiate a detailed work-up to evaluate the cause or causes of the cognitive deficit, with a special effort to discovering reversible causes of cognitive impairment. If no reversible cause of the deficit can be discovered, then additional studies should be carried out to determine the type of irreversible organic deficit (dementia) which exists, (i.e. Alzheimer's type of senile dementia, multiple infarct disease, etc.). Patients with "moderate" intellectual impairment generally can still perform many of the activities of daily living independently but they need supervision with more complex activities such as handling of money or taking of medication. Patients with "severe" intellectual impairment in most cases require continuous supervision of their activities, cannot safely live alone, and require daily assistance with many of the activities of daily living. Cases falling into the category of "mild intellectual impairment" are really in a borderland. In general, additional or continuing observation will determine whether they should be regarded as "intact" or as "moderately impaired". It is not known whether such cases constitute variants of "normal aging" or whether they constitute early cases of developing delirium or dementia. This can generally only be decided by following the patient over time.

Evaluation of Functional Psychiatric Symptomatology

It is also valuable to document the presence and the degree of functional psychiatric symptomatology in the initial contact with patients. The author has developed the Short Psychiatric Evaluation Schedule (SPES), reproduced below, for this purpose. In many ways it is analogous to the Short Portable Mental Status Questionnaire in that it, too, produces a numerical score from 0 to 15, indicating extent of psychiatric symptomatology.

The test consists of 15 questions to be answered by the patient with either a "yes" or a "no". Each question can be answered in a healthy or in a pathological direction. The pathological responses are precoded in capitals (YES, NO) while healthy responses are coded in small letters (yes, no). The number of questions answered in the pathological direction (YES, NO) constitutes the score on the SPES. Scores from 0–3 imply an absence of significant func-

SHORT PSYCHIATRIC EVALUATION SCHEDULE
Eric Pfeiffer, M.D.

Please answer the following questions *Yes* or *No* as they apply to you now. Do not skip any questions. Occasionally a question may not seem to apply to you, but please *circle* either Yes or No, whichever is more nearly correct for you. (No = 0, Yes = 1)

1.	Do you wake up fresh and rested most mornings?	yes	NO
2.	Is your daily life full of things that keep you interested?	yes	NO
3.	Have you, at times, very much wanted to leave home?	YES	no
4.	Does it seem that no one understands you?	YES	no
5.	Have you had periods of days, weeks or months when you couldn't take care of things because you couldn't "get going?"	YES	no
6.	Is your sleep fitful and disturbed?	YES	no
7.	Are you happy most of the time?	yes	NO
8.	Are you being plotted against?	YES	no
9.	Do you certainly feel useless at times?	YES	no
10.	During the past few years, have you been well most of the time?	yes	NO
11.	Do you feel weak all over much of the time?	YES	no
12.	Are you troubled by headaches?	YES	no
13.	Have you had difficulty in keeping your balance in walking?	YES	no
14.	Are you troubled by your heart pounding and by a shortness of breath?	YES	no
15.	Even when you are with people, do you feel lonely much of the time?	YES	no
	TOTAL SCORE		_____

To Be Completed by Interviewer

Patient's Name:_____Date_____

Sex: 1. Male   Race: 1. White
     2. Female   2. Black
                      3. Other

Years of Education:_____1. Grade School
                                   2. High School
                                   3. Beyond High School

Interviewer's Name:_____

---

tional psychiatric symptomatology. Scores from 4–5 constitute a borderland of uncertainty. One should be suspicious of possible significant psychopathology, but other data from the history and from the remainder of the evaluation must be used to decide whether significant psychopathology exists. Scores greater than 5 are indicative of definite psychopathology, while scores of 10 or greater indicate extensive psychopathology (Pfeiffer, 1978).

SPES scores of 5 or greater are a strong indication that functional psychopathology is present. Forms of psychopathology tapped by the test include depression, anxiety, paranoia and hypochondriasis, disorders particularly prominent in this age group.[2,9,10] The test is not capable of detecting mania in older patients, unless concomitant anxiety and delusions are also prominent. The SPES score alone is not capable of distinguishing between depression, anxiety, paranoia and hypochondriasis. Extremely high scores in the range from 12–15 are generally seen only in severely hypochondriacal patients or in floridly psychotic patients.

The SPES is sensitive to change in the patient's clinical conditions. Thus the test should be repeated at intervals (every month or every three months) to document progress being made in treatment.

ASSESSMENT OF PAST PSYCHOLOGICAL FUNCTIONING

Assessment of past psychological functioning is aimed at discovering the repertoire of coping devices available to the patient, as evidenced by his or her previous use of these devices in adapting to earlier life circumstances and adversities. It is assumed that persons who have successfully adapted in the past are more likely to continue to do so than are persons who have made poor prior adjustments. Unfortunately, a simple checklist is not available in this regard. The clinical interview must be utilized to obtain the requisite information.

The interview must first establish what adversities and life changes the patient has previously experienced. Secondly, the interview must establish how the patient has previously coped with these life changes. The range of life experiences obviously varies enormously from individual to individual, with some experiencing few, others many distressing and dislocating events. Questions to which the interviewer must seek answers include: What have been the major dislocations the patient has experienced in the past? How profoundly was the patient initially disturbed by these events? What active steps did he take to respond to the situation? What were the residual effects of his experiencing the various situations? On the assumption that the past is, to a certain extent, prolog, an examination of the specific coping devices employed by the patient will be especially illuminating. In this regard the work of Anna Freud[11] on defense mechanisms and of Vaillant[12] on hierarchies of adaptive mechanisms, is particularly valuable. Also, the magnitude of the distress experienced, short-term and long-term, and the magnitude of the dislocating event, must be compared. From this kind of examination will emerge a well-developed picture of the patient's previous adaptive style, permitting the clinician some estimate of how the patient may be able to cope with his current predicaments.

In this connection it may be stated how remarkably adaptive many older persons have proven themselves to be when the history of their past adaptation is examined. This type of review is often helpful in pointing to specific adaptations to be considered in dealing with the patient's present circumstances and in fostering optimism that older patients will once again be able to successfully adapt.

ASSESSMENT OF PRESENT SOCIAL FUNCTIONING

An assessment of present social functioning is very important. Present social functioning is, to a significant extent, a proxy indicator of both past and present psychological functioning. Thus, on the one hand, the existence of a rich network of rewarding social relationships with family members and friends is, of itself, an indication of good present, and or past psychological functioning. On the other hand, the quality of the social network is also an important factor in restoring healthy psychological functioning when this has been temporarily disturbed.

Evaluation of Quality and Quantity of Present Social Contact

In this area inquiry is made concerning a variety of issues relating to the number of social contacts the patient regularly experiences:

How frequently did he speak with someone by telephone during the past week?

How frequently did he visit someone or someone come to visit him during the past week?

How many people does he know well enough to visit in their homes?

The quality of social contacts may be ascertained by questions such as these:

Do you have someone you can trust and confide in?

Do you find yourself feeling lonely?

Do you see your friends and relatives as often as you like to?

Evaluation of Social Support Available in the Social Network

In this area inquiry is focused not so much on the moment-to-moment social contacts but rather on longer-term social commitments other persons may have towards the patient. Questions aimed at elucidating the social support structure include:

Marital status—an intact marriage is a positive social support resource.

Living arrangements—living with relatives constitutes a positive social resource.

Availability of someone to provide transportation or emergency (short-term) care in case of illness.

Availability of someone to provide ongoing care in case of illness or disability for an indefinite period of time.

The availability of caregivers in the social environment is critically important in determining whether someone can receive treatment and care on an ambulatory basis or whether hospitalization or long-term institutionalization is required.

ASSESSMENT OF PAST SOCIAL FUNCTIONING

In instances where present social functioning is inadequate, it is extremely important to ascertain the patient's past level of social functioning. Where this was abundant, pleasurable, and supportive, having become dismantled only due to outside influence (death, illness, relocation), it should be quite possible to reestablish a meaningful social network. Where the person never had good social and supportive relationships, the task will be more difficult. Psychiatric treatment attentive to uncovering the obstacles to social interaction first need to be implemented before a rewarding and supportive social network can be built.

ASSESSMENT OF INFORMAL SOCIAL SUPPORT SYSTEMS IN THE COMMUNITY

While personal social resources are important in understanding and overcoming psychological distress, informal social support structures such as exist in neighborhoods, communities, congregate housing settings, church, racial, or ethnic groups, must also be assessed and utilized in treating elderly psychiatric patients. This type of assessment cannot be easily made through an office interview with the patient. It can be done more adequately when the clinician has full knowledge of the particular community environment. It can be done most optimally through a visit to the patient's own home, either on the part of the psychiatrist or on the part of an associated nurse, social worker, medical student or resident. The friendliness/hostility, the safety/ dangerousness, the accesibility/remoteness of the environment can thus be assessed as can be the degree of recognition and/ or integration of the patient into his community. Knowledge of these factors will lead to a realistic appreciation of not only how the patient functions during his one hour in the psychiatrist's office but in the environment in which he must function 24 hours a day. Both the opportunities for support as well as the limitations inherent in the environment will then be correctly appreciated and included in the design of an overall treatment plan for the patient. For the aim is never to merely foster adaptation of a patient to a hospital or office setting but adaptation in the natural setting to which the patient will return following treatment.

COMPREHENSIVE MULTIDIMENSIONAL FUNCTIONAL ASSESSMENT OF THE OLDER PATIENT

While the above aspects of psychosocial functioning must be assessed in all older persons with psychiatric symptomatology, a still more desirable approach to older patients in general is to perform a comprehensive multidimensional functional assessment. A standardized method for such assessment has been developed under the author's leadership during his tenure at the Duke University Center for the Study of Aging and Human Development.[13] The OARS* Multidimensional Functional Assessment Methodology provides for a systematic quantitative assessment of an older person in five major areas of functioning: (1) mental health; (2) physical health; (3) social resources; (4) economic resources; (5) capacity for the activities of daily living. The OARS Methodology also inventories the patient's own perceived need for a wide range of services including his perceived need for psychotropic drugs, counseling or psychotherapy, physical health services, transportation, social and recreational services, or assistance with relocation. The full interview

* OARS: Older Americans Resources and Services

schedule requires approximately 1 and ¼ hours for its completion. Formal training (two days of training) in the use of the interview schedule is strongly recommended to assure reliable and complete data gathering. Such training is available through the Duke University Center for the Study of Aging in Durham, N.C. or through the Department of Psychiatry at the University of South Florida in Tampa, Florida.

SUMMARY

It is obvious that many more areas of psychological and social functioning could be usefully assessed. However, what has been presented here in this deliberately brief chapter is a deliberately parsimonious set of assessment techniques which successfully capture the most critical aspects of psychological and social functioning of older people. Substantially more extensive assessment methodologies are certainly available; however, these have been found to yield incomplete data sets in elderly patients with the result that "more" is actually "less." In addition, the brief procedures outlined above have been specifically standardized *on older patients,* and have a known reliability and validity. The final emphasis on *portability* (the fact that they can be administered anywhere, in the home, in the office, at the bedside) provides the practitioner with an ever-present set of techniques, enhancing the likelihood that these techniques are not only available but will actually be used.

NOTE: The section of "Communicating with the elderly patient" is reprinted from *Geriatrics* © 1978, by Harcourt Brace Jovanovich, Inc.; the article entitled "Techniques for communicating with your elderly patient" was authored by Dan Blazer, M.D.

REFERENCES

1. Eisdorfer, C. Arousal and performance: Experiments in verbal learning and a tentative theory,

in G. A. Falland (ed.) *Human Aging and Behavior*. New York: Academic Press, 1968.

2. Butler, R. N. and Lewis, M. I. *Aging and Mental Health*. St. Louis: C.V. Mosby, 1973.

3. Botwink, J. Cautiousness in advanced age. *Journal of Gerontology,* **21**: 347, (1966).

4. Verwoerdt, A. *Clinical Geropsychiatry*. Baltimore: Williams and Wilkins, 1976.

5. Butler, R. N. The life review: An interpretation of reminiscence in the aged. *Psychiatry,* **26**: 65 (1963).

6. Strain, J. J. and Grossman, S. *Psychosocial Care of the Medically Ill*. New York: Appleton-Century-Crofts, 1975.

7. Bunzel, J. H. Recognition, relevance and the de-activation of gerontophobia. *J. American Geriatrics Society,* **21**: 77–80 (1973).

8. Pfeiffer, E. A short protable mental status questionnaire for the assessment of organic brain deficit in elderly patients. *J. American Geriatrics Society,* **23**: 433–441, 1975.

9. Busse, E. W. and Pfeiffer, E. *Mental Illness in Later Life*. Washington, D.C.: American Psychiatric Association, 1973.

10. Busse, E. W., Pfeiffer, E. *Behavior and Adaptation in Late Life*. Second Edition. Boston: Little, Brown, 1977.

11. Freud, A. *The Ego and the Mechanisms of Defense*. New York: International Universities Press, 1946.

12. Vaillant, G. E. Theoretical hierarchy of adaptive ego mechanisms. *Arch. Gen. Psychiatry,* **24**: 107–118 (1971).

13. Pfeiffer, E. Ways of combining functional assessment data, in Duke-OARS: *Multidimensional Functional Assessment: The OARS Methodology*. Durham, North Carolina: Duke University Center for the Study of Aging and Human Development, 1978.

Chapter 12
Diagnostic Procedures

H. Shan Wang, M. B.

Duke University Medical Center

Objective and accurate information of the functional and structural status of the brain is indispensable in the treatment and management of elderly psychiatric patients because brain impairment is extremely prevalent in those with either organic or psychogenic psychiatric disorders. Such information will also be very useful in working with many relatively healthy elderly people in whom mild to moderate brain impairment may be present or suspected.

Organic mental disorders comprise six organic brain syndromes that are attributed to specific factors and result in transient or permanent dysfunction of the brain.[1] These brain syndromes are rather common among elderly persons. For those aged 65 years or older, it has been estimated that severe organic brain syndromes are present in about 5% of the population, and mild ones in another 10%.[2] The organic brain syndrome can be caused by a great variety of disorders originating within or outside the brain. They are classified as psychotic or nonpsychotic, according to the severity of functional impairment, and as acute or

chronic, depending on whether the underlying brain disorder is reversible or irreversible.[1] The two most common underlying brain disorders are primary degenerative disease of the brain (senile and presenile dementia of the Alzheimer's type), and the cerebrovascular disease (or multiinfarct dementia).

Regardless of the underlying etiology, the majority of organic brain syndromes are characterized by a common clinical picture consisting of disorientation, memory deficit, impairment of cognitive functioning and judgment, and labile emotion.[1] The severity of the clinical and behavioral manifestations of organic brain syndromes, as a rule, is only grossly correlated with the severity of the brain disorder.[3,4] There are considerable discrepancies between these two variables. In some cases, the clinical manifestations are more severe than what would be expected from the severity of brain disorders. Some of the clinical manifestations in these cases can be attributed to the concurrence of various psychosocial or psychogenic factors such as social isolation, depression or anxiety. These factors can often affect the patient's behaviors and cognitive functions almost in the same way as the brain disorder does. The pre-existing personality of the patient, the confronting environmental stress and the supporting system available to the patient often play an important role in the clinical manifestation, especially at the early development of brain disorder.[5,6] During this early stage, as the individual becomes aware of his mental or cognitive decline, his emotional reaction to it and his means in coping with it may contribute significantly to the final clinical picture.

Objective information about the physiological status of the brain can be derived from the many laboratory procedures currently available. An objective evaluation of the brain aims at answering the following questions: (1) Is brain disorder or impairment present? (2) Is the brain disorder a focal or a diffuse one? (3) How severe is the brain disorder? (4) What is the causative or contributory factor or factors underlying the brain disorder? (5) Can any of these factors be arrested, alleviated, corrected or completely reversed?

Among the many laboratory procedures currently available for an objective evaluation of the brain, some are too traumatic (e.g. brain biopsy), while others (such as rheoencephalography and thermography) are still in experimental stages and require further development. The following chapter will briefly describe some of the more practical and useful laboratory procedures for an objective evaluation of the aging brain, and will also review their special usefulness and limitations from a clinical point of view.[7,8,9,10]

USEFUL LABORATORY DIAGNOSTIC PROCEDURES

Skull X-Rays[7,10]

The radiographic image of the head is determined largely by the radiation absorption coefficient of the different tissues through which the x-ray beams have passed. The bony structure or calcified tissue has the highest absorption coefficient, while the air has the lowest. The absorption coefficients of the various components of the brain differ only slightly from each other and from the majority of "abnormal" tissues. Plain skull x-rays are usually normal or negative in organic brain syndrome especially when due to parenchymatous disease of the brain. For this reason, plain skull x-rays have only limited usefulness in evaluating the brain status of elderly individuals.

Plain skull x-rays, on the other hand, are the most readily available laboratory procedure. They are completely noninvasive and well-tolerated by almost all elderly patients. Therefore, they have the advantage of being used as a routine screening procedure which may occasionally provide some important clues in the planning of further diagnostic evaluation. They are particularly useful in: (1) determining the presence, location and extent of skull fracture; (2) detecting possible evidence of increased intracranial pressure (such as increased digital markings of the inner table of the skull); and (3) revealing possible indications and locations of intracranial space-occupying mass, such as the displacement of the pineal gland, the production of new bone or calcified tissue, or bone destruction.

Air Encephalography — Pneumoencephalography and Ventriculography[7,8,10,11,12]

Air has a much lower radiation absorption coefficient than the brain tissue. When it is introduced into the space within and surrounding the brain, it enhances the radiographic images of the ventricles and the cortical surface. In pneumoencephalography, after lumbar puncture, the air is slowly and fractionally injected into the spinal canal. Under special circumstances, the air can be injected directly into the lateral ventricles, after trephine openings are made in the posterior parieto-occipital regions, and needles have been inserted into the ventricles. This procedure is referred to as ventriculography. After the introduction of air, the position of the head and the posture of the patient can be manipulated in order to move the air from one part to another part of the ventricle and from one ventricle to another. A series of x-rays are then taken from different angles.

The purpose of air encephalography is to demonstrate the size and shape of the ventricles and the distribution of air within the ventricular system and around the cortical surface. A marked generalized ventricular dilatation and cortical atrophy (which can be inferred from the atrophy of cerebral gyri and the widening of cerebral sulci) are usually the characteristic findings of diffuse degenerative disease of the brain parenchyma (for example, Alzheimer's dementia). Focal cortical atrophy or focal ventricular dilatation, on the other hand, may indicate a mass lesion (such as tumor or cerebral infarction).[13] Normal pressure hydroencephalus often responds favorably to surgery, much attention has been given to the pneumoencephalographic characteristics of this condition. Unfortunately, no specific pneumoencephalographic criteria have been established for the diagnosis of normal pressure hydroencephalus nor for the prediction of its surgical outcome. Dilated ventricles, enlarged basal cistern and a relative lack of air filling the subarachnoid spaces over the cortex strongly suggests normal pressure hydrocephalus.

Air encephalography, especially the ventriculography, is invasive, traumatic, and involves considerable risks. Some patients with organic brain syndrome may show marked deterioration after the air study. With the improvement and progress made in angiography and the availability of computerized tomography in recent years, the use of pneumoencephalography and especially ventriculography has been drastically reduced. Ventriculography is employed only when there is a high risk of tonsillar herniation which may develop after the

lumbar puncture; that is, in the presence of increased intracranial pressure resulting from an obstruction of the foramen of Monro, third ventricle, aqueduct or fourth ventricle.

The interpretation of the pneumoencephalogram and the ventriculogram at times can be a difficult one, especially when the ventricular dilatation is not very marked. This is due to the fact that there is considerable variation in normal ventricular size and that there is little objective information currently available with regard to the upper normal limits of the ventricular size. As a rule, the evidence of cortical atrophy is less reliable than that of ventricular dilatation.

Electroencephalography[8,9,14,15]

This is the second most widely used procedure in evaluating the brain status of elderly persons because it is noninvasive and readily available in most medical facilities. In evaluating the clinical significance of the EEG, it is essential to keep in mind those brain wave changes that frequently occur in late life and have little or no clinical significance. A common characteristic of EEG changes after the age of 65 years is the progressive slowing of the dominant alpha frequency and the appearance of slow waves in the theta or delta range. Elderly subjects in good health are found to have a mean occipital frequency which is almost a full cycle slower than that found in healthy young adults. A slight slowing of the alpha waves is not pathognominic for any particular brain disorder.

Throughout adult life fast waves are more frequent in women than in men and tend to increase in females. Fast activity is present in 23% of females age 60 to 79 years but in only 4% of elderly males. Focal abnormalities of EEG, slow waves, and sharp waves over the anterior temporal areas have been repeatedly observed on 30 to 40% of apparently healthy elderly people. The left anterior temporal area is primarily involved (75 to 80%). In approximately 25% of temporal foci, the mid and posterior temporal leads are active. Bilateral focal patterns are found in 18 to 20, and in 4 to 5% the disturbance is more on the right. A study of healthy volunteers between the ages of 20 and 60 reveals that only 3% of normal adults under the age of 40 years have temporal lobe EEG changes. This percentage increases so that in the 20 years between 40 and 60, 20% of the subjects show temporal lobe irregularities. After age 60, the severity of the focal disturbance tends to stabilize, but new foci are found likely to appear in women. Hence, a higher percentage of women have the change as compared to men.[14,15] The electroencephalographic (EEG) changes in most organic brain syndromes are neither specific nor pathognomonic, except in a few cases where the brain disorder is associated with seizures. In diffuse degenerative disease of the brain, the EEG abnormality is usually characterized by diffuse slowing. The slowing may be greater in degenerative disease of early onset (presenile dementia) than that of late onset (senile dementia). In slowly progressing degenerative disease, the EEG not infrequently appears normal and thus cannot be clearly differentiated from that of an elderly person in relatively good health. In the latter group, the EEG may show some slowing with advanced age.[16] The EEG slowing may be aggravated in the presence of acute metabolic disorders. On the other hand, normal EEG's are not uncommon in the presence of lesions affecting the brain stem or the deep subcortical region.

The reliability of EEG findings is dependent on many factors; these include the placement of electrodes, prior medication, level of arousal, and cooperation of the subject. It is estimated that the usual arrangement of scalp electrodes employed will cover only one-fourth of the cortex. Many medications are known to affect the EEG, and in elderly persons, the EEG abnormality caused by a drug may persist for several months after the medication is discontinued. The usefulness of the information obtained from one single EEG examination at times is often limited. Serial EEG examination may be of greater value, particularly in following the course of the patient suspected of having a brain disorder.

Cerebral Angiography[7,8,11,13,17,18]

In this procedure, a radiopaque contrast medium is injected into the cerebral vascular system and a series of radiographic pictures are then taken as the contrast medium is passing through the arterial, capillary and venous system of the brain. A great variety of techniques have been developed to obtain a specific type of needed information, and to cope with many variations of the cerebral vascular system observed in different individuals.

In general, the contrast medium can be introduced into the cerebral vascular system in one of the following three ways. (1) Direct puncture: The contrast medium is injected directly into a carotid artery. (2) Retrograde brachial angiographic: The contrast medium is injected into either one or both of the brachial arteries under pressure and is forced to flush backwards to the aortic arch and its cerebral branches. (3) Catheterization method: A puncture of one of the main branches of the aorta (such as femoral, brachial, axillary, or brachiocephalic artery) is performed. With a guide wire, a catheter is advanced to reach the ascending aorta and the contrast medium is then injected to the aortic arch and its major branches, including subclavian, brachiocephalic, carotid and vertebral arteries. This is called arch aortography. The catheter can be further advanced into a selected cephalic artery, such as the right or left carotid. This is selective angiography.

The incidence of complications in cerebral angiography is rather high. In reviewing 3,300 consecutive patients who had angiography, Olivecrona found that 26% of these patients developed one or more complications.[19] A total of 1200 complications were observed: 22% were local, 5% were general, and 4% were neurological. The majority of complications were relatively minor or transient. Serious complications including death and permanent neurological deficits were observed in 1.4% of these patients. Olivecrona's findings were quite comparable with others reported in the literature.

For organic brain syndrome resulting from diffuse degenerative disease of the brain parenchyma, angiography provides little help in the diagnosis or evaluation of the brain status. The angiographic findings are indistinctive in organic brain syndrome or dementia due to degenerative or normal pressure hydrocephalus. Analysis of the position and arrangement of the deep veins may provide an estimation of the ventricular size. The main purpose of angiography is to evaluate the cerebral vascular system and to detect mass lesions, especially subdural hematoma and other intracranial tumors.

Because of the high incidence of complications and the complicated techniques involved, angiography should not be used as a screening procedure. The indication for cerebral angiography should be carefully evaluated with consideration of the risks involved.

Radioisotope Brain Scan[7,8,20]

Following the intravenous administration of a gamma-emitting radioisotope compound such as ^{99}m-technetium pertechnetate or chlormerodrin labeled with ^{203}Hg or ^{197}Hg, the distribution of radioisotope in the brain is scanned by an externally placed radiation detection system which can be stationary or moving. Because the radioisotope compound tends to accumulate in the abnormal areas in or near the brain, certain brain lesions can be localized by such scanning. The increased radioisotope is believed to be resulting from a change in the blood-brain barrier or in the increased vascularity in the lesion.

Brain scan is therefore very useful in screening patients suspected of having either primary brain tumor or cerebral metastatic lesions. It is also useful in the evaluation of cerebral infarction, arterio-venous malformation, brain abscess, subdural hematoma, or other cerebral injuries due to trauma.

Based on the arrival time and distribution of the radioisotope immediately following the intravenous administration, certain information about the cerebral vascular system can be obtained. The delay in arrival and the abnormal distribution of the radioisotope may help to identify severe stenosis or occlusion in the extra-cranial aortocephalic vessels. The brain scan, however, is usually normal in diffuse degenerative disease of the brain.

Radioisotope-Cisternography[8,10,11,12,20]

Radioisotope (for example ^{131}I-labeled human serum albumin) mixed with a few cc's of cerebral spinal fluid may be reinjected into the lumbar subarachoid space. This provides valuable information regarding cerebral spinal fluid dynamics. The radioisotope can also be injected into the cisterna magna or directly into the lateral ventrical.

After intrathecal injection, the radioisotope normally reaches the basal cistern in 1 hour, the frontal poles and sylvian fissures in 2 to 6 hours, the cerebral convexities in 12 hours, and the arachnoid villi in the sagittal sinus area in 24 hours. For normal pressure hydrocephalus, the most characteristic finding is ventricular stasis—accumulation of the radioisotope in the ventricular system and its persistence there for 24 to 48 hours or more. The cisternography is usually normal in Alzheimer's and multi-infarct dementia.

This procedure is usually less physically stressful than the pneumoencephalography to the patient. Rarely, aseptic meningitis may develop as a complication of such procedures.

Cerebral Blood Flow[8,9,21,22]

Among the many methods that are currently available for the evaluation of cerebral blood flow, the three most widely used are the nitrous-oxide inhalation method, the carotid injection and the inhalation method, the latter two using a radioisotope. This is due to the fact that these three methods all use a freely diffusable tracer and can provide a relatively reliable quantitative estimation of the blood flow to the brain.

In the nitrous-oxide method developed by Kety and Schmidt,[23] the subject inhales a nitrous-oxide gas of low saturation for 10 minutes. During this period, arterial and jugular venous blood are sampled at regular intervals for the analysis of the nitrous oxide concentration in the blood. The latter are then used, according to the Fick principle, to calculate the saturation rate which yields an estimation of the average blood flow to the brain taken as a whole. In the carotid injection method, as developed by Lassen and Ingvar,[24,25] xenon-133 or krypton-85 dissolved in saline is injected directly into the internal carotid artery after the artery has been punctured by a needle or catheterized. The clearance of radioactivity from the brain after the injection is monitored continuously by several NaI scintillation detectors placed externally over different regions of the brain. The clearance curve from a given region of the brain can then be analyzed manually or mathematically by a computer to yield two components. The fast component represents the flow to the gray matter; the slow component the flow to white matter. This method therefore can provide the flow values to gray and white matter separately for a small region of the brain. This carotid injection method and the nitrous inhalation method both involve considerable trauma and risk because a puncture or catheterization of a major artery or the jugular vein are necessary. Routinely the injection method only yields the information of the blood flow of one hemisphere.

In 1963 Mallett and Veall[26] introduced a noninvasive method for determining regional cerebral blood flow by having the patient inhale the radioactive inert gas xenon-133. This method has been further evaluated and developed by Obrist and his coworkers.[27,28,29] Many studies based on this method have been reported during the last decade and were reviewed in a recent article.[30] In this method the subject inhales a mixture of air and xenon-133 for one or two minutes. The clearance rate of radioactivity is monitored continuously by several NaI scintillation detectors placed over different regions of the brain. The clearance curves are then subjected to a two-compartment exponential analysis using a computer, and a correction for arterial recirculation is included based on the estimate of the radioactivity in the end tidal respired air sampled from the face mask. In this analysis the first compartment provides an estimate of blood flow in the fast-clearing gray matter while the second compartment represents the slow-clearing white matter and the extracerebral tissue.

The advantages of this inhalation method are complete noninvasiveness, its ability to provide a simultaneous evaluation of both cerebral hemispheres and its safety for repeat uses. The inhalation method, however, has two inherent problems. During the inhalation period the body and the extracerebral tissue are also loaded with radioactive xenon. The clearance curve obtained from a given region of the brain contains a slow component attributable to the extracerebral tissue. It also has a slight distortion as a result of recirculation of the radioisotope during the washout period. The results obtained from the inhalation method are quite comparable to those obtained by the carotid injection method. Nevertheless, the sensitivity and reliability of the inhalation method in detecting minor regional differences or changes still need further evaluation.

A reduction of cerebral blood flow is common among elderly persons, both with or without apparent neuropsychiatric disorders. The reduction of cerebral blood flow may result from (1) a depression of the cerebral metabolic activity, (2) cerebral vascular insufficiency, most likely due to arteriosclerosis, or (3) a combination of these two conditions. Depressed metabolic activity of the brain is usually related to diffuse degenerative disease of the brain, either primarily involving the brain, or secondary to a disease originating outside the brain. In the early stage of a mental disorder the differentiation between diffuse degenerative disease and cerebral vascular disease is important. Cerebral vascular disease is suggested: (1) when the blood flow is significantly reduced in one region of the brain as compared with other regions of the ipsilateral hemisphere or with the homologous region of the contralaterial hemisphere, or (2) where there is a marked reduction in cerebral blood flow without clear evidence of cognitive impairment or marked EEG abnormality, or (3) there is an impairment of vascular reactivity to change of the carbon dioxide concentration in the arterial blood.

Because the xenon inhalation method is safe for repeat use, it is most helpful in follow-up of a patient with respect to the change of the brain status over time or a reduction of cerebral blood flow related to medication such as antidepressants and tranquilizers. These medications have a tendency to lower the systemic blood pressure. In many elderly persons, due to the presence of significant arteriosclerotic change in the cerebral vascular system which leads to impairment of the autoregulatory mechanism, the cerebral blood flow becomes dependent on the systemic blood pressure. The cerebral blood flow may be significantly reduced in the presence of a drop of 10 to 20 mm. in systemic blood pressure, even though the pressure is still within normal limits.

Echoencephalography[9,31,32]

This is a relatively new diagnostic procedure utilizing ultrasonic waves for the evaluation of the internal structures of the brain. The ultrasonic waves ranging from 1 to 5 MHz are generated by activating a quartz, barium titanite, lithium sulfate or other piezoelectric crystal with an electric current. When these waves are passing through the brain, a portion will be reflected whenever they encounter an interface between components of the brain that differ significantly in density or acoustic impedence. The reflected waves are then transmitted back to the crystal and converted to electrical impulses (or echoes) that can be displayed on an oscilloscope and recorded permanently by a Polaroid camera. The horizontal scale on the oscilloscope is calibrated to correspond to the depth of the structure in the brain. The spatial relationship between different structures of the brain can therefore be inferred from the location of different electrical impulses on the oscilloscope.

One of the most prominent echoes is that from the midline structures of the brain. For this reason, echoencephalography was originally used primarily for the detection of localized space-occupying lesions such as hematoma and neoplasm which tend to displace the midline echo. Many attempts have been made recently to use the echoencephalography to determine the size of ventricles. As a rule echoes from the two walls of the third ventricle can be more readily obtained than those of the lateral ventricles.

Echoencephalography has the advantage that it is completely atraumatic and noninvasive and that the instrument involved is relatively inexpensive and simple to operate. The difficulty in this procedure is to obtain the correct echoes or to interpret them correctly. Until the development of computerized tomography, echoencephalography was a very promising method for providing structural information about the brain.

Computerized Tomography of the Brain[10,12,33,34,35,36]

This newest diagnostic procedure, which combines the advanced technology of radiography and computers, was developed by G. N. Hounsfield and introduced into clinical use by James Ambrose, both of England. Since the report of the initial results in 1972 which were subsequently published,[33,34] the use of this diagnostic procedure has been drastically increased and has had a tremendous impact on the practice of neuroradiology, neurology and psychiatry. In the meantime, the equipment or instrument has also undergone considerable modification and further development. This procedure is often also referred to as computerized transverse axial tomography, computerized axial tomography, CAT scan or CT scan. The basic theory, the special equipment and the techniques or methods involved have been described in detail by many publications.[33,34,35,36]

In brief, the scanning system consists of an x-ray tube and two collimated sodium iodide scintillation detectors. The latter are fixed on a common frame and in linear alignment with the x-ray tube across the patient's head. The common frame moves first linearly, and the narrowly collimated x-rays beam thus makes a linear scanning of a "slice" of brain tissue (normally 13 mm. in thickness by each detector). During each linear scanning, the x-rays transmissions through the head are recorded by the detectors and a total of 160 readings are obtained. At the end of a linear scanning, the common frame is then rotated one degree and the linear scanning as described above is repeated. This continues for 180 degrees and yields 180 x 160 or a total of 28,800 readings of x-rays transmissions which are stored in a computer. In the original system, the brain is looked at as a matrix of 80 by 80 or 6,400 small cubes. The readings from the input and both output detectors are used to solve 28,800 formulas simultaneously to yield 6,400 absorption coefficients—one for each cube in the matrix. The absorption coefficients are given numerical values on an arbitrary scale (for example, calcification has an absorption value ranging from 30 to 300; blood, 25 to 45; cortical gray matter, 18 to 30; white matter, 10 to 20; cerebrospinal fluid, 0 to 2). The numerical values can either be printed out directly by a line printer or displayed by a cathode ray oscilloscope as a gray-scale picture (whiteness for high density, darkness for low density) which is in turn recorded permanently by a Polaroid camera. When the scanning of a "slice" of brain tissue is completed, the scanning sys-tem is then moved to a different level of the head to scan another "slice" of brain tissue. A routine examination involves three or four scans and provides six or eight contiguous transverse axial "slices."

Computerized tomography is safe and harmless. It can demonstrate the internal structures—both normal and abnormal—of a "slice" of brain tissue without subjecting the patient to any hazard or trauma. Due to the low absorption values of cerebrospinal fluid as compared with these of brain tissue, CT scanning is particularly useful in providing an accurate assessment of the shape and size of ventricules. The cortical sulci can also be clearly identified in CT scan. For this reason, CT scan has become the procedure of choice in the diagnosis of ventricular dilatation and cortical atrophy. CT scan is also very useful in detecting focalized change of absorption values which can be attributed to the presence of an isolated mass lesion (e.g. tumor, infarction, hematoma) or multiple foci (e.g. metastatic lesions, multi-infarct). This procedure is therefore extremely helpful in differentiating the Alzheimer's dementia, multi-infarct dementia, normal pressure hydrocephalus and in separating diffuse disorder from focal disorder. It can also distinguish, in the majority of patients, the cerebral hemorrhage from cerebral infarction.[37,38] The need of pneumoencephalography and angiography has been greatly reduced since the availability of CT scan. Nevertheless, there are still some limitations of the CT scan. First, the availability of CT scan, though increasing steadily, is still relatively limited due to the high cost of its equipment and the sophisticated technology involved. The procedure itself still requires further evaluation for its reliability and validity in spite of the vast amount of clinical experience that has been accumulated during the last five years.

The requirement of keeping the head still for 20 or more minutes to complete a routine CT scan also limits its use in some agitated or confused patients. The time required to complete a scanning has greatly been reduced by the recent development of a much faster scanning system. Another limitation is that each cube in the matrix in the original model is 3 x 3 x 13 mm. A small lesion and a lesion having an absorption value that is very close to its surrounding brain tissue can be missed. The recent use of a 160 x 160 matrix and a narrower collimation to reduce the thickness of a "slice" to be scanned to 8 mm. decreases the size of each cube considerably and therefore increases its sensitivity in detecting small lesions or changes in the brain. The intravenous administration of an iodide containing contrast medium (as for IV pyelography) can increase the absorption value of the blood. By this means, the image of blood-containing tissue (hemorrhage, arteriovenous deformity, aneurysm or tumor with increased vascularity) becomes accentuated and more readily identified.

CONCLUSION

In ordering a given laboratory procedure for the evaluation of the brain, we should consider the following questions: (1) What specific information can we obtain from this laboratory procedure? (2) What do we gain from this specific information in the diagnosis, management or follow-up of a given patient? (3) Does the gain from this specific information justify the risk and trauma involved in this particular procedure?

From a clinical point of view, electroencephalography, determination of regional cerebral blood flow using the xenon-133 inhalation method and computerized tomography of the brain are probably the three most useful and practical laboratory procedures especially when used together to supplement each other.

These three procedures are all noninvasive and atraumatic. They can provide sufficient information about both functional and structural status of the brain as a whole as well as of a region of the brain. The information obtained from these three procedures is very helpful in differentiating the two most common brain disorders in the aged (Alzheimer's dementia and multi-infarct dementia) and the follow-up of their courses. The presence of significant diffuse slowing in electroencephalogram, reduction of blood flow over all regions of the brain with a relatively intact vascular reactivity, and the demonstration of marked ventricular dilatation and cortical atrophy in computerized tomography are common findings in Alzheimer's disease. In contrast, the presence of focal abnormalities (slowing or sharp waves) in electroencephalogram, and marked reduction of blood flow in only one or few regions or one hemisphere of the brain especially associated with a marked impairment of vascular reactivity strongly indicate multi-infarct dementia. This can be further confirmed by the tomographic findings of multiple foci of decreased density (or absorption value) in the brain with only slightly enlarged ventricles and mild cortical atrophy. When a localized lesion is suspected especially if it is potentially amenable to surgery or other treatment (such as normal-pressure hydrocephalus, extra-cranial carotid stenosis, subdural hematoma and certain tumors), more aggressive diagnostic evaluation using pneumoencephalography, cisternography, angiography become justified in spite of the risk and trauma involved.

PSYCHODIAGNOSTIC TECHNIQUES

Friends and relatives of the patient and not infrequently the patient himself will want to know if he is "slipping" mentally. The patient as well as interested others will want to know if it is likely that he will make some unfortunate decision seriously disrupting his long-standing personal and family relations, or will he squander his financial resources or perhaps lose the capacity to make a valid last will and testimony, a legal status called testamentary capacity.

If it does seem that there is an intellectual decline, the next question is, can it be arrested, slowed, or reversed? This involves the clinical skill of determining the underlying cause of the organic change. Perhaps the most serious problem is that of the so-called pseudodementia that accompanies some depressive reactions. (See Pseudodementia below). For obvious reasons the clinician will want to be able to measure the degree of incapacity and if appropriate follow the patient to determine improvement or further declines. Tests have been devised which can be utilized by the clinician, while there are other procedures which are complicated and require the administration and interpretation of a professional trained in psychodiagnostic techniques. The mental status examination that has been taught to medical students for many years has included a series of questions and observations which were intended to ascertain the presence or possibility of organic brain disease. These questions were usually designed to ascertain impairment of orientation for time, place, and person. Other questions were directed towards memory, short term and long term. Some questions were occasionally utilized to ascertain ability to recognize similarities, to properly identify inanimate objects, and other neuropathological manifestations such as aphasia, apraxia, alexia, etc. Quite properly attention is given emotional responses as in many organic patients these responses are easily elicited and are disproportionate or inappropriate to the stimulus.

Standardized Clinical Evaluations

Numerous attempts have been made to systematize these questions so that a relatively brief procedure would be available to the busy physician. One of the earliest attempts was published in 1953.[39] A few years later this procedure was refined by Robert L. Kahn and Max Pollack[40] and popularized by Goldfarb as it provided a simple yet relatively reliable method of evaluating large numbers of patients.[41] This revised procedure is given below and consisted of ten questions.

1. Where are you now?
2. What is this place?
3. What day is this?
4. What month is it?
5. What year is it?
6. How old are you?
7. When is your birthday?
8. In what year (or where) were you born?
9. Who is President of the United States?
10. Who was the President before him?

This test is scored as follows: 0 to 2 errors indicate no or mild organic impairment; 3 to 8 errors, moderate impairment; and 9 to 10, severe.

Short, Portable Mental Status Questionnaire. In 1974 the questionnaire was further refined, thus developing the "short, portable mental status questionnaire." This copyrighted questionnaire took into account both educational and race influence on performance and seemed to be capable of separating mild intellectual impairment from intact intellectual functioning.[42]

Bender's Face-Hand Test. Another procedure that has been in common use for many years is what has become known as the Bender's Face-Hand Test of Orientation.[43] This test is a double simultaneous stimulation of the cheek and hand of the patient who then reports where he has been touched. The patient sits opposite the examiner, resting his hands on his knees. The Face-Hand Test is done first with the patient's eyes closed; then the series is repeated with the eyes open. The examiner touches the patient simultaneously on the cheek and the dorsum of the hand, contralaterally and ipsilaterally in a specific order so as to include at least 10 trials.

In the four initial-demonstration trials the patient becomes familar with the procedures, but the examiner does not respond to the patient's answers. In trials five and six, the examiner does respond, and since the patient usually responds correctly, it serves as a reinforcement to the patient. The final trials which are a repetition of one to four are the critical steps, as errors are considered to be presumptive evidence of brain damage. Responses that are considered errors include not reporting the touch to the hand, localizing the hand touch to the cheek, the knee or elsewhere (displacement), pointing to the examiner's hand rather than to his own or pointing out in space, right or left.

Interestingly, very anxious patients make more errors with eyes open than with eyes closed. However, in 80% of persons who make errors with eyes closed, there is no improvement with eyes open. Although it seems necessary to do several trials with the patient to demonstrate the procedure, there does not seem to be a practice effect for those with organic brain disease. This procedure was originally developed for the examination of children, and consequently the modification procedure presented in Table 12-1 appears to be more useful for evaluating the geriatric patient.

Psychological Laboratory Procedures

The clinician will often request the assistance of a psychologist or a psychological laboratory in order to determine the existence or extent of mental impairment. An excellent detailed review of the psychodiagnostic procedures can be found in the 1977 publication of Bernal et al.[44]

Measures of Intelligence

As would be expected intelligence tests are administered differently to geriatric patients than to young or middle-aged adults. It is very likely that the older patient will approach the test with less confidence and with more apprehension than the younger patient. This performance anxiety may interfere with many procedures including memory and problem-solving. Hence it is recommended that such complex tasks be avoided as a first measure of the assessment battery.

Not infrequently it is very difficult to determine if the patient's defects in test procedures are the result of aging, pathological change, or represent a cohort effect. In addition, so-called intelligence tests are influenced by two major sets of influences. These include the social-cultural effect—an individual with a very enriched social-cultural environment may demonstrate a higher level of intellectual performance than an individual of equal natural ability living in a less stimulating and favorable environment. Physiological influences are the second set—the existence of physiological impairment reflects itself in intellectual performance. There are numerous reasons for such physiological impairments including nutrition, illness, and drugs. Elderly individuals seem particularly vulnerable to these two sets of influences. There is a further caution to be considered, and that is that although a number of intelligence tests are widely employed, norms on many of these instruments are adequate for young and middle-aged adults but are inadequate for the aged.

Table 12-1. Bender's Hand-Face Test Order of Stimulation.

Initial Trials and Demonstration	1. Right cheek—left hand 2. Left cheek—right hand 3. Right cheek—right hand 4. Left cheek—left hand
Teaching Trials with Examiner Response	5. Right cheek—left cheek 6. Right hand—left hand
Final Trials with Examiner Response	7. Right cheek—left hand 8. Left cheek—right hand 9. Right cheek—right hand 10. Left cheek—left hand

See text for procedural instructions and interpretation of responses.

The Wechsler Adult Intelligence Scale.
The WAIS has been widely used for over 30 years.[45] The obvious need for well-standardized norms is demonstrated by the defects that have emerged in utilizing the WAIS. The original norms were established on the basis of utilizing a defined population in an urban center. The limitation of this standardization was to a limited degree recognized, but it was not until 1959 that its shortcoming became very obvious.[46,47] These studies conducted in a very different region of the country indicated that there were consistent differences among subjects of varying ages depending upon sex, race, and economic class. However, although shortcomings still exist, the WAIS continues to be probably the best measure of intelligence for use with the aged.

Siegler, in her chapter in this handbook, describes in some detail the structure of the Wechsler Adult Intelligence Scale. The WAIS is organized into two major components, verbal and performance intelligence, with seven subtests, six verbal and five nonverbal. In her chapter Siegler concludes that verbal intelligence tends to increase until the sixties and then falls off gradually. Performance intelligence increases until the forties, with a gradual decline until the sixties, and a sharp decline thereafter (page 181). She reviews in some depth the contributions of Botwinick who utilizes multiple sources for evaluating intelligence throughout the life span and concludes that Botwinick's views are basically correct. The data indicate a maintenance of intellectual abilities through late middle age up to the sixties in most cases with declines increasing in frequency through old age; that is, after the age of 65. Verbal abilities are maintained considerably longer than nonverbal abilities, an almost two decades difference. In contrast, the abilities which require speed for optimal performance are related to aging processes which are manifest much earlier in life, as some of these declines are seen in the two decades between age 30 and age 50. However, there are always individual differences, and some individuals seem to maintain many skills into late life.

Bernal *et al.* describe several intelligence tests which are less time-consuming than the WAIS and are designed to be a more effective substitute. Such tests are often derived from the Wechsler but are supplemented by other material.

The Quick Test. This test was developed by Ammons and Ammons.[48] Apparently this procedure should be used with caution, as the vocabulary score contained in the Quick Test is a recognition vocabulary that may decline more slowly than that included in Wechsler's verbal items.

The Shipley Institute of Living Scale. Another verbal intelligence measure was developed by Mason and Ganzler in 1964.[49] This procedure also is open for serious questions as it has not been standardized on a broad spectrum of subjects. The data collected were on Veterans Administration hospital patients between the ages of 25 and 75, and education, socioeconomic status, and geographic consideration were ignored.

Group Tests. As to group measures of intelligence, the procedure does not seem to be useful for geriatric subjects as the group situation is seriously influenced by the limitations as they apply to elderly patients which have been previously noted.

Other Tests. There are other tests that are used, but not extensively. These included the Progressive Matrices Test,[50] the Geriatric Interpersonal Evaluation Scale, a screening device for evaluating the cognitive and perceptual functioning of geriatric patients,[51] and another instrument which was developed by Williams which drew upon material from a number of other procedures.[52] None of these procedures is recommended, as validity data for these instruments either are not available or are extremely difficult to locate.

Tests for Organicity

In addition to intelligence testing, psychologists have attempted to develop standardized procedures to assess specific organic impairment. Many of these procedures are particularly applicable to geriatric patients. Although the Wechsler intelligence test which has been previously discussed is frequently utilized as a measure of organic impairment, it is said to have its limitations. The estimate of organic impairment utilizing the Wechsler intelligence scale is usually based on a discrepancy between the verbal scale and the performance scale. Although it is true that many elderly patients show differences between verbal and performance tasks, it is quite possible that these differences can to a large measure be accounted for by current occupation, hobbies, and other social and economic responsibilities affecting persons in different phases of their lives. It appears that older persons who spend their lives working with their hands and utilizing perceptual data retain the ability to deal with perceptual and constructual problems, while these individuals will perform poorly on tests requiring verbal skills. In elderly people, the opposite is usually the case, as the verbal skills exceed the performance capabilities.

Halstead-Reitan. In the experience of many clinicians, the Halstead-Reitan tests have been particularly useful. This is a battery of several tests including the Halstead Neuropsychological Battery and the Reitan's Trailmaking Test (TMT). A Halstead Impairment Index can be derived from a score based on 10 discriminating tests in the Halstead battery. Even this impairment index has some limitations, as it has not been clearly standardized on a basis that includes age as a determining factor. The Trailmaking Test is one of the scales included in the Halstead Impairment Index, but it has also been used alone as an index of brain damage. This test is useful in young adults, but also must be viewed with caution in older people, as age does affect its outcome.

The so-called Goldfarb Test (MSQ) was previously mentioned. This procedure is occasionally used in the psychological laboratory particularly as the initial procedure. There are other relatively short tests for organicity. A few of the more useful ones include the Memory for Designs (MFD), the Wechsler Memory Scale, Benton's Revised Visual Retention Test, the Hooper Visual Organization Test (VOT), and the very well known Bender Gestalt. The Memory for Designs Test is an evaluation of visual memory, but the fact that there is a normal aging decline with this test and a low score fails to adequately discriminate organic and function mental disorders in the aged.

Benton's Revised Visual Retention Test. This procedure is aimed at detecting organic brain damage and focuses upon visual perception, visual memory, and visuoconstructive skill. This is an interesting test that does show a progressive progression until midlife where it has plateaued, and it is followed by a decline in efficiency of performance. Unfortunately, the corrective factor stops at age 64 so additional normative data are very much in order.[53]

The Hooper Visual Organization Test. The VOT was designed to differentiate organic from functional disorders and hopefully to diagnose organic brain pathology. Its first objective seems to have been demonstrated in differentiating organic patients from these with functional disorders. As to the second objective, and that is to ascertain the existence and the degree of organic impairment, this apparently needs considerably more study.[54]

The Bender Gestalt. A test familiar to most clinicians is the Bender Gestalt. This is one of the most commonly used perceptualmotor tests for assessing organic function. This procedure has been augmented by the Background Interference Procedure

(BIP) which seems to increase the sensitivity of the Bender Gestalt in discriminating organic brain damage from functional problems.[55]

It is evident from the material so far presented that additional attention should be given to psychological testing to determine organic brain disease in the elderly. Some of the difficulties have been recently cited by Fuld. She states that there are limitations as to what can be learned from existing tests about the specific abilities that deteriorate, in particular, dementias. She states that there are no tests of judgment or insight and no adequate procedure for evaluating attention without including memory. She also cites the problem of obtaining postmortem diagnoses for patients who are first studied earlier during the long course of a disease.

Pseudodementia.   In concluding this section it is important to return to the very serious problem of the clinician. That is to distinguish dementia from depression. A recent report by Foldstein and McHugh focuses upon this problem.[57] These authors agree that there is a mild form of cognitive disorder found in many patients prior to treatment and recovery from depression. Usually these patients do not show any evidence of disorientation, and their powers to learn are not completely lost. A more severe disorder in thinking with disorientation and memory deficit is seen in manic depressive disorders when they occur in late life. This apparent organic deficit also is relieved with proper antidepressant treatment. These cognitive changes have been termed "pseudodementia." Although these patients do not appear obviously different in their cognitive symptoms from those with irreversible changes, the terminology is considered unsatisfactory, as it may cloud the fact that there may be underlying physiological changes which would help us to understand those who recover and those who continue in their dementing trend. This objective would be consistent with the findings of Busse and Gianturco who on the basis of longitudinal studies have demonstrated that evidence of mild to moderate organic brain disease can undergo remissions and exacerbations over an extended period of time. Hence it can be an episodic disease prior to becoming a chronic disorder.

DISCUSSION

Intelligence and Cognition

As in all sciences semantic problems exist which can be troublesome to the clinician who does not accept the fact that words can be used differently; for example, the terms *cognition* and *intelligence.* The English language dictionaries are not consistent in defining these two terms, but generally speaking, *cognition* is said to be "the mental process or faculty by which knowledge is acquired" and that *intelligence* is the capacity to acquire and apply knowledge. Therefore, cognition is a component of intelligence. This how Guilford utilizes the term.[58] He utilizes a structure-of-intellect model with three components made up of operation, product, and content. The first parameter, operation, is made up of three subcomponents which include cognitive abilities, memory abilities, divergent-production abilities, convergent-production abilities, and evaluative abilities. Some psychologists are likely to use the terms cognition and intelligence synonymously. Siegler in her chapter in this book gives the following definition. "Intelligence represents the sum of the cognitive abilities generally assessed in omnibus tests which have been shown to be dependent upon and related to learning, memory, problem solving, reasoning, thinking, and the abilities required to deal with both verbal and nonverbal (or spatial-pictorial) information." This definition problem has existed for years, and in 1957 Wechsler said, "Intelligence, operationally defined, is the aggregate or global capacity of the individual to act purposefully, to think rationally, and deal effectively with his environment."[59] These differences will not be resolved; hence the clinician should understand the nuances of the various definitions.

Additions and Problems of Measuring Intelligence in Late Life

In addition to the negative influences associated with the administration of tests, there are other factors that may adversely affect the performance of elderly people on psychological testing. First, most of the test materials are geared to the young, and much of the knowledge and abilities that are included are closely associated with the academic situation. Many of the questions and the tasks that are included in intelligence tests are seen by elderly persons as "silly, dull, or nonsensical." Also elderly people are not accustomed to exposing themselves to the test situation. Eisdorfer has demonstrated that older people tend to withhold answers, particularly on time tests. They respond more frequently and most accurately when they are given additional time. This additional time may actually not be necessary but represents the conservative attitude of older people.[60]

Many elderly are less willing to guess items about which they are uncertain unless the test is set up in such a way that it is clearly to the older person's advantage to guess. Young people are willing to guess. Therefore they make errors of omission, while the reverse is true of old people who simply do not respond, and their nonresponse is an error of omission. Cautiousness may be a reflection of a psychosocial change in old people, and it is sometimes believed to be a personality change which is characteristic of late life.

Fluid and Crystallized Intelligence

Appropriately the chapter of Psychological Changes with Age discusses conceptual issues as they relate to psychological evaluation. One intriguing conceptual approach is seen in the work of Horn and Cattell.[61] They believe that they have demonstrated that intellectual ability includes two separable factors. One is fluid and the other is crystallized intelligence. Both of these important factors decline at different rates with advancing age.

Fluid ability seems to be related to physiological characteristics of the organism such as discrimination and identification of stimuli and appropriate responses. Crystallized abilities depend upon the acquisition of certain kinds of information and skills which are transmitted by the culture which are not available to the individual simply by virtue of his characteristics as a human being. Schaie, on the basis of extensive analysis of cross-sectional and longitudinal data, has concluded that the crystallized abilities show very little change in intellectual function for an individual throughout adulthood. Furthermore, he believes that the declines of intellectual abilities in old people who are reasonably healthy may not be true and irreversible but rather that their information and methods of thinking have become obsolete. Therefore he believes that something can be done about the situation such as providing continuing educational opportunities.[62]

PERSONALITY TESTING

In addition to testing of intelligence and organic mental impairment, psychologists have devoted considerable attention to the development of psychometric instruments useful in assessing personality functioning. These tests may be divided into the structured tests, such as the Minnesota Multiphasic Personality Inventory, which are directed at measuring personality traits and syndromes, and the projective tests which provide ambiguous stimuli and measure subsequent responses. Considerable attention has been directed to changes in personality structure over the life cycle. However, there continues to be a lack of reliable norms for older individuals in our current diagnostic techniques. It is the projective tests that suffer the most from the lack of these norms.

Saltzman, et al.[63] has outlined some of the

difficulties in using rating scales with elderly patients. His concerns may be applied to many personality tests. Very few scales have been developed for geriatric use specifically. With the present battery of tests available, cognitive and neurological deficits often make ratings on these tests difficult. In addition, many of these scales contain items of little relevance to the geriatric patient and may bias the response of the remaining potentially relevant items. Perhaps most important of all is the length of most multiple need scales and personality scales which greatly limits their usefulness in the geriatric population. The Rorschach, the Minnesota Multiphasic Personality Inventory (MMPI) and the Thematic Appreception Test (TAT) are the most commonly used for personality inventory. A review of these instruments as they specifically relate to the elderly will highlight some of the guidelines and problems in the use of these instruments in the diagnostic work-up of the mentally impaired older adult.

The Rorschach Test

The Rorschach Test is probably the most frequently used individual psychological test for personality assessment. It is a standard set of 10 inkblots that provide stimuli for associations. The administrator keeps a verbatim record of the patient's responses along with initial reaction time and total time spent on each card. At the completion of a "free association," the examiner systematically inquires about important aspects of each response. Some of the variables used to score the test include location, form, shading, color, movement, and either animal or human responses. Klopfer, in 1946,[64] suggested that the trend for older individuals is one of constriction, a decrease in the number of responses, a decrease in the number of human figures and movement, an increase in animal responses and a decrease in the form level ratings. Eisdorfer[65] has suggested that earlier assessments of elders' responses to the Rorschach, such as Klopfer, may have been biased by a lack of control

for intelligence. He found that the decreased fraction of whole responses was secondary to a decrease in IQ (as measured by the WAIS). In addition, the paucity of responses in the section of human movement and the increase in animal responses were more related to IQ than age. The reliance on form and color did not show any age changes. Eisdorfer concluded that the pathological signs of aging on the Rorschach may be artifacts of institutionalization or of the IQ of older individuals. In another study, Eisdorfer[66] suggested that hearing loss was related to poorer Rorschach scores.

Oberleder[67] criticized the use of the Rorschach in the elderly on the basis of psychological factors not usually considered. For example, the constriction observed in older persons may reflect excessive caution or a fear of risks that results in excessive concern with accuracy or what may be regarded as a safe response. If older people have a more heightened need for arousal than young subjects, the Rorschach inkblots may be too ambiguous a stimulant. The poor form responses of older subjects may not reflect poor ego control or reality control, but rather detachment from a rejecting and uncaring environment. Yet Oberleder suggested that the Rorschach was a non-threatening psychological test for older adults and one that is easily administered.

The Minnesota Multiphasic Personality Inventory

The Minnesota Multiphasic Personality Inventory is a widely used inventory made up of 566 questions that are either answered yes or no. In scoring the MMPI, these items are condensed into 3 validity scales and 10 clinical scales. The clinical scales include scales of depression, psychasthenia, hysteria, paranoia, schizophrenia, psychopathic deviation, mania, hypochondriasis, masculinity-femininity and social introversion. Individual scale scores as well as a profile and narrative summary are the output of this procedure. Aaronson[68] is one of a number of authors who have found that aged individuals have higher elevations on the hysterical, hypochondriacal and social introversion scales than the younger adults. He also found a lowering on the character disorder and psychotic scales. In general, older individuals tend to endorse more neurotic pictures than younger individuals on this test. Hardyck[69] found that the elderly have lower scores on the masculine-feminine scale and the manic scales.

Bernal,[70] among others, has pointed out that the MMPI is a long and tedious test for older adults especially if attention span is short and visual problems are present. It is also a particularly difficult test for the seriously ill in its self-administered form. Veker[71] specifically advises against the use of the MMPI for personality assessment of elderly brain damaged patients because of the lack of re-test reliability. Therefore attempts have been made to standardize a shorter version of the MMPI, such as Kincannon's Mini-Mult.[72] This is a 71-item test in which the items chosen are representative of the content questions tapped by the 3 standard validity scales and 8 of the 10 clinical MMPI scales.

Thematic Apperception Test

The Thematic Apperception Test (TAT), designed by Henry Murray and Christina Morgan, consists of 30 pictures and one blank card. Individual cards are chosen for any given examination based on the individual subject's age, sex, etc. Less than 20 pictures are generally used by examiners today. The TAT is probably the most frequently used projective technique by researchers to distinguish personality changes over the life cycle. Neugarten[73] found that younger individuals seemed to see themselves possessing energy congruent with the opportunities perceived in the outer world. Boldness and risk taking are rewarded by the environments for these individuals. For older persons, the outer world takes on a different meaning. The world is complex and somewhat dangerous. It cannot be reformed according to the personal

wishes of an individual but instead the individual must conform and accommodate to demands of this environment. Ego function is turned inward, yet the ego appears to be less in contact with and less perceptive in controlling and channeling internal impulses. LeBlanc[74] found that the TAT scores from people age 10–90 changed at about the age of 45 to a greater emphasis on the past. Veroff[75] determined fewer high scores on need achievement among older subjects.

One interesting development in the use of TAT is the appearance of a number of variants of this projective technique. One variation is the Geriatric Apperception Test (GAT).[76] The development of such instruments is important because it highlights the necessity of custom-made projective techniques for the elderly. This particular technique consists of 14 cards where scenes frequently encountered by older people are depicted. There has not been enough study of these instruments in the literature to date to assess their usefulness, however.

REFERENCES

1. American Psychiatric Association: Diagnostic and Statistical Manual of Mental Disorders (3rd ed. page A-1). Washington, D.C.: American Psychiatric Association, 1977.
2. Wang, H. S. Dementia of old age. In W. L. Smith and M. Kinsbourne (eds.) Aging and Dementia. New York: Spectrum Publication, pp. 1-24, 1977.
3. Wang, H. S., Obrist, W. D. and Busse, E. W. Neurophysiological correlates of the intellectual function of elderly persons living in the community. Am. J. Psychiatry, 126: 1205-1212 (1970).
4. Wang, H. S. Cerebral correlates of intellectual function in senescence. In L. F. Jarvisk, C. Eisdorfer, J. E. Blum (eds.) Intellectual Functioning In Adults, Psychological and Biological Influences. N. Y. Springer Publishing, pp. 95-106, 1973.
5. Busse, E. W. and Wang, H. S. The multiple factors contributing to dementia in old age. In Excerpta Media Intern. Congr. Series No. 274. Proceedings of the V World Congr. of Psychiatry. Amsterdam: Excerpta Medica, 1974.
6. Wang, H. S. Dementia in old age. In C. E. Wells (ed.) Dementia, 2nd edition. Philadelphia: F. A. Davis, pp. 15-26, 1977.
7. Peterson, Harold O. and Kieffer, Stephen A. In-

troduction to Neuroradiology. Hagerstown, Md.: Harper & Row 1972.

8. Pearce, J. Clinical Aspects of Dementia. Williams & Wilkins, Baltimore, pp. 66–82, 1973.

9. Wang, H. S. Special diagnostic procedures—the evaluation of brain impairment. In E. W. Busse and E. Pfeiffer (eds.) Mental Illness in Late Life. Washington, D.C.: American Psychiatric Association, pp. 75–88, 1973.

10. Lowry, J., Bahr, A. L., Allen Jr., J. H., Meacham, W. F. and James, A. E. Radiological techniques in the diagnostic evaluation of dementia. In C. E. Wells (ed.) Dementia. Philadelphia: F. A. Davis, pp. 223–245, 1977.

11. Adapon, B. D., Braunstein, P., Lin, J. P. and Hochwald, G. M. Radiologic investigations of normal pressure hydrocephalus. Radiol. Clinics of North America, 12: 353–369 (1973).

12. Katzman, R. Normal pressure hydrocephalus. In C. E. Wells, (ed.). Dementia. Philadelphia: F. A. Davis, pp. 69–92, 1977.

13. Gado, M. Localization of intracranial masses by pneumography and angiography. In E. J. Patchen (ed.) Current Concepts in Radiology. New York: C. V. Mosby, pp. 249–299, 1972.

14. Busse, E. W. and Wang, H. S. The value of electroencephalography in geriatrics. Geriatrics, 20: 906–924 (1965).

15. Wilson, W. P., Musella, L. and Short, M. J. The electroencephalogram in dementia. In C. E. Wells (ed.) Dementia. Philadelphia: F. A. Davis, pp. 205–221, 1977.

16. Wang, H. S. and Busse, E. W. EEG of healthy old persons—a longitudinal study 1. dominant background activity and occipital rhythm. J. Gerontol., 24: 419–426 (1969).

17. Meschan, I. Roentgen signs of abnormality in cerebral angiograms. In J. F. Toole (ed.) Special Techniques for Neurologic Diagnosis. Philadelphia: F. A. Davis, pp. 94–137, 1969.

18. Janeway, R.: Current techniques for aortocranial angiography. In J. F. Toole (ed.) Special Techniques for Neurologic Diagnosis. Philadelphia: F. A. Davis, pp. 140–170, 1969.

19. Olivercrona, H. Complications of cerebral angiography. Neuroradiol., 14: 175–181 (1977).

20. Maynard, C. D. and Janeway, R. Radioisotope studies in neurodiagnosis. In J. F. Toole (ed.) Special Techniques for Neurologic Diagnosis. Philadelphia: F. A. Davis, pp. 72–91, 1969.

21. McHenry Jr., L. C. Cerebral blood flow. New England J. Med., 274: 82–91 (1966).

22. Mathew, N. T. Clinical application of regional cerebral blood flow measurements. In J. S. Meyer, (ed.) Modern Concepts of Cerebrovascular Disease. New York: Spectrum Publ. pp. 63–86, 1975.

23. Kety, S. S. and Schmidt, C. F. Nitrous oxide method for quantitative determination of cerebral blood flow in man: Theory, procedure and normal values. J. Clin. Investigation, 27: 476–483, 1948.

24. Lassen, N. A. and Ingvar, D. H. The blood flow of the cerebral cortex determined by radioactive Krypton. Experientia, 17: 42 (1961).

25. Lassen, N. A., Hoedt-Rassmussen, K., Sorensen, S. C., Skinhoj, E., Cronquist, S., Bodforss, B., and Ingvar, D. H. Regional cerebral blood flow in man determined by Krypton[85]. Neurology, 13: 719–727 (1963).

26. Mallett, B. L. and Veall, N. Investigation of cerebral blood flow in hypertension, using radioactive xenon inhalation and extracranial recording. Lancet, 1: 1081–1082, 1963.

27. Obrist, W. D., Thompson, H. K., King, C. H. and Wang, H. S. Determination of regional cerebral blood flow by inhalation of 133-xenon. Circulat. Res., 20: 124–135 (1967).

28. Obrist, W. D., Thompson, H. K., Wang, H. S. and Cronqvist, S. A simplified procedure for determining fast compartment rCBF's by xenon-133 inhalation. In R. W. R. Russell (ed.) Brain and Blood Flow. Proceedings of 4th International Symposium on Regulation of Cerebral Blood Flow. London: Pitman, pp. 11–15, 1971.

29. Obrist, W. D., Thompson, H. K., Wang, H. S., and Wilkinson, W. E. Regional cerebral blood flow estimated by 133-xenon inhalation. Stroke, 6: 245 (1975).

30. Memory, J., McHenry, L. C. and Toole, J. F. The xenon-133 inhalation method for the measurement of regional cerebral blood flow. Intern. J. Neurol., 11: 179–193 (1977).

31. McKinney, W. M. Echoencephalography. In J. F. Toole (ed.) Special Techniques for Neurologic Diagnosis. Philadelphia: F. A. Davis, pp. 195–210, 1969.

32. Tenner, M. S., Wodraska, G. and Adapon, B. D. new ultrasound techniques in the evaluation of neurological disorders. Radiol. Clinics of North America, 12: 283–295 (1974).

33. Ambrose, J. Computerized transverse axial scanning (tomography), part 2, clinical application. Brit. J. Radiology, 46: 1023–1047 (1973).

34. Hounsfield, G. N. Computerized transverse axial scanning (tomography), part 1, description of system. Brit. J. Radiology, 46: 1016–1022 (1973).

35. New, P. F. J., Scott, W. R., Schnur, J. A., Davis, K. R. and Taveras, J. M. Computerized axial tomography with the EMI scanner. Neuroradiology, 110: 109–123 (1974).

36. Gawler, J., Bull, J. W. D., du Bonlay, G. and Marshall, J.: Computerized axial tomography with the EMI scanner. L. H. Krayenbu et al. (eds.) Advances and Technical Standards in Neurosurgery, Vol. 2, pp. 3–32. New York: Springer-Verlag, 1975.

37. Naidich, T. P. and Chase, N. E.: Use of computerized axial tomography in evaluation of

cerebrovascular disease. Current Concepts of Cerebrovascular Disease, *Stroke,* **10:** 19–24 (1975).

38. Constant, P., Renou, A. M. Caillé, J. M., Vernhiet, J. and Dop, A. Cerebral ischemia with CT. *Computerized Tomography,* **1:** 235–248 (1977).

39. Hopkins, B. and Roth, M. Psychological test performances in patients over 60. *J. Ment. Sc.,* **99:** 146, (1953).

40. Kahn, R. L., Goldfarb, A. I. and Pollack, M. Brief objective measures for the determination of mental status in the aged. *Am. J. Psychiatry,* **117:** 326 (1960).

41. Goldfarb, A. I. Psychiatric disorders of the aged, symptomatology, diagnosis, and treatment. *J. Am. Geriatrics Soc.,* **8:** 698–707 (1960).

42. Pfeiffer, E. A short portable mental status questionnaire for the assessment of organic brain deficit in elderly patients. *J. Am. Geriatrics Soc.,* **23:** 433–441 (1975).

43. Bender, M. B., Fink, M. and Green, M. A. Patterns in perception on simultaneous tests of face and hand. *Arch. Neurol. and Psychiat.,* **56:** 355 (1951).

44. Guillermo, A. A. B., Brannon, L. J., Belar, C., Livigne, J. and Cameron, R. Psychodiagnostics of the elderly. In Gentry, W. D. (ed.) *Geropsychology.* Cambridge, Mass.: Ballinger Publishing Company, pp. 43–77, 1977.

45. Wechsler, D. *Manual for the Wechsler Adult Intelligence Scale.* New York: Psychological Corporation, 1955.

46. Eisdorfer, C., Busse, E. W. and Cohen, L. D. The WAIS performance of an aged sample: The relationship between verbal and performance IQs. *J. Gerontol.,* **2:** 197–201 (1959).

47. Eisdorfer, C. and Cohen, L. D. The generality of the WAIS standardization for the aged: A regional comparison. *J. Abn. Psych.* **62:** 520–527 (1961).

48. Ammons, R. B. and Ammons, C. H. The quick test: Provisional manual. *Psychological Reports,* **11:** 11–161 (1962).

49. Mason, C. F. and Ganzler, H. Adult norms for the Shipley Institute of Living scale and Hooper visual organization test based on age and education. *J. Gerontol.,* **19:** 419–424 (1964).

50. Raven, J. C. *Guide to Using the Coloured Progressive Matrices.* London, Great Britain: Lewis and Company, 1965.

51. Plutchik, R., Conte, H. and Lieberman, M. Development of a scale (GIES) for assessment of cognitive and perceptual functioning in geriatric patients. *J. Am. Geriatrics Soc.,* **19:** 614–623, 1971.

52. Williams, M. Geriatric Patients. In P. Mittler (ed.) *The Psychological Assessment of Mental and Mental Handicaps.* London: Methuen and Company, 1970.

53. Benton, A. L. *The Revised Retention Test, Clinical and Experimental Application.* New York: The Psychological Corporation, 1963.

54. Hooper, H. E. *The Hooper Visual Organization Test Manual.* Los Angeles: Western Psychological Services, 1958.

55. Canter, A. A. A background interference procedure to increase sensitivity of the Bender-Gestalt organic brain disease. *J. Consult. Psychol.,* **30:** 1–97, 1966.

56. Fuld, P. A. Psychological testing in differential diagnosis of the dementias. In R. Katzman, R. D. Terry, and K. L. Bick, (eds.) *Alzheimer's Disease, Senile Dementia and Related Disorders.* New York: Raven Press, pp. 185–193, 1978.

57. Folstein, M. F. and McHugh, P. R.: Dementia syndrome of depression. In R. Katzman, R. D. Terry, and K. L. Bick (eds.) *Alzheimer's Disease, Senile Dementia and Related Disorders.* New York: Raven Press, pp. 87–93, 1978.

58. Guilford, J. P. *The Nature of Human Intelligence.* New York: McGraw, Hill Book Company, 1967.

59. Wechsler, D. *The Measurement and Appraisal of Adult Intelligence.* Baltimore: Williams, and Wilkins, (4th ed) p. 7, 1958.

60. Eisdorfer, C. Intelligence and cognition in the aged. In E. W. Busse, and E. Pfeiffer, (eds.) *Behavior and Adaptation in Late Life,* (2nd ed) Boston: Little, Brown, pp. 212–227, 1977.

61. Horn, J. L. and Cattell, R. B. Age differences in fluid and crystallized intelligence. *Acta Psychol* (Amst), **26:** 107 (1967).

62. Schaie, K. W. Age changes in adult intelligence. In D. S. Woodruff, and J. E. Birren (eds.) *Aging, Scientific Perspectives and Social Issues.* New York: D. Van Nostrand Company, pp. 111–124, 1975.

63. Saltzman, C., Cochansky, G. E., Shader, R. T. and Cronin, D. M. Rating scales for psychotropic drug research with geriatric patients. II. The Need Ratings. *Journal of the American Geriatrics Society,* 20: 215 (1972).

64. Klopfer, W. G. Personality patterns of old age. *Rorschach Research Exchange,* **10:** 145 (1946).

65. Eisdorfer, C. Rorschach performance and intellectual functioning in the aging. *Journal of Gerontology,* **18:** 358 (1963).

66. Eisdorfer, C. Rorschach rigidity and sensory decrement in a senescent population, In E. Palmore (ed.) *Normal Aging.* Durham, N.C.: Duke University Press, pp. 232–237, 1970.

67. Oberleder, M. Effects of psychosocial factors on test results of the aging. *Psychological Reports,* **14:** 383 (1964).

68. Aaronson, B. S. Age and sex influences on MMPI profile peak distribution in an abnormal population. *Journal of Consulting Psychology,* **22:** 203 (1958).

69. Hardyck, C. B. Sex differences in personality changes with age. *Journal of Gerontology,* **19:** 78 (1964).

70. Bernal, G. A., Brannon, L. J., Belar, C., Lavigne,

J. and Cameron, R. Psychodiagnostics of the elderly. In W. D. Gentry, (ed.) *Geropsychology: A Model of Training and Clinical Service.* Cambridge, Massachusetts: Ballinger Publishing Company, pp. 43–77, 1977.

71. Veker, A. E. Comparability of two methods of administering the MMPI to brain damaged geriatric patients. *Journal of Clinical Psychology,* **25:** 196 (1969).

72. Kincannon, J. Predictions of the standard MMPI scale scores from 71 items: The Mini-Mult. *Journal of Consulting and Clinical Psychology,* **32:** 319 (1968).

73. Neugarten, B. L. Personality and the aging process, in R. H. Williams, C. Tibbits, and W. Donahue, (eds.) *Processes of Aging* (Volume I). New York: Atherton Press, 1963.

74. LeBlanc, A. F. Time orientation and time estimates, a function of age. *Journal of Genetic Psychology,* **115:** 187 (1969).

75. Veroff, J., Atkinson, K. W., Feld, S. C. and Berin, B. The use of the TAT to assess motivation in a nationwide interview study. *Psychological Monograph* **74** (12), No. 499, (1960).

76. Wolk, R. L. and Wolk, R. B. *Manual of the Gerontological Apperception Test.* New York: Behavioral Publications, 1972.

Chapter 13
The Organic Mental Disorders

Murray A. Raskind, M.D.

University of Washington

Michael C. Storrie, M.D.

University of Washington

INTRODUCTION

The organic mental disorders are the most prevalent psychiatric disorders of later life. The majority of epidemiologic surveys find definite organic mental disorder in 4 to 6% of persons over age 65,[1] and 20% or more of those over age 80.[2] If persons with mild organic mental disorder are included, the prevalence rate is even higher.[1,3] The behavioral and social consequences of these disorders will become even more important as the proportion of elderly persons in the population increases. Although the clinical management of the organic mental disorders has often been associated with pessimism and even therapeutic nihilism, such a stance is no longer tenable. Many organic mental disorders are treatable and even the patient with an irreversible dementia can benefit from a well-conceived therapeutic regimen. The goal of this chapter is to provide a guide for the recognition and management of the organic mental disorders in a manner both helpful to the practicing clinican and compatible with present knowledge of the phenomenology and pathophysiology of these disorders.

CLASSIFICATION: DSM-III

The classification of the organic mental disorders in this chapter attempts to conform with the new Diagnostic and Statistical Manual of Mental Disorders, 3rd edition (DSM-III)[4] prepared by the task force on nomenclature and statistics of the American Psychiatric Association. The DSM-III will enable clinicians and research investigators to diagnose, treat, and communicate about the organic mental disorders in a more valid and reliable manner. To this end DSM-III clearly describes diagnostic entities and provides inclusion and exclusion criteria for precision of diagnosis. The diagnostic system for the organic mental disorders in this chapter differs from DSM-III in some respects for the specific purpose of simplifying its use in clinical geriatric psychiatry.

For those familiar with DSM-II,[5] the new system may at first appear confusing and/or incomplete. An obvious change is the absence of the psychotic versus nonpsychotic dichotomy, which was an important part of the DSM-II system. The use of this dichtomy in reference to the organic mental disorders has previously been criticized by Raskind[6] and Lipowski.[7] In DSM-II an organically impaired patient was diagnosed "psychotic" on the basis of severity of dysfunction. The patient with mild intellectual impairment was considered "nonpsychotic," whereas the person with qualitatively similar but more severe intellectual dysfunction was considered "psychotic." Defining psychosis by severity of dysfunction lacks precision and may even be therapeutically misleading. For instance, an antipsychotic drug such as a phenothiazine would probably not be indicated for a patient who was defined as "psychotic" (by DSM-II criteria) because of severe memory impairment and resultant inability to meet the demands of everyday life. In fact, an antipsychotic drug might actually be contraindicated for such a "psychotic" patient. In contrast, DSM-III uses the term "psychotic" to imply the presence of delusions, hallucinations, or schizophreniform thought disorder. Psychotic signs and symptoms can be present in both mild and severe organic mental disorders as well as in organic mental disorders of various kinds. This latter definition of "psychotic" is compatible with current psychopharmacologic concepts, and has clear therapeutic implications.

The separation of organic mental disorders into "acute organic brain syndromes," and "chronic organic brain syndromes" has also been deleted from DSM-III. Although less confusing than the psychotic versus nonpsychotic dichotomy, the division between acute and chronic organic brain syndromes also lacked precision. In this chapter "dementia" is roughly equivalent to "chronic organic brain syndrome," and "delirium" is roughly equivalent to "acute organic brain syndrome."

The essential feature of the organic mental disorders is transient or permanent brain dysfunction attributable to specific organic (pathophysiological) factors judged necessary for the dysfunction. Such factors are potentially demonstrable by currently available laboratory procedures (such as electroencephalogram or measurement of circulating hormone levels), physical examination, or medical history. The organic factor may be a primary brain disease, a systemic disease secondarily affecting the brain, or a drug or toxin which is currently deranging brain function or has damaged the brain in the past. Differentiation of the "organic" mental disorders from the so-called "functional" mental disorders does not imply that the latter disorders are somehow independent of brain processes. It is assumed that all psychological processes, both normal and abnormal depend on underlying physiologic processes, and it is quite conceivable that many of the "functional" mental disorders will be reclassified as organic mental disorders as new laboratory techniques are developed and the pathophysiology of the "functional" mental disorders is elucidated.

The organic mental syndromes are clusters of signs, symptoms and other features which are the clinical manifestations of the organic mental disorders. Four of these organic brain syndromes are of primary importance in geriatric psychiatry. These are:

1. dementia
2. delirium
3. amnestic syndrome
4. organic affective syndrome

Each syndrome will be described, and the specific organic mental disorders will be discussed under their appropriate syndrome.

Dementia

Primary Features. The hallmark of dementia is a deterioration of previously acquired intellectual abilities of sufficient severity to interfere with social or occupational functioning. Memory impairment is the most prominent feature and is of primary importance to the disorder. Other central features include impairment of abstract thinking and use of symbolic logic, impaired judgment, loss of impulse control and personality change. Memory loss is usually the first sign of dementia, and often remains prominent until deterioration progresses to the point at which memory is no longer testable. Remote events tend to be better preserved than those of the recent past, but this pattern of loss is variable. Impairment in abstract thinking is manifested by reduced capacity for generalizing, synthesizing, differentiating, logical reasoning, and concept formation. Impaired judgment is often an early sign of the disorder and may cause great consternation to family members and other associates, especially if the presence and nature of the underlying disorder is not yet fully appreciated. Personality change may be even more distressing to those living with the patient. Control of aggressive and sexual impulses is reduced and the capacity for empathic understanding of, or concern with, significant others gradually deteriorates. A previously nurturant, caring, and responsive spouse, parent, or friend often becomes extremely self-centered and oblivious to the needs of others.

Associated Features. Language disorder typically occurs as the disease progresses although the type of language disorder differs in the different types of dementia. In multi-infarct dementia classic aphasias occur if the areas of infarcted brain involve speech centers. In progressive idiopathic dementia (senile dementia of the Alzheimer's type) early paraphasic and anomic features progress to severe failures of comprehension and meaningful expression. Apraxias are common and cause inability to perform basic activities of daily living despite intact motor function. Disturbed sleep patterns with insomnia and nocturnal wandering, and incontinence of urine and feces are troublesome features which frequently precipitate institutional placement.

Other associated features resemble behaviors common to the "functional" psychiatric disorders. Although by no means present in all demented patients, when they occur these features demand the clinician's at-

tention. Depression may occur at any point in the course of dementia. Depression is particularly common in patients with multi-infarct dementia who often retain insight into the devastating nature of their cognitive impairment. Paranoid features also may appear. Some paranoid phenomena are clearly related to memory loss. The patient will forget the location of some object or forget having eaten a meal. When the misplaced object is perceived as missing or the food eaten at a forgotten meal is discovered to be absent from the refrigerator, accusations of theft result. Such delusions of theft based on defective memory are quite common and are frequent causes of interpersonal turmoil. Also common are delusions and hallucinations of a schizophreniform nature. These may have a bizarre quality involving plots to molest or harm the patient. Another important associated feature is the constellation of irritability, agitation, and hostility. This group of behavioral signs and symptoms is accompanied by dysphoria in both the patient and those responsible for his or her care.

Differential Diagnosis. Chronic schizophrenia in an eldery patient, particularly one who has spent many years in an institution, may superficially resemble dementia. Difficulties in examining a withdrawn, socially impaired, and sometimes uncooperative schizophrenic patient may further cloud the diagnostic issue. A history of longstanding psychiatric illness, together with the presence of schizophrenic thought disorder and grossly intact memory confirm the diagnosis of schizophrenia. It should be emphasized that the possibility of organic brain deterioration in late chronic schizophrenia is still an unsettled issue; and that both schizophrenia and dementia may co-exist in the same patient. Delirium may also be mistaken for dementia, as both manifest impairment in intellectual abilities. Furthermore the patient with dementia may be suffering from a superimposed delirium. In delirium the core features are disturbance in attention span and level of consciousness, which features are not present in uncomplicated dementia. Furthermore, the course of delirium is usually brief. Significant cognitive dysfunction lasting more than a month suggests dementia rather than delirium. Although both dementia and delirium may develop acutely, such onset favors the diagnosis of delirium.

Depression in the elderly can be mistaken for dementia, an error more commonly made in the United States than in the United Kingdom.[8,9] Intellectual function is often impaired in elderly depressives. The depressed patient often notes difficulties in thinking, concentration and memory and may exhibit actual decrements in cognitive performance.[10] Furthermore, standard psychological tests are frequently interpreted as compatible with "organicity." Such depressive "pseudo-dementia"[11] is usually distinguishable from true dementia by history and clinical examination. The most helpful diagnostic tool is a careful history of the development of the illness as described by friends or relatives. Depression begins with dysphoric mood, loss of interest and pleasure in the environment, decreased energy and activity level, changes in appetite and sleep pattern, and increased somatic complaints. Cognitive changes rarely occur before the symptoms and signs of depression have become obvious. In contrast, the patient with dementia will have exhibited memory loss and other cognitive deficits before signs and symptoms of depression appear. Clinical evaluation will also help distinguish between depressive pseudo-dementia and true dementia. The depressed patient is more likely to give "don't know" answers than to demonstrate clear gaps in memory. If the depressed patient can be motivated to attempt intellectual tasks, performance often improves dramatically. Even if some doubt remains as to the true nature of the disorder, depression should be treated vigorously. Good responses to antidepressant therapy occur in both primarily depressed patients and in demented patients with superimposed depression. It should be emphasized that rigorous longitudinal studies have demonstrated that a depressive illness in an elderly person is only rarely the prodrome of progressive dementia. Followup of elderly depressed patients has confirmed that they develop subsequent dementia at no higher a frequency than do matched populations of nondepressed elderly.[12]

Many disorders present as dementia in later life, the most common of which are degenerative neurologic diseases. These disorders will be discussed individually as to etiology, course, and specific treatment if available. General treatment modalities for the dementia syndrome will be discussed later in the chapter.

Degenerative Neurologic Disease

Progressive Idiopathic Dementia (senile dementia of the Alzheimer's type) is the most common cause of dementia in later life. The essential features of this disorder are the insidious onset of dementia with a progressive deteriorating course. The diagnosis is made by excluding other known causes of dementia. Progressive idiopathic dementia usually begins in the seventies, but may begin before the age of 65. The latter is often referred to as "presenile dementia" or classic Alzheimer's disease, but is neuropathologically indistinguishable from progressive idiopathic dementia.[13,14] Most authorities now consider the presenile and late onset forms of this disease to be the same basic entity. Post mortem examination usually reveals brain shrinkage with a weight of less than 1000 grams being not uncommon.[15] However, the clinical picture and classic histologic changes of progressive idiopathic dementia can occur in patients whose brains are of normal weight and appearance at autopsy. This latter fact must be kept in mind when evaluating the diagnostic utility of neuroradiologic tests such as computerized axial tomographic (CAT) scan. Cortical atrophy is usually prominent and widespread with particular involvement of the frontal and temporal lobes. Atrophy of the hippocampus, parahippocampus, and hippocampal gyrus are also prominent. The histologic hallmarks of the disease are senile plaques, neurofibrillary tangles, and granulovacuolar degeneration.[16] Although all of the above histologic changes may occur in normal aging, their presence in appreciable quantity is strongly correlated with the antemortem presence of dementia.[17] Neuronal loss is probably present but specific confirmation of neuronal loss is hampered by problems in cell counting technique.[18]

Although most patients have a fairly uniform downhill course, many patients will demonstrate plateaus of cognitive dysfunction which can last from months to years. The behavioral picture is essentially that of a dementia (see above). The average length of time from onset to death is often stated as 5 years, but this figure is difficult to document given the insidious onset of the disorder. There is no question, however, that this disease has poor prognosis and significantly shortens life expectancy. In a followup study of hospitalized dementia patients, over 80% were dead at the end of 2 years.[19] In a longer (20 year) followup study,[20] Kay found a mean life expectancy of 2.6 years for men and 2.3 years for women. No dementia patient survived to the end of the followup period. In the control group of nondemented elderly persons, mean survival was 8.7 years for men and 10.9 years for women, and 17 patients were still alive after 20 years. Women with dementia had only 25% of the life expectancy of comparable nondemented women and men 34% of that of nondemented men. Similar acceleration of mortality rate has been demonstrated in dementia patients in an American nursing home.[21] Given that patients with dementia are admitted to a hospital or nursing home facility only after the disease has progressed to at least moderate degree, and frequently not until the disease has been complicated by a medical disorder, the question arises as to whether dementia patients still well enough to reside in the community might have a better prognosis. Unfortunately, studies of community residents with dementia are also discouraging. A 2–4 year followup of community residents suffering from both progressive idiopathic dementia and multi-infarct dementia revealed a 75% mortality at the end of the follow-up period compared to only a 26% mortality in a normal control group.[22] Even mild dementia appears to carry considerable risk of increased mortality. Gilmore[23] recently reported a 3-year follow-up of patients with dementia who were living at home at the initial evaluation. Mildly demented patients were those who demonstrated intellectual deficits on memory and information tests but remained well-integrated into society with relatively intact social habits and retention of ability to care for themselves. Moderately demented patients had more severe cognitive impairment and were unable to care for themselves without frequent supervision and assistance from friends and relatives. Such problems as nocturnal wandering and urinary incontinence were common in the moderately demented group. Severe cases were incapable of coherent or sustained speech and led totally dependent existences. Of 12 mildly demented subjects, 9 were dead at 3-year follow-up, one was hospitalized, and only 2 were unchanged. Of the 13 moderately demented patients 5 were dead, 5 were hospitalized and 3 were unchanged. Two of the three severely demented subjects had died and one remained unchanged. Although the sample size was small, the mortality rate of the mildly demented patients is particularly discouraging. The etiology of progressive idiopathic dementia is unknown. Possible viral[24] and immunologic[25] mechanisms are currently being investigated. Specific treatment is not available.

Multi-Infarct Dementia

This illness, the second largest cause of dementia, can be attributed to underlying vascular disease. Neuropathologic studies consistently find vascular disease to be responsible for only 10–20% of dementias.[26] In these cases, the pathologic process is multiple cerebral infarction. The large majority of demented patients are suffering from progressive idiopathic dementia without significant vascular involvement. Occasionally, multi-infarct dementia and primary idiopathic dementia will coincide.

The essential features of multi-infarct dementia are stepwise deterioration of intellectual function that early in the course leaves some intellectual functions relatively intact; focal neurologic signs and symptoms; and often a history of cerebrovascular accident. Associated features include pseudobulbar palsy with emotional lability, dysarthria, dysphasia, and convulsive seizures. Characteristically the patient will have a history of hypertension and will exhibit abrupt ischemic episodes which lead to weakness, slowness, hyperreflexia, and extensor plantar responses. Fluctuation in level of cognition is common, and discrete confusional episodes (delirium) occur, presumably following new vascular episodes. Multi-infarct dementia is probably more common in men than in women, and the course of progression is highly variable depending on the occurrence of new lesions. The most important predisposing factor is arterial hypertension. Whether treatment of hypertension in an effort to prevent future cerebrovascular accidents is an effective treatment modality in this population remains to be determined. Normalization of blood pressure in younger patients with moderate to severe hypertension reduces long-term vascular complications including cerebrovascular accident. However, studies are not available in which an elderly population has been evaluated, especially one already suffering from multi-infarct dementia. Possible advantages of controlling hypertension must be weighed against the risk of adverse effects of antihypertensive medications and the risk of precipitating cerebral ischemia if blood pressure is lowered too vigorously.[27,28]

Other degenerative neurologic diseases may also produce dementia. Huntington's chorea is an autosomal dominant disorder producing a progressive dementia with onset in adult life. This disorder is associated with choreiform movements and a high incidence of severe psychiatric symptomatology including depression, paranoid states, and impulse control disorders. The caudate nucleus is the site of severe neuropathologic change, but other areas of brain including the cortex are involved. Symptomatic treatment of the movement disorder and the paranoid and aggressive behavioral symptomatology with antipsychotic drugs is occasionally helpful. Genetic counseling of family members may prevent occurrence of the disease in future generations.

Although dementia in Parkinson's disease has been recognized since 1885, its occurrence in this common disorder is receiving renewed attention. In a long-term follow-up study of patients with Parkinson's disease who received chronic levodopa therapy, dementia was found in approximately one-third of patients throughout a 6-year treatment period.[29] These investigators speculated that the high incidence of dementia in patients with Parkinson's disease who take levodopa reflected prolongation of the course of the illness rather than a direct effect of the medication. Levodopa therapy has been associated with temporary improvement in mentation in patients with the dementia of Parkinson's disease.[30,31]

Creutzfeldt-Jacob disease is a rapidly prograssive, diffuse disorder of the nervous system involving severe neurologic impairment with marked dysfunction. There is increasing evidence that Creutzfeld-Jacob disease is caused by slow virus infection.[32] Treatment with antiviral drugs is experimental at this time.

Structural Neurologic Abnormalities

Normal pressure hydrocephalus was first described by Hakim and Adams,[33] and has resulted in much diagnostic and therapeutic activity during the past decade. This entity has recently been reviewed by Katzman.[34] Although initial therapeutic enthusiasm has been somewhat dampened by experience, normal pressure hydrocephalus remains a potentially treatable cause of dementia. In its classic form a communicating hydro-cephalus is associated with gait disturbance, progressive dementia and urinary incontinence. The likelihood of discovering this disorder is higher in early onset (less than 65 years old) dementia patients than in late onset dementia patients.[35] A good response to shunt therapy occurs in approximately 50% of patients. Impairment of gait is a hallmark of the typical syndrome and patients with typical gait disturbance are the best surgical candidates. Pneumoencephalo-gram and computerized axial tomography will typically demonstrate dilated ventricles without gyral atrophy, and intrathecal cisternography with radioactive iodinated serum albumin (RISA) should demonstrate the altered cerebrospinal fluid dynamics. The latter test is helpful in differentiating hydrocephalus ex vacuo seen in primary idiopathic dementia from normal pressure hydrocephalus. Chronic subdural hematoma can cause dementia or exacerbate cognitive deficit in an already demented patient. Computerized axial tomography and brain scan will detect most significant hematomas. Surgical removal of the clot may reverse cognitive impairment, although results of treatment are highly variable. Brain tumors, either primary or metastatic can present as dementia. Some benign primary tumors such as meningiomas may be removed with partial or complete restoration of mental function. More commonly, brain tumors are not fully "curable," but surgical or radiation therapy can be palliative in some cases.

Metabolic Disorder

Although metabolic disorders most commonly produce the organic brain syndrome of delirium, they can also present as dementia. In hypothyroidism, irritability, paranoid ideation, and depression often accompany the dementia. Treatment with thyroid hormone is probably more effective in reversing the depressive and paranoid signs and symptoms than it is the cognitive deficits, but the dementia may improve or even resolve.[36] Pernicious anemia (vitamin B-12 deficiency) can present with dementia even in the absence of megaloblastic hematologic findings.[37] Serum B-12 assays are now widely available. Again, cognitive improvement with vitamin B-12 replacement therapy once dementia has developed is variable. Dementia has also been attributed to folic acid deficiency,[38] although it is more likely that decreased folate levels found in demented patients are secondary to the inadequate dietary intake of an already demented patient.[39] Hypercalcemia with slowed thinking, impaired memory, and motor retardation can closely mimic early progressive idiopathic dementia. Hyperparathyroidism, multiple myeloma, sarcoidosis and several other treatable entities can cause hypercalcemia.[40] A metabolic cause of dementia which should receive greater emphasis is multiple hypoglycemic episodes. This disorder is usually secondary to iatrogenic hypoglycemia in patients treated for diabetes mellitus with either insulin or the sulfonyl-urea derivatives. There is little evidence that any theoretic advantages of rigid blood glucose control outweigh the risks of hypoglycemic neuronal damage in elderly patients.

Systemic Illness

Congestive heart failure and/or low cardiac output states can cause or exacerbate dementia. Cognition frequently improves with an appropriate cardio-tonic regimen. Cardiac pacing may improve cognitive function in patients with bradycardia or other rhythm disturbances which impair cardiac output.[41] Renal failure, hepatic failure, and pulmonary failure can also exacerbate or be the primary cause of dementia, and treatment is again directed at the underlying disease entity. Dementia from tertiary syphilis (general paresis) is less common than in earlier years, but new cases continue to appear, particularly in elderly patients with psychiatric disorder.[42] The dementia may occur 10 to 20 or more years after the primary infection. Many elderly persons continue to be sexually active, and the risk of developing syphilis should not be dismissed solely on the basis of a person's age. Chronic meningitis, either tuberculous or fungal, may also present as dementia. These patients appear systemically ill with fever, headache, and focal neurologic signs. As with tertiary syphilis, diagnosis of chronic meningitis depends on examination of the spinal fluid.

Toxins

Bromide intoxication may present as dementia and can have an insidious onset as well as a chronic course. The elderly patient can develop cognitive impairment at relatively low blood bromide levels.[43] Bromide is still present in some currently available pharmaceutical preparations. The cortical depressant sedative and hypnotic drugs, particularly the barbiturates, may present as dementia. Behavioral toxicity from the antipsychotic or antidepressant medications is more commonly an atropine-like delirium. Mercury and lead intoxication can also present as dementia. Urine and blood assays for these drugs and heavy metals will make the diagnosis, and treatment is directed at removing the offending agent.

DIAGNOSTIC EVALUATION OF DEMENTIA

A careful evaluation of the patient presenting with dementia will often uncover a potentially correctable etiology, and will define treatable behavioral problems complicating the underlying disorder. Recent studies suggest that 10–30% of dementia patients have a potentially correctable underlying disorder.[44,45,46,47] Correctable causes are more commonly found in younger demented patients (below age 65), but advanced age by no means excludes the discovery of a correctable lesion. Common correctable disorders include depression, chronic drug toxicity, normal pressure hydrocephalus, subdural hematoma, and hypothyroidism. Resectable tumors, neurosyphilis, systemic disease, and pernicious anemia also accounted for a smaller number of correctable dementias in the above series. Unfortunately, finding a

potentially treatable cause for dementia does not mean that treatment will always be successful. Studies which report treatment results suggest that moderate or excellent improvement occurs in approximately 50% of cases. Fox[45] reported good results following treatment of patients with hypothyroidism or pernicious anemia. In a larger series, Freeman[46] reported good results following shunting in three of seven patients with normal pressure hydrocephalus. All five patients with chronic drug toxicity showed good improvement with discontinuation of the causative medication, and patients with depression and bilateral subdural hematoma also responded well to therapy. One patient with neurosyphilis responded poorly as did single patients with hepatic failure and hypothyroidism. The noninvasive diagnostic evaluation outlined in Table 13–1 should reveal most treatable causes of dementia. Even if the presence of a noncorrectable disorder is confirmed, this type of thorough evaluation helps assure both the patient and the patient's family that a reasonable attempt to uncover a correctable disorder has been made.

The basic clinical evaluation includes a careful history both from the patient and

Table 13–1.   Evaluation of the Patient with Dementia.

History from patient *and* relative or friend
Mental status exam
Physical and neurologic exam
Medication inventory
Electrocardiogram
Chest and skull x-ray
Computerized Axial Tomographic (CAT) Scan
Complete blood count
Urinalysis
Urine toxicology screen
Cerebrospinal fluid pressure, protein, sugar, cells, VDRL or STS
Serum VDRL or STS
Serum bromide
Serum sodium, potassium, chloride, bicarbonate, calcium
Serum BUN, creatinine, bilirubin, SGOT, albumin/globulin
Serum B_{12}
Serum Thyroxine
Serum glucose (fasting)

from friends or relatives who can accurately describe the onset and progression of the disorder; a careful mental status examination; and a careful physical examination. A drug inventory of current and past medications should also be obtained, along with a urine specimen for drug toxicology screen. Mental status examination should not only focus on intellectual areas such as memory, calculations, abstraction, and judgment; but must also assess mood, presence of hallucinations and delusions, impulse control, and sleep pattern. Physical exam must be directed toward systemic illnesses which can impair mental function. Cognitive tests and behavioral ratings scales can be helpful to the clinician in the initial evaluation and ongoing management of the demented patient. These instruments are more often supplementary than central to the differential diagnostic process.[48,49] They find their greatest clinical utility in quantifying the degree of cognitive impairment; delineating selective areas of cognitive and functional disturbance; and providing reliable data for evaluating progression of the disorder. These instruments systematize the type of observations obtained by a good mental status assessment. Rather than being redundant, however, they add reliability and quantification to the clinical examination. A convenient instrument which can both aid in the diagnosis of organic mental disorder as well as provide some quantification of the degree of intellectual impairment is the Short Portable Mental Status Questionnaire (SPMSQ) developed by Pfeiffer.[50] This instrument has modified and elaborated upon the Mental Status Questionnaire of Kahn and Goldfarb,[51] a widely used instrument since its introduction in 1960. The SPMSQ uses 10 brief items to test short-term memory, long-term memory, orientation, fund of knowledge, and both attention span and calculation ability as assessed by a serial mathematical subtraction test. The validity and reliability of this instrument in the detection of dementia have been demonstrated by the author[50] and independently by Schuckit.[52] This is not a highly sensitive instrument, and may fail to detect mild impairment. Its ability to delineate discreet areas of cognitive dysfunction is also limited. However, its brevity, ease of administration, validity, and reliability, are strong assets in clinical practice. A more comprehensive albeit still brief instrument is the Mini-Mental State (MMS) developed by Folstein et al.[53] This instrument assesses orientation, registration of information, attention and calculation (again with a serial subtraction test) and information recall; and also tests for aphasia, an area not evaluated by the SPMSQ. The validity and reliability of this instrument have also been established, as well as its ability to differentiate between dementia and depression with secondary cognitive impairment in hospitalized patients. The MMS provides more information concerning cognitive function than does the SPMSQ, but the increased difficulty of administration may weigh against its adoption by the busy clinician. Another convenient instrument which quantifies mental status data in a brief format has been developed by Jacobs et al.[54] for use on a general hospital medical service. This instrument focuses on detection of impaired attention span and is thus very sensitive to the presence of delirium. It also assesses memory, orientation and the ability to use abstraction and symbolic logic in a simple manner. This instrument, the Cognitive Capacity Screening Examination, deserves further evaluation in clinical settings. The above three instruments all require the active participation of the patient, participation which may not be obtainable from some severely impaired or behaviorally disturbed patients with organic mental disorder. Furthermore, they do not evaluate activities of daily living or "functional" type behavioral pathology such as affective disturbance, delusions, agitation, and impulse disorders.

Rating scales which do not require active participation by the patient have been developed to meet these latter needs. These instruments can be used to document and roughly quantify impairment in performance in activities of daily living such as dressing, eating, bowel and bladder function, and other aspects of self care. They can

also be used to assess mood, unusual ideation or behavior, social relations, and even
give a rough estimation of cognitive function. Such rough estimates of cognitive
function as rated by an outside observer are
far less valid than the results of the active
tests of cognitive function described above,
but may be the only estimate available for a
given patient. The Sandoz Clinical Assess-
ment-Geriatric (SCAG) is a recently developed observer rated scale with good reliability and validity.[55] It assesses mood, behavior
and observed gross cognitive dysfunction,
but does not evaluate activities of daily living except for one global "self care" item.
The Geriatric Rating Scale (GRS) developed
by Plutchik, et al.[56] emphasizes activities of
daily living behaviors, but does not assess
mood. The dementia scale of Blessed, Tomlinson, and Roth[57] does provide an instrument which combines an active test of information, memory, and concentration together with an observer rated scale of activities
of daily living. This scale has much to
recommend it and is also of historical note
in that it was used in the classic studies
defining the relationship between neuropathologic changes and behavioral functioning in progressive idiopathic dementia. Including one or more of the above instruments in the initial evaluation and on
periodic follow-up examinations helps the
clinician follow the progression of the
disorder and response to treatment regimens.

Some discussion is in order of the more
comprehensive psychometric and neuropsychological tests useful in both research
and intensive investigation of selected patients. Unfortunately, these tests are often
inapplicable to the moderately or severely
impaired patient with dementia because of
inability to comply with instructions or complete the tasks, nor are they more sensitive
or specific for diagnosing early dementia
than is a careful history taken from relatives
combined with a careful clinical assessment
of the patient. The Wechsler Adult Intelligence Scale (WAIS), which was developed to
quantify intellectual ability in a normal

adult population, is sometimes useful in
detecting early organic mental disorders.
The discrepancy between verbal IQ and performance IQ suggests organic mental disorder, but the WAIS often fails to distinguish between organic mental disorder
and such entities as depression with secondary cognitive impairment. The Halstead-
Reitan Neuropsychological Test Battery is a
sensitive and specific neuropsychological instrument for the detection and delineation
of brain impairment.[58] Unfortunately the
test is complex and takes hours to complete
in its standard form. Several investigators
have developed abbreviated versions of the
Halstead-Reitan Battery but length of time
for administration still approximates 1 hour,
and degree of task complexity is often
beyond the capacity of the patient with
dementia. However, the Halstead-Reitan
Battery and its modifications can be useful
in pinpointing discrete areas of cognitive dysfunction in patients with mild
dementia.[59]

Utilizing micro-computer systems for the
administration of dementia screening batteries appears feasible.[60] Test material can
be presented visually or audibly and patient
response may be either verbal or nonverbal.
Such factors as rate of stimulus presentation, response accuracy, and reaction time
may be analyzed on line with preliminary
results available by the end of the testing
procedure. The precise quantification of
reaction time may prove to be particularly
helpful in the assessment of dementia.[61]
Another promising area involves the adaptation of developmental scales utilized in normal childhood development and in assessment of the mentally retarded.

THE TREATMENT OF DEMENTIA

Treatment of Behavioral Complications of Dementia

The secondary behavioral features of dementia are the most treatable aspects of this
disorder. Paranoid states, nocturnal delirium, agitation, hostility, impulsivity, depres-

sion, sleep disturbance and many other behaviors are responsive to treatment. The psychopharmacologic approaches to the treatment of these disturbances will be discussed first. Psychosocial therapies which also are clearly useful, will be discussed subsequently.

The antipsychotic medications are effective in the treatment of schizophreniform psychotic symptoms such as delusions and hallucinations, nocturnal conceptual disorganization, and the behavioral "syndrome" manifested by agitation, irritability, hostility and impulsivity. Other than for the last "syndrome," the antipsychotic medications are specifically useful in conditions which meet the concept of psychosis in DSM-III. They are not helpful for impaired memory or other intellectual deficits or for impaired activities of daily living secondary to intellectual deterioration, and may even be deleterious for these latter problems.[6] The more acutely disturbed the patient, the more likely that the drugs will be helpful. Although reports of well-designed clinical studies in this area are few, a review of some of the studies is instructive. Tsuang et al.[62] compared haloperidol (average dose 2.0 mg/day) to thioridazine (average dose 113 mg/day) in a group of "acutely psychotic" geriatric patients, which included both demented and chronic schizophrenic patients. The drugs were effective in decreasing hallucinations, hostility, excitement, anxiety, and grandiosity. No improvement in memory impairment, confusion, or other intellectual deficits was noted. Seager[63] found chlorpromazine (average dose 150–200 mg/day) significantly more effective than placebo in acutely disturbed patients with dementia. Sugerman et al.[64] found haloperidol to be significantly more effective than placebo in alleviating agitation, hostility, and hyperactivity in patients with dementia. Not all studies have been positive, however. Robinson[65] found chlorpromazine no better than placebo for the control of nonschizophreniform behavioral symptoms in female elderly patients with dementia and noted that the active drug group actually deteriorated at a significantly higher rate than did the placebo group. Most of this deterioration was attributed to increased inertia in the active drug group. Both Altman et al.[66] and Barton and Hurst[67] have reported clinical improvement in patients during the "clearance period" preceding institution of a study drug. This clearance period is the time following discontinuation of previous psychotropic medications, many of which were antipsychotic medications. These latter studies suggest that adverse drug effects such as lethargy, central anticholinergic toxicity with increased confusion, and extrapyramidal side effects may adversely affect the dementia patient who lacks specific indications for the antipsychotic drugs.

The choice of an antipsychotic medication for an individual patient depends on the side-effect profile of a particular drug and the behavioral and medical status of the individual patient. There is no evidence that any antipsychotic drug is more effective than another in treatment of psychotic symptomatology. Adverse effects of the antipsychotic drugs include peripheral and central anticholinergic toxicity, extrapyramidal signs and symptoms, sedation, and orthostatic hypotension. Anticholinergic effects include urinary retention, constipation, dry mouth, blurry vision, and delirium with exacerbation of cognitive impairment. The high dosage antipsychotics such as chlorpromazine and thioridazine are more anticholinergic than the low dosage antipsychotics such as haloperidol, thiothixene, and trifluoperazine.[68] One of the latter medications would be preferable in a patient susceptible to anticholinergic drug effects. In contrast to the situation with anticholinergic activity, the low dosage antipsychotic medications such as haloperidol, thiothixene, and trifluoperazine are more likely to cause extrapyramidal signs and symptoms than are the high dosage medications such as thiodiazine and chlorpromazine. Parkinsonian or extrapyramidal side effects commonly seen in the elderly include a reversible parkinsonian syndrome, akathisia, and tardive dyskinesia. Akathisia, a syndrome of motor restlessness and a subjective discomfort can be confused with agitation and motoric hyperactivity secondary to the underlying disorder. In the patient with pre-existing parkinsonism or a low threshold for developing extrapyramidal toxicity, a drug such as thioridazine would be preferable. Thioridazine and chlorpromazine are more sedating than the low dosage medications. This effect can be helpful in a severely agitated patient or in one with sleep disturbance, but may cause problems in a patient with social withdrawal or lethargy. Although overdoses of antipsychotic medications have been associated with disturbances in cardiac rhythm and conduction, these effects have not been documented at normal dosage levels. However, the electrocardiogram should be monitored when the antipsychotic medications are being instituted.

The pharmacologic treatment of depression in the demented patient is more difficult than in the nondemented depressed patient, but can be extremely helpful in selected patients. The tricyclic antidepressants have been demonstrated effective in nonelderly depressed patients and are widely used in the elderly. Unfortunately, data from placebo-controlled clinical studies of tricyclic antidepressant therapy in depressed dementia patients are not available. Indications for using these medications in such patients rest on inferences from their use in young or elderly nondemented patients. The tricyclics are most effective if depression is manifested by decreased appetite, weight loss, psychomotor retardation, and sleep disturbance with early morning awakening.[69] Insidious onset also favors the use of these medications. Because depression in the elderly is often manifested by somatic complaints or hypochondriasis which "mask" the depressed mood, the antidepressant drugs are frequently effective in seemingly hypochondriacal patients. De Alarcon[70] found hypochondriacal symptoms to be the first manifestation of depression in 29% of 152 elderly depressed patients admitted to the Bethlehem Royal Hospital. These somatic complaints typically preceded the appearance of overtly depressive symptoms by 2–3 months. As many as 64% of the elderly patients in this series had hypochondriacal symptoms at some time during their illness. Comparison with younger depressed patients confirmed a significantly higher incidence of hypochondriacal symptoms in the elderly. Furthermore only 20% of these elderly hypochondriacal depressed patients had a history of excessive bodily preoccupation during earlier life. The various tricyclic antidepressants have equal therapeutic efficacy but differ in profile of adverse effects. Of particular importance are differences in anticholinergic and sedative activity. These drugs rarely produce extrapyramidal effects, but are more likely to interfere with cardiac rate or rhythm than are the antipsychotic drugs. Cardiac toxicity of these drugs has been documented in the acute postmyocardial infarction period[71] and in cases of overdose with exceedingly high drug plasma levels.[72] These drugs should be used cautiously in patients with cardiac disease.

A reasonable starting dose of the commonly used tricyclic antidepressants (doxepin, amitriptyline, imipramine, desipramine, or nortriptyline) in the elderly depressed patient is 25 mg/day. The drug should be increased by 25 mg/day every 4 to 5 days until the patient begins to show a therapeutic response, side effects become troublesome, or a total daily dosage of 150 mg/day (in divided doses) is reached. Higher doses are advisable only if low plasma drug levels can be documented. It is important to educate the patient, the nursing staff and the family that although adverse effects can occur rapidly, therapeutic response is often delayed 1 to 2 weeks after a therapeutic dosage level has been attained. Failure to increase dosage above the starting level is a common cause of drug failure. Once a therapeutic response occurs the patient should be maintained at the same dose of medication for 3 months, after which time the dose may be tapered gradually. If signs and symptoms recur the patient should receive maintenance therapy with subsequent trials of drug reduction at periodic intervals.

Unfortunately, demented patients who develop depression are often unable to tolerate the tricyclic antidepressants because of anticholinergic toxicity, excessive sedation, or hypotension. Several other pharmacologic agents have antidepressant activity and although probably less effective than the tricyclics are also less likely to produce severe adverse effects. Furthermore, in some situations nontricyclics are specifically indicated. Several of the antipsychotic medications have demonstrated antidepressant efficacy. These include thiothixene,[73] and thioridazine.[74] They are especially useful in patients who have both depression and schizophreniform psychotic symptoms or severe agitation. The psychostimulant drugs (methylphenidate, the amphetamines, and magnesium pemoline) are also useful in some demented patients suffering from depression. A recent placebo-controlled study[75] demonstrated that methylphenidate was significantly more effective than placebo in alleviating withdrawn, apathetic and depressed behavior in a group of elderly patients with dementia. Lithium carbonate, an antimanic drug is sometimes indicated in the patient with dementia and associated manic features such as hyperactivity, irritability, assaultiveness, and pressured speech. The manic syndrome is usually well disguised in the demented patient but should be suspected if a reasonable dose of antipsychotic medication is not effective in treating the above signs and symptoms, or if the antipsychotic medications must be used in such high dose that significant side effects occur. Lithium carbonate must be used conservatively in elderly patients, who tend to develop central nervous system and neuromuscular toxicity at lower serum levels than do young patients.[6] The half-life of lithium increases with age, particularly if glomerular filtration rate is seriously impaired. The therapeutic level (and also toxic level) for certain older individuals may therefore be reached quickly and low dosage levels (300–900 mg/day) together with careful monitoring of blood lithium levels and clinical status are in order. Lithium is particularly problematic in the elderly patient who becomes sodium depleted either because of a sodium restricted diet, increased sweating in a warm environment or the use of sodium depleting diuretics.

Sleep disturbance in the elderly demented patient is often treatable and this problem is of critical importance in maintaining elderly dementia patients at home.[76] Increasing daytime activity and limiting napping as much as possible are general approaches which should always be instituted if possible. Educating family and patient to the fact that sleep in the elderly normally contains increased awakening episodes and decreased deep sleep (stage 4 slow wave sleep) can be reassuring to those disturbed by any change in sleep pattern. However, many patients with sleep disturbance superimposed upon dementia will need pharmacologic intervention. If sleep disturbance is secondary to pain, congestive heart failure, or pulmonary insufficiency, these problems should be addressed with the appropriate medical regimen. If the sleep disturbance is a symptom of depression, the more sedative tricyclic antidepressants such as amitriptyline or doxepin are indicated. If nocturnal delirium with schizophreniform features is the cause of impaired sleep, the antipsychotic medications are the treatment of choice. The traditional hypnotics and sedatives such as the barbiturates, benzodiazepines, and similar agents are of only limited usefulness. They will improve sleep during an acute episode of situational anxiety but lose their effectiveness with chronic administration. Unfortunately, these agents can paradoxically increase agitation and confusion in a few susceptible patients. The sedative antihistaminic drugs such as diphenhydramine or hydroxyzine may also be useful and are relatively free of side effects.

Cognitive Acting Drugs

The most effective of the "cognitive acting" drugs were originally evaluated in dementia patients because of their activity as vasodilators, although it is unclear that this property is related to reported therapeutic efficacy. Furthermore, the drugs appear to affect a broad range of behaviors other than cognitive function *per se*. Three of these drugs, Hydergine, cyclandelate, and papavarine have appeared effective in enough clinical trials to warrant their discussion.[6] It should be emphasized that in most reported clinical studies of these agents, the population has been composed of heterogeneous "organic brain syndrome" patients. It is likely however, that the majority of subjects were suffering from progressive idiopathic dementia given the preponderance of this disorder in the type of residential settings in which the studies were conducted.

Dihydroergotamine (Hydergine), a combination of three hydrogenated ergot alkaloids may be the most effective of these drugs. Positive effects on behavior of demented patients compared to placebo have been demonstrated in most studies. Metabolic studies on animal brain preparations suggest that Dihydroergotamine may specifically normalize neuronal metabolism in the aging brain.[77] Most studies find improvement in such areas as activities of daily living, somatic complaints, mood, attitude, and sense of well-being. It has been suggested that part of the therapeutic activity of Dihydroergotamine is related to antidepressant efficacy. However, a recent study by Gaitz *et al*. revealed that positive changes in cognitive function could not be accounted for merely as a reflection of "halo" effect of improved mood and general sense of well-being.[78] Dihydroergotamine appears to alleviate a broad range of behavioral symptoms associated with dementia in selected patients although it is difficult to demonstrate changes in memory performance using active psychometric assessment.

Papaverine, an alkaloid derivative of opium with vasodilator properties has also been demonstrated superior to placebo in ameliorating symptoms associated with organic brain syndrome in several studies.[6] Although general improvements in behavior and in the performance of activities of daily living have been reported, it has again been difficult to clearly document significant intellectual improvement. A recent study by Branconnier and Cole[79] in a group of mild to moderately demented outpatients revealed significant treatment effects for papaverine on several tests of cognitive function.

Cyclandelate, another drug with vasodilator activity, has also been demonstrated more effective than placebo in treating patients with "organic brain syndrome."[6] Again, mildly impaired patients appear to be the most suitable candidates for a trial of this drug. A recent carefully evaluated study of cyclandalate in patients with either moderate dementia or depression with cognitive impairment failed to support the positive results found in earlier studies.[80] However, this latter negative study did not include mildly impaired demented patients.

Walsh[80a] has advocated the use of anticoagulant therapy for the treatment of presenile dementia. Though he reports excellent results, his studies are anecdotal and have not been replicated to date.

In summary, the above cognitive-acting drugs are probably effective for ameliorating adverse behavioral signs and symptoms in at least some patients with dementia. Improvement is usually of mild degree and the drugs must be administered for a considerable length of time before therapeutic results occur. It is not possible at this time to predict with any degree of certainty how a particular individual with dementia will respond to therapy with one of these agents. Future studies should focus on this latter problem and should rigorously define homogeneous groups of demented patients with specific organic mental disorders, with particular attention to separation of progressive idiopathic dementia from multi-infarct dementia.

Systematic investigations of two initially

exciting agents have dampened enthusiasm concerning their efficacy. Jacobs et al.[81] reported the effectiveness of pure oxygen administered under high pressure (100% at 2.5 atmosphere absolute, 3 hours per day for 15 days) in improving memory and other cognitive functions. Other investigators using protocols similar to that of Jacobs have been unable to confirm these initial findings.[82,83] Gerovital-H3, the active ingredient of which is procaine, has long been touted as an effective treatment for the aging process by Rumanian investigators. The large literature on Gerovital has been reviewed by Ostfeld et al.,[84] and Jarvik and Milne.[85] Both reviewers conclude that there is no satisfactory evidence that Gerovital can reverse the "aging process" or improve cognition in dementia. The mild monoamine oxidase inhibitor activity of Gerovital suggests possible antidepressant efficacy, although such action has not been well documented.

Three currently active areas of investigation into the neurochemistry of dementia and memory disorders may provide leads for specific psychopharmacologic interventions for cognitive dysfunction. Recent studies suggest deficiencies in cholinergic enzyme systems in brains of deceased patients with primary idiopathic dementia (Alzheimer's disease).[86,87] The most striking deficiencies were found in hippocampal, temporal, frontal and parietal cortex, the same brain regions showing the most extensive pathological changes characteristic of progressive idiopathic dementia. Supportive studies suggest that cholinergic neurons are particularly vulnerable to loss in progressive idiopathic dementia.[88] An open pilot study of Deanol,[89] a substance assumed to increase brain acetylcholine content, suggested improved behavior in cognitively impaired patients, although memory effects could not be specifically documented. Further research with agents acting upon brain cholinergic systems is indicated. Another exciting area of investigation involves the relationship of brain peptide hormones to memory processes. DeWied and his colleagues have demonstrated that both vasopressin and adrenocorticotropic hormone (ACTH) are involved in memory function in animals.[90] Legros[91] et al. recently demonstrated a positive effect upon learning and memory in nondemented men ages 50–65 treated with exogenous vasopressin. Case reports also suggest that vasopressin may be helpful in treating memory impairment.[92] Adolfsson, Gottfries and Winblad have demonstrated reduced levels of dopamine in the brains of patients with dementia and report cognitive improvement with the use of L-dopa combined with a peripheral decarboxylnse inhibitor.[92a]

Psychosocial Therapies

Interpersonal and environmental therapeutic techniques and strategies have become increasingly important in the treatment of the patient with dementia. The major therapies will be discussed and studies evaluating their efficacy when available, will be reviewed.

Reality Orientation. This therapy was developed by Taulbee and Folsom at the Veterans Administration Hospital in Tuscaloosa, Alabama.[93] Anecdotal reports have suggested that this treatment modality is useful in improving behavior in elderly populations with mixed diagnoses of chronic schizophrenia and organic mental disorders. The group sessions have a structured format. They are limited to four members, meet for 30 minutes 5 days a week, and utilize the same room for each session. The central tool in the therapy session is a large board constructed so that oversize letters may be used to spell out the date, time, place, patient's name, weather report, next meal and other discrete every day events. The leader utilizes visual and auditory reinforcement to gain the patient's attention and to elicit active responses indicating that the information has been memorized, even if only transiently. The formal sessions are supplemented on a 24-hour basis by ward personnel and family members who provide essential reality orientation information to the patient when a conversation or other interaction is initiated. A few controlled evaluations of reality orientation are now available and results of these studies have been mixed. Brook et al.[94] found improvement in ward behavior rating scales in an experimental group receiving reality orientation compared to a control group who received only exposure to the physical reality orientation setting. Improvement in the experimental group persisted throughout the entire 16-week study. These investigators modified standard reality orientation technique by gearing activities to the level of social and intellectual functioning of the individual patients. For instance, patients with only mild impairment participated in such activities as writing a diary and recounting their current thoughts and activities. More seriously impaired patients were treated in a standard fashion and tasks consisted of such things as identifying their therapist by name and identifying the objects in the room. Of interest is the fact that improvement could only be demonstrated for mildly impaired patients who (presumably) received the modified type of activities. The patients with marked impairment did not significantly benefit from reality orientation compared to the control group. Citrin and Dixon[95] reported improved performance on a test of orientation items following reality orientation therapy, but could not document changes in ward behavior as assessed by the Geriatric Rating Scale. Because orientation items tested were identical to those rehearsed in the Reality Orientation classes, these results were not surprising. Whether improvement in residents' frequently rehearsed responses generalized to a wider range of cognitive behavior was not determined. Harris and Ivory[96] evaluated reality orientation in a state mental hospital. Unfortunately, it is doubtful that their patients were suffering from dementia given that the mean age of the treatment group was 66.6 years and the mean length of current hospitalization was 23.0 years. Although diagnostic categories in this study were not rigorously described, the above age and length of hospitalization

characteristics suggest that the population was composed predominantly of patients with chronic functional disorders who had grown old during their hospitalization. These authors demonstrated increased verbal behavior and decreased bizarre verbalization in the treatment group.

Negative studies of reality orientation have also appeared. Barnes[97] could not demonstrate improvement in memory or orientation in a small group of dementia patients treated with reality orientation. MacDonald and Settin[98] compared reality orientation to participation in a sheltered workshop. Subjects were relatively young, mean age 64.4 years with a range of 40–74 years and severely impaired patients were excluded. Sheltered workshop therapy encouraged meaningful task participation with reinforcement for task completion. The tasks selected involved constructing gifts for residents of a nearby school for children. The reality orientation session included standard reality orientation techniques as well as enrichment aspects such as reading and discussing newspaper articles. The reality orientation subjects actually showed a trend toward deterioration in affect as measured by the Life Satisfaction Index. On the other hand, the sheltered workshop patients demonstrated a significant increase in Life Satisfaction Index scores. Cognitive function was not specifically assessed in this study. Informal observations suggested that the type of subject exposed to reality orientation in this study may have been too intact for the treatment modality. Complaints that the sessions seemed boring and useless were common. A second study by Dennis[99] reached similar discouraging conclusions. A group of hospitalized geriatric patients showed increased depression and decreased life satisfaction following treatment with remotivation therapy, a derivative of reality orientation.

On balance, reality orientation is probably effective for certain patients with dementia. Best results can be anticipated from a program in which the specific content of therapy is tailored to the individual attributes and needs of the patient. Enthusiastic and regular interaction of staff members with patients probably contributes a great deal to the success of treatment, and may be the critically important factor.

Other interpersonal therapies of a less formally structured nature have also been used with demented patients. Burnside has conducted group therapy in several formats and at least transient beneficial impacts on mood, motivation and intention have been described.[100] Individualized treatment for "excess disabilities" of dementia patients has been demonstrated effective by a group from the Philadelphia Geriatric Center.[101,102] The term "excess disability" describes the discrepancy which exists when an individual's functional incapacity is greater than that warranted by the actual physical or mental impairment, and implies the presence of treatable physical, psychological and/or social factors. Highly individualized treatment programs have been demonstrated more effective than standard residential treatment programs as assessed by blind observers.

Milieu therapy has been adapted to the treatment of dementia patients in a residential setting. Milieu therapy for the institutionalized elderly has received much impetus from work at the University of Michigan Institute of Gerontology. This area has recently been reviewed by Coons.[103] Milieu therapy uses the total environment as the therapeutic modality. It places a large amount of responsibility on the individual patient for his or her own therapeutic program, and structures the environment to offer opportunities and experiences for the individual to approximate the social roles normally available in the outside community. A structured series of meaningful behavioral expectations are formulated by both staff and patient, and positive reinforcement for appropriate behavior is emphasized. Homogeneous groupings of individuals according to their needs, degree of independence, and degree of disability is helpful.

Family involvement is important in the management of the patient with dementia. The family are the primary therapists while the patient lives at home. These family members are under great stress. Caring for a family member with a progressive dementing illness has some unique problems which are not shared by those caring for a family member afflicted with a severe or even terminal illness which leaves cognitive function intact. Group sessions with spouses and other close relatives of dementia patients have been conducted at the Seattle/Tacoma VA Geriatric Research, Education, and Clinical Center. These relatives are able to share the problems peculiar to their situation and help each other devise practical approaches to management.

DELIRIUM

Delirium includes the spectrum of clinical pictures of diverse organic etiologies whose most prominent feature is a disorder of attention. Essential features are rapid onset of fluctuating disturbances of attention, memory, and orientation. Also present are reduced wakefulness or insomnia, perceptual disturbances, and changes in psychomotor activity. This organic brain syndrome is synonymous with "metabolic encephalopathy" and roughly equivalent to the terms "acute brain syndrome" and "acute organic brain syndrome".

The disorder of attention is manifested by impaired ability to sustain attention to environmental stimuli, to engage in goal directed thinking, or to perform goal directed behavior. The patient is unable to carry on a conversation without becoming distracted and can barely sustain attention long enough to watch television or read. Thinking may be either slowed or accelerated and can become completely disorganized. The patient frequently loses his or her train of thought, switches from subject to subject, and may become completely incoherent. In contrast to dementia, disorders of memory and orientation are secondary rather than primary. Because the patient cannot attend to stimuli, he or she is unable to register and retain new information. There is often little if any recall of the delirious episodes once the delirium has resolved, although patients may report the episode as a "bad dream." Level of consciousness can vary from drowsiness or stupor in conditions such as hepatic or renal failure, to excessive alertness and severe insomnia in sedative drug or alcohol withdrawal. Vivid dreams and nightmares are common and may merge with hallucinations occuring in periods of wakefulness. Perceptual disturbances include misinterpretation, illusions, or hallucination. Delusions and hallucinations are commonly visual, but can frequently be auditory or occur in other modalities of sensation. Acute paranoid episodes can present serious management problems and endanger the safety of the patient.

Associated features include the range of affective responses. Fear, anxiety and anger commonly accompany delusional ideation and may precipitate attempts at escape from the immediate environment or destructive rage episodes. Less frequently euphoria is present. Depression may also occur, raising the risk of suicidal behavior. It is common for sensory misperceptions and fearfulness to reach greatest intensity at night.

The onset of delirium is usually rapid and duration brief. An episode of delirium can last for hours or days but rarely persists for greater than 1 month. In the absence of complications, clearing of the delirium leaves the patient's previous level of functioning intact. In some cases, depending on the etiology of the delirium, a dementia may persist after the delirium has cleared. Cognitive impairment often fluctuates, and lucid intervals may occur, especially during the daytime hours.

Etiologic factors are numerous. They include acute brain events, general medical illness, drug ingestion, drug withdrawal in a dependent person, postoperative states, and less well-understood phenomena such as sensory deprivation and the coronary care unit syndrome. See Table 13-2.

Differential diagnosis includes acute functional psychoses such as manic disorder, depressive disorder psychotic type, schizophrenia, and schizoaffective disorder. Ab-

Table 13-2.   Etiologies of Delirium.

SYSTEMIC ILLNESS	NEUROLOGIC DISORDERS
Congestive heart failure	Cerebrovascular accident
Pulmonary insufficiency	Head trauma
Renal insufficiency	Subarachnoid hemorrhage
Hepatic insufficiency	Meningitis (acute and chronic)
Lupus erythematosus	Intracranial mass lesion
Infection	Neurosyphilis
Burns and multiple trauma	Seizure (ictal or post-ictal)

METABOLIC DISORDERS	TOXIC
Hypothyroidism	Bromide
Hyperadrenalcorticism	Levodopa
Hypoadrenalcorticism	Digitalis
Hypercalcemia	Anticholinergic drugs
Hypoglycemia	antipsychotics (phenothiazines, etc.)
	tricyclic antidepressants
MISCELLANEOUS	antispasmodics (Belladonna, etc.)
Withdrawal from addiction to alcohol, sedatives, hypnotics	antiparkinsonian anticholinergics
Post-operative state (particularly cardiac surgery)	Corticosteroids
Intensive care unit syndrome	

sence of an organic cause, history of past psychiatric illness, and the pattern of onset of the present illness episode are helpful in differential diagnosis. Furthermore, signs and symptoms of delirium are typically shifting, poorly systematized and accompanied by fluctuations in level of awareness and impaired memory and orientation. The electroencephalogram often demonstrates generalized slowing of background activity in delirium, a finding not present in psychotic disorders. Differentiating dementia from delirium is usually straightforward, but delirium can be superimposed upon a pre-existing dementia even if only for a period of hours, and the clinical picture may be confusing. Furthermore the elderly patient with dementia is at increased risk for the development of delirium from any of a number of causes.

The treatment of the delirious patient must be based on the treatment of the underlying disorder. Frequently, however, symptomatic treatment is necessary especially if agitation, anxiety, perceptual distortions, delusions, or other behavioral features are interfering with diagnostic evaluation or treatment of the underlying disorder, or are endangering the patient's safety. Mild agitation and anxiety sometimes respond to reassurance, especially from a family member, a nurse regularly caring for the patient, or a physician whose role is clear to the patient. Structuring the environment so as to provide constancy of stimulation at a moderately low level (but not so low as to cause sensory depriviation) is also helpful. A night light can make a major difference in some patients whose delirium is exacerbated by darkness. The importance of a physically secure and carefully monitored environment cannot be overemphasized.

Although psychotropic medication should be avoided if possible, agitation, severe anxiety, insomnia, hallucinations, and delusions often necessitate pharamocologic intervention. If the delirium is secondary to withdrawal from central nervous system depressant drugs such as alcohol, barbiturates, or benzodiazepines, treatment with a sedative/hypnotic suppressant drug is indicated. The clinician may use a medium duration barbiturate such as pentobarbital or secobarbital, a benzodiazepine such as chlordiazepoxide, or paraldehyde. Dosage must be titrated for the individual patient. Treatment with these agents is most effective if started before delirium has progressed to an advanced stage. If delusions and/or hallucinations are prominent, careful use of an antipsychotic medication is indicated. In delirium not secondary to withdrawal from depressant drugs, antipsychotic medications are the treatment of choice. The antipsychotic medications with lowest anticholinergic activity and those least likely to cause seizures or hypotension are preferable. Haloperidol given p.o. or IM in 1 mg or 2 mg doses 2 to 4 times a day has proved effective. The goal of using psychotropic medication in delirium is to control symptoms without adding to disturbed brain function with sedative or anticholinergic drug effects.

AMNESTIC SYNDROME

The essential feature of this disorder is a disturbance in short-term memory but not in immediate recall in a patient who is neither delirious nor demented. Impairment in short-term memory implies that the individual is either unable to consolidate memory into permanent memory storage or cannot retrieve memory from storage. New information cannot be retained for more than a brief interval and new memories cannot be laid down. DSM-III chooses an arbitrary time of 25 minutes as the criterion for transfer of information from immediate memory into memory storage. Associated features include some impairment in remote memory and some degree of disorientation. Associated symptoms such as lack of initiative, and emotional blandness may occur. Confabulation; i.e. filling memory gaps with inventive stories is variably present.

The most common type of amnestic syndrome is Korsakov's psychosis, an amnestic syndrome secondary to thiamine deficiency, most commonly in alcoholics. This disorder almost always follows one or more episodes of Wernicke's encephalopathy, and pathologically involves the diencephalon and medial temporal lobes. Causes of the amnestic syndrome include anoxic encephalopathy, cerebral infarction, and encephalitis.

The amnestic syndrome is differentiated from dementia in DSM-III, although given the nonmemory intellectual impairments noted in at least Korsakov's psychosis, this differentiation is one of degree. Factitious illness may be confused with the amnestic syndrome, but careful memory testing will point toward the correct diagnosis.

Although often believed an irreversible and untreatable disorder, a careful study of patients with Korsakov's psychosis has demonstrated that treatment results are often good. Treatment consists of long-term abstinence from alcohol, and parenteral thiamine during the acute episode of Wernicke's encephalopathy and/or upon admission to hospital after a bout of excessive drinking. Approximately 25% of patients with Korsakov's psychosis recover fully, and another 25% recover to a significant degree.[104] The time course of recovery is highly variable, ranging from weeks to years.

ORGANIC AFFECTIVE SYNDROME

The essential feature is a disturbance of mood resembling a depressive or a manic episode. This syndrome can be attributed to a clearly defined organic factor and does not meet criteria for delirium or dementia. The depressed type of organic affective syndrome is far more common than the manic type. The possible etiologic factors of the organic affective syndrome overlap those for delirium, and both syndromes may coexist in a specific patient. Causes of the organic affective syndrome, depressed type, are listed in Table 13-3. Hypothyroidism frequently causes a depressive syndrome, and the thyroid function of depressed older persons should be routinely evaluated, especially in patients with previous thyroid surgery, thryoid irradiation, or those on maintenance lithium therapy. Cushing's syndrome is also associated with depression although a manic syndrome can also occur. Hypoparathyroidism with hypercalcemia classically presents with features of retarded depression, as do many other medical illnesses causing hypercalcemia. Drugs used to

Table 13-3. Etiologies of Organic Affective Disorder, Depressed.

SYSTEMIC ILLNESS	NEUROLOGIC DISORDERS
Congestive heart failure	Parkinson's disease
Pulmonary insufficiency	Intracranial mass lesion
Renal insufficiency	Huntington's chorea
Hepatic insufficiency	
Lupus erythematosus	**TOXIC**
Acute intermittent porphyria	Reserpine
Viral infection	Alpha methyldopa
Pancreatic carcinoma	Clonidine
	Propranolol
METABOLIC DISORDER	Bromide
Hypothyroidism	Ethanol
Hyperadrenalcorticism	Barbiturates
Hypokalemia	Diazepam
Hypercalcemia	Glucocorticoids
Pernicious anemia	Digitalis
Acute intermittent porphyria	

treat hypertension are particularly prone to cause a depressive syndrome. Reserpine has long been known to precipitate depression in older persons, particularly those with a previous history of primary depression. Although reserpine induced depression was more common in the era of high-dose reserpine therapy, even low-dose reserpine can precipitate depression in a susceptible individual. Depression secondary to alpha methyl dopa, Clonidine, and more recently propranolol[105] has also been reported. Although diuretics such as the thiazides and furosemide do not in themselves affect mood, secondary hypokalemia can present as depression. Alcohol commonly precipitates a depression in heavy drinkers, particularly toward the end of a binge drinking episode. The barbiturates, benzodiazepines, and the other sedative/hypnotic agents have also been implicated. The antipsychotic agents occasionally precipitate depressive signs and symptoms. This phenomenon is particularly common in patients treated with depot prolixin preparations.[106]

Treatment of the organic affective syndrome is directed toward correcting the underlying medical disorder or by removing the causative toxic agent. Sometimes, of course, this is not possible. In other cases the depression will persist despite removal of the offending agent or what appears to be adequate treatment of the underlying disorder. This problem is common in depression associated with Parkinson's disease or other neurologic disorders. In such cases treatment with one of the tricyclic antidepressants is sometimes effective. These drugs have been demonstrated to improve both mood and motor function in Parkinson's disease.[107,108]

The manic type of affective syndrome is far less common than the depressive type. Hyperthyroidism may present as a hypomanic or even manic syndrome as can hyperadrenocorticalism either from Cushing's disease or from the administration of exogenous steroids. Excessive use of the psychostimulant drugs such as the amphetamines, methylphenidate, or magnesium pemoline can produce hypomanic or rarely manic features. Delirium from anticholinergic drugs may have a strong manic component. Levodopa may also precipitate a manic syndrome. Treatment of the underlying cause of the manic organic affective syndrome is almost always effective in terminating the affective disturbance, and lithium therapy is rarely necessary. If manic symptoms present a short-term management problem, an antipsychotic agent such as chlorpromazine or haloperidol may be used.

REFERENCES

1. Kay, D. W. K., Beamish, P. and Roth, M. Old age mental disorders in Newcastle upon Tyne. *Br. J. Psychiat.* **110:** 146–518 (1964).
2. Kay, D. W. K. Epidemiological aspects of organic brain disease in the aged. In C. M. Gaitz (ed.) *Aging and the Brain.* New York: Plenum Press, pp. 15–27, 1972.
3. Slater, E. and Roth, M. (eds.) *Clinical Psychiatry,* 3rd Ed. Baltimore: Williams and Wilkins, p. 545, 1969.
4. The Task Force on Nomenclature and Statistics of the American Psychiatric Association, *Diagnostic and Statistical Manual of Mental Disorders, 3rd. Ed.* Washington D.C.: American Psychiatric Association, 1978.
5. The Committee on Nomenclature and Statistics of the American Psychiatric Association, *Diagnostic and Statistical Manual of Mental Disorders, 2nd Ed.* Washington, D.C.: American Psychiatric Association, 1968.
6. Raskind, M. A. and Eisdorfer, C. Psychopharmacology of the aged. In L. L. Simpson (ed.) *Drug Treatment of Mental Disorders.* New York: Raven Press, pp. 237–266.
7. Lipowski, A. J. Organic brain syndrome: Overview and classification. In Benson, D. Frank, and Blumer, Dietrich (eds.) *Psychiatric Aspects of Neurological Disease.* New York: Grune & Stratton, pp. 11–35, 1975.
8. Post, F. The outcome of mental breakdown in old age. *Br. Med. J.* **1:** 436–448 (1951).
9. Zubin, J. and Fleiss, J. Current biometric approaches to depression. In R. R. Fieve (ed.) *Depression in the 1970's: Modern Theory and Research.* The Hague: Excerpta Medica, pp. 7–21, 1971.
10. Teasdale, J. E. and Beaumont, J. G. The effect of mood on performance on the Modified New Word Learning Test (Walton-Black). *Br. J. Soc. Clin. Psychol.* **10:** 342–345 (1971).

11. Post, F. Dementia, depression, and pseudodementia. In D. Frank Benson and Dietrich Blumer, (eds.) *Psychiatric Aspects of Neurologic Disease.* New York: Grune & Stratton, pp. 99-120, 1975.

12. Post, F. The management and nature of depressive illnesses in late life: A follow-through study. *Br. J. Psychiat.* 121: 393-404 (1972).

13. Katzman, R. The prevalence and malignancy of Alzheimer disease: A major killer. *Arch. Neurol.* 33: 217-18 (1976).

14. Terry, R. D. Dementia: A brief and selective review. *Arch. Neurol.* 33: 1-2 (1976).

15. Tomlinson, B. E. The pathology of dementia. In Charles Wells (ed.) *Dementia, 2nd Ed.* Philadelphia: F. A. Davis, pp. 113-153, 1977.

16. Roth, Martin. Classification and aetiology in mental disorders of old age: Some recent developments. In D. W. K Kay (ed.) *Recent Developments in Geriatrics.* London: British Journal of Psychiatry, pp. 2-18, 1970.

17. Tomlinson, B. E. Morphological changes and dementia in old age. In W. Lynn Smith and Marcel Kinsbourne, (eds.) *Aging and Dementia.* New York: Spectrum Publications, pp. 25-56, 1977.

18. Corsellis, J. A. N. Observations on the neuropathology of dementia. *Age and Ageing* 6 (Suppl): 20-29 (1977).

19. Roth, M. The natural history of mental disorder in old age. *J. Ment. Science* 101: 281-301 (1955).

20. Kay, D. W. K. Outcome and cause of death in mental disorders of old age: A long-term follow-up of functional and organic psychoses. *Acta Psychiat. Scand* 38: 249-276 (1962).

21. Peck, A., Wolloch, M. A. and Rodstein, M. Mortality of the aged with chronic brain syndrome: Further observations in a five-year study. *J. Am. Geriatr. Soc.* 26: 170-176 (1978).

22. Kay, D. W. K., Bergman, K., Foster, E. M. *et al.* Mental illness and hospital usage in the elderly: A random sample followed up. *Comp. Psychiatry.* 11: 26-35 (1970).

23. Gilmore, A. Brain failure at home. *Age and Ageing* 6: 56-60 (1977).

24. Gajdusek, D. C., and Gibbs, C. J., Jr. Slow virus infections of the nervous system. In D. B. Tower (ed.) *The Nervous System, Vol II.* New York: Raven Press, pp. 113-135, 1975.

25. Terry, R. D. and Wisniewski, H. M. Structural and chemical changes of the aged human brain. In Gershon, Samuel, and Raskin, Allen (eds.) *Aging: Genesis and Treatment of Psychologic Disorders in the Elderly,* Vol, II. New York: Raven Press, pp. 127-141, 1975.

26. Hachinski, V. C., Lassen, N. A. and Marshall, J. Multi-infarct dementia: A cause of mental deterioration in the elderly. *Lancet* II: 207-209 (1974).

27. Jackson, G., Mahon, W., Pierscianowshi, T. A. *et al.*: Inappropriate antihypertensive therapy in the elderly. *Lancet* II: 1317-1318 (1976).

28. Graham, D. I. Ischaemic brain damage of cerebral perfusion failure type after treatment of severe hypertension. *Br. Med. J.* 4: 739 (1975).

29. Sweet, R. D., McDowell, F. H., Fiegenson, J. S. *et al.*: Mental symptoms in Parkinson's disease during chronic treatment with levodopa. *Neurology* 26(4): 305-310 (1976)

30. Loranger, A. W., Goodell, H., Lee, J., *et al.* Levodopa treatment of Parkinson's syndrome: Improved intellectual functioning. *Arch. Gen. Psychiatry* 26: 163-168 (1972).

31. Loranger, A. W., Goodell, H., McDowell, F. H., *et al.* Parkinsonism, L-dopa and intelligence. *Am. J. Psychiatry* 130: 1386-1389 (1973).

32. Gibbs, C. J., Gajdusek, D. C., and Asher, D. M. Creutzfeldt-Jacob disease (spongiform encephalopathy): Transmission to the chimpanzee. *Science* 161: 388-389 (1968).

33. Adams, R. D., Fisher, C. M. and Hakim, S. Symptomatic occult hydrocephalus with "normal" cerebrospinal fluid pressure: A treatable syndrome. *N. Eng. J. Med.* 273: 117-126 (1965).

34. Katzman, R. Normal pressure hydrocephalus. In C. E. Wells (ed.) *Dementia,* 2nd Ed.. Philadelphia: F. A. Davis pp. 69-92, 1977.

35. Chandrasekaran, S. and Reynolds, R. E. Occult hydrocephalus in the elderly. *J. Am. Geriatr. Soc.* 18: 481 (1970).

36. Whybrow, R. A. and Wilson, R. A. Mental changes accompanying thyroid gland dysfunction. *Arch. Gen. Psychiat.* 20: 48-65 (1969).

37. Strachan, R. W. and Henderson, J. G. Psychiatric syndromes due to avitaminosis B_{12} with normal blood and bone marrow. *Quart. J. Med.* 34: 303-309 (1965).

38. Reynolds, E. H., Rothfield, P., and Pincus, J. H. Neurological disease associated with folate deficiency. *Br. Med. J.* 2: 398-400 (1973).

39. Sneath, P., Chanarin, I., Hodkinson, R. M. *et al.* Folate status in a geriatric population and its relation to dementia. *Age and Ageing* 2: 177-181 (1973).

40. Eisdorfer, C. and Raskind, M. A. Aging, hormones and human behavior. In B. Eleftheriou, and R. Sprott (eds.) *Hormonal Correlates of Behavior: Vol. I: A Lifespan View.* New York: Plenum Press, pp. 369-394, 1975.

41. Laforet, E. G., Sidd, J. J. and Waterman, W. E. The relationship of heart rate to mood in patients with heart block: Effect of pacing. *J. Gerontol.* 29(6): 643-644 (1974).

42. Raskind, M. A. and Eisdorfer, C. Screening for syphilis in an aged psychiatrically impaired population. *West. J. Med.* 125: 361-363 (1976).

43. Raskind, M. A., Kitchell, M. and Alvarez, C. Bromide intoxication in elderly. *J. Am. Geriatr. Soc.* 26: 222-224 (1978).

44. Marsden, C. D. and Harrison, M. J. G. Outcome of investigation of patients with presenile dementia. *Br. Med. J.* 2: 249-252 (1972).

45. Fox, J. H., Topel, J. L. and Huckman, M. S. Dementia in the elderly—a search for treatable illnesses. *J. Gerontol.* **30(5):** 557–564 (1975).

46. Freeman, F. R. Evaluation of patients with progressive intellectual deterioration. *Arch. Neurol.* **33:** 658–659 (1976).

47. Victoratos, G. C., Lenman, J. A. R. and Herzberg, L. Neurological investigation of dementia. *Br. J. Psychiat.* **130:** 131–3 (1977).

48. Wells, C. E. and Buchanan, D. C. The clinical use of psychological testing in evaluation for dementia. In: Charles E. Wells (ed.) *Dementia.* Philadelphia: F. A. Davis, pp. 189–204, 1977.

49. Wells, C. Chronic brain disease: An overview. *Am. J. Psychiat.* **135:** 1–11 (1978).

50. Pfeiffer, E. A Short Portable Mental Status Questionnaire for the assessment of organic brain deficit in elderly patients. *J. Am. Geriatr. Soc.* **23:** 433–441 (1975).

51. Kahn, R. L., Goldfarb, A. I., Pollack M. *et al.* Brief objective measures for the determination of mental status in the aged. *Am. J. Psychiat.* **117:** 326 (1960).

52. Haglund, R. M., and Schuckit, M. A. A clinical comparison of tests of organicity in elderly patients. *J. Gerontol.* **31:** 654–659 (1976).

53. Folstein, M. F., Folstein, S. E. and McHugh, P. R. "Mini-Mental State": A practical method for grading the cognitive state of patients for the clinician. *J. Psychiat. Res.* **12:** 189–198 (1975).

54. Jacobs, J. W., Bernhard, M. R., Delgado, A. and Strain, J. J. Screening for organic mental syndromes in the medically ill. *Ann. Int. Med.* **86:** 40–46 (1977).

55. Shader, R. I., Harmatz, J. S. and Salzman, C. A new scale for clinical assessment in geriatric populations: Sandoz Clinical Assessment—Geriatric (SCAG). *J. Am. Geriatr. Soc.* **22(3):** 107–113 (1974).

56. Plutchik, R., Conte, H., Lieverman, M. *et al.* Reliability and validity of a scale for assessing the functioning of geriatric patients. *J. Am. Geriatr. Soc.* **18(6):** 491–498 (1970)

57. Blessed, G., Tomlinson, B. E. and Roth, M. The association between quantitative measures of dementia and of senile change in the cerebral gray matter of elderly subjects. *Brit. J. Psychiat.* **114:** 797–811 (1968).

58. Doppelt, H. E. and Wallace, W. L. Standardization of the Wechsler Adult Intelligence Scale for Older Persons. *J. Abnorm. and Soc. Psychol.* **51:** 371–381 (1955).

59. Filskov, S. B. and Goldstein, S. G. Diagnostic validity of the Halstead-Reitan neuropsychological battery. J. Consult. Clin. Psychol. **42:** 382–390 (1974).

60. Perez, F. J. Neuropsychological aspects of Alzheimer's Disease and multi-infarct dementia. Presented at "Biomedical Aspects of Senile Dementia and Related Disorders," March 22–23, St. Louis, Missouri, 1978.

61. Ferris, S., Crook, T., Sathananthan, G. *et al.* Reaction time as a diagnostic measure in senility. *J. Am. Geriatr. Soc.* **24:** 529–533 (1976).

62. Tsuang, M. M., Lu, L. M., Stotsky, B. A. and Cole, J. O. Haloperidol vs thioridazine for hospitalized geriatric patients: Double-blind study. *J. Am. Geriatr. Soc.* **19:** 593–600 (1971).

63. Seager, C. P. Chlorpromazine in treatment of elderly psychotic woman. *Br. Med. J.* **1:** 882–884 (1955).

64. Sugarman, A. A., Williams, B. H. and Adlerstein, M. A. Haloperidol in the psychiatric disorders of old age. *Am. J. Psychiat.* **120:** 1190–1192 (1964).

65. Robinson, D. B. Evaluation of certain drugs in geriatric patients. *Arch. Gen. Psychiat.* **1:** 41–46 (1959).

66. Altman, H., Mehta, D., Evenson, R. and Sletten, I. W. Behavioral effects of drug therapy on psychogeriatric patients. I. Chlorpromazine and thioridazine. *J. Am. Geriatr. Soc.* **21:** 241–248 (1973a).

67. Barton, R. and Hurst, L. Unnecessary use of tranquilizers in elderly patients. *Br. J. Psychiat.* **112:** 989–990 (1966).

68. Snyder, S., Greenberg, D. and Yamamura, H. I. Antischizophrenic drugs and brain cholinergic receptors. *Arch. Gen. Psychiat.* **31:** 58–61 (1974).

69. Bielski, R. J. and Friedel, R. O. Prediction of tricyclic antidepressant response. *Arch. Gen. Psychiat.* **33:** 1479–1489 (1976).

70. De Alarcon, R. Hypochondriasis and depression in the aged. *Gerontol. Clin.* **6:** 266–277 (1964).

71. Coull, D. C., Crooks, J., Dingwall-Fordyce, I. *et al.* A method of monitoring drugs for adverse reactions: II. Amitriptyline and cardiac disease. *Europ. J. clin. Pharmacol.* **3:** 51–55, 1970.

72. Petit, J. M., Spiker, D. G. and Biggs, J. T. Psychiatric diagnosis and tricyclic plasma levels in 35 hospitalized overdose patients. *J. Nerv. Ment. Dis.* **163:** 289–293 (1976).

73. Kiev, A. Double-blind comparison of thiothixene and protriptyline in psychotic depression. *Dis. Nerv. Syst.* **33:** 811–816 (1972).

74. Hollister, L. E. and Overall, J. E. Reflections on the specificity of action of antidepressants. *Psychosomatics* **6:** 361–365 (1965).

75. Kaplitz, S. E. Withdrawn, apathetic geriatric patients responsive to methylphenidate. *J. Am. Geriatr. Soc.* **23(6):** 271–276 (1975).

76. Prinz, P. and Raskind, M. A. Aging and sleep disorders. In R. Williams, and I. Karacan, (eds.) *Sleep Disorders.* New York: Wiley and Sons (in press).

77. Meier-Ruge, W., Engz, A., Gygax, P., Huntziker, O., *et al.* Experimental pathology in basic research of the aging brain. In Samuel Gershon, and Allen Raskin (eds.) *Aging: Genesis and Treatment of Psychologic Disorders in the Elderly,* Vol. II. New York: Raven Press, pp. 55–126, 1975.

78. Gaitz, C. M., Varner, R. V. and Overall, J. E.

Pharmacotherapy for organic brain syndrome in late life. *Arch. Gen. Psychiat.* **34**: 839–845 (1977).

79. Brannconnier, R. J. and Cole, J. O. Effects of chronic paparverine administration on mild senile organic brain syndrome. *J. Am. Geriatr. Soc.* **25**: 458–462 (1977).

80. Davies, G., Hamilton, S., Hendrickson, E., *et al.* The effects of cyclandelate in depressed and demented patients: A controlled study in psychogeriatric patients. *Age and Ageing* **6**: 156–162 (1977).

80a. Walsh, A. C., Walsh, B. H. Presenile dementia: Further experience with an anticoagulant-psychotherapy regimen. *J. Am. Geriatric. Soc.,* **22**: 467, (1974).

81. Jacobs, E. A., Alvis, H. J. and Small, S. M. Hyperoxygenation: A central nervous system activator? *J. Geriatr. Psychiat.* **5**: 107–121 (1972).

82. Goldfarb, A. I., Hochstadt, N., Jacobson, J. H. *et al.* Hyperbaric oxygen treatment of organic mental syndrome in aged persons. *J. Gerontol.* **27**: 212–217 (1972).

83. Thompson, L. W. Effects of hyperbaric oxygen on behavioral functioning in elderly persons with intellectual impairment. In S. Gershon, and A. Raskind (eds.) *Aging,* Vol. II. New York: Raven Press, pp. 169–177, 1975.

84. Ostfeld, A., Smith, C. M. and Stotsky, B. A. The systemic use of procaine in the treatment of the elderly: A review. *J. Amer. Geriatr. Soc.* **25(1)**: 1–19 (1977).

85. Jarvik, L. F. and Milne, J. F. Gerovital-H3: A review of the literature. In Samuel Gershon and Allen Raskin (eds.) *Aging: Genesis and Treatment of Psychologic Disorders in the Elderly,* Vol. II. New York: Raven Press, pp. 203–227, 1975.

86. Davies, P. and Maloney, A. J. F. Selective loss of central cholinergic neurons. *Lancet* **II**: 1403 (1976).

87. Perry, E. K., Gibson, P. H., Blessed, G., Perry, R. H. and Tomlinson, B. E. Neurotransmitter enzyme abnormalities in senile dementia. *J. Neurol. Sci.* **34(2)**: 247–265 (1977).

88. White, P., Goodhardt, M. J., Keet, J. P. *et al.* Neocortical cholinergic neurons in elderly people. *Lancet* **I**: 668–670 (1977).

89. Ferris, S., Sathananthan, G., Gershon, S. *et al.:* Senile dementia: treatment with deanol. *J. Am. Geriatr. Soc.* **25**: 241–244 (1977).

90. de Wied, D., Bohus, B., Gispen, W. H. *et al.* Hormonal influences on motivational, learning, and memory processes. In Edward J. Sachar (ed.) *Hormones, Behavior, and Psychopathology.* New York: Raven Press, pp. 1–14, 1976.

91. Legros, J. J., Gilot, P., Seron, X. *et al.* Influence of vasopressin on learning and memory. *Lancet* **I**: 41–42 (1978).

92. Oliveros, J. D., Jandali, M. K., Timsit-Berthier, M. *et al.* Vasopressin in amnesia. *Lancet* **I**: 42 (1978).

92a. Adolfssen, R., Gottfries, C. G., Winbald, B. Substitution therapy with L-dopa and dopamine against in-dopamine disorders of Alzheimer type. Paper presented at XIth International Congress of Gerontology, Tokyo, Japan, August, 1978.

93. Taulbee, L. and Folsom, J. C. Reality orientation for geriatric patients. *Hosp. Community Psychiatry* **175**: 135–137 (1966).

94. Brook, P., Degun, G. and Mather, M. Reality orientation, a therapy for psychogeriatric patients: A controlled study. *Brit. J. Psychiat.* **127**: 42–45 (1975).

95. Citrin, R. S. and Dixon, D. N. Reality orientation: A milieu therapy used in an institution for the aged. *Gerontologist* **17(1)**: 39–44 (1977).

96. Harris, C. S. and Ivory, P. B. C. An outcome evaluation of reality orientation therapy with geriatric patients in a state mental hospital. *Gerontologist* **16(6)**: 494–503 (1976).

97. Barnes, E. K. Effects of reality orientation classroom on memory loss, confusion and disorientation in geriatric patients. *Gerontologist* **14**: 138–144 (1974).

98. MacDonald, M. L. and Settin, J. M. Reality orientation versus sheltered workshops as treatment for the institutionalized aging. *J. Gerontol.* **33(3)**: 416–21 (1978).

99. Dennis, H. Remotivation therapy for the elderly, a surprising outcome. Paper presented at Gerontological Society 30th Annual Scientific Meeting, San Francisco, California, 1977.

100. Burnside, I. M. (ed.) *Working with the Elderly: Group Processes and Techniques.* Duxbury Press: North Scituate, Mass., 1978.

101. Brody, E. M., Kleban, M. H., Lawton, M. P. *et al.* Excess disabilities of mentally impaired aged. Impact of individualized treatment. *Gerontologist:* Summer: Part 1: 124–133 (1971).

102. Kleban, M. H., Lawton, M. P., Brody, E. M. *et al.* Characteristics of mentally impaired aged profiting from individualized treatment. *J. Gerontol.* **30(1)**: 90–96 (1975).

103. Coons, D. Milieu therapy (the social-psychological aspects of treatment). In William Reichel, (ed.) *Clinical Aspects of Aging.* Baltimore: William and Wilkins, pp. 115–127, 1978.

104. Victor, M., Adams, R. D. and Collins, G. H. *The Wernicke-Korsakoff Syndrome.* Philadelphia: F. A. Davis, 1971.

105. Waal, H. J. Propranolol-induced depression. *Br. Med. J.* **2**: 50 (1967).

106. Alarcon, R. and Carney, M. W. P. Severe depressive mood changes following slow release intramuscular fluphenazine injection. *Br. Med. J.* **3**: 564–567 (1969).

Chapter 14
Paranoia and Schizophrenic Disorders in Later Life

Carl Eisdorfer, Ph.D., M.D.

University of Washington

INTRODUCTION

Among the variety of symptoms exhibited by older persons in cognitive and emotional distress, paranoia as it involves suspiciousness and persecutory ideation, is among the most disturbing, not only to friends and relatives, but also to those professionals charged with the responsibility for the patient's care.[1] Paranoid symptoms may range from mild querulousness to an unswerving conviction in the reality of a delusional system. Unfortunately the empirical data on paranoid symptomatology and course is remarkably sparse for so disquieting a problem.

In clinical settings paranoia in the elderly is often identified as a symptom of dementia. In rarer instances, in association with the other signs of the disorder, it may also be seen as the manifestation of a late onset schizophrenia. Most often perhaps it is observed among the aged as a symptom cluster in its own right with varying degrees of intensity.

The variations in onset and course, as well as the prognosis and tractability of symp-

toms of suspiciousness and paranoia in the aged warrant a closer inspection of their distinguishing features. There is a range of clinical patterns involving paranoia which require delineation for a useful differential diagnosis. Since the data base remains sparse, particularly in the United States, some of the speculative discussion in this paper should be considered as proposals for empirical clinical investigation rather than as confirmed scientific data.

BACKGROUND

The prevalence of paranoid behavior among the aged is not well documented in the United States, although clinicians working with older people indicate that it is a frequent occurrence.[2] Fiske-Lowenthal[3] and her colleagues have reported that in their sample of psychiatrically impaired elderly living in San Francisco, 17% exhibited the symptoms of "suspiciousness" at least to some degree. Kay and Roth[4] studied a group of patients from Great Britain and Stockholm whom they diagnosed as late paraphrenia. These (99) patients represented 10% of the admissions of all (psychotic) patients aged 60 or older from hospitals involved in the study. Kay[5] has also estimated that about 4% of all schizophrenic illness in males and 14% in females occurs after age 65. This accounted for 5–6% of all first admissions in Britain of patients with psychoses (in 1966). Fish[6] reports that 9.4% of all inpatient admissions aged 60 or older to four hospitals in Edinburgh (in 1957) showed paranoid ideation. Schizophrenia and organic psychosis accounted for the great majority of the admissions, but a quarter to a third of late onset paranoia was not related to either diagnosis.

While the epidemiologic data identify paranoia as a problem of considerable magnitude, they also point up the difficulties associated with the lack of clarity or precision in the diagnosis. The scaling of a subjective behavioral variable such as paranoia or suspiciousness is a particularly complex diagnostic problem because it has such a broad scope and may be regarded as a symptom cluster rather than a unitary behavioral sign. The examiner must determine the pervasive scope of the symptom focus, i.e., is it a relatively minor suspicion in the life of the patient with the content limited to suspected theft or rearrangement of property, or does the "victim" believe that there is a widespread pattern of interference involving major alterations in the environment and/or affecting his or her bodily organs. Are there outside forces or agents (e.g., the FBI, CIA, foreign governments) operating in some conspiratorial or malevolent manner, or supernatural beings—the devil—involved? It may also be quite important to establish the individual's perception and belief in how powerful the distortion and malevolence are and what they believe is the consequence of what is going on about them. A belief can be upsetting and socially irritating, or so threatening to one's being that the individual is found in a rather profound social crisis.[7] It is necessary to explore whether the victim feels compelled to some action and whether hallucinations are present and if so, the form they take, i.e. are they voices only or are odors, visions and other sensory events prominent?

For the purpose of this report we will distinguish (more or less arbitrarily) between four degrees of intensity of paranoid ideation. These are:
(1) suspiciousness; (2) transitional paranoid reaction; (3) paraphrenia (late onset paranoia without other evidence of schizophrenic illness); and (4) paranoia associated with schizophrenia of late onset. The last two will be discussed together in this report.

SUSPICIOUSNESS

It is highly probable that most older persons with heightened suspiciousness never see a mental health professional. Although the data here are not directly the product of investigating the epidemiology of paranoia in the community, the work of Lowenthal and her colleagues[3] and the epidemiologic report of Kramer and his associates[8] would appear to support this contention. A paper by Savage and his colleagues[9] reported that 11% of their aged community sample were felt to be "perturbed" in view of their pattern of answers to items on the paranoia scale.

The suspicious patient is one who has vague complaints about external forces controlling his/her life. These beliefs may be generalized, may become more focal with one or a limited number of targets developing. Such targets may, to some degree, have some peer group social sanction, e.g., landlords, bosses, nursing aides (particularly when the individual is of a different racial or ethnic background from the patient), but they may also relate to someone close to the individual, e.g. a grandchild (making noise to disturb the individual), or a son- or daughter-in-law (who wishes they were living elsewhere and speaks to them in hostile tones). Generalized feelings of desertion (by God), of being abused by the younger generation, by the government, or by negative outside forces may also play a prominent role in the life of the individual for whom suspiciousness is a conspicuous trait. In such instances the symptoms are poorly formed, troublesome rather than disabling, do not involve the body or "mind," are not accompanied by disturbed reality, i.e. hallucinations, and do not involve outside organizations in any systematic pattern of behavior.

There are a number of possible bases underlying suspiciousness as a pattern.[10,11] For some individuals suspiciousness is a lifelong (personality) style which becomes exaggerated as a result of situational changes in his/her later years. It has been proposed that a precondition which disposes older individuals to heightened suspiciousness includes a long-standing propensity for using the psychological defense mechanism of projection.[2] Since projection is among the earlier defense mechanisms, its presence among persons of all ages is not unusual. It is clear that for most individuals, however, aging is associated with a variety of traumatic changes involving loss, and that such losses involve psychosocial as well as physical factors. Such losses may include specific or nonspecific somatic alterations, leading, in turn, to a range of perceived changes in functional capacities, as well as increased medical problems in the older person. Of particular importance in this regard is the loss of perceptual ability, hearing in particular, and poorer cognitive capacity with associated attentional and mnemonic deficits.[12] Other losses may involve interpersonal contacts, often through change in occupational roles, or as a result of retirement, loss of friends (secondary to relocation, retirement and/or death), loss of loved ones, (e.g. spouse); loss of income; loss of access to one's children (secondary to their moving away). These may all contribute to a heightening of anxiety and paranoid ideation.

What characterizes many of these losses is that they are not under the control of the individual; furthermore, in some instances they are so subtle in their development as to be imperceptible to the victim (at least for some time). Thus while some traumata are readily apparent, e.g. loss of a friend, relative, etc., other losses and their early impact may be subliminal and gradual. Some physical, auditory and even economic changes (which may develop through inflation) are quite insidious as they diminish the capacity of the individual to be independent and lead inexorably to a progressive loss of control over the environment.

It is not at all improbable that this progression of losses challenging the person's mastery over the world may lead to a search for some explanation to account for the loss(es). In the absence of clear targets, and given certain predispositions in character structure, individuals often resort to the mystical, or regress to primitive interpretations of their world in a reasonable effort to reduce the ambiguity of the unknown.[13] Thus the etiology of one's problems could well reside in the machination of some outside person, group of persons, or force(s) and consequently there is good reason to be on guard and suspicious of others.

In a recent reformulation of the Learned Helplessness model of depression, Abrahamson, Seligman and Teasdale,[13] have employed an attribution theory approach which may be as appropriate to paranoid ideation as to depression. In the face of a significant loss of control, individuals find a causal agent to which they can attribute that loss. Such attributional mechanisms may be personalized as in depression, externalized where environmental cues and checks are possible, or they may be dysfunctional in the case of unusual sensory (e.g. somatic) or cognitive experiences. Sparacino[15] stresses the value of an attributional approach in dealing with the aged since their interpersonal losses lead to impaired use of social concensus, a major factor in causal attribution. Thus, according to Sparacino[15] anomalous events may "be accounted for through bizarre or delusional explanatory systems." (p. 415)

While depression and depressive illness are frequent concomitants of traumatic loss, suspicion, particularly in early stages, may be an alternative or co-existing reaction to unexplained, unconsciously perceived or progressively subtle losses. In this context the loss of sensory acuity, particularly auditory loss, has been associated with paranoia at many stages in the lifespan, including the aged.[12,16] Although supporting data are only suggestive, it has been proposed[16] that paranoid ideation is a frequent accompaniment of social hearing loss since the individual senses the impaired communication between himself/herself and others, and projects to others the basis for the difficulty. Since hearing loss is so much more frequent among the aged than among the young, suspiciousness verging on paranoia may indeed by anticipated with greater frequency among older persons. Less mature thinking and perception have also been associated with hearing loss among nonpsychiatrically labeled older men and this could serve as a framework for projection.[12]

It seems important for the clinician to keep in mind that the suspiciousness of the older person may not always be unrealistic, however. An evaluation of the reality of the situation being reported is a crucial factor always to be considered in the assessment of suspiciousness. Butler has suggested that there is a rather pervasive form of bias against the aged and the aging.[11] To the extent that "ageism" does exist, the aged individual may indeed perceive something akin to social discrimination, and suspicious behavior may be reactive. Thus certain suspicions may need to be examined for accuracy of the ideation prior to clinical assumptions as to the pathologic nature of the symptoms, e.g. that physicians are less likely to give them careful examination and treatment, that bank officials are reluctant to give them loans, that landlords would like to evict them in order to raise the rent, that children would like to spend less time with them, that nursing home staff or other patients are removing possessions, and that they are less likely to be employed. The accuracy or overgeneralization of these problems must inevitably become an issue for careful scrutiny by the examining clinician.

Clinical Management of Suspiciousness

Where an individual reports considerable concern about intrusion affecting his or her property, e.g. the inspection and rearrangement of closets, the suspicion of minor thefts, and even in the absence of hallucinations, somatic distortions or an organized plot specifically directed toward them (by some specified individual, group or agent of government), suspiciousness of clinical note may be present. The person said to be clinically suspicious reports events such as losses or intrusions for which there is no basis. Care should be taken to distinguish unwarranted suspicions from a realistic fear that individuals or groups will steal Social Security checks (in regions where this may be a genuine problem), or fear of assault on life and limb.

Where we find unwarranted suspiciousness it is clear that such a condition may become disabling, particularly over time, and thus require careful attention, including evaluation and the prompt initiation of treatment. The management of suspiciousness and paranoia is probably best treated by considering four intervention categories: (1) situational and environmental manipulations; (2) identification and replacement of loss; (3) observation; (4) psychopharmacologic strategies.

1. Mild suspiciousness is often a function of the physical and social context in which individuals find themselves. Frequently it is precipitated by percieved awareness of events and lack of control. Attempts to restore control and decision making to the individual, i.e., helping to regain mastery over his or her life, to the greatest extent possible, may be quite valuable. In institutional settings, greater decision-making activity on the part of the older person is often salutory. Thus opportunities to select and structure visiting hours, and access to information, are options that facilitate the gen-

eral restoration of dignity to the individual, so that once again they may "feel like real people" rather than identify themselves as inmates, clients or patients. Counseling with other members of the family may also be quite helpful for both the patient at home and the one in an institution.

2. Restoration and prevention of loss is an extremely important treatment approach. In the case of hearing loss, the use of appropriate hearing aids, in conjunction with individual discussions (counseling) as to the value of the hearing aid and early concern with the adaptation to the new quality of hearing, may be crucial in helping a person deal with this loss. Programs of exercise, physical fitness, alternative hobbies, occupations and the like may be similarly helpful. Here it is quite likely that the clinician will need the help of other professionals who may provide specialized help to the older patient and increase social interaction with the patient.

Loss of memory and attention are often associated with difficulty in locating (i.e. retrieving) objects and the suspicion of theft or belief that someone intentionally moved them. Specific help with organizing possessions and recognition on the part of members of the staff or family concerning the nature of the problem can be of help. The reduction in tension between the staff and a patient when the staff learns to accept and deal with the patient's accusations as related to his or her psychopathology rather than as a manifest attack on their own honesty can be quite salutary. It reduces the hostility and social isolation directed toward the patient and can involve the staff in a therapeutic strategy. The possibility of memory enhancement techniques should not be discarded (nor should the possibility that another individual inadvertently removed the object(s) for the sake of safety or good housekeeping be ignored).

3. Observation. Major environmental change, particularly when the change is associated with other psychological trauma, e.g., giving up one's home following the death of a spouse and shifting to a new environment, or being moved from one nursing home to another, may precipitate a problem. This phenomenon may be associated with paranoid beliefs, even in the young where culture shock and associated paranoid ideation are reported among young persons such as Peace Corps volunteers in reaction to a major environmental change.[32,33]

Suspiciousness may occur independently of other illnesses, but may be associated with dementia. It has been suggested that this pattern may be particularly characteristic of aged persons with domineering personalities who strive to deny their failing memories through projecting their problems to others. Careful differential diagnosis is therefore indicated.

Often supportive help and a willingness to observe the older person over a period of time without over concern can be of help. Counseling with the children (parent surrogate) may be helpful to alleviate their anxiety and reduce the pressure they are likely to bring to bear on the parent. This can also do much to defuse a potentially serious familial situation.

4. Psychopharmacology. Psychopharmacologic therapy is not indicated for the mildly suspicious patient. The use of antianxiety medications may be the most reasonable strategy for the more seriously upset individual, but this should be limited to a relatively brief period and used only in conjuction with other psychosocial strategies. Research on pharmacotherapeutic strategies for this condition is seriously lacking.

TRANSITIONAL PARANOID REACTION

Post[17] has described the condition of Paranoid Hallucinosis in which the individual may present with a relatively focal complaint. These complaints are often narrow and situational, but may nonetheless be quite disturbing both to the individual and to his/her environment. These reactions may be associated with frank hallucinations, both visual and auditory (primarily auditory), and may focus upon a relatively narrow problem, e.g., theft, interfering voices, perceived desire to get the patient to move from his/her domicile or to rearrange their personal possessions. The external locus is usually in relatively close proximity, e.g. next door, the landlord or the manager of the housing project. There is no evidence that the patient believes in the existence of an organized plot or where he or she overhears him or herself being referred to in the third person, or feels possessed by spirits or extraterrestrial forces.

A conspicuous feature of this pattern includes the social isolation of the individual, typically a woman, and the relatively narrow nature of the complaints, as well as their disturbing depth of intensity. Hearing difficulties or other impairments in communication may also be noted. The patient often has recently moved or been cut off from friends and neighbors. Interestingly enough, the paranoid syndrome exacerbates this problem. Post's[18] descriptions of "paranoid illness associated with sensory and cerebral defects" (Chapter 3, p. 112) largely fits this category. The paranoia associated with confusional states or other impairments in awareness may also be diagnosed as transient. Such individuals are markedly anxious in the face of persecutory feelings.

The treatment of such transient paranoia consists principally in intervening into the process creating the social and cognitive isolation of the individual. Relocation of the older person may be quite helpful. Restitution of a pattern of social communication which may require attention to auditory loss or social contact is often required. The symptom often disappears without further problem subsequent to such social intervention. Where delirium is secondary to some physical (e.g. metabolic) disruption, appropriate treatment is, of course, indicated.

Short-term psychopharmacologic treatment with antipsychotic medications in small doses may be helpful,[7,19] but is not indicated in the absence of the other intervention strategies.

PARAPHRENIA AND PARANOID SCHIZOPHRENIA

Roth[20] and Kay and Roth[21] distinguish paraphrenia from paranoid schizophrenia. They indicate that in the former condition paranoid delusion and hallucinations are prominent, but the more severe cognitive, affective and personality attributes of schizophrenia (including impairment of volition of the individual), are not present, nor does the deterioration which typifies schizophrenia occur. The distinction between paraphrenia, which has its onset in later adult life, and paranoid schizophrenia of late onset is unclear according to Post,[17] although late onset feelings of persecution with profound ideation components are usually readily determined. Post[18] recommends that in the absence of organic confusional or affective symptomatology, and where the persecutory beliefs are not transitory, that the term Functional Paranoid Psychoses be employed. This idea has considerable merit, but in later papers Post[17,22] changes his terminology to distinguish between paranoid hallucinosis (relatively mild and transient), schizphreniform illness and schizophrenia. Unfortunately the inconsistent terminology leads to some confusion, particularly in view of the current trend to redefine schizophrenic illness as process, or nuclear schizophreniform psychosis,[23] reactive psychosis,[24] and in terms of good and poor premorbidity.[25] A wide range of specialized terms is also used, e.g. conjugal paranoia, prison psychosis and the like,[26] further compounding the confusion. On the other hand, the distinction between the more inclusive and severe schizophrenic symptoms with onset in middle age and late onset often seems clear;[6,27] and separation of the two states, i.e., paraphrenia and paranoid schizophrenia, seems warranted at this time.

A 5-year follow-up of 42 patients (39 women and 3 men) aged 60 and over in Britain was combined with a study of the records of 57 patients (48 women and 9 men) in Stockholm in a study conducted by Kay and Roth.[21] All patients had been diagnosed as paraphrenic; the group in Britain had been seen between 1951 and 1955 (inclusive), the patients in Stockholm from 1931 to 1937.

In both hospitals these patients represented about 10% of those admitted over age 60, their mean age was 70 years, and women clearly outnumbered men. The onset of the disorder was always after age 55 (though this was undoubtedly influenced by the nature of the selection). In only one case, however, was there a hospital admission prior to the age of 60. Half of the women were unmarried and 40% of all patients were living alone. This was more than twice the rate found for persons with organic psychoses (16% of whom had been living alone, and over three times the rate found for affective illness, i.e. 12%). Clinical follow-up showed that these patients were indeed isolated socially as well as physically, that prognosis was poor for their psychological state although they showed no particular worsening of their disorder, no increased incidence of organic psychiatric disease and no shortening of life. The authors concluded that the disease represented an incomplete form of schizophrenia modified by age.

The usual physical health of these patients had been quite good, with the notable exception of hearing, which was impaired in 40% of the British patients. 15% had "marked" hearing loss. The Stockholm sample only recorded the more severe cases and these numbered 16% of their sample. Thus two variables, social isolation and hearing impairment, were quite prominent in this group.

Cooper and colleagues[28,16] investigated the role of deafness in paranoid disorders in a group of hospitalized patients. One hundred and thirty-two consecutive patients over age 50 diagnosed as either paranoid or affective psychosis with no prior history of psychiatric illness and no sign of dementia at the time of the diagnosis comprised the sample. Audiometric examinations were conducted and social deafness assayed in 111 of the 132 (54 paranoid and 54 affective). Those not examined were reported to be too ill, had refused, or died (but were reported not to differ in social characteristics from those studied).

Those diagnosed as manifesting paranoid illness showed, to a statistically significant extent, lower social class, greater likelihood of being divorced or separated, greater likelihood of living alone, and more social deafness. Depressed patients were more likely to have two or more living children, a family history of affective disorder in the first degree relatives, and the presence of a precipitating factor. The premorbid personality, while difficult to define precisely, was significantly correlated with paranoia.

In a subsequent evaluation of the deaf patients in this group, more patients were added. When the total of 69 paranoid and 68 affective disorders were obtained, 27 paranoid and 18 affectives were diagnosed as socially deaf by the authors.[27] Analysis of their data is reported as giving "limited support" to the contention that there is a psychosis associated with deafness and that it is of the paranoid rather than affective type. It was also suggested that those paranoid patients also suffering from deafness were perhaps less schizophrenic in personality than were the nondeaf. The possible additional problem of cataracts was cited, but the data are only suggestive.

Schizophrenia in the elderly nearly always is associated with a delusional system more or less well organized, and the presence of hallucinations. Prodromal signs, according to Kay,[5] usually follow a pattern of irritability, suspiciousness and seclusion, as well as odd behavior which may appear for months or even years before they become of professional concern.

In more severe illness delusional ideas of wide range may be elaborated and may vary from persecutory to grandiose. Frequently, however, landlords, nursing home staff and neighbors (i.e., persons in relatively close proximity) are implicated as interfering in one's life. Typically, however, they are organized into a delusional system and part of some delusional plot which may be quite widespread. While auditory hallucinations are most common, other modalities may be involved and affect is usually appropriate to the content of what is reported. Orientation and memory are typically unimpaired in the uncomplicated case. Post[29] reports on a sample of 93 patients with paranoid symptoms but no marked affective component. As indicated above in Post's schema,[22] late onset paranoia is divisible into three categories: (1) paranoid hallucinosis; (2) schizophreniform symptomatology; and (3) schizophrenic symptomatology.

Post[17] feels that older patients (with initial onset of schizophrenia) only manifest some of the Schneiderian first rank symptoms,[30] e.g., thought intrusions, depersonalization, experiences of influence and voices discussing him/her in the third person. In contrast to the other two forms of paranoid states for the schizophrenic patient, these processes do not disappear even in a protective environment, and continue indefinitely without treatment. Herbert and Jacobson[31] reported successful prognosis for their sample of paraphrenic women who received phenothiazine therapy on an inpatient basis. Long term follow-up was lacking, however. Post[29] also reported successful treatment with phenothiazines although a proportion (18 of 65) remained psychotic throughout the three-year follow-up.

Raskind and his colleagues (in manuscript) compared the results of prescribing oral antipsychotic medication in an outpatient group of paraphrenic patients with the effectiveness of very low doses of depot (intramuscular) medication (prolixine enanthate). There was a significant degree of improvement among the group receiving depot antipsychotic medication which Raskind, et al. attribute to differences in compliance. Outpatient management of these patients was characterized by a tripartite program of antipsychotic medication, resocialization and "shuttle diplomacy." The latter involved contacting individuals living in close proximity to the patient and indicating to those aware of the patient's condition that the "illness is now being treated" and that prognosis is good. Many of those in the patient's environment had been caught up in the delusional system and accused publicly of a variety of heinous activities. Resocialization involves planned visits by members of the outreach team. The results of the program described by Raskind and his colleagues are promising.

CONCLUSION

Our knowledge of the etiology, course and prognosis of paranoid illness with onset in late life is scant. Salient variables such as genetic endowment, a variety of losses, social isolation and sensory impairment all appear to play a role in the etiology of the symptom cluster, although their specific influence is only speculative. Therapy is largely symptomatic with antipsychotic medication, social intervention and replacement of loss playing important roles. Clinical and basic investigations are very much needed to develop a base of information on which patient care may rest.

REFERENCES

1. Stotsky, B. Nursing home or mental hospital: Which is better for the geriatric mental patient? *J. Genetic Psychology,* III, 113–117 (a) (1967).
2. Busse, E. W. and Pfeiffer, E. *Behavior and Adaptation in Late Life.* Boston: Little Brown, 1975.
3. Lowenthal, M. F. *Lives in Distress: The Paths of the Elderly to the Psychiatric Ward.* New York: Basic Books, 1964.
4. Kay, D. W. K. and Roth, M. Environmental and hereditary factors in the schizophrenias of old age ("late paraphrenia") and their bearing on the general problem of causation in schizophrenia. *J. Mental Science,* 107: 649 (1961).
5. Kay, D. W. K. Schizophrenia and schizophrenia-like states in the elderly. *British J. of Hospital Medicine,* October, 369–376 (1972).
6. Fish, F. J. Senile paranoid states. *Geront. Clin.,* 1 (1959).
7. Raskind, M., Alvarez, C. and Herlin, S. Fluphenazine enanchate in the outpatient treatment of late paraphrenia. (In manuscript).

8. Kramer, M., Taube, C. A. and Redick, R. W. Patterns of use of psychiatric facilities by the aged: past, present and future, In C. Eisdorfer and M. P. Lawton (eds.) *The Psychology of Adult Development and Aging*. Washington, D.C.: American Psychological Association, pp. 428–528, 1973.

9. Savage, R. D., Gaber, L. B., Britton, P. G., Bolton, N. and Cooper, A. *Personality and Adjustment in the Aged*. New York: Academic Press, 1977.

10. Eisdorfer, C. Mental health in later life, In S. Golann and C. Eisdorfer (eds.) *Handbook of Community Mental Health*. New York: Appleton-Century-Crofts, p. 952, 1972.

11. Butler, R. *Why Survive? Being Old in America*. New York: Harper and Row, 1975.

12. Eisdorfer, C. Rorschach rigidity and sensory decrement in a senescent population. *J. Geront.*, **15**: 188 (1960).

13. LaBarre, W. *The Ghost Dance: Origins of Religion*. New York: Doubleday (Delta), 1972.

14. Abramson, L. Y., Seligman, M. E. P. and Teasdale, J. D. Learned helplessness in humans: Critique and reformulation. *J. of Abnormal Psychology*, **87**: 49 (1978).

15. Sparacino, J. An attributional approach to psychotherapy with the aged. *J. of the Am. Geriatrics Soc.*, **XXVI**, 9 (1978).

16. Cooper, A. F., Kay, D. W. K., Curry, A. R., Garside, R. F. and Roth, M. Hearing loss in paranoid and affective psychoses of the elderly. *The Lancet*, (October 12, 1974).

17. Post, F. Paranoid disorders in the elderly. *Postgraduate Medicine*, **53**, 4:52 (April 1973).

18. Post, F. *The Clinical Psychiatry of Late Life*. New York: Pergamon Press, 1965.

19. Langley, G. E. Functional psychoses, In J. G. Howells (ed.) *Modern Perspectives in the Psychiatry of Old Age*. New York: Brunner/Mazel, pp 326–355, 1975.

20. Roth, M. The natural history of mental disorder in old age. *J. Ment. Sci.*, **101**: 281 (1955).

21. Kay, D .W. K. and Roth, M. Schizophrenias of old age, In C. Tibbetts and W. Donahue (eds.) *Processes of Aging*. New York: Basic Books, 1963.

22. Post, F. Schizo-affective symptomatology in late life. *Brit. J. Psychiat.*, **118**: 437 (1971).

23. Langfeldt, G. The erotic jealousy syndrome. A clinical study. *Acta Psychiatr. Neurol. Scand.* (Suppl. 151) (1961).

24. Faergeman, P. *Psychogenic Psychoses*. London: Butterworths, p. 199, 1963.

25. Freedman, A. M. and Kaplan, H. I. *Comprehensive Textbook of Psychiatry*. Baltimore: Williams and Wilkins, 1967.

26. Tanna, V. L. Paranoid states: A selected review. *Comprehensive Psychiatry*, **15**, 6:453 (1974).

27. Kay, D. W. K., Cooper, A. F., Garside, R. F. and Roth, M. The differentiation of paranoid from affective psychoses by patients' premorbid characteristics. *Brit. J. Psychiat.*, **129**: 207 (1976).

28. Cooper, A. F., Garside, R. F. and Kay, D. W. K. A comparison of deaf and non-deaf patients with paranoid and affective psychoses. *Brit. J. Psychiat.*, **129**: 532 (1976).

29. Post, F. *Persistent Persecutory States of the Elderly*. Oxford: Pergamon Press, 1966.

30. Schneider, K. Primare and sekundare symptoms bei schizophrenie. *Fortschr. Neurol. Psychiat.*, **25**: 487 (1957).

31. Herbert, M. E. and Jacobson, S. Late paraphrenia. *Brit. J. Psychiat.*, **113**: 461 (1967).

32. Alexander, A. A., Workneh, F., Klein, M. H. and Miller, M. H. Psychotherapy and the foreign student, In P. Pederson and R. Wintrob (eds.) *Cross-cultural Counseling*. Honolulu: Cultural Learning Institute, University of Hawaii, 1976.

33. Chu, H-M, Yeh, E-K, Klein, M. H., Alexander, A. A. and Miller, M. H. A study of Chinese students' adjustment in the U.S.A. *Acta Psychologica Taiwanica*, **13**: 206–218, 1971.

Chapter 15
Affective Disorders

William W. K. Zung, M.D.

Duke University Medical Center

I. ETIOLOGY AND PREDISPOSING FACTORS

In this chapter, we will examine the intricate factors which when interlaced, display a clinical picture of the elderly person with a mood disorder. We will perlustrate the mesh of the canvas upon which life has splashed its hues, drawn its conclusions, and tinged it with tell-tale blues. To understand depression of the elderly is to know the very fiber out of which the warp and woof of man's nature and destiny is woven.

A. Biological Aging and Basic Life Functions

Aging can be defined as the reversal of the basic functions of life which man experiences from birth. The adult person is not a static entity, and development in its fullest sense does not cease with the completely matured adult. Aging can also be defined as a continuous process with progressive loss of functions, which with the passage of time results in the deterioration of the mature adult and ultimately leads to his death. In order to understand aging and its effect on man with respect to mood disorders, we must first look at what are the basic functions of life. These can be listed as: (1) Behavior; (2) Growth; (3) Metabolism; (4) Reproduction; (5) Movement; (6) Responsiveness; and (7) Adaptation.[1] Progressive loss of life's basic functions in man as a result of aging could result, although it is not always inevitable or inexorable, in the following conditions as listed in Table 15–1. We will return to these basic life functions and look at them again as they relate to other factors that influence mental illness and mood disorders in the elderly.

Biological aging, basic life functions and mood disorders intersect at a point distinguished within the past two decades by research in the areas of neuroanatomy, neurophysiology, neurochemistry and neuropharmacology. Of immediate interest are the findings relating certain naturally occurring amines to the pathogenesis of mood disorders. These are: norepinephrine (NE), dopamine (DA), and serotonin (5-HT), all biogenic amines intimately involved with the

Table 15-1. Effect of Aging on Basic Life Functions.

	BASIC LIFE FUNCTION:	AGING PRODUCES, FOR EXAMPLE:
I. 1.	BEHAVIOR	I. Withdrawal, disinterest
II. 2.	GROWTH	II. Decrease in weight, sleep, energy,
3.	METABOLISM	impaired function of all body
4.	REPRODUCTION	systems, diminished libido with
		loss of secondary sexual characteristics
III. 5.	MOVEMENT	III. Decreased motor and joint mobility
IV. 6.	RESPONSIVENESS	IV. Decreased tolerance for stress,
7.	ADAPTATION	disturbance of reality testing,
		diminution of impulse control,
		increased dependency

centers of the central nervous system such as the limbic structures that regulate drives and emotions. Based upon knowledge of anatomic structure and sites of nerve tracts mediated by these biogenic amines, the effect of disturbances of these systems has been postulated or identified. Noradrenergic tracts are believed to have a major role in mood disorders. Dopaminergic tracts have been identified to be involved in the pathophysiology of Parkinson's disease. Serotonergic tracts have a major role in producing sleep disturbances. From these investigations, a catecholamine hypothesis of mood disorders had been proposed: there appears to be a significant disturbance in the metabolism of NE in patients with mood disorders, with the evidence indicating either an absolute or a relative deficiency of NE in depressives, and an excess of NE in manics.[2]

In general, biogenic amines including 5-HT and the catecholamines, NE and DA, are metabolized to biologically inactive compounds by oxidative deamination by the enzyme monoamine oxidase (MAO). It has been reported that MAO activity appears to increase with advancing age.[3] According to the data reported, there is an increase of the MAO enzyme activity, with a peak rise starting at about 45 years old, and steadily increasing with age. The importance of this finding can be understood in the light of the biogenic amine theory of mood disorders, and our understanding of the pharmacology of psychotropic drugs. Evidence from psy-

chopharmacology points to the fact that many of the drugs used in the treatment of depressive disorders are known to increase the available neurotransmitters such as NE. It has been inferred that their antidepressant effect is related in some way to their ability to increase NE levels. For example, the tricyclic antidepressants inhibit the reuptake of NE released at the synapse, thus increasing the available NE at receptor sites. The monoamine oxidase inhibitors (MAOI) increase the supply of available NE by inhibiting the degradation of NE within the presynaptic nerve ending.

Much of this work is based on animal studies and most of the postulates have heuristic value, still lacking the necessary chain of evidence that could translate theories into clinical practice. We must therefore be cautious about interpreting these findings as causal effects and not assume that the primary defects in depression of middle and late life are results of these changes in the MAO mechanism. Thus no biogenic amine theory could explain the etiology of mood disorders, and in fact, altered biogenic amine metabolism in all likelihood is secondary to other biochemical events.[4]

B. Psychosocial Aging and Adaptation

The attainment of the chronological age of 65 years old by man is most often used as the definition of: Who is elderly? T. S. Eliot in his poem "Gerontion," a title that comes from the Greek word from which geriatrics is derived, geras (γηρασ) meaning old age, gave the poet's concept of the aged when he wrote,

> "Here I am, an old man in a
>   dry month,
> Being read to by a boy, waiting
>   for rain."

The elderly is old in years, but he is complete, capable, and competent to take care of his own needs and wants. To age successfully means to live life to its fullest, to the end. It means that each of the following stages of aging must be completed: (1) Realization of the human reality that loss and/or separation is a continuous process; (2) Resignation to the occurrence of the process. (3) Resolution of the process/event by acceptance of its finality. Painting a picture of an ideal aged person, we would envisage a person who: maintains continuity with the past in terms of goals and interests; is confident in his capacity to deal with the problems of everyday living, can resolve conflicts in a culturally acceptable manner; and is patient, tolerant, rational, considerate, cooperative, self-reliant and self-disciplined.

When the necessary stages of psycho-sociological aging as enumerated above are not completed successfully at any step of the way, the path over which the elderly must travel leads toward the royal road to a mood disorder. Envision now the antithesis of the ideal aged person, the person who instead has inadequately adapted to the aging process and who has lost contact with time, and by living exclusively in the past becomes disoriented and disorganized; has failed to adapt to biological aging with its physical limitations and has developed increased demands on others; is unable to deal with the problems of everyday living and resolves conflicts in socially disturbing ways with frequent displays of anger, mistrust and suspicion; and is impatient, irritable, intolerant, dogmatic, irrational, uncooperative, restrictive, rigid and regressive in behavior.

C. Stress and Basic Life Functions

Aging is a continuous process punctuated in life by events and/or processes which often produce stress. Stress refers to all such events or processes whether they originate from within the person, or from without in the environment, and results in a situation which requires the person to resolve the stressful event or process. Stress can and does occur at any age, but with aging stress can become a greater risk factor for disease since the elderly's vulnerability to the vicissitudes of life are increased. Stress as a force on the vital balance between health and sickness can produce its own effects on the basic functions of life as summarized in Table 15-2.

D. Classification of Stress

Stress as a contributing factor to the development of mood disorders can be classified as object losses of the following kinds:[5]

1. Loss of a loved person, such as death of a family member, friend, or associate, or the separation from such a person.

2. Loss of health through loss of or damage to the body or body functions. In addition to the loss of physical health, the loss of physical attractiveness and appearance are significant when they involve emotionally invested parts of the body, such as the face.

3. Loss of job from which a person earned a livelihood and enjoyed status as a productive member of society. For the elderly, this particular object loss in the form of retirement looms realistically in the background for years and makes its phantasmagorical appearance at the age of 65. Here is a change in status that relegates a person into obsolescence, as if an ultimate computer within the person, with its programmed senescence, has begun to print the last lines of its output. Retirement has its positive aspect in that the person who has been successful sees it as a well-earned cessation

Table 15-2. Effect of Stress on Basic Life Functions.

BASIC LIFE FUNCTIONS:	FUNCTIONAL SPHERES OF PERSON:	STRESS PRODUCES:
I. 1. BEHAVIOR	I. PSYCHIC-AFFECTIVE	I. Unpleasant affect, anxious, depressed, helpless, hopeless
II. 2. GROWTH 3. METABOLISM 4. REPRODUCTION	II. PHYSIOLOGIC	II. Accelerate, precipitate, uncover pre-existing pathology at some level (cellular, organ, system)
III. 5. MOVEMENT	III. PSYCHOMOTOR	III. Inappropriate, un-realistic, repetitive actions
IV. 6. RESPONSIVENESS 7. ADAPTATION	IV. PSYCHOLOGIC	IV. Generalized confusion, disinterest, indecisive-ness, irritability, dissatisfaction
		Loss of coping and adaptive mechanisms, personal devaluation, suicidal rumination

from work which allows him/her to enjoy his remaining years in an unharried, unhurried and dignified way. The man or woman who has not achieved a measure of success, and who was not content with his/her work, will increasingly feel a sense of failure and frustration. As time goes by, the feeling gradually becomes one of annihilation, that life is over and it is the end of the line. The prospect of achieving his/her life's goal is remote, if not past, and retirement is but a pyrrhic victory over age and long years. Failures during this period are doubly damaging to the man or woman who has not achieved, and increases the likelihood of an experience which leads to a mood disorder.

For the woman, her life as she ages is affected largely through changes in the pattern of her husband's life and economic status. In addition, the woman who has devoted the largest part of her life and efforts as a mother and homemaker first gradually and then suddenly finds herself relatively less occupied, less needed and heir to the "empty nest"[6].

4. Loss of valued personal possessions (home, property, memorabilia) which are vested with memories, these losses involving more than the material value of the object. The elderly especially cling to the old, where familiarity provides comfort and security.

5. Changes in way of life and living such that an established and comfortable mode of living no longer exists.

6. Failures of plans or ventures where investments of time and effort have failed.

7. Loss of membership or status in a group (social, political, professional, idealogical) means loss of personal acceptability by a group that shared common goals and activities.

8. Loss of pets as significant objects that filled a unique role to which the owner may have ascribed many qualities. For the elderly, for whom a pet can be the most important living object, the loss of a pet is profoundly felt.

Loss as an etiological factor in producing stress can be of three kinds, all of which are equally important as stressors:

1. Real loss: the change in status here is irrevocable and the object lost no longer has

real existence in the real world. The loss has occurred and the lost object is unavailable and inaccessible.

2. Threatened loss: when the loss has not occurred but there exists in reality a potential loss. The anticipation that it will or might take place requires the person to deal with the loss before it actually takes place.

3. Imaginary or fantasized loss: where the person experiences a sense of loss or anticipates a loss for which no basis in reality exists. Such a fantasy may originate from a misinterpretation or exaggeration of the environment to mean loss or separation when in actuality none was present.

E. The Measurement of Stress as Life Events

One approach to determining the effects of loss or life events as stressful factors that affect the health/disease balance in a person has been that of Holmes and Rahe.[7] They constructed the Schedule of Recent Experience which is a self-rating questionnaire. In addition to general biographic information, the items question the respondent about 42 life-change situations for a specified period of time prior to answering the questionnaire. Areas of life events measured include: health, work, home and family, personal and social, and financial. Each life-change situation has been assigned a numerical score previously determined by the authors.

It is apparent from a perusal of the list that although empirical values for "at risk" have been developed, individual variations must be taken into account. It is necessary to know the meaning of the event for the person in terms of: (1) His past experiences and personal development; and (2) His current psychological state with respect to the dynamic equilibrium between resources and vulnerabilities.

Whether or not a particular situation is experienced as stressful thus depends on both qualitative and quantitative aspects of the event. Qualitatively, events may or may not be experienced as stressful depending on whether or not that person has in the past developed adequate means of adaptation to it. Quantitatively, for every person there is a range which defines the capacity of his system to respond successfully to change, without tipping the balance toward the sickness end. The fact that stressors are highly individualistic dictates that judgment cannot be made from the nature of the stimulus event, but requires knowledge of the response as well.

A number of attempts have been made to correct for the use of life events as a meaningful factor in the etiology of affective disorders, by assigning labels which have more specificity for events as provoking or precipitating factors. Examples include: (1) Exits—Entrances; (2) Desirable—Undesirable; (3) Intrapersonal—Interpersonal; (4) Active—Passive; (5) Major—Minor; (6) Controlled—Uncontrolled; (7) Upsetting—Not-Upsetting; (8) Threatening—Not-threatening; (9) Expected—Unexpected; and (10) Short-term—Long-term.

In summary, resolution of stressful life events depends upon: (1) Genetic predisposition; (2) Prevailing early life experiences and adequacy of previous adaptive and coping mechanisms; (3) Patterns and profiles of premorbid personality; and (4) Presence and absence of supporting systems.

II. ESSENTIAL SIGNS AND SYMPTOMS CHARACTERISTIC OF DEPRESSIVE DISORDERS

A. Varieties of Emotions

Starting from the time of earliest recorded medicine, the classification of the etiology of disease has been divided into outer and inner "influences" by the Chinese, which has its counterpart in Western medicine in the Cartesian dichotomy of environment versus heredity. The inner influences of Chinese medicine and cosmology are the emotions, of which there are seven: (1) Joy; (2) Grief; (3) Anger; (4) Fear; (5) Love; (6) Hate; and (7) Desire. It was said by the Chinese that if the emotions were kept within normal limits, no disease would come. If the emotions were so powerful as to be uncontrollable and governed the life of the person, then they would injure the body.

Tomkins proposed that affective responses are the primary motives of human beings.[8] He listed as the primary affects, the following eight with alternative words denoting moderate and high intensity of the affect, respectively: (1) Enjoyment—Joy; (2) Interest—Excitement; (3) Surprise—Startle; (4) Distress—Anguish; (5) Fear—Terror; (6) Shame—Humiliation; (7) Contempt—Disgust; and (8) Anger—Rage. Other authors writing on the varieties of affective disturbances listed the primary affects as: elation, depression, fear, anxiety, anger, confusion, bewilderment, suspicion, amourousness, awe, awfulness, jealousy, hatred, lack of feelings, guilt, and pain.[9,10]

Common illnesses are more often seen and the disturbance of affect most commonly encountered is depression. This pervasive mood disturbance becomes the glasses through which the person sees and feels the world around him. Wearers of rose-colored glasses see a rosy world, whereas wearers of blue-colored glasses see only a blues-colored world.

B. Classification of Depressive Disorders

The diagnosis of depression as an affective disorder has been of great interest for decades, as evidenced by the extensive literature available on this subject. The establishment of a classification of depression which is jointly inclusive and mutually exclusive and which brings order where order is now lacking, or the establishment of an operational definition of depressive disorder commanding wide agreement among clinical practitioners and investigators in all countries, constitutes one of the most pressing needs of present day psychiatry. We need operational definitions and the diagnostic dialectic as avenues toward understanding and investigating the etiology and treatment of depressive disorders.

Starting with nosology, which is the science of classification of diseases, let us look to see how descriptive psychiatry has helped us toward understanding depression as an emotional disorder. Kraepelin[11] classified depressive disorders using the etiological approach as those which have an endogenous origin, contributed by genetic and constitutional factors. These are described as internal factors such as degenerative or metabolic changes, and are intrinsic processes of nature. The other category are those depressions caused by exogenous factors, such as bacterial infections or chemical toxins. These are external factors that come from the environment or life events and situations, and as such are part of the nurturing process. The nature-nurture concept of depressive disorders has been investigated by Sandifer et al.[12] who supported the existence of these two types. Lange[13] used the term "reactive" for the endogenous depression which was preceded by an environmental stress. Today, endogenous and reactive depressions in word and concept still persist and choices of treatment reflect these original etiological concepts. An endogenous depression being organic in etiology is said to respond best to treatments which are somatic and alter the internal milieu such as electroconvulsive therapy and drugs. Exogenous or reactive depression, being a psychogenic disorder, responds best to psychotherapy, and methods which are directed towards altering the external environment, such as family, group, or milieu therapy.

The diagnostic dilemma of depressive disorders theorized as either being two separate entities (endogenous and reactive) or as a continuous process, has a long history. Investigators who conceptualized depression as a continuum in a unitarian model include Mapother,[14] Lewis,[15] Hill,[16] and Kendell.[17] Investigators who conceptualized depression in terms of the endogenous-reactive types in a dichotomous model include Kiloh and Garside,[18] and Fahy et al.[19] A summary of the usual characteristics attributed to endogenous and reactive depressions is found in Table 15-3.

The classification of depression into the

Table 15-3.   Characteristic Diagnostic Distinctions between Endogenous and Reactive Depressions.

ENDOGENOUS DEPRESSION	REACTIVE DEPRESSION
1. Age: older, 40 & over	Younger
2. Family history of depression	No family history present
3. Premorbid personality: normal	Neurotic: inadequate, hysterical, obsessional
4. Precipitating factor: absent	Present
5. Affect: pervasive depression	Less severe or as pervasive
6. Physiological symptoms	Fewer symptoms, less severe
A. Decreased appetite	
B. Decreased weight	
C. Decreased libido	
D. Increased fatigue	
E. Sleep disorder: middle of night, and early a.m. wakings	Difficulty in falling asleep
F. Diurnal variation: present, depression worse in a.m.	Diurnal variation: absent, depression worse in p.m.
7. Psychomotor activity: retardation, agitation	Less severe
8. Psychological symptoms:	
A. Loss of interest in life	Less severe
B. Self-reproach, guilt, remorse	Self-pity, less guilt
9. Response to ECT: yes	Response to ECT: no

psychotic-neurotic severity model was originally used as an expediency for commitment purposes. A psychotic depression is presently defined as having impaired mental functioning, which interferes grossly with the person's capacity to meet the ordinary demands of life. Thus, in addition to the severe pervasive alteration of mood, there is decreased cognitive functioning, distortion, misinterpretation, and decreased reality testing. A neurotic depression is defined as having some impaired mental functioning, but the neurotic patient is aware of this fact. Thus, reality testing is present, while distortions and misinterpretations are absent (see Table 15-4).

There is an erroneous tendency to use the terms endogenous as synonymous with psychotic, and reactive as synonymous with neurotic. From the definitions presented above, we can see that one set of terms is based on etiological concepts, while the other is based on a concept of severity of the psychopathology present. These sets of terms are not synonymous, nor are they mutually exclusive. Thus, a patient can have a reactive depression of psychotic proportion, or have an endogenous depression of a neurotic severity.

Nosology based on the age of the patient (childhood, adolescence, young adulthood, middle age, involutional, and senile depressions) draws attention to the ongoing emotional growth, development, and maturational processes which are unique to each age group and alerts the clinician to their special problems. Paykel[20] used a classification of four typologies which are partially age dependent. He demonstrated that with respect to response to tricyclic antidepressants, the "psychotic" depressives respond best, the "anxious" respond worst, and the "hostile" and "young depressives with personality disorders" respond somewhere in between. He described the psychotic as being the oldest in age, most severely depressed, with the presence of delusions. They score high on the variables measuring guilt, retardation, anorexia, and insomnia and score low on variables measuring precipitating factors and premorbid neuroticism. The anxious depressed are mid-

Table 15-4. Characteristic Diagnostic Distinctions Between Psychotic and Neurotic Depressions.

PSYCHOTIC DEPRESSION	NEUROTIC DEPRESSION
1. Mood disturbance: pervasive, and severely depressed	Minimal, mild, or moderate
2. Physiological functions: (appetite, weight, libido, energy, sleep) markedly decreased	Fewer symptoms, less severe
3. Psychomotor activities: severe retardation or agitation	Minimal, mild, or moderate
4. Psychological functions: markedly disturbed, may appear to be organic with decreased intellectual and cognitive functions	Fewer symptoms, less severe
5. Loss of capacity to meet ordinary demands of life	Less severe
6. Reality testing: disturbed	Usually intact
7. Delusions, hallucinations: may be present	Absent

dle aged, with presence of anxiety and depression. In addition to fatigue, they have obsessional symptoms and feelings of depersonalization. They score high on premorbid neuroticism. The hostile depressives are described as younger in age and they manifest hostility and self-pity. The young depressives with personality disorders are characterized as being mildly depressed and they manifest marked fluctuations of mood which are related to the environment.

Another dimension which is clinically useful in describing depressed patients is their psychomotor activity, as being either agitated or retarded. These descriptive terms are independent of the etiological or severity distinctions, but reflect the predominant presenting feature of the depression.

Extending this typology to include a third group called hostile depressions, Overall et al.[21] have shown that response to drug treatment can be predicted based on these three types. Thus, in a study using tricyclic antidepressants, the retarded group responded best to the drug studied, while the agitated-anxious patients responded worst. The anxious group responded best to phenothiazines, while there was no response with the other two groups with this compound.

Other approaches to understanding depressive disorders through nosology include that proposed by Blinder, which he considered to be a pragmatic classification.[22] All depressions are classified under one of five types: (1) physiologic retardation depression; (2) tension depression; (3) schizo-depression; (4) depression secondary to problems in living; and (5) depression symptomatic of organic illness.

Pollitt[23] suggested a classification of depression based on physiological disturbances. These include the "S" or somatic type where symptons are called collectively, the functional shift, and result from alterations in biological rhythms, metabolism, and autonomic balance. The second or "J" type is a justified type, where the illness is understandable in terms of the patient's predicament.

Van Praag et al.[24] have divided the depressions into vital and personal. Vital depressions are primarily affective in sphere, in the presence of endoreactive dysthmia with somatic concomitants of the affect. Personal depressions are primarily in the sphere of psychical feeling and the existence of the depression is experienced as something rational by the patient.

A more recent classification of depressive disorders has been proposed by Woodruff et al.[25] in which the authors attempted to avoid etiologic or symptomatic implications. A primary depression is defined as a depressive episode occurring in a patient whose previous history is either well psychiatrically, or a previous episode of mania or depression and no other psychiatric illness. A secondary depression is defined as a depressive episode occurring in a patient who has had a pre-existing, diagnosable psychiatric illness other than a primary affective disorder (such as organic brain syndrome, schizophrenia, or personality disorders). There are several obvious problems with this schema. For example, a patient can have pre-existing symptoms that suggest a nonaffective psychiatric disease, but since it was not documented, does the patient still have a primary depression? Thus, the endogenous-reactive or nature-nurture etiological concepts of depression come up again and again, in various guises and schemata.

Leonhard[26] proposed a classification which has been extensively researched by Perris.[27] Depressions are classified as unipolar or bipolar. Unipolar are episodes of affective illnesses involving only mania or only depression. Bipolar depressions include both phases with mania and depression occurring in the same patient (see Table 15-5).

Another commonly used term classifies a certain type of depression which is called masked depression. Synonyms for these include: depression sine depression, depressive equivalent, depression in disguise, and occult depression. Depressed adult patients who present themselves to the physician for complaints other than feeling depressed, can be categorized as usually manifesting: (1) hypochondriasis; (2) drug dependence, of which alcohol is the most frequent; and (3) psychosomatic disorders. The most frequently seen and reported psychosomatic illnesses involving the various organ systems are: central nervous system (CNS)—headache; CV—hypertension; respiratory—asthma; gastrointestinal—peptic ulcers; genitourinary—enuresis; musculoskeletal—low back pain; and skin—various dermatoses such as eczema. Masked depressions of childhood manifest in the following ways: (1) hyperactivity; (2) aggressive behavior; (3) delinquency; (4) hypochondriasis; and (5) psychosomatic illness.

A unique classification of depression has been proposed by Pare et al.[28] Here the classification is based upon genetic background and drug response to the monoamine oxidase inhibitors (MAOI) and tricyclic antidepressants. From their findings, they differentiated responders and nonresponders and predicted that the response of depressed patients to MAOI and tricyclic

Table 15-5.   Characteristic Distinctions between Unipolar and Bipolar Psychoses.

	UNIPOLAR PSYCHOSES	BIPOLAR PSYCHOSES
1. Affective disturbance:	Characterized by recurrent depressions (or manias) of stereotyped symptomatology, and without phases of the opposite polarity.	Characterized by the occurrence of both depressive and manic phases.
2. Median age at onset:	About 45 years	About 30 years
3. Family history:	Specific heredity for the same form of illness and low for the other within each group. More dominant in bipolar than unipolar.	
4. Premorbid personality:	Predominance of substable or syntonic personality Active, social	Predominance of subvalid or asthenic personality.
5. Precipitating factor:	No significant differences	Tendency to more frequent "somatic" factors.
6. Clinical ratings:	No significant differences either in anxiety-depression.	

antidepressants would be similar in succeeding illnesses, and that responses of first-degree relatives who are treated for depression using these drugs would be in the same direction.

A complete compendium of the existing known classification of mental disorders official, semiofficial, national, and individual has been compiled by Stengel.[29]

Depression as an affect or feeling tone, is a ubiquitous and universal condition which as a human experience extends on a continuum from normal mood swings to a pathological state. Thus, depression can be used to describe: (1) an affect which is a subjective feeling tone of short duration; (2) a mood, which is a state sustained over a longer period of time; (3) an emotion, which is comprised of the feeling tones along with objective indications; or (4) a disorder which has characteristic symptom clusters, complexes, or configurations.

The nomenclature of depression as it appears in the *Diagnostic and Statistical Manual of Mental Disorders. Second Edition*[30] has classified the disorder using several conflicting dimensions. First, by presumed etiology: depression is considered to be a disorder not attributed to physical conditions, as opposed to the organic brain syndromes, which are disorders caused by or associated with impairment of brain tissue function. Second, by severity: it is listed under psychoses and also as one of the neuroses. The distinction is based upon degree of impairment of reality testing or functional adequacy. Third, by age of onset: there is a separate nomenclature for depression occurring in the involutional period. Fourth, by environment: manic-depressive illnesses are diagnosed when there is no obvious precipitating event, while psychotic depressive reaction is used when the illness is attributable directly to a precipitating life experience. Fifth, by history: patients are classified as manic-depressives according to the subtypes of manic, depressed or circular. The lack of clarity of such a classification leaves much to be desired. In fact, uncertainty about the basic or essential criteria for

classification has shown to contribute to the unreliability of psychiatric diagnosis. In addition, from the results of recent studies on the present diagnostic state, it is apparent that comparative studies of depressive disorders based on clinical diagnosis is tenuous because of the lack of uniformity among clinicians.[31,32] To make diagnosis and studies comparable, systematic methods for both using a standardized approach is necessary.

The following figure shows in a flow diagram the relationship of various approaches to the diagnosis of depressive disorders (see Fig. 15-1).

In the cells numbered 8, 10, 12 and 14, we have the various diagnostic categories which are used today, diagnostic categories being those depressions that have been given names as a disorder, illness, syndrome or symptom complex, and have been perpetuated because they continue to have some value. Cell 8 represents the American Psychiatric Association Diagnostic and Statistical Manual (DSM) nomenclature, which in its present DSM-II form will be replaced by DSM-III. This revision of classification by the APA of its DSM within the space of less than a decade does not reflect progress in psychiatry as much as dissatisfaction with this classification.

Cell 10 represents those diagnostic categories which have some presumed etiological basis for their labels, such as the endogenous-reactive depressions.

Cell 12, called clinical typology, are those diagnostic categories whose labels reflect the clinical profile of the patient as he or she is perceived by the clinician. These include the agitated-retarded depressions.

Cell 14 includes what I call the statistical typology of diagnostic category of depressive disorders. This would include such types as those generated by multivariate analysis of multiple-item rating scales, such as hostile depression.

Cell 16 includes what I call the biological typology. In this method of categorizing subgroups of patients with depressive disorders, biological measurements are

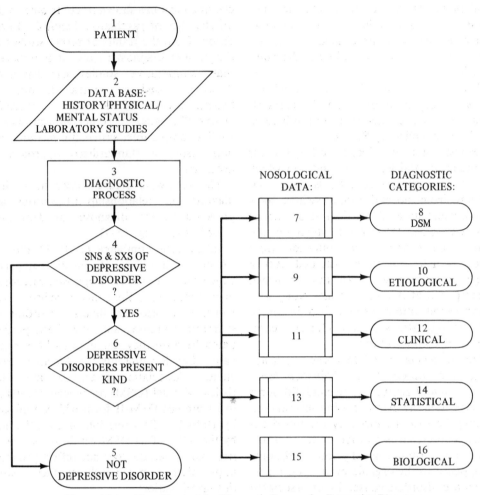

Figure 15-1.   Flow Chart of the Diagnostic Process for Depressive Disorders.

made and patients are classified according to the results on these variables. The newer biological subgroups include those most recently proposed by Maas through the use of biochemical and pharmacological variables.[33] Two groups A and B are based upon urinary levels of 3-methoxy-4-hydroxyphenyl glycol (MHPG), and clinical response to psychotropic drugs. Group A depressed patients show: (1) low pretreatment urinary MHPG; (2) favorable response to treatment with imipramine or desipramine; (3) elevation of mood following dextroamphetamine; and (4) modest or no increment in urinary MHPG level following treatment with imipramine, desipramine, or dextroamphetamine. Group B depressed pa-

tients are characterized by: (1) normal or high urinary MHPG at pretreatment; (2) failure to respond to imipramine but response to amitriptyline; (3) no mood change following dextroamphetamine; and (4) decrease in urinary MHPG following treatment with imipramine, desipramine, or dextroamphetamine.

Older uses of pharmacological methods to categorize diagnostic groups include the works of Shagas[34] with sedation thresholds using barbiturates, while Gellhorn and Loofbourrow[35] have summarized work using mecholyl and noradrenaline tests.

Meldman has attempted to bring the findings of many investigators in the field of attention and arousal to bear on clinical psychiatry, with an attempt to categorize disorders as "attentional diseases."[36] Emotional disorders then, including depression, are categorized by the biological phenomena of activation, arousal, and selective attention. Affective disorders, for example, show emotional hyperattentionism, cognitive hypoattentionism, and actional hyper- or hypoattentionism. Although decrease in arousal seems apparent in severely depressed patients with associated loss of interest and decreased psychomotor activity, neurophysiological studies using electromyography (EMG) and electroencephalography (EEG) indicate the presence of increased arousal in depression. It may be that the clinically apparent slowing and retardation is a function of increase in arousal beyond the point of optimal functioning. Specific studies to support this method of categorizing patients using the attention model are those reported by Whatmore and Ellis[37] using EMG measures; by Wilson and Wilson,[38] Paulson and Gottlieb,[39] and Zung[40] using photically elicited EEG arousal responses; and by Zung, Wilson and Dodson[41] using auditory responses during all-night sleep EEG recordings.

Using the results of these tests as the nosological data base (No. 15), the diagnostic category labeled biological (No. 16) could conceivably have nomenclature such as hypothalamosis, or diencephalic diatheses. More specifically, the subcategories could reflect dysfunctions of the arousalstat, appestat, or libidostat.

Returning to the dialectical dilemma of sorting out diagnostic categories, we can see from the figure that each category requires a nosological data base (cells 7, 7, 11, 13). The construction of the Affective Disorder Diagnostic Sheet or ADDS provided a systematic method of recording the necessary data which is common to all the categories. Fig. 15-2 summarizes the use of the ADDS as a nosological data base for categorizing depressive disorders.

The question now is this: If we can define the diagnostic categories and systematize the nosological data base upon which the diagnoses are made, can we agree on what is the core psychopathology found in depression in the first place? This takes us to Cell 4 in the figure. If we can standardize the operational definition for this decision process, then we are much closer to understanding what depression is.

C. Diagnostic Criteria for Depressive Disorder

The first problem in planning an operational definition or classification is that of choosing the measurement characteristics that are going to be used as a basis for the empirical identification of the underlying population. The variables chosen are such that they are: (1) Relevant for distinguishing among different types of psychiatric patients (depressed or not depressed); (2) Relevant for distinguishing between psychiatric patients and normals; (3) Able to produce homogeneity within groups, defined so that patients who are grouped together are similar enough that for most practical purposes they can be treated as if they are alike (all depressed); (4) Useful in assigning individuals according to the definition developed so that the operational definition will have some general applicability.

Examining the above typologies for the classification of depressive disorders, it becomes clear that for every method of classification, there are Linnaean-like binomial nomenclature such as: *Depression endogenous, Depression psychotic, Depression unipolar, Depression agitated,* or *Depression hostile.* The word depression is equivalent to the "genus," and the modifying label to the "species" of the binomial nomenclature. The modifiers determine the typology and subtypologies, while the genus denotes depression as the disorder with common characteristics. The core signs and symptoms of depression are thus universally recognized and accepted, and are listed in Table 15-6.

The classification and definition of depressive disorders can be painted in many styles using large strokes of helplessness and

Figure 15-2. Diagnosis of Depressive Disorders by Typology using the Affective Disorder Diagnostic Sheet.

AFFECTIVE DISORDER DIAGNOSTIC SHEET (ADDS)	APA DSM II	ETIOLOGICAL TYPOLOGY		CLINICAL TYPOLOGY		STATISTICAL TYPOLOGY
		Endogenous- Reactive	Unipolar- Bipolar	Psychotic- Neurotic	Primary- Secondary	
A. DEMOGRAPHIC						
1. Age	x	x	x			x
2. Sex						x
3. Race						x
4. Marital status						x
5. Education						x
6. Occupation						x
B. PRESENT ILLNESS						
1. Precipitating factor?	x	x				x
2. Sxs of depression?	x	x	x	x	x	x
3. Sxs of mania?	x		x		x	x
4. Psychotic?	x	x		x		x
5. Duration of P.I.?						x
6. Previous tx for P.I.?						x
C. PAST MEDICAL HISTORY						
1. Premorbid personality		x	x			x
2. Previous psychiatry hx?	x				x	x
a. Depression?	x		x		x	x
b. Mania?	x		x		x	x
c. Other dx?					x	x
d. Hospitalization?						x
e. Previous tx?						x
f. Age initial onset?						x
D. FAMILY HISTORY						
1. Depression-Mania?		x				x
2. Other?						x

hopelessness on the canvas or using fine petite points of MHPG determinations. Heuristically, using Occam's razor, we can reduce the observed signs and symptoms of a depressive disorder and correlate these to the most basic core functions we know, that of life itself. If we use as a basic working hypothesis that every activity of a human being is the result of understandable psychic, physiological, psychomotor, and psy-chological processes, then we could postu-late and view depression as involving a dys-function of the basic functions of life (see Table 15-7).

D. Associated Features of Depressive Disorder

In order to determine what associated features of psychopathology were present in

Table 15-6. Criteria for the Diagnosis of Depressive Disorder.

1. PERVASIVE AFFECT
1. Depressed, sad
2. Tearful

2. PHYSIOLOGICAL DISTURBANCES
1. Diurnal variation
2. Sleep: early and frequent waking
3. Appetite: decreased
4. Weight: decreased
5. Libido: decreased
6. Fatigue, unexplainable
7. Constipation
8. Tachycardia

3. PSYCHOMOTOR DISTURBANCES
1. Agitation
2. Retardation

4. PSYCHOLOGICAL DISTURBANCES
1. Confusion
2. Emptiness
3. Hopelessness
4. Indecisiveness
5. Irritability
6. Dissatisfaction
7. Personal devaluation
8. Suicidal rumination

the elderly depressed, we conducted a longitudinal study to investigate this.[42] We used the Interviewer-rated Psychiatric Inventory List (IPIL), and its self-rated form called the Self-rating Psychiatric Inventory List (SPIL)[43] which measures the following clinical dimensions: (1) Psychoticism, as manifested by the presence of paranoid delusions, delusions of reference, derealization, and auditory, olfactory, and visual hallucinations; (2) Elation, both affective, psychomotor and psychological symptomatology; (3) Depression; (4) Anxiety; (5) Neuroticism, as measured by the quantitative presence of: obsessive-compulsive thoughts and behaviors, hypochondriasis, and phobias; and (6) Emotional Status, as measured by: (a) The person feels that he has control over himself at the intrapersonal level, and is able to make decisions about his own life, and is able to use coping and adaptive mechanisms for problem-solving. (b) The person feels that he has available and accessible meaningful relationships with others at the interpersonal level, and he feels satisfaction with his role within his particular social system. The depression ratings in the IPIL and SPIL were based upon the

Table 15-7. Manifestations of Disturbance in Basic Life Function in Depressed Patients.

BASIC LIFE FUNCTIONS:	FUNCTIONAL SPHERES OF PERSON:	DISTURBANCES IN PERSON WITH DEPRESSIVE DISORDER MANIFESTS:
I. 1. BEHAVIOR	I. PSYCHIC-AFFECTIVE	I. Mood change: sad, depressed, tearful
II. 2. GROWTH 3. METABOLISM 4. REPRODUCTION	II. PHYSIOLOGIC	II. Decreases in appetite, weight, sleep, energy, libido, dysautonomias
III. 5. MOVEMENT	III. PSYCHOMOTOR	III. Agitation or restlessness, Retardation or withdrawal
IV. 6. RESPONSIVENESS 7. ADAPTATION	IV. PSYCHOLOGIC	IV. Generalized disinterest, confusion, indecisiveness, irritability, dissatisfaction, emptiness, hopelessness Loss of coping and adaptive mechanisms, personal devaluation, suicidal rumination

previously reported Depression Status Inventory[44] and the Self-rating Depression Scale.[45] The anxiety ratings were based upon the previously reported Anxiety Status Inventory and the Self-rating Anxiety Scale.[46]

In order to compare these clinical dimensions obtained from elderly patients with depression-only, this same battery of evaluations was given to three other study groups: patients with dementia-only, patients with depression-and-dementia, and a group of elderly healthy volunteers. Table 15-8 summarizes the results obtained from the four study groups.

We can see from Table 15-8 that the psychoticism index for the four groups was similar and not statistically different from each other, and all have an index below the morbidity cut-off score of 45. On the clinical dimension of elation, there were no interviewer-rated differences, while the self-rating did show significant differences among the four groups. The normal healthy group scored higher than did the three patient groups on this dimension. Patients with depressive disorders rated higher on the depression dimension on both interviewer-rating and self-ratings, with both indices

above the morbidity cut-off score of 50. We can see from the table that depressed patients have significant anxiety concomitantly as part of the clinical feature of their illness. Thus, on both interviewer- and self-ratings, patients with depression-only scored significantly higher on anxiety than did the other three study groups, with their anxiety indices above the established morbidity cut-off score of 45. On the neuroticism dimension, all three patient groups scored higher than did the normal elderly volunteer groups. Lastly, on the measure of emotional status, patients with depression-only scored higher than did any other group, at a statistically significant level, indicating that this group felt a significant lack of available emotional resources.

E. Depression in the Elderly is Different

We have thus far examined the human person, starting with his basic life functions, and explored the effects of aging in terms of the four functional spheres of: (1) Psychic-affective; (2) Physiologic; (3) Psychomotor; and (4) Psychologic. We have seen that stress as a factor, whether it be from within

Table 15-8.   Comparison of Interviewer-rated Psychiatric Inventory List and Self-rated Psychiatric Inventory List results for four study groups of elderly subjects as measured by the various clinical dimensions.

VARIABLE	DEPRESSION ONLY		DEMENTIA ONLY		DEPRESSION & DEMENTIA		HEALTHY NORMAL		P
	MEAN	S.D.	MEAN	S.D.	MEAN	S.D.	MEAN	S.D.	
INTERVIEWER:									
Psychoticism	25.6	1.2	26.9	6.0	26.7	3.3	25.0	0.0	—
Elation	27.6	6.0	28.6	7.7	27.9	8.4	28.4	6.4	—
Depression	65.8	11.4	51.4	12.5	58.6	8.4	31.6	6.2	0.01
Anxiety	51.1	11.1	40.0	6.6	46.4	8.6	31.2	6.7	0.01
Neuroticism	43.2	12.5	41.8	10.9	46.1	9.3	28.2	5.8	0.01
Emot. Status	46.9	9.0	36.1	8.8	38.2	7.1	28.1	3.7	0.01
SELF:									
Psychoticism	28.2	4.0	27.7	5.2	27.7	4.6	25.8	1.7	—
Elation	34.0	9.0	35.0	12.5	37.3	16.8	51.5	15.3	0.01
Depression	62.2	11.9	50.6	13.8	53.3	10.8	35.1	7.3	0.01
Anxiety	52.1	11.3	37.8	7.9	42.8	7.6	30.0	7.6	0.01
Neuroticism	46.3	9.2	46.5	9.9	48.0	13.0	34.7	6.9	0.01
Emot. Status	44.5	9.1	37.2	9.3	39.8	10.6	31.2	5.7	0.01

the person, or from outside the person, produces additional changes in the basic life functions. Lastly, we have probed at depth, the disturbances that a person with a depressive disorder manifests in terms of a core of signs and symptoms. Taking now into account our earlier discussion on the nature of aging, stress and stressors, life events and losses, and human needs, we are now ready to see how depression in the elderly is different from depression in the non-elderly. If we accept the criteria for health and normality as a person's ability to work and produce, to love and play, and to enjoy life, then we can see that the realities of life do not provide this for the elderly. Instead, real life events take place that impair the ability of the elderly to be normal. Table 15-9 demonstrates how these events lead to personality changes, which clinically manifest themselves as symptoms of depression which are part of the core of depression in the elderly. We can see that our previous

explorations into the meaning of life events as stressors had a single purpose: to understand their role in the etiology of depression in the elderly.

Several authors have commented that depression in the aged tends to take a form which is different from that usually found in younger persons.[47-49] Table 15-9 illustrates the sequence of events and processes that evolve in the aging process and contribute towards these differences. Starting with the right-hand column entitled: *Real Life Events that Occur,* and then moving towards the left, to the next column headed: *Personality Changes as*; and followed by *Manifested in the Elderly Depressed as*, we can see how biological, and psychosocial aging processes affect the four functional spheres of a person.

The elderly are characterized by their states of being anxious, preoccupied with physical symptoms, fatigued, withdrawn, retarded, apathetic, inert, disinterested in

Table 15-9.   Real Life Events as Factors in the Development of Depressive Disorders in the Elderly.

FUNCTIONAL SPHERES OF PERSON:	MANIFESTED IN THE ELDERLY DEPRESSED AS:	PERSONALITY CHANGES AS:	REAL LIFE EVENTS THAT OCCUR:
I. Psychic-affective	I. Anxiety	I. Feeling of inferiority, fear, panic	I. Loss of status via retirement
II. Physiologic	II. Preoccupation with physical symptoms, fatigue, hypochondriasis	II. Denial of emotional impact, greater dependency needs	II. Physical illness, physical disabilities
III. Psychomotor	III. Withdrawal, retardation, placation	III. Loss of motivation, Tendency to suspiciousness	III. Social isolation Loss of love objects
IV. Psychologic	IV. Irritability, rejection, rumination, preoccupation. Disturbed reality testing, confabulation, distortion Loss of self-esteem, personal devaluation, worthless, helpless, Feelings of emptiness, hopelessness, apathy, disinterest	IV. Conservatism of outlook and action Feelings of anger, Development of over-independence, over-compensation	IV. Role changes, Biological aging with: decrease in vibratory and sensory acuity Reduction of recent memory

their surroundings, and lacking drive. In one reported study of depression in the normal aged,[50] the Self-rating Depression Scale was used and results of the factor analysis obtained from the scale indicated the following: Four factors were identified, with Factor 1 clustered around items that measured personal devaluation, emptiness, indecisiveness, dissatisfaction, hopelessness, psychomotor retardation, suicidal rumination, and confusion. On the basis of these items with the highest factor saturations, this factor was called "Loss of self-esteem." The most important saturations in the second, third and fourth factors were weighted in the direction of the biological symptoms and these included: sleep disturbance, decreased appetite, weight loss, decreased libido, diurnal variation, constipation, tachycardia, fatigue, psychomotor agitation, and retardation. Thus, pathological aging may be an extension of normal aging, and the necessary matrix has already been laid down. The importance of this factor in the etiology of depression in the aged was underscored by one report.[51] The authors found in their experience that guilt and introjection of hostility or introjection of unacceptable impulses were relatively unimportant factors with elderly people, and not the major cause of feelings of depression. Instead, they suggested that depression was more related to feelings of inferiority and the loss of self-esteem.

The predictive but changing environmental circumstances to which the elderly are subject, such as loss of status as a result of retirement, loss of physical health with physical disabilities, social isolation and role changes contribute to the decrease in one's self-esteem, and the growth of pessimism. Pessimism is so common in the aging population that it is frequently considered the "normal neurosis" of the aged. Though a certain degree of pessimism may be considered a normal or predictive response to aging, the gloomy outlook may be magnified and distorted to such a degree that the individual develops nihilistic ideas leading to severe depression and suicide. The antidote for lack of self-esteem is not high self-esteem, but to feel good just by being a person and accepted for being a person.

In addition to the physical and social real-life events that occur in the aging process and contribute to the development of a depressive disorder, the physiological changes as real-life events also contribute in a detrimental fashion. In the aged, the central nervous system may be marginally operational and thus there is an increasing potential for perceptual distortion of external stimuli. If one misperceives the stimulus, then the response will be inappropriate, and the environment reacts negatively to the inappropriate responses. We may see either an overt negative reaction or the more passive isolationism. Both will increase feelings of insecurity, which lead to anxiety, anger, or agitation. We all tend to resort to or rely on patterns of behavior that we have found to be successful in earlier life, but such a pattern becomes a characteristic of psychological adjustment. The more rigid the behavior pattern, the less successful it tends to be in satisfying one's needs, and the resultant depression tends to further compromise the rather tenuous physiological and psychological functions.

F. Physical Illness and Mental Health

The primary sign of aging is loss of physical health. Results of this are physical illnesses, physical disabilities, increased vulnerability to disease, infection, accidents, malnutrition, debilitation, discomfort and malaise. The primary symptom of aging is fatigue. This is a result of physical illness, as well as a denial mechanism. There is a shift from acknowledgment of the emotional impact and turmoil to the psyche caused by the physical illness to focusing on the physical illness itself. Typically, the person claims that "nothing's wrong with me, it's just that I have a (whatever-physical-disorder), and I feel tired, that's all." With the onset of physical illness, there develops a greater dependency need, followed by the preoccupation with physical symptoms, which is so often encountered as hypochondriasis and dismissed as clinically insignificant.

In my previous discussion of stressors, life events and losses, I pointed out that loss as an etiological factor in producing stress can be either real losses, threatened losses, or imaginary losses. In one study that was conducted and reported, the role of physical health and medical illnesses as an etiological factor in depression of the elderly was investigated.[42] Four groups of elderly subjects, who were diagnosed as having depression-only, dementia-only, depression-and-dementia, and normal healthy volunteers, were given a questionnaire that recorded their past medical history. Results of this study are found in Table 15-10. All the sub-

jects were asked to rate themselves as to how their health was from birth to 30 years old, from 31 years old to the present, and their health right now. This was done on a 4-point scale with 1–excellent, 2–good, 3–fair, and 4–poor. There were no statistically significant differences among the four groups for physical health for the period of birth to 30 years old. When we came to the period from 31 years of age until the present, the depression-only group scored their global health as fair, while the other three study groups scored their health as good, at a statistically significant level. When asked how their health is right now, all three patient groups rated themselves significantly worse, with the depressed-only group scor-

Table 15-10. Comparison of Past Medical History as: 1. Global rating of health from birth to 30 y/o, 31 y/o to present, and health right now, using a 4-point scale (1 = excellent, 2 = good, 3 = fair, 4 = poor). 2. Number of hospitalizations and operations in a lifetime. 3. Number of visits to M.D., number of days sick at home, or in hospital or nursing home, and number of actual illnesses. 4. Number of health problems, medicines taken, and problems with performing activities. 5. Global assessment of health-sickness on a 10-point scale (1 = worst, 10 = best) for the present, 5 years ago, and 5 years in the future.

VARIABLE	DEPRESSION ONLY		DEMENTIA ONLY		DEPRESSION & DEMENTIA		HEALTHY NORMAL		P
	MEAN	S.D.	MEAN	S.D.	MEAN	S.D.	MEAN	S.D.	
1. *Past Med. Hx*									
Before 30	1.8	0.7	1.6	0.7	1.8	0.7	1.6	0.7	—
After 30	2.7	0.8	2.0	0.6	2.2	0.7	1.8	0.7	0.01
Now	2.9	0.9	2.6	0.8	2.7	0.7	1.8	0.4	0.01
2. *PMHx: Life-time*									
# Hospital	5.2	2.2	2.9	2.3	4.6	2.9	4.4	2.9	—
# Operations	2.8	1.5	1.0	0.6	2.1	1.5	2.3	2.2	—
3. *PMHx: Past Yr*									
# See MD	6.5	2.9	2.0	1.4	4.0	2.5	2.0	2.4	0.01
# Sick at home	1.9	1.5	0.7	1.0	0.6	1.1	0.3	0.5	0.01
# Sick H/NH	1.1	1.0	0.5	0.9	0.6	0.7	0.1	0.3	0.01
# Illnesses	1.1	1.2	1.1	0.9	1.1	1.3	0.3	0.5	—
4. *PMHx: Past Month*									
# Problems	3.5	2.3	2.3	1.5	2.5	2.3	1.1	0.8	0.01
# Meds	3.9	3.2	2.0	2.8	2.3	1.7	1.1	1.2	0.01
Activity prob	2.6	2.7	0.6	0.7	2.6	2.6	0.1	0.5	—
5. *Health Ladder*									
Health Now	4.9	2.4	5.8	1.9	5.9	2.1	8.8	1.9	0.01
Health 5YA	7.0	2.4	6.1	2.3	6.3	2.5	8.8	2.1	—
Health 5YF	5.7	2.2	5.0	0.6	5.6	2.3	8.7	1.7	0.01

ing the worst of all. Patients were next asked to check the total number of hospitalizations and operations they have had in their lifetime. Results of this showed no significant difference in these two health indices among the four groups. The next set of questions asked the subjects about their health history in terms of the past year. It is of interest to note that the total number of medical illnesses among the four study groups was not significantly different, whereas the use of direct support systems associated with health care was significantly different. The depression-only group made more visits to see their doctors, spent more days sick in bed, or in a hospital or nursing home. Using a time period of the past month, the subjects were asked to rate themselves on the following variables: number of health problems, number of medications taken, and number of troubles with performing activities such as lifting, stooping, walking, dressing, and eating. All three patient groups scored themselves significantly less able to perform than did the healthy elderly volunteers, with the depression-only group having the highest number of health problems. Lastly, we can see from Table 15-10 (Health Ladder) that when all four study groups were asked to assess their own health on a global 10-point scale, with 1–worst, and 10–best, the depressed-only scored their present health as being worse than the other three groups. Finally, the depression-only group rated their projected health 5 years in the future lower than the healthy volunteer group, which is most likely a reflection of their current psychological state, that of feeling depressed and hopeless about the present and future.

III. DIFFERENTIAL DIAGNOSIS

A. Depression and Dementia

The symptoms of a depressive disorder are most often confused with those of dementia. Dementia is defined differently by different users of the term, and we are faced with a similar dialectical dilemma as with the meaning of the term depression. Post suggested that in order to escape the terminological jungle, all organic brain syndromes be referred to as cerebral failures.[52] Cerebral failures are divided by Post into those with rapid acute onset, and those with gradual onset which can lead to either depression, dementia, or both in combination.

The state of the art today with reference to differentiation between dementia and depression can be summarized by Table 15-11. Not all of these features are applicable to every patient, and unfortunately, they are not always as definite and crystal clear in their manifestations. In order to make use of these differential clinical features, it is imperative to obtain a thorough history of the present illness in terms of its chronological development from an independent source. This significant-other person may be a family member, a friend, an associate or other workers in the health care role. It is the time course of the *onset* of these diagnostic features, as well as the time course of their *remission* which becomes the diagnostic key to the puzzle of differential diagnosis between depression and dementia.

B. Pseudodementia

Pseudodementia is a term applied to the clinical condition appearing in elderly patients with depression who manifest transient cognitive impairment. Madden[53] *et al.* reported 300 patients in a psychiatric unit of a general hospital over the age of 45 who exhibited behavior suggestive of organic brain syndromes when first seen. Ordinarily the clinical findings would invalidate a favorable prognosis and seriously weigh against an active therapy program. However, in retrospect, they found that none of the 300 patients really suffered from irreversible organic syndromes as the basis for their presenting illness. The authors made the observation that the requirements of a somewhat inflexible nomenclature and

Table 15-11.   The Differential Diagnosis between Dementia and Depression.

DEMENTIA	DEPRESSION
1. AFFECT: Labile, fluctuating from tears to laughter, not consistent or sustained; may show apathy, depression, irritability, euphoria or inappropriate affect. Normal control impaired, can be influenced by suggestions.	1. Depressed, feelings of despair which are pervasive, persistent. Anxious, hypomanic. Affect not influenced by suggestion.
2. MEMORY Decreased attention. Decreased for recent events. Confabulation. Perseveration.	2. Difficulty in concentration. Impaired learning of new knowledge. Decreased attention, with secondary decrease in recent memory.
3. INTELLECT: Impaired, decreased, as tested by: serial 7's, similarities, recent events.	3. Impaired, but can perform serial 7's, remember recent events.
4. ORIENTATION: Fluctuating with varying levels of awareness. May be disoriented for time, place.	4. May have some confusion, not as profound as in dementia.
5. JUDGMENT: Poor judment with inappropriate behavior, dress. Deterioration of personal habits, and personal hygiene. Loss of bladder and bowel control.	5. May be poor.
6. SOMATIC COMPLAINTS: Fatigue. Failing health complaints, with vague complaints of pain in head, neck, back.	6. Typical complaints as: decreased sleep decreased appetite decreased weight decreased libido decreased energy constipation
7. PSYCHOTIC BEHAVIOR: Mainly visual, hallucinations, delusions	7. May occur in psychotic depressions, with mainly auditory hallucination; delusions.
8. NEUROLOGICAL SYMPTOMS: dysphasia, apraxia, agnosia	8. Not present.

the ominous specter of tradition seem to have obscured our recognition of disturbances easily identified in younger patients.

Pseudodementia was described by Madden as a nondementing psychosis with the following clinical features: disorientation; defects in recent memory, retention, calculation, and judgment. These features disappeared with alleviation of the psychotic picture by means of short-term intensive therapy. These patients would also exhibit intellectual impairment which is typified by the inability for new learning. Previous investigations of memory impairment in depressed patients have documented this defect, which on psychological testing would suggest the presence of an organic brain syndrome.[54] We had postulated that this specific deficit of ability for new learning as found in depressive disorders is based upon a disturbance of the reticular activating system, and its inability to screen incoming sensory signals efficiently.[40,41,55]

C. Central Anticholinergic Syndrome

Occasional patients present with confusion states that are clinically indistinguishable from organic brain syndromes or with depressive disorders, but in fact are iatrogenically induced. Psychotropic drugs such as tricyclic antidepressants, antipsychotic agents, and antiparkinsonian drugs produce anticholinergic side effects. These toxic side effects occur intermittently appearing as confusional states which have been called central anticholinergic syndrome.[56] It is characterized by the presence of a marked disturbance of: short-term memory, impaired attention, disorientation, anxiety, visual and auditory hallucinations, and increased psychotic thinking. Elderly patients are most susceptible to this atropine-like toxicity and develop this syndrome. Physostigmine has been demonstrated to reverse these target symptoms.

IV. PREVENTION AND TREATMENT

A. The Treatment of Depression: A triadic approach

In the treatment of depression, therapeutic outcome is the main concern of the medical practitioner. Equipped with old and new treatment modalities, and knowledge of their individual and combined capabilities, the practitioner nevertheless faces therapeutic failures along with his successes, and we need to understand both. The proposed model is not meant to be reductionistic by narrowing the complex phenomena of treatment response to a single schema, instead it represents a holistic attempt to emphasize the interrelationship between the various factors.

Starting with *Treatment* (1—all numbers refer to cells in Fig. 15-3), we can see that by itself treatment does not cause a patient to be *Improved* (10). Treatment would include psychotherapy, drugs, electroconvulsive therapy and the physical and occupational therapies. Treatment does, however, affect the patient's biological systems and *Internal Milieu* so as to produce *Changes in Cerebral Activities* (2). Regardless of one's approach to the mechanism underlying the pathogenesis of depression (such as neurophysiological, biochemical, neuroendocrinological or psychoanalytical), his concern should be: what is the ultimate action of the treatment on the somatic substrate? In drug treatment,

we have come closest to a one-to-one hypothesis relating the molecular structures of the antidepressant compounds with the molecular structures of the neurones.

If we conceive of depression as a psychiatric disorder which manifests itself in the three areas of *Affective Changes* (3), *Physiological Changes* (4) and *Psychological Changes* (5), we can predict that changes in cerebral activities will affect all three areas. The end result of treatment manifests itself as *Behavioral Changes* (6). These changes may be positive and therapeutic with obvious symptomatic relief exhibited clinically, or they may include adverse reactions and complications.

Notice that the result of our treatment so far is the symptomatic changes produced in our patient, and we still have not reached our goal: that of an improved patient. Behavioral changes effected by our treatment constitute only one process of three which all together eventually will lead to a therapeutic outcome. Thus, although cerebral actions and changes are necessary conditions, they are not regarded as sufficient. The crucial point of this model is at this junction. It is here that the other two of the three trichotomies *Premorbid Personality* (7) and *External Milieu* (8) enter into the schema. Premorbid personality includes the usual demographic data about the patient: his age, sex, race, marital status, education and socioeconomic status. It also includes factors such as his attitudes and expectations, which are results of the psychodynamic factors which make that patient "himself." External milieu factors include: the doctor-patient relationship, with its implications of suggestability and faith on the part of the patient, the regard the doctor has for his patient, and for the treatment method itself (and placebo effect). It cannot be emphasized enough that it is the doctor who treats, and not the treatment. A compassionate, responsive, sympathetic physician showing tender loving care may be the best treatment. Encompassed within the external medical milieu are the nurses, attendants and other ancillary helpers. Their

THE TREATMENT OF DEPRESSION: A HOMEOSTATIC MODEL

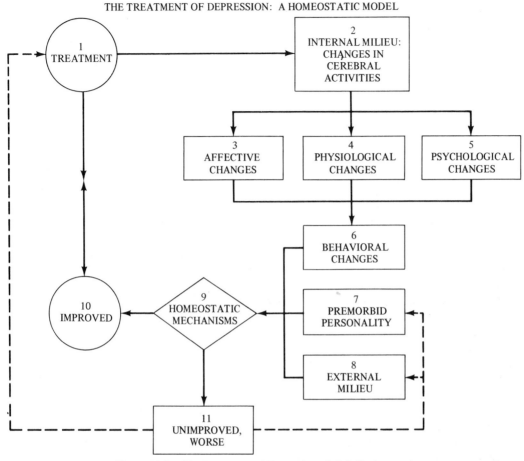

Figure 15-3.   The Treatment of Depression: A Triadic Approach.

warmth, interest, continuing efforts and contacts (or lack of it) contribute to the larger society in which the patient finds himself. Additionally, there is the non-medical milieu: the society of family, friends, community and the physical environment.

The three simultaneous processes influence *Homeostatic Mechanisms* (9) to produce a patient who is either *Improved* (10) or *Unimproved* or *Worse* (11). Any understanding of the therapeutic outcome is the understanding of all three: treatment, premorbid personality and external milieu. If the outcome is unsuccessful, the practitioner must look to all three (as indicated by the dotted lines and arrows) in order to understand the nature of the therapeutic failure. Similarly, the evaluation of the prognosis of any therapeutic program must

also take all three processes into consideration. As the patient's physician, we must be prepared not only to understand but also to influence all three, at the same time, when necessary.

B. Physical Health and Mental Illness

Most aged patients, whatever their primary diagnosis, are most likely to have multiple health problems, both medical and psychiatric. It cannot be emphasized enough that consideration of this fact must be taken into account when we discuss prevention and treatment of the elderly depressed patient. A direct method physicians can follow to help prevent mental illness in their elderly patients is to treat and improve the patients' general physical illnesses. By decreasing the severity of physical illness, we improve mental health, and we also decrease the high risk of suicide in this population. Suicide occurs with alarming frequency among the aged, with the highest correlation of suicide among those with physical illnesses, and depressive disorders. When patients have multiple diseases, the physician has more avenues of approach toward helping the total sick person.

C. Pharmacotherapy

Detailed descriptions concerning the use of pharmacological agents in the treatment of mood disorders can be found in standard textbooks on psychopharmacology,[57,58] and more specifically in the elderly in articles and books.[59-61]

It would be helpful to keep in mind the following age-related changes when using psychotropic agents to treat the elderly; changes that have a direct bearing on the pharmacology of the drug being used. The elderly have:

1. Diminished physiological functions including: (a) Decreased protein synthesis and binding—most drugs act by being protein-bound. When less plasma protein is available, the conjugation of a drug with the body protein will proceed at a slower rate, resulting in more active molecules of drugs available for action. The implications are that lower dosages of drugs need to be used in the elderly. (b) Decreased liver function—the majority of the drugs we prescribe today are metabolized and detoxified in the liver. When liver enzyme induction is diminished, more free drug is available with the consequence that usual dosage of most drugs has a more intensive effect and longer duration of action in the system. (c) Decreased gastric acid production—certain drugs like the barbiturates require an acidic substrate to dissolve; when there is decreased gastric secretion, there is decreased total absorption of acid-requiring drugs. (d) Decreased intestinal motility—the result of this is that more of a given drug will be available for a longer time since its transit time in the intestinal tract has increased.

2. Elderly have a different fat/muscle ratio with more fat and less muscle tissue so that absorption of any fat-soluble drug will be greater. In addition, when fat deposition increases, the amount of intracellular water is reduced, resulting in decreased excretion and increased duration of drug action.

In the decision process to determine the pharmacological treatment of depressed patients, the following factors should be kept in mind: (1) General health history and status; (2) Nutritional history and status; (3) Drug history and status; and (4) Laboratory results of selective tests. In selecting the drug to treat the patient's present illness, the following factors need to be kept in mind: (1) If there is a history of previous depressions, what treatments were used and what was the efficacy of previous drug therapy? If there is a history of a positive response to a particular drug, that should be the drug selected for further treatment. (2) If there is a history of negative response, a review of the dosage and duration of treatment is necessary before deciding that the patient was refractory to the particular medication used, since underdosage and inadequate duration of clinical trial are common. (3) History of previous treatment response to psychotropic drugs by relatives.

Tricyclic Antidepressant Drugs (TAD). These compounds are the usual drugs used when initiating pharmacotherapy of patients with depressive disorders. Amitriptyline or imipramine are used as follows: (1) Start with low dosages and progress to a therapeutic dosage which should be as high as the patient needs clinically, and can tolerate. The nonelderly adult maximum total daily dosage is 300 mg, but the elderly patient may not be able to tolerate a total daily dosage higher than half of that. Start with low dosages (especially if there is a history of sensitivity to drugs in general, and the patient reports a number of side effects with the TAD), and progressively increase to the maximum by the end of the third week. (2) There are differences of opinions as to whether the TADs should be given in divided daily doses, or in single bed-time doses as used with elderly depressed patients. Those favoring divided doses do so on the basis of better control over side effects in the event of their occurrence, avoidance of peaking of blood levels, and the need for pill taking and the placebo effect on the elderly patient who is actively doing something to help his own condition. Those favoring single bed-time doses do so on the basis of minimizing day-time side effects such as orthostatic hypotension, maximizing the sedative side effects of the TAD, and increasing drug compliance and drug taking. A suggested program is to start the patient with 40–50 mg, total daily dosage (divided, or single h.s.), for several days and then increase to 75 mg by the end of week 1. Increase the total daily dosage to 100 mg by the end of week 2, and to 150 mg by the end of week 3. Dosages are increased if therapeutic effects are not seen, and if the previous dosage regimen has been adequately tolerated.

It is important that the patient and the family are informed that there may be no visible sign of improvement for 2 to 3 weeks, or else there is a great likelihood the patient will refuse to continue with the medication. A 4-week trial of medication is necessary before deciding whether or not the TAD is effective or ineffective. After the patient has achieved a clinical remission of his depression, the TAD should be continued for an additional 6 months of treatment. Again, the patient and the family need to be informed of the importance of the continuation of TAD therapy, or else there is a great likelihood that the patient will discontinue taking the medication.

If the TAD used appears to be ineffective after an adequate clinical trial of at least 4 weeks, and if the patient clinically can tolerate being drug free for a period of a week, then the use of another class of antidepressant drugs, such as the monoamine oxidase inhibitors, should be considered.

Monoamine Oxidase Inhibitors (MAOI). Phenelzine (Nardil) is the most effective member of the hydrazine class of monoamine oxidase inhibitors, and is reported to have fewer incidences of hypertensive crisis. At this time, it is also the only MAOI available to the prescribing physician. The nonelderly adult maximum total daily dosage is 75 mg, and as with the TADs, the elderly depressed patient may not be able to tolerate the same maximum dosage. The same principals used with TADs are used in the prescribing of MAOIs with respect to: starting with low dosages, gradually increasing and titrating for maximum clinical effect versus possible side effects, and use of maintenance therapy after clinical remission of depression for 6 months.

The use of MAOIs may be contraindicated in the elderly because of the likelihood of drug-drug interaction. There is a greater possibility of the elderly depressed patient taking a number of other medications for other conditions. Rabin, in his review of prescribed and nonprescribed medication usage, found that the elderly (65 years of age and over), although comprising only 9% of the population, receives 22% of all prescribed drugs.[62] In addition to the problem of polypharmacy in this group, there is also the problem of maintaining the restrictions of a necessary tyramine free diet. Patients on MAOI need to be instructed as to their dietary restrictions, and a sample instruction sheet can be made up and given to all patients on this medication.

Lithium. The use of lithium for the treatment of manic states is well documented, whereas the use of lithium as the drug of choice for the treatment of depression is not. Thus, lithium is indicated for treating the bipolar manic attack, and for prevention of recurrence of bipolar mania and depression. It does not seem to be useful in unipolar depressive disorders.

As with the TADs and the MAOIs, the elderly are more liable to its pharmacological effects and toxicity may occur at a serum level (such as 1.0 meq/1), which is lower than the recommended level for nonelderly depressed patients of 1.2 to 1.5

meq/1. Again, start with low dosages, increase gradually, and titrate dosage for maximal clinical improvement with minimal side-effects and therapeutic serum blood levels. The half-life of lithium is longer in the aged and often a patient may achieve an adequate blood level on smaller doses than is suggested for nonelderly adults. For example, to achieve the recommended therapeutic serum level of 1.2 to 1.5 meq/1, a younger patient might receive a daily total dosage of 1500 mg lithium, but an elderly patient might only need 600 to 900 mg total daily dosage to achieve the same blood level.

Since there is a lag time of several weeks before the therapeutic effects of lithium are apparent, the immediate and concomitant use of antipsychotic drugs, such as haloperidol or phenothiazines may help gain a more rapid control of the manic episode.

As with the use of MAOI, and TAD, the dangers of polypharmacy must be kept in mind as concomitant use of diuretics and low salt diets increase the liability to toxic side effects. Therefore, when lithium is used in the elderly, lithium and electrolyte levels should be frequently monitored. Increasing confusion is one of the predominant signs of lithium toxicity and the patient and family need to be instructed to be alert for this change in behavior.

D. Electroconvulsive Therapy (ECT)

Detailed descriptions concerning the use of ECT such as: examinations prior to ECT, preparation of the patient, use of muscle relaxant drugs, present techniques of ECT, spacing of treatments, prognostic tests for ECT, complications, contraindications, indications and results may be found in standard textbooks on somatic treatment.[63]

The clinical effectiveness of ECT has been summarized in a number of studies.[64-68] A comparison of the effectiveness of ECT in producing significant improvement with antidepressant drugs (TADs, and MAOIs), and with placebo (PBO) indicate the following, reported in mean percent of patients showing significant improvement.

In addition to the increased overall effectiveness of ECT over pharmacotherapy, improvement using ECT is also more rapid over time, and the follow up studies show that 85% of these patients have remained well without further symptoms.[69-71] The differences of efficacy between ECT and antidepressant drugs may be a result of inadequate drug dosages and insufficient duration of treatment in the use of antidepressants.

ECT is indicated for the treatment of all typologies of depressive disorder, whether it be one of the APA DSM-II, etiological, clinical, or any of the other typologies discussed in the previous section on classification of depressive disorders. Data from Greenblatt indicated relative effectiveness of ECT of 77%, 78%, and 85% for psychoneurotic depressive reaction, manic-depressive, depressed, and involutional melancholia, respectively.[64] The main criteria for selecting ECT as the treatment of choice is *not* on the type of depression, but rather the severity of the depression, and the necessity for an immediate response.

There are no lower or upper age limits when ECT is to be considered. Kalinowsky and Hippius consider depression in the elderly to respond well to ECT. They recognize that pronounced intellectual impairment, disorientation and other clinical ex-

TX MODALITY	GREENBLATT[64]	LEHMANN[65]	MRC[66]	WECHSLER[67]	ZUNG[68]
ECT	76%	80%	71%	72%	86%
TAD	49%	60%	52%	65%	67%
MAOI	50%		30%	50%	
PBO	46%		39%	23%	

pressions of arteriosclerotic changes make them less reluctant to treat such patients in view of their post-treatment organic like changes. They support the view that except when there is a questionable psychiatric diagnosis, they never exclude a patient in definite need of ECT because of any simultaneous disease. They report treating patients with ECT who were in their eighth and ninth decades of life, even in the presence of marked neurological pathology secondary to cerebral arteriosclerosis.

Several investigators have attempted to identify clinical signs and symptoms which would predict response to ECT.[72-74] Results of these studies indicate that depressives with characteristics most often ascribed to patients with endogenous depressions respond best. However, such results may reflect the circular thinking involved in selecting patients for treatment using ECT to begin with.[74]

A number of studies have reported favorable results using unilateral ECT with depressed patients with the advantage of less memory impairment. These results have been reviewed and summarized by D'Elia and Raotma.[75] The finding of less confusion and less memory impairment is an important consideration when ECT is considered for use in the elderly, for whom the least amount of organic impairment produced would be a desirable factor. However, the goal of recovery within the shortest period of time should not be jeopardized by relying on unilateral ECT until its therapeutic efficacy has been demonstrated to be as good as bilateral ECT.

The effectiveness of ECT in the treatment of mania and hypomania is not as well investigated or documented as its use in the treatment of depression. One recent retrospective study compared groups of patients in the same institution before and after introduction of ECT and reported that the group of patients who had received ECT were significantly better on discharge than those not treated with ECT.[76] Kalinowsky stated that the manic phase of the manic-depressive psychosis differs from the de-

pressive phase in its response to ECT. Treatments given twice or three times a week are frequently ineffective, whereas treatments given at closer intervals, such as 2 or 3 per day, have produced better results.[63]

E. Non-somatic Treatment Modalities

The wide array of psychologically oriented treatment methods available to the practitioner makes it possible for the physician treating an elderly depressed patient to be innovative, direct, and effective. The vast possibilities are outlined as follows:

1. PSYCHOTHERAPY

Individual	*Group*
a. Psychoanalytic	a. Supportive
b. Supportive	b. Insight-oriented
c. Insight-oriented	c. Family
d. Crisis intervention	d. Marriage
	e. Sensitivity
	f. Encounter
	g. Psychodrama

2. BEHAVIOR THERAPY

Individual, or Group

a. Systematic desensitization
b. Aversion
c. Token economies
d. Biofeedback

3. SOCIAL THERAPY

a. Milieu therapy—environmental manipulation
b. Occupational—vocational and avocational
c. Recreational

4. HYPNOSIS

The therapeutic goal of these various methods are the same: to help the depressed patient deal with his symptomatology related to the depressive disorder, and to help the depressed elderly patient deal with the psychological disturbances that have evolved from the aging process, from stress, from life events, and from all the significant losses that have occurred. The objectives of the therapy are to overcome the withdrawal, denial, projection, and somatization which the depressed elderly have by strengthening their self-reliance, self-awareness and self-esteem; decreasing their internal stress and anxiety; and learning to adapt to the here and-now situation. The elderly depressed patient has within the general sense of the word increased dependency, and has specific needs such as help with activities of daily living, nursing care, nutritional requirements, and input from personal contacts with helping-caring people. The greatest concern for the physician treating an elderly depressed patient is that of unqualified acceptance of the patient as a person, an open and direct approach to the patient's problems, and a realistic setting of treatment goals. The science of medicine includes the increased use of methods and results of scientific studies such as those we have described. Unfortunately, the more laboratory tests that are used, the more some doctors seem to become preoccupied with them, and spend less time with the patient. In this age of automation, there is more science and less concern with the whole person. Yet, we must remember that the treatment of depression is more than using drugs or psychotherapy or social therapy. Rather, it is the triadic approach we described above: the treatment process, the patient, and the physician. His effectiveness as a significant part of the nondrug treatment of his patient is determined by his own personality, his charm, his presence, his confidence, his ability to allay a patient's fears and concerns, and his not letting a patient become unduly discouraged. In summary, his effectiveness as a physician is dependent upon his ability to practice the art of medicine.

THE DIAGNOSIS AND TREATMENT OF MANIC DISORDERS IN LATE LIFE

Depressive illness is certainly the most prominent affective disorder in late life, but manic disorders do occur. Langley[76] suggests that they make up only 5% to 10% of all referrals for affective disorder and Roth[77] found 13% of 220 patients hospitalized for affective disorders to be suffering predominately from manic symptomatology. The essential features of a manic episode is a distinct period when the predominant mood is either elevated, expansive, or irritable and associated with hyperactivity, excessive involvement in activities without recognizing the high potential for painful consequences, pressure of speech, flight of ideas, inflated self-esteem, decreased need for sleep and distractibility.[78] It may appear as a manic or as a bipolar affective disorder.

Yet manic episodes are frequently atypical in the elderly.[76] Overactivity may not be as pronounced and the condition may be mistaken for the symptomatology of an agitated depression. This is especially a problem when manic and depressive features are intermixed in the patient (a not uncommon occurrence in late life). Speech will tend to demonstrate circumstantiality and even obsessive thought patterns as opposed flight of ideas. Paranoid delusions are much more common than at other stages of the life cycle. The patient may show evidence of a mild organic mental syndrome and appear to be most confused about his or her environment. Irritability and anger are much more common than the feelings of gaiety typically experienced in younger patients. The same etiological features discussed previously in this chapter regarding depression also apply to mania (which has been labeled the mirror image of depression).[79]

The patient who demonstrates evidence of mania should be hospitalized. Such patients are very difficult to manage as outpatients and often place considerable pressure on their families. Compliance in taking medications is poor and pharmacologic management is the basis of effective therapy. Lithium carbonate has greatly improved the treatment and prognosis for relapsing cases of mania at all stages of the life cycle. Dosage should begin 900 to 1800 mgs per day, depending on body weight, during the

acute manic phase. A lithium level of from
.8 mEg/1 to 1.2 mEg/1 is usually required
to control an acute attack and from .5
mEg/1 to 1.0 mEg/1 for maintenance
therapy. Special precautions must be taken
in monitoring the electrolyte mixture in
older patients because fluid balance may be
disrupted in patients with marginal cardiac
and renal function.[80] The phenothiazines
and buterophenones (especially haloperidol)
may be most helpful in controlling the acute
episodes of mania until a therapeutic level of
lithium is reached (usually after 3 or 4 days).

REFERENCES

1. Hardin, G.: *Biology: Its Human Implications,* San Francisco: Freeman, pp. 9-11, 1954.

2. Schildkraut, J. The catecholamine hypothesis of affective disorders: A review of supporting evidence, *Am. J. Psychiat.* **122:** 509-522 (1965).

3. Robinson, D., Davis, J., Niles, A., Ravaris, C. and Sylvester, D. Relation of sex and aging to monoamine oxidase activity of human brain, plasma and platelets, *Arch. Gen. Psychiat.* **24:** 536-539 (1971).

4. Shopsin, B.: Catecholamines and affective disorders revised: A critical assessment, *J. Nerv. Ment. Dis.* **158:** 369-383 (1974).

5. Engel, G.: *Psychological Development in Health and Disease,* Philadelphia: Saunders, pp. 294-297, 1962.

6. Lidz, T.: *The Person: His Development Throughout Life Cycle,* New York: Basic Books, pp. 476-495, 1968.

7. Holmes, T. and Rahe, R.: The social readjustment rating scale, *J. Psychosom. Res.* **11:** 213-218 (1967).

8. Tomkins, S. and McCarter, R. What and where are the primary affects? *Percept. Motor Skills* **18:** 119-158 (1964).

9. Hohman, L. and Wilson, W. P. The varieties of affective disturbances, *South. Med. J.* **55:** 307-309 (1962).

10. Gallemore, J. and Wilson, W. P. The complaint of pain in the clinical setting of affective disorders, *South. Med. J.* **62:** 551-555, 1969.

11. Kraepelin, E.: *Manic-Depressive Insanity and Paranoia,* May Barclay trans-ed, Edinburg: E. & S. Livingstone, 1921.

12. Sandifer, M. G., Jr., Wilson, I. C. and Green, L.: The two-type thesis of depressive disorders, *Am. J. Psychiat.* **123:** 93-97 (1966).

13. Lange, J. The endogenous and reactive affective

14. disorders and the manic-depressive constitution, in Bumke (ed.) *Handbook of Mental Diseases,* Berlin: Springer, 1928, vol. 6.

14. Mapother, E. Opening paper of discussion on manic-depressive psychosis, *Br. Med. J.* **2:** 872—876, 1926.

15. Lewis, A. J. Melancholia: A clinical survey of depressive states. *J. Ment. Sci.* **80:** 277-378 (1934).

16. Hill, D. Depression: Disease, reaction, or posture? *Am. J. Psychiat.* **125:** 445-457 (1968).

17. Kendell, R. E. *The Classification of Depressive Illnesses,* Maudsley Monograph No. 18 OUP, 1968.

18. Kiloh, L. G. and Garside, R. F. The independence of neurotic and endogenous depression, *Br. J. Psychiat.* **109:** 451-463 (1963).

19. Fahy, T. J., Brandon, S. and Garside, R. F. Classification of depressive illness, *Proc. Roy. Soc. Med.* **62:** 331-336 (1969).

20. Paykel, E. S. Depressive typologies and response to amitriptyline, *Br. J. Psychiat.* **120:** 147-156 (1972).

21. Overall, J. E., *et al.* Nosology of depression and differential response to drugs, *J.A.M.A.* **195:** 946-948 (1966).

22. Blinder, M. G. Classification and treatment of depression, *Int. Psychiat. Clin.* **6:** 3-26 (1969).

23. Pollitt, J. D. Suggestions for a physiological classification of depression, *Br. J. Psychiat.* **111:** 489-495 (1965).

24. Van Praag, H. M., Uleman, A. M. and Spitz, J. C. The vital syndrome interview, *Psychiatr. Neurol. Neurochir.* **68:** 329-346 (1965).

25. Woodruff, R. W., Murphy, C. E. and Herjanic, M. The natural history of affective disorders: I. Symptoms of 72 patients at the time of index hospital admission, *J. Psychiatr. Res.* **5:** 255-263 (1967).

26. Leonhard, K. Aufteilung der endogenen, *Psychosen Berlin, 2nd Ed.,* 1959.

27. Perris, C. A study of bipolar (manic-depressive) and unipolar recurrent depressive psychoses. *Acta Psychiatr. Scan.* **42:** 1-89 (1966).

28. Pare, C. M. B., Rees, L. and Sainsbury, J. J. Differentiation of two genetically specific types of depression by the response to antidepressants, *Lancet* **2:** 1340-1397 (1962).

29. Stengel, E. Classification of mental disorders, *Bull. WHO* **21:** 601-663 (1959).

30. *Diagnostic and Statistical Manual of Mental Disorders,* 2nd Ed. Washington, D.C.: American Psychiatric Association, 1968.

31. Sandifer, M. G., Jr., *et al.* Similarities and differences in patient evaluation by US and UK psychiatrists, *Am. J. Psychiat.* **126:** 206-212 (1969).

32. Gurland, B. J., *et al.* Cross-national study of diagnosis of the mental disorders: Some comparisons of diagnostic criteria from the first investigation, *Am. J. Psychiat.* **125** (suppl.): 30-39 (1969).

33. Maas, J. Biogenic amines and depression, *Arch. Gen. Psychiat.* **32:** 1357-1361 (1975).

34. Shagas, C. and Jones, A. A neurophysiologic test for psychiatric diagnosis: Results in 750 patients, *Am. J. Psychiat.* **114:** 1002-1009 (1958).

35. Gellhorn, E. and Loofbourrow, G. *Emotions and Emotional Disorders,* New York: Harper & Row, 1963.

36. Meldman, M. *Diseases of Attention and Perception,* Oxford: Pergamon Press, 1970.

37. Whatmore, G. and Ellis, R. Some neurophysiologic aspects of depressed states: An electromyographic study, *Arch. Gen. Psychiat.* **1:** 70-80 (1959).

38. Wilson, W. and Wilson, N. Observations on the duration of photically elicited arousal responses in depressive psychoses, *J. Nerv. Ment. Dis.* **133:** 438-440 (1961).

39. Paulson, G. and Gottlieb, G. A longitudinal study of the electroencephalographic arousal response in depressed patients, *J. Nerv. Ment. Dis.* **133:** 524-528 (1961).

40. Zung, W. W. K. Photic arousal response in depressed patients during ECT, *Acta Psychiat. Scand.* **45:** 295-302 (1969).

41. Zung, W. W. K., Wilson, W. P. and Dodson, W. E. Effect of depressive disorders on sleep EEG responses, *Arch. Gen. Psychiat.* **10:** 439-445 (1964).

42. Zung, W. W. K. and Wang, H. S. Depression and dementia in the aged: A model for psychosomatic medicine, Costa Mesa, CA: Academy of Psychosom. Med., 1977.

43. Zung, W. W. K. The Self-rating Psychiatric Inventory List, 1978.

44. Zung, W. W. K. The Depression Status Inventory: An adjunct to the self-rating depression scale, *J. Clin. Psychol.* **28:** 539-543 (1972).

45. Zung, W. W. K. A self-rating depression scale, *Arch. Gen. Psychiat.* **12:** 63-70 (1965).

46. Zung, W. W. K. A rating instrument for anxiety disorders, *Psychosom.* **12:** 371-379 (1971).

47. Levin, S. Depression in the aged: A study of the salient external factors, *Geriatrics,* **18:** 302-307 (1963).

48. Mayer-Gross, W., Slater, E. and Roth, M. *Clin. Psychiat.,* London: Cassell, 1960.

49. Foulds, G. Psychotic depression and age, *J. Ment. Sci.* **106:** 1394-1397 (1960).

50. Zung, W. W. K. Depression in the normal aged, *Psychosom.* **8:** 287-292 (1967).

51. Busse, E. and Reckless, J. Psychiatric management of the aged, *J.A.M.A.* **175:** 645-648 (1961).

52. Post, F.: Dementia, Depression, and Pseudodementia, In D. F. Benson and D. Blumer (eds.) *Psychiatric Aspects of Neurological Disease,* New York: Grune and Stratton, 1975.

53. Madden, J., Luhan, J., Kaplan, L. and Manfredi, H. Nondementing psychoses in older persons, *J.A.M.A.* **150:** 1567-1572, 1952.

54. Zung, W. W. K., Rogers, J. and Krugman, A. Ef-

fect of electroconvulsive therapy on memory in depressive disorders, In J. Wortis (Ed.) *Rec. Adv. Biol. Psychiat.* **10:** New York: Plenum Press, pp. 160-178, 1968.

55. Wilson, W. P. and Zung, W. K. Attention, discrimination and arousal during sleep, *Arch. Gen. Psychiat.* **15:** 523-528, 1966.

56. Davis, J., Fann, E. W., El-Yousef, K. and Janowsky, D. Clinical problems in treating the aged with psychotropic drugs, In C. Eisdorfer, and E. W. Fann, (eds.), *Psychopharmacology and Aging,* New York: Plenum Press, 1973.

57. Ban, T. *Psychopharmacology,* Baltimore: Williams & Wilkins, 1969.

58. Klein, D. and Davis, J. *Diagnosis and Drug Treatment of Psychiatric Disorders,* Baltimore: Williams & Wilkins, 1969.

59. Hall, M. Drug therapy in the elderly, *Brit. Med. J.* **4:** 582-584 (1973).

60. Lamy, P. Drugs and the geriatric patient, *J. Am. Ger. Soc.* **19:** 23-33 (1971).

61. Davis, R. *Drugs and the Elderly,* University of Southern California, Ethel Percy Andrus Gerontology Center, 1973.

62. Rabin, D. L. Use of medicine: A review of prescribed and non-prescribed medicine use, USPHS, DHEW, Washington, D.C., 1972.

63. Kalinowsky, L. and Hippius, H. *Pharmacological, Convulsive and Other Somatic Treatments in Psychiatry,* Grune & Stratton, New York, 1969.

64. Greenblatt, M., Grosser, G. and Wechsler, H. Differential response to hospitalized depressed patients to somatic therapy. *Amer. J. Psychiat.* **120:** 935-943 (1964).

65. Lehmann, H.: The pharmacotherapy of the depressive syndrome, *Canad. Med. J.* **92:** 821-828 (1965).

66. Medical Council Report: Report by Clinical Psychiatry Committee. Clinical trial of the treatment of depressive illness, *Brit. Med. J.* **1:** 881-886 (1965).

67. Wechsler, H., Grosser, G. and Greenblatt, M. Research evaluating antidepressant medications on hospitalized mental patients: A survey of published reports during a five-year period, *J. Nerv. Ment. Dis.* **141:** 231-239 (1965).

68. Zung, W. W. K. Evaluating treatment methods for depressive disorders, *Amer. J. Psychiat.* **124** (suppl.): 40-48 (1968).

69. Abrams, R. Recent clinical studies of ECT, *Sem. Psychiat.* **4:** 3-12 (1972).

70. Lippincott, R. Depressive illness: Identification and treatment in the elderly, *Geriatrics* **23:** 149-152 (1968).

71. Tait, C., Jr. and Burns, G. Involutional illnesses. A survey of 379 patients, including follow-up of 114, *Amer. J. Psychiat.* **108:** 27-36 (1951).

72. Hamilton, M. and White, J. Factors related to the outcome of depression treated with ECT, *J. Ment. Sci.* **106:** 1031-1041 (1960).

73. Carney, M., Roth, M., and Garside, R. The

diagnosis of depressive syndromes and the prediction of ECT response, *Brit. J. Psychiat.* **111:** 659–674 (1965).

74. Zung, W. W. K. and Wonnacott, T. Treatment prediction in depression using a self-rating scale, *Biol. Psychiat.* **2:** 321–329 (1970).

75. D'Elia, G. and Raotma, H. Is unilateral ECT less effective than bilateral ECT? *Brit. J. Psychiat.* **126:** 83–89 (1975).

76. Langley, G. E. Functional psychoses, In J. G. Howells, (ed.) *Modern Perspectives in the Psychiatry of Old Age.* New York: Brunner/Mazel, pp. 326–355, 1975.

77. Roth, M. The natural history of mental disorder in old age. *J. Ment. Sci.,* **101:** 281 (1955).

78. *Diagnostic and Statistical Manual-III.* Draft of April 15, 1977, American Psychiatric Association, 1977.

79. Pfeiffer, E. *Disordered Behavior: Basic Concepts in Clinical Psychiatry.* New York: Oxford University Press, 1968.

80. Show, A., Amdisen, A., Trap-Jensen, J. Lithium poisoning. *Am. J. Psychiatry,* **125:** 520 (1968).

Chapter 16

Anxiety, Dissociative and Personality Disorders in the Elderly

Adrian Verwoerdt, M.D.

Duke University Medical Center

ANXIETY DISORDERS

Anxiety and Coping in Old Age

Anxiety, the distressing affect which is subjectively experienced as worry similar to fear of a real danger or the anticipating of danger, is sometimes felt to be the central emotional experience in modern society. Before reviewing the clinical anxiety disorders, it is useful to distinguish several basic types of anxiety. Primary anxiety is the response to an overwhelming influx of external or internal stimuli. Secondary (depletion) anxiety refers to the anticipation of loss of external supplies; developmentally it is analogous to separation anxiety. Tertiary (guilty) anxiety is the warning signal in response to unacceptable impulses or fantasies; psychodynamically, it corresponds to superego anxiety. In old age, depletion anxiety appears to play a more significant role than the other two forms of anxiety.

Specific types of stress produce specific psychobiological states of distress (anxiety) which in turn, mobilize mental mechanisms and behavior patterns aimed to deal with the stress. These mechanisms are a function of the ego, which is conceptualized as a set of regulatory principles whose main task is to balance pressures originating from inner needs and drives, external opportunities and constraints, as well as the guidelines of one's conscience. Ego functions, including defense mechanisms, require energy to function effectively. For example, with less energy being available to the ego, it may become difficult to maintain repression. In such a case, there are several possible developments. First, some of that which was repressed may emerge into conscious awareness; and, if this repressed mental content is threatening or unacceptable to the individual, anxiety will be the result. Or, with repression itself being unable to do the job, auxiliary defenses are called into action, e.g., denial or projection. Third, there is the possibility of acting out. One of the earliest ego functions is to interpose a time lag between stimulus and response, so that a behavioral response is no longer an automatic reflex. During this delay of gratification, there is opportunity for selecting those behavioral responses which are likely to be maximally effective. Regression of this ego function may result in "the geriatric delinquent," dominated by the pleasure principle, and oriented toward immediate gratification, often at the expense of long-range plans.[1]

Coping is that state between the organism and his environment which allows the organism to conform to the reality of the external world while at the same time allowing activity directed toward change. The proper use of psychological defense mechanisms is essential to coping.

Whether coping is adaptive or maladaptive depends on the type and intensity of the defense as well as on its appropriateness to the situation. *Adaptive* coping techniques imply a re-establishment of an equilibrium that was disturbed due to the loss. In the case of coping with physical illness, for example, adaptive devices presuppose some amount of cognitive awareness regarding the illness, a willingness to seek medical help and a realistic adjustment to the sick role. *Maladaptive* defenses aggravate the patient's suffering, deplete his resources and weaken his resistance. The *selection* of a particular defense frequently results in certain characteristic behaviors. This has definite implications, not only for the individual's adjustment, or lack thereof, but also for clinical management. The various defense techniques and the behavioral patterns commonly associated with them can be grouped into three main categories, i.e., those aimed at (1) retreat and conservation of energy (e.g., regression, withdrawal); (2) exclusion of the threat from awareness (e.g., denial, suppression); and (3) mastery and control (e.g., reaction formation; compulsiveness).[2] The first group of defenses represent low-energy patterns, while the third group comprises high-energy patterns. The latter include reaction formation, counterphobic defenses, overcompensation, compulsive defenses, the "manic" cluster (denial; hyperactivity; suppression through diversion), as well as the "paranoid" cluster (projection; hostile aggression against or fleeing from the externalized threat). As the years go by, the high-energy defensive patterns become more vulnerable, due to physical illness or aged-related decline in energy production.[3]

In addition to these age-related ego changes there are two other dimensions of the personality that can be affected by aging. One of these pertains to drives and needs; the other, to the superego (conscience).

Typical of the senescence of living systems is the progressive decline in ability to produce energy.[4] Therefore, it is plausible to assume that with aging, the strength of the drives declines. This will be particularly true of the active drives (e.g., genital sexuality; generativity in the areas of work and parenthood). Another characteristic of aging is that the resting level of a biological function may show no significant change with age, but after stress, return to the baseline level is prolonged (e.g., displacements in electrolytes, blood glucose levels). With advancing age, more time is needed to restore the organism, which, on the psychological level, is experienced as an increase in needs. Thus, the needs for stability, shelter, rest, etc. will become relatively more important. These needs have a quality of being relatively more "narcissistic," self-oriented, and aimed at self-preservation. Important in this context is the fact that, because of declining strength and resources, the aged person has less power to bring about the fulfillment of his particular needs.

Finally, the *superego,* or conscience, may also be involved in age-related changes. Favorable changes are related to the phenomenon of mellowing and can come about in various ways. First, vis-à-vis less urgent drives, the superego may no longer have to be as alert or on guard. A relaxed superego may be inwardly experienced as a sense of freedom. Whatever energy has been freed, may now become available for other, possibly creative, purposes. Secondly, a person who has been "on good behavior" most of his life, may come to feel that now it is time for a reward, e.g., the experience of leisure during retirement. Unfavorable developments occur when, in the course of aging, needs or impulses emerge which are unacceptable to the superego. For example, a disabled person needing to accept help from others, may consider such dependency gratifications inconsistent with his self-concept, so that feelings of shame and guilt develop, or an attitude of rebellious protest.

Pathogenesis and Phenomenology

Anxiety disorders in the elderly may be grouped depending on their phenomenology and pathogenesis, as follows:

Acute traumatic anxiety
Chronic neurotic anxiety
Helplessness anxiety
Anxiety-depression
Phobic disorders
Obsessive compulsive disorder
Anxiety associated with psychosis

Acute Anxiety Reactions may develop as an acute adjustment reaction of late life; or they may result from a weakening of the ego's stimulus barrier. Normally, the ego is able to screen and ward off unwanted stimuli through various mechanisms, e.g., selective inattention or turning to external diversions. In conditions of moderate to severe regression, however, the ego boundary becomes more penetrable, as it were, and the patient is vulnerable to a barrage of unwanted stimuli. This type of anxiety arises any time when the psyche is overwhelmed by an influx of external or internal stimuli too great to be mastered. It is characteristic of infancy, when the ego is immature, but may occur whenever the ego is relatively weak, for example, in old age. Clinically, it is manifested by a primitive response of diffuse painful unpleasure. Milder cases show restlessness, tension, and irritability; more severe cases, outbursts of rage, or defensive attempts to re-establish a stimulus barrier by way of withdrawal.

Chronic Neurotic Anxiety is usually a carry-over from earlier years; the behavioral

patterns and symptoms have become ingrained in the character although they are usually not ego-syntonic. The patient suffers from tension and agitation, but is unable to explain why. Varying degrees of depression are usually present as well. The physiological concomitants of anxiety are often more prominent than the subjective feelings of anxiety. The agitation due to chronic anxiety should be differentiated from agitated depression; from akathisia, a side effect of antipsychotic drugs; and from the tremors that can be a side effect of lithium. Therefore, prior to starting pharmacotherapy it is useful to have a drug-free baseline.

Helplessness Anxiety arises due to (a) anticipation of loss of external supplies, or (b) fears of loss of control and mastery. (a) *Depletion Anxiety:* In elderly individuals, the nature of anxiety is not usually in terms of a danger signal pertaining to unacceptable impulses from within, but to loss of external supplies (object loss). Since the patient is not always aware of the source of his anxiety, a careful exploration of his life situation is in order. For example, the patient's anxiety may be based on the assumption that, when he will be in need of help, others will not be available or accessible. Frequently, this is experienced as anxiety about becoming a burden on others as well as fears of abandonment and loneliness. (b) Anxiety also may be generated by *loss of control and mastery*. This may be acute (as in sudden physical illness) or slowly progressive (due to accumulating losses in the area of personal competence and autonomy). Anxiety associated with this is felt as loss of self-confidence and shame.

Anxiety-Depression is frequent among middle-aged and elderly patients. Several factors may contribute to the development of mixed anxiety and depression. First, anyone who is depressed, but not yet at the point of hopelessness, will be fearful in the anticipation of yet additional misfortunes. Conversely, patients with anxiety symptoms may become more and more discouraged about their painful handicap.

Another type of anxiety-depression originates from guilty anxiety. Part of the superego is the idealized self concept, the *ego ideal,* which includes one's aspirations and life goals. At some point in middle age, a person may wonder if he will reach his goals. Some people will feel that they have arrived; others, that they have fallen short of their aspirations. The phrase "having arrived" is commonly used to refer to a sense of status in life, or the attainment of a plateau on which success comes in one's grasp. Once attained, this succession into the ego ideal will serve as insurance against the risks of loss of self-esteem that would result from "being over the hill." The sense of "not making it," or having missed the boat is at the center of experience from which evolve the severe involutional grief reactions, anxiety-depression mixtures, and agitated depressions.

Simple Phobia. Anxiety may be relieved by projection and externalization. This is accomplished by displacement onto objects and situations which serve as an external symbol of inner concerns or feelings. Once the internal problem has become an external threat, i.e., a phobia, the patient may feel in a position to cope, either by flight from the external threat, or, as in the case of counterphobic defenses, by fighting it. The latter vicissitude shows how counterphobic mechanisms can contribute to the development of certain paranoid states. Conversely, the breakdown of counterphobic defenses is one of the causes of phobia: due to decompensation of this mastery mechanism, the original phobic anxiety returns.

Obsessive-Compulsive Disorders. Although obsessive-compulsive symptoms are not infrequently associated with major mental illness in late life, obsessive-compulsive neurotic disorder as a separate disease entity apparently is rare.[5] Obsessive-compulsive disorder apparently predisposes to depressions, and can be a contributing factor in the

pathogenesis of senile dementia.[6] In again other cases, the neurosis may be alleviated due to intrapsychic factors responsible for the phenomenon of mellowing. Finally, a "pseudo-cure" may present itself when the patient has found acceptable ways and means of regression, e.g., through the sick role.

Not infrequently, obsessive-compulsive phenomena occur in the context of depression. Their psychodynamic significance may involve attempts to maintain control over unacceptable aggressive or sexual impulses. In other cases, obsessive doubt and compulsive rituals may serve an ulterior motive, e.g., avoiding painful decisions. Compulsive rituals may emerge as a last effort to prevent the life space from decaying into a micro-slum. In such cases we see the evidence of breakdown scattered all over the place, with the individual concentrating on keeping one tiny detail straightened out. One octogenerian, for example, with serious senile dementia, developed a compulsive habit of washing the tip of his cane.

Anxiety Associated with Psychosis. Delusional phobias, persecutory anxieties, and paranoid fears may occur in the context of chronic paranoid schizophrenia, paranoid states, or, at some point along the final common path toward senile dementia. This type of anxiety disorder is nonspecific with regard to age, except of course in the case of senile dementia.

Treatment

Clinical management involves a comprehensive approach in which drugs, psychotherapy, medical treatment, socioeconomic measures and environmental manipulation are fitted into a therapeutic program which will suit the needs of the individual patient. The promotion of appropriate dependency is therapeutically useful because it takes attention away from anxiety-provoking concerns, and when the motive of anxiety is absent, maladaptive defenses may be prevented from developing. An attempt should be made to prevent, eliminate or treat anxiety-provoking factors, which in the aged, often pertain to loss of external supplies, role uncertainty, intrafamilial strife, borderline economic resources, relentless progress of physical disability, drastic changes in the body image, etc. Antianxiety agents should be employed promptly to interrupt any vicious cycle of anxiety-depression, physical illness and other stresses.[7]

Acute Anxiety. For milder cases, the benzodiazepines can be used first; if the symptoms persist, or in more severe cases, antipsychotic agents may be tried. It is in the nature of an adjustment reaction to be transitory and responsive to counseling or guidance; this should focus on the patient's reactions to the precipitating event and resolving the environmental stress. Medication should be limited to a few weeks since chronic reliance on drugs may provide just enough relief to keep the patient from seeking a decisive solution.

While in milder cases, it is appropriate to try adjusting the patient to the environment (an approach typical for patients in younger age groups), in more severe cases, one attempts to accomplish precisely the opposite: to adjust the environment to the patient. One radical form of environmental support involves providing an "ego prosthesis." When the severe regression breaks down ego organization, leading to diminished resistance to external stimuli, a regimen can be provided that serves as an "ego prosthesis." Such an artificial ego implies organizing the patient's environment for him, with the spatiotemporal relations of his milieu kept constant. The principle is that of "sameness;" by keeping the milieu constant, the sense of loss of mastery in the patient is minimized. Constancy can be applied to arrangement of furniture, temperature, light, procedures, as well as visiting times.

Chronic Neurotic Anxiety. After a lifetime of behavioral patterns based on neurotic anxiety, an etiologically based insight therapy is not indicated. Generally, such patients do not respond well to therapeutic attempts aimed at insight, without drug therapy. In addition to the use of antianxiety drugs, the symptoms of anxiety, agitation, insomnia and tension, often can also be alleviated by increasing the level of activity. In planning programs of activities, some basic points must be kept in mind.

• The need for an individualized approach is pointed up by the fact that for each individual, sick or healthy, the pattern of age decrements is characteristic and the rate of decline varies from one function to another.

• Activity is to be more than passive participation in time-filling work. Therapeutic activity has purpose; the more completely it absorbs the patient's energies, the more beneficial it will be. When activities bring about contacts with other people, isolation is reduced.

• In designing an activity program, find out patient's interests; make a list of potential activities (indoors, outdoors) appropriate for the season; determine patient's attention span for each activity; preferred time of the day and preferred sequence of activities; arrive at a mutually agreed regimen of daily activities, covering about one month at the time; have patient return to report on regimen; review and make changes as needed.

• These patients frequently like simple, mechanical work, which does not require problem-solving or a dead-line, e.g., gardening.

• In many cases, maintenance drug therapy is needed to alleviate discomfort interfering with the optimal participation in the therapeutic program. If tension continues, one should consider the possibility of mixed anxiety-depression and add an antidepressant drug.

Helplessness Anxiety. Antianxiety drugs will alleviate the subjective experience of apprehension, protect the patient from the associated physiological stress, and facilitate the process of gathering information about the patient's life situation. One should quickly explore the possible causes of the anxiety before it becomes chronic. In addition to these immediate goals, there is the long-term therapeutic goal to re-establish the patient's equilibrium on a lasting basis. This involves several procedures, including:

• Necessary support in the areas of concern, e.g., financial assistance, homemaker services, legal aid, social contacts.

• In some cases, a permanent relationship with the patient. Continuation of medications represents an implicit contract to follow him at regular intervals.

• If proper support has been provided it is useful to take the patient off the medications, and observe how he is doing. When anxiety continues, after the alleged deficiencies in his life situation have been corrected, chances are that it has multiple origins, and that the original complaint was only the tip of the iceberg.

In the case of anxiety due to *loss of control,* the initial goal is to develop an optimal physician-patient relationship, and reduce anxiety by medication. Once the patient feels more secure in the relationship with the therapist, specific concerns can be identified. Usually it is more difficult to obtain this information than in depletion anxiety where the patient can simply point to an external problem. When the deficiency is more personal (pertaining to neuromuscular, mental, and social capacities that represent basic instrumentalities in the areas of love, play and work), it is more embarrassing to verbalize. The patient is gently but firmly advised to get whatever medical examinations are in order. Elderly patients often resist having alleged physical or mental defects examined; they may fear getting lost in the labyrinth of the modern hospital, or finding out that theirs is a hopeless case. It may be necessary to provide arrangements to make sure that the patient will not get lost in the maze of the hospital. After medical evaluation, it is frequently also a problem to get the patient to accept the recommended treatment. Here again, the "positive transference" element can serve its purpose. In

spite of appropriate treatment, a residue of decreased physical, mental or social competence may keep the anxiety going. Supportive therapy then should be maintained indefinitely. The goals of therapy include to help the patient adjust to the appropriate level of functioning, and to provide for corresponding changes in the environment: the more helpless the patient, the more helpful the environment must become.

A few more points with regard to therapeutic management:

• Generally, to reduce helplessness and enhance a sense of control, an "obsessive-compulsive" behavioral style may be encouraged: preference for predictability, avoidance of uncertainty and emphasis on regular routines.

• Relatives can be advised that feelings of helplessness in the aged family member can be alleviated by anticipating some of his needs. This fosters a subjective sense of control and may prevent angry frustration, depression or shame. Patients handicapped by memory loss often have a relationship with a relative who serves as a prosthetic memory device. In contacts with such patients and their relatives, one can observe that whenever the patient's memory fails him, he sends out a nonverbal signal (a quick look) toward the relative, who then responds by filling in the necessary details.

• It is essential to remind the patient of remaining assets, and encourage mobilization and diversions consistent with remaining potential. Premature or undue support has an adverse effect, by promoting regression. Thus, it is often difficult to stay on an intermediate course, avoiding on the one hand, insufficient support (which would create more anxiety) and, on the other hand, too much support (which would promote regression).

• The importance of sustaining activity is emphasized by the fact that decreased physical activity can cause significant changes in the distribution, metabolism, and excretion of drugs.[8] Motivation for activity must include a goal that seems worth the effort. A patient may learn to walk following a stroke, but, unless, he has a motive for walking, he may soon abandon the attempt. The milieu of the average institution frequently offers little incentive to activity thus fostering regression and deterioration. Self-care and independence have appeal only to the extent that there is something to live for. The therapist and other members of the treatment team can become sources of incentive, by appropriately rewarding the patient's efforts.

Anxiety Associated with Psychosis. Clinical management includes the use of antipsychotic agents, in addition to whatever medical, social, and environmental intervention is indicated. In many such patients, anxiety and helpless panic respond well to an approach which consists of: providing a structured relationship or environment; being generously supportive, while firmly insisting on suppression of psychotic thoughts, and focusing on the realities of the here-and-now.

DISSOCIATIVE DISORDERS

Dissociative disorders (as listed in DSM III) include amnesia, fugue and depersonalization. Their common denomination is a specific disturbance in conscious awareness.

Amnesia

Memory includes the ability to register, store and retrieve information; memory disturbances may be due to impaired functioning of any or all of these capacities. The ability to register, store or retrieve information depends, among other things, on the state of consciousness and the intactness of abstract capacity. A disturbed sensorium leads to a disturbance in attention, e.g., inability to concentrate, distractibility. Attention may also be affected by intense emotional states. In severe depression, for example, there may be intense preoccupation with depressive thought content. This points out that amnesia can be psychogenic (e.g., hysterical) or organic in origin.

Confabulations, a form of paramnesia, are products of fantasy being substituted for memory gaps and frequently colored by wishful thinking, which occur in Korsakov's syndrome and certain types of senile dementia. Kahn and Goldfarb[9] introduced a Mental Status Questionnaire consisting of 10 questions that pertain to orientation of time, place and person; recent and remote memory; and general information. Performance is scored in terms of the number of wrong answers; the error scores indicate the degree of organicity.

The capacity for abstract thought includes the specific function of apperception: a mental scanning process of comparing incoming stimuli and images with those already stored in memory. The actual fact of a loss or stress cannot be undone by the ego, but it is possible for the ego through its defense mechanisms, to try to prevent the loss from reaching conscious awareness. The situation may become rather complex, when ego functions themselves are changing as well, e.g., in organic mental disorder. In these instances the ego's ability to perceive reality is impaired and the impact of losses may be blunted. Reality perception may also be diminished through a process of withdrawal which prevents the individual from feeling the pain that would have come with clear awareness of having suffered a loss.

Fugue (Functional Brain Syndrome)

Orientation is the process by which a person uses sense data (from internal and external origins) to gain information about the spatiotemporal characteristics of his whereabouts, the position he occupies in his milieu, and how and why he came to be there. For orientation to be intact, the sense organs must provide a minimum of sensory input, to be integrated centrally in an intact brain; apperception is the mental scanning process of comparing incoming stimuli with those already stored in memory. Thus, disorientation can be caused by peripheral or central factors, or by a combination of both.

Because of difficulties in perception, comprehension, memory, as well as slowness in psychomotor skills, aged persons become more sensitive to *environmental changes.* Relatively minor alterations, such as a shift in household arrangements or family relationships, can cause serious psychological upsets. The brain is the "organ of adaptation," and whether it is in a state of compensation or decompensation, depends on the demands made on it. Cardiac status, by way of analogy, may decompensate when the input presented or the output demanded, exceeds the heart's potential for work. Likewise, the brittle brain status of an old person may decompensate because of changes in the input or the output.

1. *Abnormal Sensory Input* may be quantitative or qualitative in nature. *Quantitative* input changes include sensory overload, i.e., an increase in the amount of stimuli reaching the aged brain, e.g., chronic overcrowding of a three-generational family in a small dwelling; and sensory underload, i.e., an undue decrease in the number of afferent stimuli reaching the central nervous system. These quantitative changes can be chronic or acute, abrupt or insidious, or of minor or major proportions. Sensory deprivation or social isolation may be imposed on the individual (e.g., being alone in the hospital room; having the eyes covered following cataract surgery); they may be the outcome of life-long character traits (e.g., the isolation of the schizoid person); or, they may be due to major psychopathology (e.g., self-absorption in severe depression).

Qualitative changes in the input pertain to exposure to unfamiliar stimuli, e.g., sudden transfer to elderly persons from their homes to an institution. The aged person should not as a rule, be moved out of his familiar habitat without his prior knowledge and approval. Ideally, the transfer to an institution or chronic care facility involves a consensus between the aged individual, the significant family members, and a third party (social worker, physician, operator of the boarding home or nursing home). A move carried out suddenly, without due preparation, may lead to a "transplantation shock" in the aged person; a relocation can amount to a dislocation.[10] In preparing him, one could arrange a series of preliminary visits to the boarding home prior to the move. When the move takes place, the individual should be encouraged to take some of his (most personal) possessions with him.

2. It is also possible for the brain to decompensate because of *changes in the output.* These include quantitative or qualitative changes pertaining to the individual's behavioral activities or motor patterns; changes in the demands of performance and work, and, modifications in coping techniques (e.g., exhaustion due to manic hyperactivity).

3. In as much as the brain, in our cybernetic schema, is interposed between the sensory input and the motor output, the phrase *throughput* can be used to refer to the "black box" function of the CNS. Disturbance in the throughput (apart from organic brain changes) may develop on the basis of progressive accumulation of disturbing emotions. Accumulating anxiety and tension may reduce the homeostatic and information processing capability of the brain. When the status of the brain is already borderline, any further decrease of its efficiency is enough to tip the balance toward decompensation. The clinical manifestations of such cerebral decompensation appear to be similar to those of an acute organic mental disorder. When, however, such acute confusion states have been precipitated by environmental changes or transient internal pressures, it would be appropriate to speak of a "functional brain syndrome," rather than an organic mental disorder.

Depersonalization

The ego boundary is a dynamic structure that functions *like* a membrane. It is the subjective demarcation between self and not self, inside and outside. The term body image refers to a person's subjective image of his own body. In addition to this inner mental picture, the body image includes a set of personal values, assigned to parts of the body, and to the body as a whole (pride in physical prowess; shame about physical shortcomings, etc.). The role of the body image is particularly relevant with regard to somatic expressions of psychiatric illness (e.g., conversion, hypochondriasis). Depersonalization is a mechanism that involves a protective blurring of ego boundaries and impaired reality testing. The usual distinction between self and not self becomes less clear and the result is a sense of estrangement from reality. The protective quality of depersonalization lies in the individual's feeling that "this experience is not really happening to me—it is just like a dream."

PERSONALITY DISORDERS

These disorders are characterized by deeply ingrained, maladaptive patterns of behavior that are recognizable by the time of adolescence, or even earlier. There are numerous types, including paranoid, asocial, schizoid, compulsive, hysterical (histrionic), narcissistic, antisocial, borderline, avoidant, dependent and passive-aggressive personality. Of particular interest in this review is the relationship between aging and personality disorders: How does the aging process influence the various lifelong patterns of personality disorder? What are the adaptational assets and liabilities of various personality disorders vis-à-vis the stress of aging? Which types of behavioral disturbances can arise, for the first time in senescence?

Effects of Aging on Personality Disorders

1. Statistical data from mental hospitals and community mental health centers show that the diagnosis of personality disorders occurs most frequently in the 25–44 age range (about one out of every three admissions), while the incidence of personality disorders in the two adjacent age groups (18–24, and 45–64) is slightly less.[11] In contrast, the frequency in the 65+ age group drops below 5%. These cross-sectional studies, however, do not tell us what happens to particular individuals, over a period of many years. The statistical finding that the incidence of personality disorders decreases after middle age does not justify the conclusion that such disorders ameliorate with advancing age. Although a favorable development is possible, it is just as possible that a personality disorder may progressively decompensate. An alcoholic, for example, may develop an organic mental disorder; a compulsive personality, an involutional depression; and, a schizoid type, schizophrenia. Some people with personality disorders simply may not survive until old age: they become the victims of their deficient adaptation, and succumb due to accidents, or lack of proper self-protection. Thus, in as much as personality disorders are thought to originate in early life, a pattern of repeated failure and maladjustment increasingly takes its toll as the individual is confronted with the tasks of adulthood.

On the other hand, certain impulse disorders may settle down after the midpoint in life. This is probably due to an interaction between intrapsychic shifts and social changes. The former include changes in the drives (lesser intensity); in the ego (belated mastery of skills) and superego changes (e.g., mellowing). Social-interpersonal developments can further contribute to the amelioration of behavior disorders. An alcoholic may come to the point where the satisfactions of the group experiences of Alcoholic Anonymous, or of religious conversion, are felt to be more rewarding than the euphoric oblivion from alcohol. And, an individual with a long history of breaking the law, may find himself at a point where he can use his inside familiarity with delinquency as the very basis for efforts aimed at rehabilitating law-breakers. In such instances, intrapsychic shifts and social opportunities interact, and complement each other, to bring about the behavioral improvements.

The life histories of character disorders frequently show a life-long pattern of deficient personality functioning, and the individual "losing out" all along without clearly realizing this. The losses are not the usual kind (loss of something of value), but missed opportunities: the individual is missing out on basic elements in the spectrum of human experience. Since what is being missed, are opportunities, he tends not to know about such a loss, and not to feel like a loser. But when such a person arrives in old age, he has little to show for, there is a paucity of external objects, and a poverty of external support systems. Now awareness grows that something is amiss. In keeping with the life-long pattern of not seeing the deficiency as self-related, the patient is aware only of the deficiencies around him: somebody else must be responsible, somebody else is not giving him enough. Thus, a variety of personality disorders end up in late life as losers, blaming the environment for being a have-not. Their clinical symptomatology is characterized by hapless complaining and persistent bitterness; accusations are directed at whatever people happen to be around or various community agencies. These individuals show no evidence of organicity, schizophrenia, or recurrent depressions. Their past history reveals lack of significant achievement in education, marriage, parenthood, work, and social relationships; failure to learn from experience; increasing impoverishment of self and milieu; and the absence of recognizable depression.

2. Regarding the *adaptational assests and liabilities* of personality disorders vis-à-vis the stress of aging, the following points may be considered:[12]

a. *General Aspects. Effects of Aging on Coping Patterns.* Character disorders relying largely on coping patterns requiring little energy, may be relatively better equipped to deal with the stresses of aging. These low energy patterns (see above) apply to inade-quate, dependent and schizoid personalities; they may feel quite comfortable with the regressive modes of adaptation, frequently encountered in old age. Persons using primarily high-energy defense patterns (see above) are likely to be more vulnerable. For example, the paranoid personality who reacts with hostility and aggression, and the compulsive personality who requires much time and energy for pursuing perfectionism or repeating his rituals, run out of the energy required to maintain such coping techniques. In personalities with inadequate impulse control (e.g., borderline and histrionic personality) life may act as a therapist, in as much as the strength of the drives declines with age. However, this is still a far from simple proposition: active and aggressive impulses may well decrease in intensity, while passive needs become more prominent. In personalities who are action-prone or tend to act out, age-related illness interferes with their habitual activity patterns; anxiety, depression, and regressive behavior may be the result, especially if action had been used to ward off intrapsychic tension.

b. *Specific Personality Disorders and Reaction to Age Related Stresses.* The *schizoid* personality avoids close involvement with others and has difficulty in being normally assertive; he is seclusive and sometimes eccentric. The paranoid individual has certain schizoid traits and a tendency to use projection which results in suspiciousness. Emotional stress, including age-related losses, may increase the tendencies toward withdrawal and projection, resulting in overt symptomatology; and a severely schizoid person may become a recluse living in marginal circumstances. On the other hand, in the loneliness of old age, individuals with mild schizoid tendencies may well feel relatively comfortable: such persons have traveled lightly through life, with a minimum of belongings. They had not much to begin with, and have not much to lose in the end.

Schizoid and avoidant personalities may

view illness as a secure bridge leading toward another human being. They may wish to hang onto their illness, or their sick role, because the contacts with nurses and physicians provide them with closeness which, however, does not necessarily involve true intimacy. In the course of an illness, they may develop an attachment to the hospital or clinic in general, rather than to specific members of the staff.

Lonely, inwardly isolated persons tend to view the world as a cold, inhospitable place, and for some of them work served defensively as a way to avoid intimacy and to build a personal bastion of strength from which they could deal at a safe distance with others. Upon retirement such a person will again face the original fear of intimacy, and thus need to develop other distancing techniques (e.g., social withdrawal).

The *histrionic personality* is excitable, dramatic and attention-seeking. These individuals are immature, vain, egocentric, and tend to eroticize relationships, but their emotions are shallow. Underlying this changeable surface behavior, there are often strong dependency needs. What suffers due to age-related decline in energy and attractiveness is the individual's ability to effectively use dramatization, seductiveness, and over-reactivity. The aging process may predispose them to involutional depressions, hypochondriasis, and hysterical exaggeration of physical illness. Prior to the onset of a depression, there may be periods of heightened sexual inclinations and romantic activities, or attempts to deny the existence or significance of involutional processes. On the other hand, it is possible that age-related improvement occurs in terms of decreased excitability and dramatization provided such behavioral changes are felt to be egosyntonic, and are reinforced by the environment.

Narcissistic personalities operate on the premise that they are exceptional. Life's inevitable losses deflate their undue self-esteem and make it progressively more difficult to maintain belief in one's special status. When their sense of invulnerability is punctured by the discovery of the "Achilles heel," such persons react with depression (due to unresolved involutional grief); hypochondriasis; or more severe psychopathology (manic-like conditions, paranoid decompensation).

The *dependent* personality may not fare too badly, in the course of life. If the dependency features are out in the open, the issue is at least unambiguous. Some people, for whatever reasons of their own, may feel attracted to a passive, dependent person; a strong marital partner may provide the needed gratifications. And if the latter should die, various substitutes may be available (children; the security of a home or hospital, etc.). A dependent individual may welcome illness as a means of permitting him to gratify his dependency needs. When bolstered by a supportive environment, dependent, inadequate and immature personalities may maintain themselves for a long time. They may feel quite contented about retirement (often an early or forced retirement), because they do not have to cope with the demands of work any more. Likewise, illness may provide a welcome escape from adult role responsibilities. Many such persons depend for their happiness on the support from social service and other agencies.

The *compulsive* personality is characterized by undue concern with conformity and adherence to standards of conscience. They are rigid, inhibited, and unable to relax. Those who were able to make a virtue out of necessity and use their compulsiveness adaptively, may in old age, draw the benefits from this orderliness and regularity. But, if the emphasis was on rigidity and inhibition, the losses in old age may precipitate an involutional depression. This personality disorder is considered to have more than average susceptibility to involutional depressions and a greater tendency to react maladaptively to the stress of intellectual decline in later years.[6]

In the area of work, the *perfectionist* pays more attention to the detail than the overall pattern. He works in order to do things right, at the right time, in the right place; it is more important how he does it, than what he does. When, however, the details can no longer be attended to, he feels at a loss and his productivity comes to a halt. In senescence, the decline in the energy required to live up to high standards, may result in feelings of helplessness, and shame. Thus, physical illness may bring about anxiety and depression in these personalities. On the other hand, sometimes physical illness is the lesser of two evils. For example, an ambitious, hard-striving, middle-aged man who discovers that he has fallen short of the goals set by his ego-ideal, may find in illness an alibi that covers his shortcomings, be they real or imagined.

The mental mechanisms of reaction formation and/or over compensation may produce, in a basically dependent person, a facade which is precisely the opposite: undue self-reliance and aggressiveness. The *passive-aggressive* personality is characterized by passive as well as aggressive behavior. The latter is expressed by passive means: e.g., obstructionism, procrastination, and a tendency toward brooding and cherishing of old hurts. Passivity applies not only to the method of expressing aggressive impulses, but also to underlying dependent wishes. Conflicts develop because the aggressiveness and independence are not genuine, and therefore difficult to maintain. In addition, the surface of strength has had the effect of attracting others who are passive or dependent, and this adds to the strain. The day of reckoning comes, when there is no longer enough energy to maintain the independent facade. The patient will fight the loss of face, first by way of an increase in the very aggressiveness or appearance of self-reliance, then often suddenly giving way to helpless dependency and regression.

Individuals whose premorbid personalities showed prominent reaction formations may react to physical illness in a surprising way. The *emotionally distant* personality, whose coldness is the result of reaction-formation against tender feelings, may use the illness situation for the expression of emotional warmth and experience in intimacy. Thus, physical illness may come to be the currency that permits the exchange of emotional warmth between persons who otherwise have a distant relationship. The same constellation may develop in the case of *avoidant* personalities who have deepseated fears of rejection. Physical illness may be used in a similar way by patients who are *overly self-reliant*. They may publicly protest but secretly enjoy being sick, because the illness "forces" them temporarily into a position of dependency and receptivity.

Age Related Determinants of Behavior

Certain behavior disorders arise for the first time in old age, and reflect the pathogenetic effect of aging. This category includes three types of psychopathological constellations: (1) changes in the personal time perspective; (2) regressive ego changes leading to (re-)activation of latent conflict and acting out; and (3) behavior disturbances secondary to other age-related mental illness.

(1) *Time Perspective.* With advancing age, there are specific alterations in the *time perspective*. Some individuals feel that time is running out and want to make the most of whatever time remains. Those who discover that they have missed out on this or that subjectively important experience, may want to catch up. Depending on many factors (ego strength, appropriateness of belatedly attaining overdue goals, situational opportunities and constraints, etc.), such endeavors will succeed or fail. Persons who have been "on good behavior" all of their lives may feel that now the time has come for a reward. This may reflect a process of genuine mellowing, but it can also be a caricature of it. The latter happens when the individual used to resent being on good behavior. His resentment may have betrayed itself through getting irritated at people who did indulge without qualms in those pleasures which our patient had renounced. In such cases, the old person will reach for his reward with a vengeance as though in

finally doing what he wants, he is getting back at the authority that had kept him so long in line.

The altered time perspective may be associated with a decline in the ability to delay gratification. This regressive ego change may result in acting out of socially undesirable behavior.

(2) *Ego Changes* in old age may activate psychological conflicts which, throughout life, had remained latent. Due to age-related stresses, the ego may function less effectively and ego strength may decompensate. Due to weakening of repression or reaction formation, impulses that used to be kept in check, now come to the fore, and find expression in specific behavior patterns. These tend to be the opposite of what used to be the life-long dominant ego style.

In the case of acting out, we deal with a specific wish, or a cluster of wishful fantasies, which used to be repressed. When the ego's capacity to maintain repression is diminished, these wishes can gain access to the motor apparatus and be acted upon. Related to this, and often an essential part, is the reactivation of a childhood neurosis.

(3) *Behavioral Disturbances Secondary to Senescent Psychopathology.* In these cases the behavior disorder emerges, not as a carry-over from the past, but as the result of specific late life psychopathology.

In Organic Mental Disorder, behavioral disturbances can develop due to profound regression; unlearning of previously acquired skills; loss of impulse control; impaired judgment, etc. Examples include deviant sexual behavior, combativeness, loss of social decorum, incontinence, as well as deterioration of personal hygiene and lifespace.

Manic States. In contrast to mania in younger age groups, hyperactivity is less prominent. What may be striking, however, are behavior patterns reflecting an underlying sense of grandiosity or invulnerability (for example, expansive business transactions, inappropriate romantic pursuits).

Depressive Conditions may cause behavioral disturbances, such as self-destructive activities. In extreme depression with hopelessness, the ultimate act of despair is to take one's loved ones along in death (homicide-suicide).

Paranoid States are frequently associated with outward aggression, including tendencies toward malice, ill-will, vicious gossip, and litigation. There is a risk of combative, or even homicidal behavior.

REFERENCES

1. Wolk, R. L., Rustin, S. L. and Scotti, J. The geriatric delinquent. *J. Am. Geriatr. Soc.* **11:** 653–659 (1963).
2. Verwoerdt, A. Psychopathological responses to the stress of physical illness. *Adv. Psychosom. Med.* **8:** 92–114 (1972).
3. Verwoerdt, A. *Clinical Geropsychiatry.* Baltimore: Williams & Wilkins, pp. 31–33, 1976.
4. Calloway, N. O. The role of entropy in biologic senescence. *J. Am. Geriatr. Soc.* **14:** 342 (1966).
5. Roth, M. The psychiatric disorders of later life. *Psychiat. Annals* **6(9):** 417–445, (1976).
6. Gianturco, D. T., Breslin, M. S., Heyman, A., Gentry, W. D., Jenkins, C. D. and Kaplan, B. Personality patterns and life stress in ischemic cerebrovascular disease: I. psychiatric findings. *Stroke* **5:** 453–460 (1974).
7. Verwoerdt, A. *Clinical Geropsychiatry.* Baltimore: Williams & Wilkins Company, pp. 147–158, 1976.
8. Levy, G. Effect of bed rest on distribution and elimination of drugs. *J. Pharm. Sci.,* **56:** 928 (1967).
9. Kahn, R. L., Goldfarb, A. I., Pollack, M. and Peck, A. Brief objective measures for the determination of mental status in the aged. *Am. J. Psychiatry* **117:** 326–328 (1960).
10. Aldrich, C. K. and Mendkoff, E. Relocation of the aged and disabled: A mortality study. *J. Am. Geriatr. Soc.* **11:** 185–194 (1963).
11. U.S. Department of Health, Education and Welfare, Biometry Branch, Washington, D.C., No. 7, 1971.
12. Verwoerdt, A. *Clinical Geropsychiatry.* Baltimore: Williams & Wilkins pp. 85–88, 1976.

Chapter 17
Adjustment Disorders of Late Life: Stress Disorders

Charles M. Gaitz, M.D.
and
Roy V. Varner, M.D.

Texas Research Institute of Mental Sciences

Relating mental disorders to stress is by no means a novel idea. In fact, not many years ago, neuroses and psychoses usually were considered to be reactions, and diagnosis was not complete unless external precipitating stresses and predisposition were noted. A relationship between psychological factors and somatic disorders has long been recognized in our conceptualization of psychosomatic disorders, and certain illnesses such as asthma, peptic ulcer and hypertension have been studied intensively to determine how psychological factors may contribute to the onset of these illnesses. More recently, however, less emphasis has been placed on external influences and more on internal neurophysiological and biochemical factors in the development of emotional distress.

NOSOLOGY

We shall focus on psychiatric disorders labeled transient situational disturbances in DSM-II, the Diagnostic and Statistical Manual of Mental Disorders compiled by the American Psychiatric Association in 1968. A new edition, DSM-III, is being prepared for distribution in 1979. The preliminary version of DSM-III (January, 1978) does not include the diagnosis of transient situational disturbances. Such disorders will probably be classified under the diagnosis of adjustment disorders.

The essential feature of the disorder, whether it is diagnosed as transient situational disturbance or adjustment disorder, is "maladaptive reaction to an identifiable life event(s) or circumstances(s), which is not merely an exacerbation of one of the mental disorders previously described and which is expected to remit if and when the stressor ceases."[1] (N:6) The description of adjustment disorders in DMS-III makes clear that the stressors may be single or multiple, may be recurrent, may occur in a family setting or may be limited to the patient, or may occur in a group or community setting where the stressor involves many other people.

Some stressors are associated with specific developmental stages. The severity of the adjustment disorder is not predictable directly from the severity of the stressors. Individuals who are particularly vulnerable may have a rather severe form of the disorder when only a mild or moderate stressor is present. Personality organization, cultural or group norms and values will also contribute to the severity and manifestation of the disturbance. The manifestations of the disorder are varied and cover a range of emotional, physical and behavioral symptoms. The age at onset, of course, is variable and although it is assumed that the disorder will remit when the stressor ceases, remission may be either sudden or gradual, immediate or delayed, and the disorder may even be chronic if the stressors persist.

In DSM-II, the transient situational disturbances are classified according to the patient's developmental stage; there are subtypes for infancy, childhood, adolescence, adult life and late life. In DSM-III, adjustment disorders are also divided into several subtypes. The basis for classification, however, is on clinical manifestations, not on developmental stage. Phrases such as "with depressed mood," "with mixed emotional features," are used to define subgroups. Nevertheless, it is recognized that some stresses are associated with specific developmental stages and that the stress of an event will be different for persons in different developmental stages.

Though there is some similarity to the conceptualization of psychosomatic disorders, adjustment disorder "with physical symptoms" would be only one of several types of adjustment disorders; there might not be any demonstrable structural changes in the body. When adjustment disorders occur in late life, physical health factors become extremely important. As persons age, they are likely to have more physical impairments which, in turn, influence adjustment. The relationship between physical and emotional health is complex, however, and we cannot always determine it exactly nor can we always find out which problem came first.

STRESS AND MENTAL ILLNESS

The literature on the relationship of stress and mental illness sheds little light because of a tendency to confuse actual stress with what is "stressful." Eisdorfer[2] clarifies some of these methodological issues in a review of the literature on behavioral stress, paying special attention to the contributions of Selye, Lazarus, Lowenthal, and many others. Concluding that the multiplicity of approaches and definitions have led to confusion, Eisdorfer calls for a more unified interdisciplinary approach in which research methods, nomenclature, and the characteristics of various stressor parameters are all agreed upon. Researchers face a challenging task in cataloging and quantifying stressors and stress response in human beings, since "individuals are capable of responding to a range of physical and behavioral stimuli with a wide variety of complex and synergistic responses," Eisdorfer writes (p. 30). He points out that stress is not always a bad thing, as is usually implied in writings on the subject; stress can, in fact, lead a person to try new and more effective kinds of adaptations. In other words, stress may either represent or be a precursor to a favorable rather than an unfavorable adaptation. Stress is presumed, though not proved, to accelerate the "aging process." Since it may deplete the reserve capacity of all organisms, stress becomes a crucial interest for both psychological and medical scientists.

As applied in the physical sciences, stress dynamics refer to force directed at a physical object (stressor) to which an opposing force is exerted (strain), with subsequent temporary alteration in the structure of the object. Since behavioral scientists have been less precise and have investigated stress without always clearly differentiating between the stressor (that which induces the stressful state) and the result of stress, it has not always been easy to distinguish between precursors and consequences of stress. Behavioral scientists, for example, have not been consistent in their definitions or frames of reference. Anxiety, psychosomatic disorders, depression, other physical disease, etc., may all represent *results* of stress. Disasters, job pressures, family conflict are more appropriately called *stressors,* although the word "stress" is often applied to these as well. Results of stress may also become stressors in themselves if they are not altered or mitigated in some way. Therefore both the precursors and consequences have pathophysiological, social and psychological dimensions.

One may presume that stress intensifies the aging process, but this is difficult to prove. Somewhat to support this position, Comfort[3] believes that the aging organism shows "a decline in resistance to random stresses," and Ordy,[4] who defines organismic stresses as random deviations from a steady state, points out that two of the most prominent features of biological aging are an increased probability of death and decreasing behavioral, physiological and biochemical adaptation to external and internal environmental challenges.

Changes in adaptive capacity have been demonstrated not only for the total organism but also at the cellular level. Aging neurons may exhibit less capacity to adapt to stress. Cell loss as well as alterations in function has been demonstrated for organs including the lung, heart and kidney, but these are observed only when the organisms are subjected to challenges or stress. The cencept is echoed by Meier-Ruge.[5] Wang[6] has illustrated the relationship between alterations in physiological, psychosocial and psychological status and the precipitation or exacerbation of late-life dementia. With these concepts as a base, we can construct a paradigm of stress to help us study stressors, stress, and maladaptivity to stress, in aging human beings.

Bergman[7] reminds us of Hooke's law which states the basic equation for the concept of stress in engineering or physical science models: $S = k \times s$ where S is stress, k is the elasticity coefficient, and s is strain. This model, by presenting stress as a dynamic situation, offers us a basis for understanding psychosocial aspects of stress phenomena. The notion of k, the *elasticity of physical objects,* may be applied to the human in terms of psychological and physiological defenses and adaptive devices. *Strain* is the measurable effect of all compensatory activities, psychosocial and physiological.

Human beings are always under stress. Their situation is like that of an airplane flying in calm air. If turbulence or other stressful conditions develop, strain increases and the elasticity of the aircraft's metallic rib and skin structure is stressed even more. If elasticity is strained beyond a certain limit, the airplane may break up. In the human, an alteration of homeostasis may disrupt the ability to cope with a stressor; the consequence may be psychiatric illness, social maladaptation, physical illness, or a combination of all three.

In summary, then we may conceptualize the relationship of stress and psychiatric disorders in a manner analogous to concepts applied in the physical sciences by using the formula, $S = k \times s$, where S = stress; k = aging brain, genetic factors, concomitant disease states, social and financial resources, psychological traits and defenses; s = actual behavior, affective states, thought disorders, cognitive alterations, maladaptive behavior.

In late life especially, as Verwoerdt[8] writes, losses are frequent stressors. Perhaps one may look upon all major stressful life situations as relative loss. Verwoerdt believes that the capacity to develop or use adaptive mechanisms diminishes as one grows older. Psychological decompensation may occur as stress states hasten a process of withdrawal and lessened perception of the pain of stressful events, causing a kind of regression in a predisposed individual. The tendency, of course, is magnified if intracranial or extracranial brain disease impinges on brain function. Verwoerdt uses Holmes and Rahe's Social Readjustment Rating Scale[9] as example of an attempt to quantify some of the stressor events inherent in psycho-socio-biological loss. The Scale considers the relative impact of 43 life events. Some of these events are, of course, more likely to occur late in life, and there is also a greater likelihood of losses accumulating as one grows older (death of spouse, of close family members or friends; losses associated with changes in financial status, residence, social roles, etc.) Other stressful losses include diminished sexual gratification, physical illness, a shortened future, and age-related changes such as those in the endocrine system that affect the drive systems of hunger and sex. Psychological responses to physical illness, as well as the direct effects of illness, lead to vicious circles within this loss/stress system.

THE NEUROBIOLOGICAL MATRIX OF STRESS: THE AGING BRAIN

In the absence of unusual stress, the aging individual may have enough functional capacity to maintain normal homeostasis. But involution of all organ systems has been shown to be associated with aging, and it carries with it the potential for reduced adaptivity to a stressful state. It is particularly important to consider how changes in the brain may affect adjustment when we are concerned with adjustment disorders of late life.

Meier-Ruge[5] cites many pathophysiological observations that support the probability that involution of the brain with aging is not caused by a clearly definable pathologic process but is likely to be a problem of metabolic "homeostatic maintenance." Protein synthesis is affected in that there is increased probability of error in intracellular translation of the genetic code for protein synthesis. Increased half-life of enzyme proteins results ultimately in accumulation of insufficient or inactive neuronal proteins. In physiologic (nonstress) conditions, reduced metabolic adaptive activity is not significant. In stressful situations, however, the decline in adaptive reserve capacity may become important

regardless of whether the stressors are psychic or metabolic, and whether the metabolic disturbance is related to an intracranial or extracranial abnormality. Gradually, repeated or persistent stress results in irreversible symptoms. This mechanism may explain, at least partially, the development of senile dementia and the morphological changes associated with this condition.

One must also consider how other concomitant pathological processes may affect the aging brain. Obrist[10] explains that both intracranial and extracranial vascular diseases represent additional stresses to the aging brain. He refers to Brody's work describing the neuronal depopulation of "normal senescence" as part of the basis of normal brain involution, and speculates that the loss of cells contributes to the intellectual and also the vascular and metabolic changes associated with aging. A complex relationship probably exists between such disease processes as cardiovascular insufficiency, long-term hypertension, "microinfarcts," and processes of "normal" involution (intraneuronal metabolic alterations) described by Meier-Ruge. As we learn more about these relationships, we may be able to understand how certain phenomena are related. For example, it would be desirable to know more about the relationship of circulatory and electroencephalographic changes in old age.

Samorajski[11] reports on still other "normal" changes in the involuting, nondiseased aging brain. These include alterations in catecholamine metabolism and availability. Samorajski points out that the transition between the presumably "normal" changes described by Meier-Ruge and Brody and the traditional disease states, such as vascular disease and Alzheimer's atrophy, is not always clear, even in morphologic examinations.[12]

The aging brain is a changing brain. Anatomic and physiologic changes have been demonstrated conclusively. Conceivably these changes affect adaptation to stressors. This principle should apply generally and be independent of the nature of the stressor. That the aging brain probably is less adaptable to the neurophysiological stress induced by psychosocial stressor events is especially relevant in our consideration of adjustment disorders. How much lessened adaptivity there is may depend on the rate of aging processes in the brain and the additional concomitants of disease states.

Maladaptive states in the elderly often produce a syndrome suggesting dementia that is really not the product of a disease process, either intracranial or extracranial. Social and cultural and psychological stressors have been implicated in this form of "pseudodementia." The aging brain's lessened adaptive capacity probably increases the likelihood of a person's developing an organic brain syndrome associated with extracranial processes. Libow,[13] for example, goes so far as to call organic brain syndrome associated with extracranial processes a pseudodementia. Still another association may be the pseudodementia that accompanies affective disorders in which withdrawal and apparent cognitive impairment is closely related to the emotional state. Perhaps there is a predisposition because of the aging brain's relatively limited ability to respond to stress. Since no human feeling occurs in a "vacuum" independent of a nervous-system physiology, it would thus appear that a psychosocial stress is translated to an anxiety state, the substrate of which is a metabolic stress at the brain neuronal level. The aging brain presumably does not adapt to this stress like a younger brain. This may explain why some old persons may "look organic" under stressful situations but retain few or no manifestations of this when the stress fades or disappears.

THE PARAMETERS OF LATE-LIFE STRESS

The interaction between physiological, sociological, and psychological loss in human stress has already been described in terms of the dynamism's contribution to late-life stress decompensation and overt mental illness. The role of the less adaptive aging brain has also been discussed, as has the increased probability of losses occurring as one grows older. In the psychological dimension, Bergman[7] examined how personality types and stress adaptiveness were related. He concluded that certain personality types show a greater degree of "strain" or maladaptive response under stress, and he calls maladaptivity the "signs of strain." In other words, one's lifelong personality traits represent one of many kinds of adaptive variables which, collectively, form the k constant of the stress equation described.

Stressful events like progressive physical illness may further alter the k factor. In addition to personality traits, Bergman found that constitutional and genetic factors influence the quality/quantity of response, especially autonomic response, to stress stimuli. Some persons, for example, may be genetically predisposed to anxiety. Interestingly, personality traits labeled "paranoid," "hostile," and "aggressive" that may have been seen as maladaptive earlier, do not seem to predispose older persons to affective reactions to stress. For example, persons who are paranoid and aggressive often have learned to do without company and close relationships; they seem to live on in a self-contained and undefeated way. Persons with marked dependent traits are likely to accept placement in institutions. Conceivably, then, extremes of passivity and aggressiveness may be effective adaptive strategies in late life. It seems that one's normal aspirations at the end of the life cycle may become frustrated by unavoidable stressors (losses, prejudices, rejections, etc.) of late life. Bergman concludes that genetic factors and early environmental experiences may be of greatest importance in determining the ability of old persons to withstand the stresses of age. Social factors as stressors may be somewhat overemphasized and signs of "strain" attributed to social stressors may really be manifestations of physical illness.

The fact that more socially maladaptive aged persons tend to be institutionalized than others could give a false impression of maladaptation as the apparent result of prolonged or intense late-life stress. Kral[14] reported that the cataclysmic stress conditions of concentration camps in Europe did not increase the frequency of functional psychosis; neurotic conditions even improved, but senile psychosis occurred more often. Once again, one may assume that the aging brain cannot adapt to stress as easily as in early life. Kral also studied the relationship between frequency of late-life organic brain syndrome and the kind of stress situation caused by emotional insecurity in childhood. Individuals with this history seemed generally less adaptable throughout their lives, which suggests early developmental compromise of the adaptive arsenal, k.

Neurophysiologic changes also may be associated with persistent stressors. Busse[15] examined electroencephalograms of old people and found that people of lower socioeconomic status had a significantly higher percentage of dysrhythmic EEGs in comparison to EEGs of subjects of the same age group belonging to upper social classes. One may presume that the poorer subjects had experienced more stressful events such as inadequate diet and health care, less education, and other deprivations. These could be considered to be stress precipitators and/or compromisers of adaptive reserve capacity.

Wolffe[16] also implicates stress endured in the past as an important factor in the etiology of senile psychosis. He found that people who had undergone stressful events for a prolonged period showed the same type of impairment in certain intellectual functions as did organically brain-damaged patients. As Busse[17] observed, women are likely to employ hypochondriacal defenses if they are exposed to social stress late in life—for example, being criticized for roles of mothering and housekeeping which have been important to their self-esteem. Another example of a stressful situation in late life is nursing a sick husband who has done nothing to deserve devoted care.

Maddox et al.[18] identified five major adult-life events likely to produce stress in late life: widowhood, retirement, retirement of spouse, departure of last child, and major illness. According to Maddox et al., "resources" (the pool of adaptivity potential, or the k constant of the stress equation) including psychological, sociological, and general health resources acted as moderator variables in influencing the individual's mode of adaptation (or *strain*) to the event. Therefore, not all of these life events produced increased stress. Departure of the last child, for example, precipitated no serious problems and was often associated with an increase in life satisfaction.

Results of life-cycle stress research are somewhat inconclusive in regard to the exact role of environmentally produced stress in producing psychopathology or physical illness. Dohrenwend and Dohrenwend[19] referred to a "fascinating tangle of correlations," and they urge more research to clarify the true nature of the "adaptation syndrome." In another work, Dohrenwend, et al.,[20] challenged those who argue for rejecting Holmes and Rahe's Social Readjustment Rating Scale as a stressor model, and they proposed improvements in measuring life events. Perhaps Dohrenwend's refined investigational approach will help to correlate socioenvironmentally induced stress with precipitation or aggravation of illness.

Troyer et al.[21] examined the effects of anxiety on learning. Anxiety triggers stressful psychological events which in turn can alter cognition, another kind of psychological function. Actually, anxiety can be thought of as a psychoneurophysiological event. It appears to be facilitative up to a point but then becomes inhibitory; arousal seems to enhance the learning of simple tasks but has the opposite effect on performance of complex tasks. Techniques for gathering such psychological data (paraphernalia of psychological testing, interview) in themselves are stress stimuli that affect results, so that heightened anxiety levels induced by testing may inhibit learning or memory in the elderly. In addition to the stress of the exam, Eisdorfer mentions autonomic predisposition to maladaptive response to stress, particularly in hypertensive patients, who may have an unusually high arousal level to begin with, as influencing cognition in older persons. "In the older organism, the pathology secondary to stress may be impossible to differentiate from changes relating to age and/or preexisting disease," Eisdorfer notes (p. 36). Since prolonged stress may produce signs of physiologic premature aging in certain animal experiments, we may assume that in human beings it may aggravate psychological, behavioral, and physical decline in late life. Depression as a phenomenon may, for example, increase generally with age, impairing physical health which then becomes another stressor. Physical health seems to be an important adaptive factor in any stress situation, although repeated encounters with stress over time remain a less well-understood phenomenon.

STRESS AND LATE-LIFE PSYCHIATRIC SYNDROMES: TREATMENT CONSIDERATION

The following case illustrates the need for differentiating stress disorders in late life from those of more clearly defined psychopathologic syndromes. The latter may be stress-induced, but they are not as easily reversed by reducing the stressor and are more apt to interfere in interpersonal and occupational functioning. The patient shows many of the features compatible with a diagnosis of adjustment disorder (or transient situational maladjustment). In diagnosing adjustment disorders, the degree of severity of the stressor is not necessarily related to the degree of stress experienced nor to the amount of decompensation that the patient shows. The degree of decompensation is related to the individual's inherent adaptive strengths and potential adaptive devices, k.

An 80-year-old married female was referred to a geropsychiatric clinic because of recurrent insomniac episodes and crying spells. These began when her 88-year-old husband became ill and later had to be placed in a nursing home. There was no history of previous psychiatric illness, but questioning revealed many separations and deaths of significant others, including an early death of her mother. She had been married twice before she married her present husband 18 years ago. The third marriage had been the happiest. She was very much aware of feeling the stress induced by his lingering illness. She knew she was afraid of living alone and of being generally less able to cope than when she was younger.

Physical assessment revealed a history of successful treatment for hypertension. Blood pressure was 170/100 but her only current medication was aspirin for mild arthritic symptoms.

When first seen, the woman was carefully groomed, talkative, wore glasses, and walked with a cane. She had an appropriate interpersonal manner, seemed to be quite psychologically minded and in good contact with her feelings, which she described as mostly sad. She became extremely tearful when talking about her husband's illness, although she was able to control the affects of sadness and grief, and she did not express any guilt feelings. She showed no cognitive impairments and no evidence of a thought disorder. She reported not sleeping well, poor appetite, but no weight loss and no suicidal ruminations. She was very verbal about her feelings and agreed with the interviewer that she had begun grieving in anticipation of her husband's death and its implications.

In accord with DSM-III, the diagnosis would be as follows:

Axis I: Clinical psychiatric syndrome—adjustment disorder with depressed mood 309.00

Axis II: Personality disorder—none.
(A history of dependency conflicts in the past was obtained, but her adaptation over the years had been adequate. A current personality-trait diagnosis was not justified).

Axis III: Nonmental medical disorders—essential hypertension, mild.

Axis IV: Severity of psychosocial stressors—moderately severe.

Axis V: Highest level of adaptive functioning in the past year—very good.

One may expect this patient to respond well to brief supportive psychotherapy. Since she is functioning at a high level of emotional maturity, relates well to others, has adapted well to stressors in the past, has considerable insight, the factors suggest a k index which would be compatible with a stress situation in which current strains (the patient's anxiety, insomnia, grieving, etc.) will not result in a severe physical or psychological decompensation. A fairly strong social support system will help. In the absence of a true affective disorder, we believe that the therapeutic approach should be one of allowing the grieving process to proceed in a setting that permits verbalization between patient and therapist. Verwoerdt[9] advises that medications in such cases be limited. Drugs may afford just enough relief to interfere with the patient's need to find solutions and make decisions, as well as allaying anxiety just enough to mask the need for verbalization of affective discomfort. The clinician should remember that the patient is an elderly woman who has had lifelong conflicts with dependence vs. independence, experienced object loss, and that she dealt with these quite adequately over the years. Now, late in life, she is beginning to show signs of stress discomfort, if not early decompensation, connected with the terminal illness of her husband.

Although she was not experiencing a frank clinical depression, her case illustrates the stress dynamism in action, with what appears to be a kind of temporary decompensation, or, more to the point, *strain* which does not appear to be progressing into a true, more traditional, and more easily definable "mental illness." That she does not show pseudodementia is again probably a factor of her good physical health and overall favorable adaptivity potential. Stress leading to more severe psychopathology may require genetic predisposition in addition to less effective adaptive potential, k. With advancing age, however, the capacity to maintain an inner steady state regardless of changing external circumstances becomes compromised. The range of adjustment as well as the choices of adjustment become smaller and narrower for the aging individual. Adjustment disorders in late life thus must be treated with caution and care, with principal therapeutic strategies aimed at bolstering adaptive strengths.

CONCLUSIONS

Adjustment disorders in late life are not diagnosed as often as they should be. The concepts fundamental to this diagnosis furnish a useful rationale for treatment. Attention is focused on stressors that disturb equilibrium; interventions to neutralize these stressors may be very effective since such stress disorders are likely to be reversible. What appears to be a relatively acute disorder may, however, prove to be an early stage of another more persistent or complicated psychiatric disorder. Attention to losses as stressors is especially important. As persons age, their losses occur more frequently with cumulative effect. At the same time, biological changes reduce the person's ability to respond to stressors regardless of their nature. Early recognition and intervention to neutralize, or at least minimize, the effects of stressors carries with it the promise of avoiding or modifying the course of mental incapacity late in life. Research still needs to be done to elucidate the process by which stress, however initiated, may lead to permanent destruction of various physiological processes, and also to determine if, and how, stress may be a cause of accelerated aging.

REFERENCES

1. Diagnostic and Statistical Manual of Mental Disorders-III Draft, The Task Force on Nomenclature and Statistics of The American Psychiatric Association, Washington, D. C., 1978.

2. Eisdorfer, C. Stress, disease and cognitive change in the aged. In C. Eisdorfer and R. O. Friedel. *Cognitive and Emotional Disturbance in the Elderly:* Clinical Issues, Chicago: Year Book Medical Publishers, pp. 27–44, 1977.

3. Comfort, A. The Biology of Senescence. New York: Holt, Rinehart and Winston, 1956.

4. Ordy, J. M. and Kaack, B. Psychoneuroendocrinology and aging in man. In B. Eleftheriou and M. F. Elias (eds.) *Special Review of Experimental Aging Research: Progress in Biology.* Bar Harbor, Maine: EAR, Inc., 1976.

5. Meier-Ruge, W. From our laboratories. Triangle **14:** 71–72. East Hanover, N. J.: Sandoz, 1975.

6. Wang, H. S. Dementia in old age. In C. E. Wells (ed.) *Dementia: Edition 2, Contemporary Neurology Series,* Number 15, pp. 15–26. Philadelphia: F. A. Davis, 1977.

7. Bergman, K. Personality traits and reactions to the stresses of ageing. In H. M. Van Praag and A. F. Kalverboer (eds.) *Ageing of the Central Nervous System: Biological and Psychological Aspects,* pp. 162–182. Haarlem, Netherlands: De Erven F. Bohn N. V., 1972.

8. Verwoerdt, Adriaan. Clinical Geropsychiatry. Baltimore: Williams and Wilkins, 1976.

9. Holmes, T. H., and Rahe, R. H. The social readjustment rating scale. *Journal of Psychosomatic Research,* **11:** 213–218 (1967).

10. Obrist, W. D. Cerebral physiology of the aged: Influence of circulatory disorders. In C. M. Gaitz (ed.) *Aging and the Brain,* pp. 117–133. New York: Plenum Press, 1972.

11. Samorajski, T. Central neurotransmitter substances and aging: A review. *Journal of the American Geriatrics Society,* **25:** 337–349 (1977).

12. Samorajski, T. How the human brain responds to aging. *Journal of the American Geriatrics Society,* **24:** 4–11 (1976).

13. Libow, L. W. Pseudo-senility: Acute and reversible organic brain syndromes. *Journal of American Geriatric Society,* **21:** 112–120, (1973).

14. Kral, V. A. In geriatric psychiatry: paper presented at University of Ottawa, February, 1967. In F. C. R. Chalke and J. J. Day (eds.) *Primary Prevention of Psychiatric Disorders.* Toronto: University of Toronto Press, 1968.

15. Busse, E. W. Psychopathology. In J. E. Birren (ed.) *Handbook of Aging and the Individual,* Chicago: University of Chicago Press, pp. 364–378. 1959.

16. Wolffe, H. G., Chapman, L. F., Thetford, W. N., Berlin, L. and Guthrie, T. C. Highest integrative functions in man during stress. In *The Brain and Human Behavior.* Baltimore: Williams and Wilkins, 1958.

17. Busse, E. W. Discussion II. In C. Eisdorfer and R. O. Friedel, (eds.) *Cognitive and Emotional Disturbance in the Elderly:* Clinical Issues, Chicago: Year Book Medical Publishers, pp. 105–110. 1977.

18. Maddox, G. L., Busse, E. W., Siegler, I., Nevlin, J. B., Palmore, E., Cleveland, W. P. and Ramm, D. Stress and adaptation in later life; Symposium presented at Gerontological Society, San Francisco, 1977. Abstracted in *The Gerontologist,* **17:** 5, pt. 2, p. 139.

19. Dohrenwend, B. P. and Dohrenwend, B. S. The conceptualization and measurement of stressful life events: An overview of the issues. In J. S. Strauss, H. M. Babigian and M. Roff (eds.) *Origins and Course of Psychopathology,* pp. 93–115. New York: Plenum, 1977.

20. Dohrenwend, B. S., Drasnoff, L., Askenasy, A. and Dohrenwend, B. P. Exemplification of a method for scaling life events: The PERI life events scale. *Journal of Health and Social Behavior,* in press.

21. Troyer, W. G., Eisdorfer, C., Bogdonoff, M. D., and Wilkie, F. Experimental stress and learning in the aged. *Journal of Abnormal Psychology,* **72:** 65–70 (1967).

Chapter 18
Disorders Related to Biological Functioning

Ewald W. Busse, M.D.
Duke University Medical Center

Dan Blazer, M.D.
Duke University Medical Center

Introduction

Physical symptoms are frequently the predominating complaint of individuals with mental illnesses in later life. In addition, the geriatric clinician is less likely to encounter the classical symptom patterns of mental illness uncomplicated by physical complaints that allow an operational diagnosis to easily be made. Symptoms such as pain, lethargy, constipation, decreased appetite, sleep disturbance, etc. are often seen in the physically healthy but mentally impaired older adult. Such symptoms may be secondary to intrapsychic factors e.g., a psychological conflict is converted into a physical symptom in a conversion disorder, physical complications of mental impairment e.g., a sleep disorder in a patient suffering from an organic mental disease, or a combination of the two. Determining the relative contribu-

Preparation of this chapter was supported in part by Research Career Development Award #1 K01 MH 00115–01A1 (Dr. Blazer).

Preparation of this chapter was supported in part by Grant #5 P01 AG00364 from the National Institute on Aging (Dr. Busse).

tion of intrapsychic factors, psychosocial factors, psychosomatic factors, somatopsychic factors, and psysical factors to the development of physical symptomatology in the mentally impaired older adult is a difficult but important task for the clinician working with an older adult.

The third edition of the Diagnostic and Statistical Manual[1] classifies disorders related to biological functioning into a number of separate and diverse categories. The sleep disorders, one of the most frequent symptoms of the mentally impaired elderly, are divided into nonorganic and organic etiology. Though exaggerated concern over the normal changes in sleep that accompany aging are most prevalent, insomnia, sleep-wake cycle disturbances, and hypersomnia may also be seen. The most frequent organic causes of sleep disorder in late life are organic mental disease, depression and illness of the other organ systems (e.g., angina pectoris).

The psychosexual disorders (disorders in sexual functioning where psychological factors are of major etiologic significance) are separated from disorders of psychosocial adjustment to organic sexual dysfunction (which are classified as a form of adjustment disorder). The elderly, when considered as a group, do demonstrate gradual decline in sexual activity with increasing age. The clinician, however, will observe a wide range of sexual interest and activity, including individuals who are greatly concerned about some change in sexual functioning. A frequent problem is a lack of understanding of the changes in the sexual response with increasing years. The most frequent psychosexual disorder is secondary impotence. Adjustment disorders may arise secondary to physical impotence or reduced ejaculatory demand in the male, and dyspareunia and/or pain on orgasm in the female.

Mental impairment may present in the form of either bodily symptoms and/or pathological changes. First, the somatoform disorders are disorders for which there are no known demonstrable organic findings to explain physical symptoms and for which there is evidence that symptoms are linked to psychological factors. The two most common somatoforms disorders in late life are psychogenic pain disorder (the complaint of pain in the absence of adequate physical findings and associated with positive evidence of the etiological role of psychological factors) and hypochondriasis (the presentation of physical symptoms or complaints not explainable on the basis of demonstrable organic findings and apparently linked to psychological factors).

Chronic pain syndromes are less prevalent among the elderly than at other stages of the life cycle but remain a significant problem in management. Hypochondriacal complaints are repeatedly encountered in the elderly and the site of symptom formation is often centered on the gastrointestinal tract and/or the skin. Urinary incontinence may also be related to psychological factors.

Conditions in which psychosocial factors are judged to be contributing to the initiation, exacerbation or perpetuation of a nonmental disorder with definite tissue breakdown were formally classified as "psychophysiological disorders."[2] The former explanation for such physical symptoms (namely that they are caused by a specific psychological conflict or emotional factors exclusively) has proven to be oversimplistic. Nevertheless, psychosocial factors continue to play an etiologic role in the development of many of these conditions.[3] DSM-III therefore classifies such conditions as "psychic factors in physical conditions" and specifies these conditions according to the degree the psychological component contributes to the etiology. Hypertension is the most important of these conditions in the elderly.

For convenience, the editors have included the drug use disorders in this chapter as well. Conditions where the use of drugs affect the central nervous system and result in maladaptive behavioral changes but not those changes relating to the direct central nervous system effects of these drugs (which are covered under the Organic Mental Disorders) will be considered. The drugs most commonly misused by the elderly are alcohol, sedatives and the minor tranquilizers.

SLEEP DISORDERS

Normal Sleep Patterns in the Elderly

The elderly require less sleep, on the average, than individuals earlier in life. In fact, the requirement for sleep in the human appears to decrease gradually over the entirety of the life cycle.[4] From the age of 50 until 90, individuals require between 6 and 7 hours of sleep per night. The absolute and relative time spent in REM sleep and Stage IV sleep decreases with aging.[4] Feinberg has noted a slowing of the EEG spindle activity with increasing age.[5]

The sleep of the elderly is lighter and associated with more frequent awakenings during the night. The common geriatric symptom of nocturia in males is not the only cause of the awakenings. The older person who remains in bed throughout the night experiences a series of "awakenings" (according to the EEG), a definite change from patterns of sleep earlier in life. Yet some feel that normal aging persons distribute their sleep somewhat differently across the 24-hour cycle (such as catnapping for 15 to 60 minutes several times during the daytime hours).[6]

The normal changes in sleep with aging can be very disturbing to the elderly. Many older persons are concerned that poor sleep will lead to serious illness (the sleep problems often being related only to general anxiety or normal physiologic changes in sleep).[7] The complaints include difficulty in going to sleep, insufficient sleep, restless sleep, frequent awakenings, etc. Relatives and friends may complain that the patient in fact is sleeping too much. Contrary to most clinical impressions, however, Ginsberg did not find sleep disturbances among chronic elderly psychiatric patients to be frequent in the nonpsychotic group (only 18.6% reporting such symptoms).[8]

Sleep Disorders of Nonorganic Etiology

Temporary and even persistent insomnia may develop in the elderly who are forced to adjust to a new environment. The movement of an older person to a nursing home or into the home of a relative may force sleep habits upon the older person that are not physiological. For example, a family member may insist that the older person get a "good night's sleep" by retiring at 10 o'clock p.m. when the older person needs only 6 to 7 hours sleep. The older person may then complain of difficulty falling asleep, early morning awakening or a broken pattern of sleep. Adjusting the environment (not the patient) is the solution to this type of sleep disorder.

Anxiety disorders, especially generalized anxiety, may lead to muscle tension, cardiovascular distress, stomach upset, urinary frequency and especially insomnia. These patients will spend literally hours in bed worrying about the day's events, the anticipated problems of the morrow, physical

health, past sins, etc. The most important treatment of this form of insomnia is increasing the patient's level of activity. Judicious use of the minor tranquilizers can be of definite benefit when given before bedtime. Insight oriented and supportive psychotherapy may be of some benefit, but usually will not stand alone as an effective therapeutic modality.

Hypersomnia may be symptomatic of loneliness, grief or general life dissatisfaction. Excessive sleep is more likely to be a complaint of family members or the staff of a long-term care facility than of the patient. Careful evaluation is required to rule out an organic basis of hypersomnia. Treatment often centers around the judicious use of stimulants (methylphenidate in low doses being the preferred agent) and increasing the patient's level of activity.

Sleep Disorders of Organic Etiology

Sleep Disorders Secondary to Psychiatric Disorders: In acute mental syndromes, REM mechanisms may intrude into the waking state.[10] This happens most frequently at night because of the decreased social stimulation and more ambiguous sensory input at night.[12] The hallucinations in delirium are often of a dreamlike nature. In fact, the number of REM episodes are high in acute delirium. Additional supportive evidence that the psychological changes in delirium may be secondary to the intrusion of REM processes into wakefulness includes the fact that drug withdrawal (especially barbiturates and alcohol) may lead to REM rebound. These drugs suppress REM sleep initially but then allow it to gradually return to baseline level. Both the barbiturates and alcohol can lead to delirious episodes on withdrawal.[10]

Many sleep researchers have concluded that definite changes occur in the sleep of patients who suffer from dementia (chronic organic mental disorders). Prinz relates evidence that there is a strong correlation between decreases in WAIS performance scores and percentages of REM and slow wave sleep.[9] Feinberg has demonstrated that patients with organic mental disorders show less total sleep time and a marked increase in the time spent awake. The findings are correlated with low REM and Stage IV sleep (less than for the normal aged).[10]

If a patient with chronic organic mental disease is awakened repeatedly from REM sleep a state of extreme agitation and disorientation will develop. Similar awakenings occurring during non-REM sleep are associated with lower levels of agitation and disorientation. It is suspected that this agitation may result from REM (i.e., dream) material forcing itself into the waking state. Drugs which reduce the intensity of REM sleep (such as barbiturates) might be useful in curtailing nocturnal confusion if they did not further depress cognitive function.[10] Flurazepam has less sedative action than the barbiturates but also is less effective in decreasing REM sleep.

In spite of the changes described above, one study suggests that most patients with organic mental syndromes sleep without difficulty.[8] The sleep problems among the organically mentally impaired, for the most part, do not require clinical intervention. In many cases, intervention (especially with drugs) is contraindicated. Therefore the rather routine practice of prescribing a sedative hypnotic at night on a prn basis for the hospital or nursing home patient with a chronic pain syndrome should be discouraged.

Depression has also been noted to significantly affect the sleep patterns of the elderly.[11] Slow wave sleep has been shown to be markedly diminished in the depressed elderly. In fact, older subjects free from depressive illness in one study were found to be comparable to young, mature subjects in the percentage of slow wave sleep.[11] Researchers who have studied the "normal" patterns of sleep among the elderly must be careful in the selection of subjects for such studies. The frequency of symptoms of organic mental disorders and depression among the elderly may significantly affect the findings. Sleep in the elderly depressed is significantly improved by the use of the more sedating tricyclic antidepressants. The tricyclic antidepressants (e.g., imipramine, amitriptyline) increase slow wave sleep, but may also produce nightmares when given in large doses at bedtime. The latter side effect may be especially troublesome in the patient who has marginal cognitive function secondary to concomitant organic mental disorders.

Sleep Disorders Secondary to Physical Disorders

Acute and chronic physical illness can definitely lead to the development of disorders in sleep among the elderly. Dyspnea, regardless of etiology (e.g., chronic obstructive pulmonary disease, congestive heart failure, etc.) may cause sleep difficulties secondary to shortness of breath. Acute and chronic pain may also lead to sleep disturbances. Though psychogenic pain disorders are less common in the elderly than in midlife, certain pain syndromes are encountered more frequently in the elderly. These include pain secondary to fractures (especially fractures of the hip), arthritic pains (especially secondary to osteoarthritis) and pain secondary to cancer.

Chest pain is another cause of sleep disturbances in the elderly (as in other stages of the life cycle). Nocturnal angina is commonly associated with REM sleep.[13] Angina is less common in patients with ischemic heart disease in late life but still may certainly present as a disturbing factor in sleep. Hypothyroidism is also known to cause significant changes in the sleep patterns of the elderly. Hypothyroid patients demonstrate a marked decrease in the percentages of stages 3 and 4 sleep in late life (as opposed to younger patients who only have a decrease in stage 4 sleep). These patterns improve with treatment.[14]

The clinical management of sleep disorders secondary to physical illness naturally relies upon the treatment and management of the primary illness. However, the clinician working with the older patient must not concentrate solely on "treatment" but also should consider symptom removal. The relief of pain, regardless of its etiology, will be greatly appreciated by the older patient, even if the primary illness remains untreated (e.g., cancer).

Primary Sleep Disturbances of Organic Etiology

Narcolepsy (irresistible sleep attacks of short duration which usually last less than 15 minutes) begins in adolescence or early adult life and once begun, continues throughout the adult life cycle. The attacks are possibly less frequent in old age. Narcolepsy is often associated with catalepsy (70%), sleep paralysis (50%) and hypnagogic hallucinations (25%).[15] The sleep attacks are associated with REM sleep and these individuals appear to have the ability to proceed directly from wakefulness into REM sleep. Drugs that inhibit REM sleep, such as methylphenidate and the amphetamines, are, therefore, potentially useful therapeutic agents. The side effects of these stimulants, however, have led to the use of the tricyclic antidepressants such as amitriptyline and desipramine, which are also REM inhibiting. Desipramine is probably the preferred drug because it produces less sedative effects.[16]

Hypersomnia of organic etiology is characteristic of patients who have encephalitis lethargic, brain tumors and myxedema.[15] The specific mechanisms are unknown but pathological effects of these conditions may be related to damage of the diencephalon. Symptoms include confusion on awakening with difficulty awakening. Disorientation that follows awakening may last for as much as an hour. Therefore these patients may be confused with individuals who have chronic organic brain syndromes. REM and non-REM sleep patterns are normal in this condition. Heart rate and respiration are increased before and during sleep in these individuals (differentiating them from patients with hypersomnia from hypothyroidism). Methylphenidate and the amphetamines appear to be of benefit as therapeutic

agents and they do not usually lead to addiction.

The Treatment of Sleep Disorders

If a sleep disturbance in an individual is specifically caused by known organic pathology that might respond to medical intervention, the first step in the treatment of sleep disorders is the treatment of the underlying condition. More often than not, however, the complaints of sleep disturbances in the elderly do not stem from well-circumscribed medical or psychiatric conditions. Yet the clinician should not discount sleep disturbances of nonspecific etiology for they can be most disturbing to the elderly patient. A program of good sleep hygiene can be most beneficial.

If physical health permits, exercise in the afternoon or early evening appears to aid sleep. This type of exercise program has not been studied specifically in the elderly. Yet sleep cannot be forced on a given night by exercising during the preceding day. For most individuals, a cool rather than a warm room is more conducive to sound sleep. Many elderly individuals tend to keep their houses or apartments excessively warm. This practice may lead to frequent awakenings. Temperature should never be lowered below 60 degrees, however, for the elderly are particularly susceptible to the development of hypothermia.

A light bedtime snack, such as warm milk, may be quite beneficial in promoting sleep.[18] Not only does this practice produce a favorable psychological effect, but there is some evidence that milk mobilizes serotonin which is known to induce sleep (as described below). All stimulants should be avoided for at least 3 to 4 hours before bedtime (especially caffeine).

The patient should be encouraged to get out of the bed at the same time every morning. This regular arousal time appears to strengthen circadian cycling and therefore to lead to regular times of sleep onset. Many elderly patients spend between 9 and 12 hours per day in bed but sleep only 6½ hours to 8 hours. Decreasing time spent in bed appears to improve the quality of sleep, as these long periods in bed are thought to be related to fragmented and shallow sleep.[18] Naps should be avoided during the day, regardless of the amount of sleep the preceding night. If the patient is not successful in falling to sleep after 10 or 15 minutes, a greater effort to produce sleep onset is usually of no benefit. The patient should be encouraged to switch on the light and to do something else, such as reading or watching television. After 15 to 30 minutes, with the onset of drowsiness, the patient should return to the bed and again attempt to fall asleep. If the second attempt is to no avail, the procedure can be repeated until sleep develops with ease. This practice can be of definite benefit to individuals who feel angry, frustrated or tense about being unable to fall asleep quickly.[18]

The sleep "milieu" is of great importance in promoting satisfactory sleep in the elderly. Sheets and pillowcases should be changed regularly, the bed should be "made-up" each morning, and the bedroom should be as free from external disturbance as possible. If practical, the bedroom should not be used excessively during the remainder of the day (thus promoting the cognitive association between the bedroom and sleep). If an individual is troubled by a sleep disorder, seeing the bed frequently or constantly during the day heightens anxiety about the sleep disorder and further decreases the probability that sleep can be pleasant and satisfactory.

The chronic use of sedatives and hypnotics by the elderly to induce sleep can lead to many undesirable side effects. These include tolerance to the drug, physical dependence and toxic effects of the drugs secondary to daytime retention (producing symptoms such as delirium, drowsiness, decreased mental alertness and loss of equilibrium). The elderly do not excrete these agents as quickly as the young. In addition, they are more likely to develop an acute mental syndrome (delirium) from these medications (especially the barbitu-

rates). Regardless of the age of an individual, the sedative hypnotic agents should only be used on a temporary basis. Most of these agents have been proven ineffective and even antagonistic to sleep after 2 weeks of continual use.[18]

Flurazepam loses its potency more gradually than the barbiturates and other sedative hypnotic agents. Yet this drug in its usual therapeutic dose (15 to 30 mgs at night) has been noted by clinicians to induce states of confusion in the elderly. Triazolam, a substitute benzodiazepine, at a dose of .25 mgs is a shorter acting drug and is reported to have less effect on the electroencephalogram. In one double blind study, triazolam was considered more effective than flurazepam with no decrease in hypnotic effects over a four week period and no evidence of tolerance.[19]

Many individuals use alcohol as a nighttime sedative. Alcohol may in fact enable the tense and anxious to fall asleep more quickly, but the ensuing sleep of these individuals tends to be more fragmented.[18] If the benzodiazepines, such as diazapam and chlordiazepoxide, are substituted for alcohol, the patient may avoid a fragmented pattern during the night, but (especially with the longer acting chloridazepoxide) may develop a confusional state in the morning.

Hartmann[20] reports that as little as 1 gm. of tryptophan can clearly improve sleep in some patients. 1-tryptophan is a serotonin percursor and serotonin is known to play some role in the initiation and maintenance of sleep. The clinical effects of using tryptophan includes its propensity to reduce sleep latency and to reduce awakening time. Low doses appear to induce sleep without producing distortions of physiologic sleep. The drug is considered to be quite safe. 1-2 gms of 1-tryptophan is normally ingested in the diet and is rapidly metabolized. There are no known allergies to the drug nor is tolerance thought to develop. This drug clearly needs to be studied more thoroughly.

In the depressed, the use of antidepressant medications, especially amitriptyline and doxepin can lead to increased sleep. Both the anticholinergic and the antidepressant effects may improve the quality of sleep in the depressed individual. As mentioned previously, the tricyclic antidepressants increase slow wave sleep. Yet giving all of this medication at bedtime to an older person (as has been recommended for younger individuals) may lead to nightmares and confusion in the elderly.[21]

Of the usual sedative hypnotics prescribed for sleep disturbances, chloral hydrate (the oldest) may be the safest. 500 mg. of the drug does produce CNS depression but confusional states, tolerance and addiction rarely develop (even though it is considered a controlled drug). Chloral hydrate should not be taken on an empty stomach and definitely not be combined with alcohol (the old "Micky Finn").

The elderly may frequently self-medicate themselves for sleep difficulties with over-the-counter preparations. The most popular of these over-the-counter soporifics usually contain scopolamine, an anticholinergic agent, which may lead to confusional episodes and even a toxic delirium in the elderly. The use of such medications should be discouraged. Aspirin is also used frequently to induce sleep. The sedative effects of the salicylates may be secondary to the relief of pain and/or possible increase in brain serotonin level. Again the use of aspirin to induce sleep is poorly understood and the side effects of the salicylates are potentially harmful to the elderly patient.

Taking a medication to induce sleep has become so much a part of our modern technological society that we should not expect rapid changes in the practice of physicians or expectations of patients. Therefore, clinicians should seriously consider the deleterious vs. the beneficial effects of withdrawing a low dose of a sedative hypnotic agent from an older person who has taken these medications for many years. Low doses of the hypnotics for long periods of time probably do not produce complications and sudden withdrawal of such a hypnotic may lead to a disintegration of the doctor-patient relationship. These patients

will ultimately find a physician who will prescribe the medication for them. The careful and judicious use of these medications plus the induction of sleep hygiene techniques will eventually enable the clinician to withdraw these medications with the cooperation of the patient.

PSYCHOSEXUAL DISORDERS AND ADJUSTMENT TO ORGANIC SEXUAL DYSFUNCTION

Normal Sexual Functioning in the Aging Female

The aging female undergoes a rather dramatic change in endocrine function at menopause. Though there is no evidence that these changes significantly effect overall sexual functioning in the postmenopausal woman, the consequences of these endocrine changes remain largely unknown. The most profound change is an increase in total output of gonadotropin secondary to the decrease in estrogen at menopause. Menopause is the consequence of ovarian hypofunction routinely experienced by women at a median age of 50 years. Modern medicine has made it possible to prevent many of the normal symptoms of menopause with estrogen sulfate (or another natural estrogen) and medroxyprogesterone acetate. In later years, the progestational agent can be removed while continuing the estrogen indefinitely. Much controversy continues to surround the use of such agents because of their potential carcinogenic properties.[22]

Masters and Johnson[23] have described in detail the sexual changes in the aging female. Delayed development of vaginal lubrication upon response to sexual stimulation is one of the more prominent late-life changes. This delay in lubrication is secondary to both decrease in estrogen content and changes in the structure of the vaginal wall; namely a decrease in elasticity. Nevertheless the pleasure gained from vaginal and clitoral stimulation remain unchanged in the elderly woman. The orgasmic phase of the sexual response for the 50- to 70-year-old woman is shortened when compared to younger women, especially in the absence of estrogen replacement therapy. Orgasm itself may be associated with either a decrease in the number of uterine contractions or a spastic contraction. Complaints of recurrent abdominal pain in the elderly female may be secondary to these spasms. The resolution phase of the sexual response is more rapid in late life. The labia and breast continue to be very responsive to stimulation even in 80-and 90-year-old females, but the sexual flush decreases in intensity and extent with age.

For both sexes, sexual activity reaches a peak in the 20- to 30-year-age range and declines each decade thereafter. In the Duke Longitudinal Studies, more than 40% of the married couples between 60 and 70 were no longer having sexual relations.[24,25,26,27] Masters and Johnson[23] report that there may be a reduction in sexual interest in the elderly woman because of decreased sex steroids. On the other hand, masturbation as a means of releasing sexual tensions probably increases after menopause, at least into the 60- to 70-year-age range. This increase in masturbatory activity may be related to the unavailability of a sex partner for the aging female. In the Duke study, only one-third of the women (average age 70) reported continuing sexual interest and this proportion did not change significantly over a 10-year period. One-fifth of the females who initially entered the study continued to have sexual intercourse regularly and this proportion did not decline over the next 20 years.[24,25,26,27] These studies indicate that the level of sexual interest and activity for females in late life is less than for males. A number of reasons may be contributing to these findings. First, women in this cohort (unlike women who have grown up during a period when sexual expression was more appropriate for the female) may have always been less interested in sexual matters. As mentioned above, menopause with its accompanying decrease in sex steroids could possibly lead to some decrease in sexual interest (but this remains unproven). In the Duke study, the median age of cessation of

sexual intercourse occurred nearly a decade earlier in women than in men (60 and 68 respectively).[24] This finding is probably secondary to the average difference in age of marriage partners for this cohort of the elderly and therefore decreased sexual interest and activity might be secondary to the unavailability of a sexual partner. For a small percentage of women, there is an increase in sexual interest and activity with advancing age.[24,25,26,27]

Though these studies reveal a general decrease in sexual interest and activity for older women, they also reveal a wide range of interest and activity in sexual matters. Even if biological factors play a role in continuing sexual interest and activity, there is certainly no evidence that the gradual changes of aging prohibit pleasure in sexual relationships. Therefore, many of our prejudices about sexuality in late life for the woman are unjustified.

Normal Sexual Functioning in the Aging Male

The aging male does not experience the dramatic change in endocrine functioning seen in the aging female. However, there appears to be a decline in the ability of the Leydig cells of the testes to produce testosterone in response to gonadotropin in aging men. Both total and free testosterone levels are decreased with advancing years. Gonadotropin levels are subsequently increased. The increase in gonadotropin is less dramatic in males than in females, however. The male gradually loses his ability to produce an adequate number of viable sperm with advancing years (usually during the seventh and eighth decade). The development of infertility is highly variable and in no way is associated physiologically with a decrease in sexual satisfaction.

Masters and Johnson again have provided the most thorough information about the sexual response of the aging male. The older man tends to require a longer period of time to respond to effective sexual stimulation than the younger man. The younger man may require only seconds to achieve erection, but the older man may require minutes. Once erection has been established, the older male has far greater control of ejaculatory demand because of the increased length of the plateau phase.

The experience of orgasm in the male with ejaculation is basically similar throughout the life cycle. Yet the aging male may not experience the phase of ejaculatory inevitability that is experienced earlier in life. The volume of seminal fluid is definitely reduced with aging. Often men will become disturbed when they notice this decrease in semen and will fear that their sexual functioning is altered. There is no evidence that decreased seminal output leads to a decreased enjoyment during orgasm.[23]

The refractory period (i.e., the period following ejaculation during which time the male is physically unable to respond to sexual stimulation) may increase from minutes to hours as the male ages. The elderly male typically loses his erection very quickly following ejaculation. Erections during REM sleep continue in the older man as they do in the young. However, the erections become less full in the aging process.

The aging male also can expect to normally reach ejaculation less frequently during sexual intercourse than his younger counterpart. This reduction in ejaculatory demand may lead to ejaculation during every second or third episode of intercourse. Yet the aging male can "force" ejaculation more frequently. A clinician should remember that this freedom from the demand to ejaculate during every episode of intercourse can be relaxing and satisfactory to the sexual enjoyment of the aging male.[23]

The Duke Longitudinal Study[24,25,26,27] revealed that 80% of the men (n = 116) who originally entered the study (aged 60 to 94 at Round 1) had continuing sexual interest. It should be remembered that these men were functioning adequately in health, intellectual status and socially. Interest in sexuality did not decline significantly over a 10-year period. At the beginning of the study, 70% of the men surveyed were sexually active but this proportion dropped to 25% during a 10-year period.[24,25,26,27] 20% to 25% of the men demonstrated an increase in sexual activity with advancing age.

As can be seen from the above data, the general pattern of sexuality in the elderly male is for sexual interest to basically continue unabated until very late in life. Sexual activity appears to decline rather dramatically during the seventh and eighth decades. Yet the overall picture again is one of great variability in sexual interest and activity in the aging male. Many men continued to enjoy an active sex life well into the eighth and ninth decades.

Sexual Dysfunction in the Aging Female:

As mentioned previously, there is no physiologic basis to the common belief that the aging female cannot enjoy sexual intercourse in late life. However, a number of problems may potentially lead to sexual dysfunction. Women live longer than men and therefore are much more at risk for being without a sexual partner as they age. This lack of an available partner is probably the most common cause of declining sexual interest or frustration in the aging female. The widowed elderly woman who nurses her husband through months (and even years) of illness may find herself particularly frustrated in her wishes to express herself sexually. The physical and emotional energy required to care for the husband may have temporarily distracted her from the need to be sexually satisfied. Once the grieving process has taken its normal course, old desires and interests are coupled often with a new burst of energy. Yet she finds herself in a social environment with few physically healthy eligible men. Friends and especially the family may expect her to "be proper" or to "act her age." This "double jeopardy" often eliminates the opportunity to meet and associate with the opposite sex. Techniques for the relief of sexual tension, such as masturbation, may be substituted but this does not negate her desire to develop a meaningful heterosexual relationship.

Another complaint is that of dyspareunia (pain on coitus). Dyspareunia is most commonly caused by postmenopausal senile vaginitis. The vagina normally undergoes contraction and loses elasticity with aging. Trauma to the vaginal wall during intercourse may lead to pain and bleeding. The complaint of pain during intercourse should not be discounted by the clinician. Elderly women do not usually interject such concerns if they are not of major importance to their sense of physical and emotional well-being. Since the condition is potentially treatable, it is of added importance that such complaints not be overlooked. Embarrassment and even shame may lead the elderly woman to disguise her complaints. Whenever the clinician becomes confused about the nature of a complaint in the lower abdomen or genitourinary region, closer questioning may reveal that dyspareunia is, in fact, the major problem. Senile vaginitis is the most common cause of postmenopausal bleeding. The application of estrogen locally in the form of creams or suppositories each night for three or four weeks can be very helpful in alleviating the symptoms of senile vaginitis. The clinician should be careful that other conditions (candidiasis, diabetes mellitus, vaginal carcinoma, etc.) do not cause or contribute to the symptoms.

Occasionally the aging female will complain of abdominal pain during intercourse. This pain may be secondary to uterine spasms during orgasm.[29] As mentioned previously, these spasms are to be expected in the postmenopausal woman. Yet the onset of such pain in the aging female may be of particular concern. Her sexual partner, not wishing to inflict pain, may shorten or cease sexual intercourse. Neither partner is satisfied and emotional tension then surrounds the sexual experience. In addition, the woman may develop a particular concern that such spasms are secondary to a serious illness (e.g., cancer). Reassurance and explanation are the cornerstones of the treatment of this condition. Estrogen replacement is also a useful therapeutic adjunct.

Sexual Dysfunction in the Aging Male:

If one marital partner is referred to a physician in late life for sexual dysfunction, the probability of that marital partner being the male is 80%.[30] Though we may see a change in this ratio over the next few years (especially as a new cohort of women reach late life), the male is much more likely to openly express concern to the physician about sexual dysfunction with aging. Cultural stereotypes have been unfair to both sexes, and these stereotypes (accompanied by their characteristic expectations) contribute to the disproportion. The male is expected to remain potent or is expected to lose all interest in sex. Minor changes in sexual performance are frequently seen as pathological and the clinician is subsequently consulted. The female, in contrast, is expected first to have little interest and concern in sexuality, and, if she does, to "keep it quiet."

The most common complaint in the aging male is secondary impotence. Though erectile impotence may occur on occasion in relatively young men, it becomes increasingly prevalent as the male ages.[31] There are many possible etiologic factors contributing to secondary impotence in the aging male and the treatment of this disorder is usually dictated by the etiology. Inheritance may play some causative role,[32] but other factors are more important. The most prevalent cause of impotency in the aging male is fear of nonperformance. As mentioned above, the decrease in ejaculatory demand results in episodes of intercourse without ejaculation on a more frequent basis. The cultural belief that intercourse cannot be satisfying to the male with ejaculation may elicit considerable concern in the aging male. Each occasion of intercourse becomes a "test" of his potency. The fear of failure leads to increased emotional tension and decreased spontaniety. Successful and satisfactory intercourse becomes even less frequent and the male becomes further disturbed. A vicious cycle develops. Both partners may be so obsessed with the man's need to perform with ejaculation on every occasion of intercourse that satisfaction is rarely experienced. The fear of nonperformance may be further complicated by the mistaken belief that he cannot satisfy his sexual partner without achieving ejaculation (which is definitely not true). A willingness to listen and calm reassurance by the clinician may go a long way toward interrupting this vicious cycle.

Poor health status is another problem. For example, a number of illnesses lead to physiologic changes in erectile and ejaculatory capacity. Diabetes may lead to a weakness of erection. Obesity is often associated with impotence (though not always). Injury to the spinal cord (depending on the level of the injury) may lead to impotence. (However, it is important to remember that the paraplegic may in fact be able to maintain an erection and engage in satisfactory sexual intercourse). In addition to these specific illnesses and injuries, a general decrease in physical health functioning will often be associated with a decrease in sexual potency. For example, the patient suffering from congestive heart failure, a malignancy, chronic obstructive pulmonary disease, etc. will often manifest sexual dysfunction in his symptom picture. Urologic surgery may lead to temporary loss of sexual potency, but impotence is not an inevitable sequel to transurethral surgery or genital manipulation.

The physician who is treating the impotent male must always consider the possible role of prescribed medications or other drugs in the etiology of sexual dysfunction in late life. Hypertensive agents such as guanethidine and reserpine, partially deplete norepinephrine stores which may produce impotence (including dysfunction in erectile potency, the ability to ejaculate and the intensity of climax).[33] The phenothiazines (especially thioridazine) and other anticholinergic drugs block sympathetic and parasympathetic innervation of the sex organs.[33] Many over-the-counter sleep medications have significant anticholinergic effects. Sedative and other sleep medications (including phenobarbital and diazepam) are

also important contributors to sexual dysfunction in late life.

Alcohol remains the most important pharmacologic agent in the etiology of secondary impotency in men. Though the consumption of alcohol typically decreases in the later years, alcohol may have a particularly deleterious effect on the male whose physical health is marginal and/or who is depressed. The ability of alcohol to stimulate sexual activity in early life (mainly due to a decrease in inhibitions) declines as one ages. Alcohol is often used as an escape and men who fear poor sexual performance may escape to the bottle to avoid a confrontation with their own fears. Small quantities of alcohol intake, however, do not typically produce adverse sexual performance.

Impotent elderly males may become very distressed about their condition and therefore be susceptible to unusual and diverse pharmacologic techniques that are passed on by the lay public. The clinician should especially be concerned about the possible use of an elixir such as strychnine. The anabolic steroids have been used in therapeutic trials for the treatment of sexual dysfunction in late life, but it is uncertain whether such practices are in fact appropriate.

Another important and potentially reversible cause of impotency in males during late life is secondary impotency that may develop following an acute illness or injury. The male, for example, who has suffered from an acute myocardial infarction may be unable to engage in sexual intercourse for a period of weeks. Once his physical health permits sexual intercourse, he finds himself unsuccessful in his first few attempts following his illness. This "lack of success" in performance is then accompanied by the fear of nonperformance described above. The early re-establishment of sexual intercourse in chronic illness or injury accompanied by an atmosphere of openness and ventilation in the hospital or outpatient facility can be of great value in avoiding the progression of this psychologically induced impotence.

Physical handicaps may cause secondary impotence in aging men. Noncoital techniques (e.g., solitary or mutual masturbation) can be substituted for normal genital intercourse and thus becomes a method of sexual satisfaction. A knowledge of such techniques and a willingness to discuss their merit openly with the physically handicapped can be of great value in sexual counseling.[30] The clinician should remember that, in the paraplegic male, orgasm can occur in spite of denervation of the pelvic floor and that genital skin and smooth muscle retain their innervation.

Another common cause of impotence in the male is psychiatric disorder. In fact, blood testosterone may be significantly decreased by emotional states of tension or depression.[37] The high incidence of depression among the elderly coupled with atypical symptom patterns of presentation (often including organic complaints) impel the clinician to consider depressive illness in the different diagnosis of secondary impotence. Other psychosocial states that may result in secondary impotence include monotony and boredom, mental or physical fatigue, anxiety states, etc.

A less common, but disturbing, condition that may affect the aging male is retrograde ejaculation. Diabetes may cause damage to the nerves which control the bladder.[34] This damage may also occur secondary to prostatic surgery[35] or colon surgery.[36] The result of the denervation is a redirection of semen into the bladder instead of through the penis during normal orgasm. All other sensations of orgasm remain unchanged. The semen is later voided in the urine and may be mistaken for an infection. The elderly male may have difficulty in explaining this symptom. Whenever the clinician is having difficulty in understanding the description of genitourinary symptoms, retrograde ejaculation should be considered. Explanation and reassurance are the only interventions necessary.

Socially Inappropriate Sexual Behavior

The typical stereotypes of the "dirty old man" or the "prudish" elderly woman are examples of society's plagues upon older adults. Socially inappropriate sexual behavior is rarely encountered among the elderly. In fact, the old age group, when compared with other age groups, rarely is involved in child molestation and/or exhibitionism.[30] The elderly, however, continue to be the subject of degrading humor, suspicion or contempt when sexuality is considered. Fear among younger adults (e.g., a fear of competition in the sexual arena) is one factor that has lead to the stereotypes of inappropriateness which effectively eliminated the free expression of sexual interest and needs on the part of the elderly.

The clinician may occasionally encounter sexually inappropriate behavior in long-term care facilities, especially among men. Though such behavior is rarely a danger to staff or other patients, it can become a great concern, especially to female staff members. Typical examples include the man with organic mental disease who "pinches the nurses" or physically handicapped individuals who purposefully allow themselves to be exposed. In the latter case, such men are quite conflicted over their loss of physical mobility (which is coupled with a fear of loss of masculinity). Since a long-term care facility does not frequently allow the patient an opportunity to express his concerns openly and little, if any, potential for developing a heterosexual relationship, inappropriate behavior results. An explanation of the dynamics of the patient's concerns to staff, and encouragement of patients to discuss their concerns often eliminate the behavior.

Older women, are more at risk for a different type of problem. Interest in appearance (e.g., getting one's hair fixed), in being kissed (or even touched) by others, in male companionship, etc. is often ignored by family members and the staff of institutions. The woman may literally find herself "out of touch" with her own feminine self-image and with heterosexual interaction. Family and staff members discount requests to go to the beauty parlor, to get a new dress or to spend time with men as unimportant, or even unbecoming to their views of how the older woman should behave. The clinician should remind family and staff of the continuing needs of the aging woman to express her sexuality.

With the increasing controversy concerning homosexuality in our society, some mention should be made of the homosexual in late life. There is little evidence that being homosexual leads to particular problems in old age, contrary to the stereotypes of a lonely sexually frustrated and unhappy older homosexual. The homosexual does face certain problems, however.[38] These include the loss of people close to them, the fear of institutionalization and decreasing family and social supports. The late life homosexual may be at particular risk for institutionalization when physical or mental impairment develop because of a scarcity of social supports. Homosexuality is also less accepted among individuals 65 and over secondary to the value system of this particular cohort of elderly. The developing tolerance seen in other age groups (at least at present) may not reflect the views of the elderly.

Treatment of Sexual Dysfunction in Late Life

A number of medications can possibly benefit the elderly male and female who suffer from sexual dysfunction. The use of L-dopa, especially with elderly men, may lead to some sexual rejuvenation but these effects are generally short-lived.[33] The anabolic steroids (already mentioned) produce sexual rejuvenation in some but have also been shown to adversely affect sexual activity. There is no evidence that amyl nitrate increases the sexual functioning of the elderly. In summary, the use of medications in the treatment of sexual dysfunction in elderly males and females remains in experimental stages. Prescribing such medications requires close monitoring by the clinician for possible side effects. One must also be wary of the possible "placebo" effect of these medications.

Regardless of the etiology of sexual dysfunction in late life, a most important element in treatment is the development of a supportive atmosphere in working with the aging patient. Guidelines for developing a favorable atmosphere include the following:

1. Obtain a thorough sexual history.

2. Establish an open atmosphere for the discussion of sexual matters (at the same time respecting individual differences).

3. Intervene as early as possible when a problem is identified.

4. Encourage communication between the sexual partners.

5. When appropriate, instruct sexual partners in particular techniques that may be substituted for their usual approach to sexual expression (especially in patients with handicaps or patients with marginal physical capacities—for example, the postmyocardial infarction patient).

6. Carefully monitor medications and eliminate or decrease the dosage of drugs that may inhibit sexual activity (if possible).

7. Suggest changes in the environment when appropriate (e.g., creating an environment that allows privacy, or encouraging members of the environment to respect the sexual needs of the older patient).

8. Emphasize the broader aspects of human sexuality (closeness, touch, sensuality, being valued as a man or woman, etc.).

9. Respect individual differences.

SOMATOFORM DISORDERS

The somatoform disorders, according to the third edition of the Diagnostic and Statistical Manual[1] are disorders for which there are no demonstrable organ findings to explain the symptoms and for which there is positive evidence that the symptoms are linked to psychological factors. Symptom formation is not under voluntary control, however. DSM-III categorizes the somatoform disorders into (1) somatization disorders (Briquet's syndrome); (2) conversion disorders; (3) psychogenic pain disorders; and (4) hypochondriasis.

Somatization disorder (Briquet's syndrome) usually begins early in life and is seen infrequently among the elderly. The symptoms in the elderly patient are rarely different than those at other stages of the life cycle. Conversion reactions are seen in elderly patients, but again the presentation of symptomatology is not significantly different than among other age groups. Both of these conditions, in "pure form," are rare in the elderly. When present, they usually do not respond as promptly or effectively to treatment.

Chronic pain can be seen among the elderly but it is not as frequent as during other stages of the life cycle. Clinicians in the Pain Clinic at Duke University Medical Center have noticed that individuals with chronic pain syndromes generally develop their chronic pain in midlife with only occasional appearance of chronic unexplained pain late in life. Pain may be a more likely outcome of unsuccessful negotiation of crises in midlife than in late life (for moderately severe pain effectively removes an individual from the responsibilities of adulthood). Physiologic evidence supports the view that the elderly may not be as susceptible to the development of problems with pain as individuals in midlife. There is a sensory loss in the pain experience with advancing years.[39] The elderly also demonstrate less ability to locate a particular pain in physical illness and therefore pain is less helpful in identifying these illnesses (e.g., myocardial infarction and peptic ulcer disease).[30] Yet older patients do develop chronic pain syndromes. Those who do suffer from pain tend to respond to placebos with greater frequency than do younger patients.[40]

Clinical experience at Duke has also shown that behavioral techniques developed by Fordyce and others[41] can be as effective in treating chronic refractory pain syndromes in late life as they are with patients earlier in the life cycle. In fact, the management of chronic pain syndromes generally involve a multidimensional and interdisciplinary approach (the sine qua non of good medical care in the elderly. Pharmacologic therapy usually involves the systematic decrease in narcotic analgesic medications, coupled with the judicial use of phenothiazines and tricyclic antidepressants when appropriate. Other dimensions of therapy include physical therapy (to increase instrumental and physical activities of daily living), biofeedback and relaxation techniques (to decrease muscle tension and conscious obsession over the pain), behavior techniques on the ward (to facilitate independent behavior and to inhibit "pain behavior"), group therapy and supportive individual therapy. The clinician must coordinate the various facets of this therapeutic approach, which, once instituted, can be most effective.

Headache, an uncommon symptom to develop after the age of 55, can also be of psychiatric etiology. Less than 2% of individuals over the age of 55 experience severe headaches for the first time.[42] When headache appears in late life, the usual diagnostic considerations of migraine or muscle contraction headaches must give way to considerations of other causes. Unilateral headache may be secondary to temporal arthritis, as the prevalence of this entity rises each decade after the age of 50.[43] Other conditions that may cause headache include hypertension, mass lesions (though infrequently seen among the elderly), ischemia of pain sensitive structures, and cluster headaches (a variant of migraine).[44] Psychiatric problems that lead to headaches in late life most commonly are of affective etiology (depression) but may be secondary to anxiety. The treatment of headache in late life is similar to the treatment at other points in the life cycle. The use of biofeedback techniques, in addition to the judicious use of the minor tranquilizers form the basis of the treatment of muscle contraction headaches. Ergot preparations are valuable both in the treatment and prevention of vascular headaches. Antidepressant medications may have a dramatic effect in relieving the headache of the depressed patient.

Hypochondriasis

Patients with hypochondriasis do not have the multiplicity of symptoms or the onset in early life that characterizes the somatization disorder (Briquet's syndrome). Many feel that hypochondriasis is especially prevalent among the elderly. Clinical experience indicates that the condition is more frequent among older women.[45] The syndrome is characterized by fears or worries about the body which are grossly exaggerated.[46] There may be some tendency for a greater preoccupation with the body in late life because of chronic physical diseases which facilitate the redistribution of affect toward the body. Disengagement, flight into the sick role and decreased self-esteem may also contribute to the development of hypochondriacal symptoms.[47]

Affective disorders in late life may present with exaggerated fears and worries about the body. Depression is the most common affective condition to be masked by physical symptoms. Because depression is more common in the elderly, one might expect to see an increased prevalence of hypochondriacal symptoms. An added advantage of such symptoms is that the depressed patient may receive secondary gain in the form of attention, comfort, touching and interest which are associated with interactions between physicians, family members and the patient involving the pain.

Most studies indicate that the prevalence of "hypochondriasis" is quite high among the depressed elderly. In one study, hypochondriacal symptoms are found in 65.7% of men and 62% of women among 152 depressed patients over the age of 60. The most common presenting symptom was constipation. Hypochondriacal symptoms may be associated with overt symptoms of anxiety or depression. 24.8% of those individuals with hypochondriacal symptoms attempted suicide while among those free of such symptoms only 7.3% attempted suicide. The presence of hypochondriacal symptoms in the older patient with significant depression may present a potentially critical situation to the clinician.[48]

A community survey in Durham, North Carolina[49] revealed that approximately 10% of the elderly assess their physical health to be poorer than their health status was actually rated on an objective basis. These individuals were more depressed and had decreased life satisfaction. Though their physical health status was normal, their activities of daily living were decreased and they had an increased number of doctors visit when compared to a control group. They also reported a greater number of symptoms when asked objectively. One surprising finding was that these individuals were actually more willing to see a mental health counselor (if they demonstrated some impairment in their mental health) than the controlled population. This finding is in contrast to the general belief that the hypochondriacal patient avoids mental health services and gravitates to individuals who they feel will take interest in their physical health only. A separate study found 53.6% of the elderly surveyed who felt themselves in better health than others. 31% reported that they felt their own health about the same as others and 9.8% considered their health to be poorer than those of other persons their age.[50]

Maddox,[51] in another study of the elderly in Durham County, reported that two of three elderly subjects displayed a reality orientation in their subjective evaluation of health status. 17% assessed their health as subjectively poor when it was objectively good and 13% assessed their health as subjectively good when it was objectively poor.

When taken together, these studies indicate that between 10% and 20% of the elderly who are in the community consider their health to be poor when compared to persons their own age and view their health to be subjectively worse than it is demonstrated on objective examination. These individuals may not all deserve the label of "hypochondriacal" but the factors contributing to the development of this negative assessment of health status may form a predictable pattern. This turning into the body may (1) facilitate communication and interaction with others (via symptom communication); (2) displace anxiety; (3) form an identification with a deceased or absent loved one; (4) provide punishment for unresolved guilt feelings; and (5) control the behavior of individuals within the immediate environment. Regardless of the etiology, these individuals are quite difficult for the physician to treat.

Nevertheless, certain guidelines have been found to be most helpful in the treating of these individuals.[52] These guidelines include:

1. Never try to explain to the patient that his or her symptoms are not caused by an illness. Emphasize that the individual has a serious condition worthy of the attention of the physician but that the condition is not critical.

2. Do not attempt to treat the "illness."

3. Listen attentively to the patient describe his or her symptoms.

4. Offer whatever help is feasible but do not promise marked success.

5. Do something that helps the patient understand that an effort is being made, such as the use of certain mild medications (which may be under the control of the patient), physical therapy, biofeedback, etc.

6. Instruct the patient to return on a regular basis. Continue to see the patient regularly. The vists over time may be spaced out and the time spent with the patient may be decreased.

7. If possible, form a group of individuals who suffer from chronic complaints. Group therapy techniques may be quite valuable with such individuals if placed in the proper context.

8. Do not venture a diagnosis or prognosis of the condition.

9. Expect the patient to shift the content of the sessions to psychosocial issues over time.

10. Avoid shifting the patient from one physician to another.

11. Schedule patient visits in a medical clinic setting (as opposed to a psychiatric facility) even if the primary clinician is a mental health professional.

Patients with hypochondriacal symptoms need 15 to 20 minutes on each visit initially, but this time may be decreased to 10 minutes over time. Limits must be set on the time spent during each visit. The interval between visits should not be abused by the patient. If the patient calls between visits, the telephone conversation should be limited to brief sessions and the patient should be encouraged to elaborate on difficulties at the next appointed visit. It must be remembered that these individuals greatly desire understanding on the part of the clinician and not necessarily a cure.

Gastrointestinal Complaints

Many older people present to the clinician with gastrointestinal symptoms that are known to have prominent if not total psychiatric causation. In one study of 300 elderly people initially seen as outpatients over the age of 65 with primary complaints referrable to the gastrointestinal tract, 56% had a functional etiology.[53] Their symptoms included heartburn, ulcerlike distress, belching, nausea and vomiting, diarrhea, constipation and flatulence. Many complained of anorexia and weight loss though no organic cause could be discovered. Factors commonly recognized as related to the development of functional bowel symptoms in the elderly include emotional tension, life events producing stress, fear of disease and death, depression, cerebral arterial sclerosis and the habitual use of cathartics. Loneliness and sexual frustration were found to be particular problems among the female elderly.

Yet the clinician must remember that many symptoms thought to be functional in etiology may turn out to be serious organic conditions. Particular problems in the elderly that lead to gastrointestinal complaints include obstruction, idiopathic megacolon, drug intoxication, hypothyroidism and immobility.[54] In fact, gastrointestinal disorders in the 65 and older affect 46% of patients admitted to hospitals with chronic illnesses and 69% of the medical emergencies.[55]

Constipation is a frequent complaint of older persons who have psychiatric problems. Constipation may be caused by loss of tone in the bowel wall, diminished peristalsis and loss of strength of the abdominal musculature that normally occurs with aging. Of more importance, however, are inadequate intake of fluids, habitual use of cathartics and laxatives, and faulty eating habits. The anxiety and depression over regular bowel movements certainly contributes to the problem. In fact, a preoccupation with bowel habits may be less related to age than to the sociocultural environment of those individuals in late life (such as beliefs in the need for laxatives, food habits, the need to eliminate waste on regular basis, etc.). Treatment of constipation should be both physical and psychological. Large quantities of cooked vegetables and the regular use of whole grain cereals are most important. The irritant laxatives should be avoided if at all possible. At the same time, reassuring the patient that constipation is troublesome but not critical and therefore must be accepted can be of great help. The psychiatrist and primary care physician may have prescribed medications for emotional problems (e.g., thioridazine, amitriptyline, etc.) that have significant anticholinergic activity which in turn leads to constipation. If these medications can be avoided, constipation will be less of a problem. Patients suffering from constipation should be encouraged to exercise as much as possible (which may have the secondary effect of facilitating increased self-esteem and decreased depression and anxiety).

"Neurodermatitis" is seen frequently in the elderly, is more refractory to treatment and causes more distress than in the young. In one study of individuals 60 years of age and older, neurodermatitis was the fourth most common dermatosis in order of total visits per diagnosis.[56] Lichen simplex chronicus (localized neurodermatitis) occurs especially around the ankles and neck.[57] In addition, 12% of one series of elderly patients had "neurogenic excoriatoris" (small excoriatal, "picked" areas) especially on the accessible areas of arms, legs and face.[57] Lichenification is a pattern of response of predisposed skin to repeated rubbing. Neurodermatitis must be distinguished from the "winter itch" of normal aging (the tendency for aged skin to dehydrate and chap more easily) and from more serious physical conditions that may lead to pruritis (e.g., diabetes mellitus, kidney disease malignancy, gout, etc.).[57] Treatment includes the use of local preparations (beware of bath oils which make the bathtub quite slippery), antihistamines (diphenhydramine is preferred but should be given at night because of its soporific effect) and/or the major tranquilizers. If the onset and exacerbation of the condition is clearly related to emotional factors, psychotherapy may be of value. Relaxation techniques, including biofeedback may also be helpful.

Hereditary predisposition, moisture, incontinence, local irritation, rubbing, self-treatment, endocrine and physiological changes all contribute to the development of anogenital pruritis. The absence of a sexual partner in the female may lead to increased masturbatory activity thus producing the localized neurodermatitis. Males and females excessively concerned about bowel habits may spend much time at the toilet. Excessive "wiping" may also lead to the development of a dermatitis, further complicating the exaggerated concern with bowel functioning.

Urinary incontinence is not generally thought to be of psychiatric etiology. Yet experienced clinicians[58] have indicated that urinary incontinence may frequently be a by-product of poor emotional adjustment in the older adult. In fact, urinary incontinence may develop as a consequence of the dependency role of patients in long-term care facilities and as a means of expressing anger toward caretakers (i.e., urinary incontinence is often much more troublesome to the caretaker than to the identified patient). There is also an association between incontinence and chronic organic mental syndromes.[59] The treatment of urinary incontinence (which includes behavioral techniques) has been described in detail by Brocklehurst.[60] Yet these treatment techniques have been used infrequently in the United States. A more positive approach to the treatment of urinary and fecal incontinence is of great importance to clinicians in both home care and long-term care facilities.

Psychosomatic Reactions

The third edition of the Diagnostic and Statistical Manual[1] classifies all conditions where psychological factors are judged to be contributing to the initiation, exacerbation or perpetuation of a nonmental medical disorder as "psychosomatic reactions." The degree to which psychological components are a contributing factor to the medical illness is indicated as probable, prominent, unknown, etc. In the second edition of the Diagnostic and Statistical Manual, these entities were classified as the "psychophysiological disorders" (i.e., physical symptoms that are caused by emotional factors and involve a single organ system, usually under autonomic nervous system innervation). In the last 10 years, it has become evident that psychic factors play only a contributory role in the development of these conditions and must be considered in the context of genetic and physiologic predisposition.[3] Some of the classic psychosomatic illnesses will be considered below. Each presents certain unique problems in the aging population. So few studies to date have considered these conditions in a life-cycle perspective that few answers to the obvious questions have evolved.

Hypertension is by far the most common of the psychosomatic reactions in late life. Many have outlined the dynamic pattern of essential hypertension as involving hostile competitive and aggressive tendencies which are in conflict with passive tendencies and dependent longings. These inferiority feelings lead to a reactivation of the hostile competitiveness which in turn leads to anxiety secondary to the fear of losing approval and security if the impulses are expressed. Personality characteristics of such individuals include insecurity, restlessness, hypervigilance, obsessive-compulsive behavior and suspicion of the environment.

Though there is little evidence that these personality characteristics have any etiological relationship to essential hypertension, one is struck by the prevalence of many of these characteristics in the mentally impaired elderly. This results in inhibition of aggression, anger and resentment. The ultimate outcome of these inhibited tendencies is "essential hypertension."[61,62,63]

Donnison[64] attributed the increased prevalence of high blood pressure among the elderly in our society to a failure of older persons to adapt to the revolutionary changes in the mode of living and to the elderly's inability to transmit appropriate modified social patterns to the young. Cruz-Coke[68] introduced the concept of the "ecological nitch" to explain the consistently low blood pressure of groups living in isolated regions and enjoying an unchallenging and unchallenged tradition handed over from one generation to another. When the nitch is disturbed, there is a change in the culture. Some adapt to this change and some do not. These theories could be consolidated into a theory that would consider our society as one that not only decreases the status of older people but inhibits their ability to express their emotions (including hostility). With the loss of social role, the older person also loses the privileges associated with such a role (including the privilege of becoming angry). The repressed anger in the predisposed individual, may be transduced into central nervous system lowering of renal artery blood flow and the release of renin or a disinhibition of the kidneys inhibiting actions on extrarenal pressure mechanisms.[3] The cumulative effect is a sustained elevation of blood pressure.

Yet many questions remain unanswered concerning hypertension in the elderly. The typical rise in blood pressure with advancing years may be physiologic for some individuals who require increased cerebral blood flow in a restrictive vascular system. In fact, the failure of blood pressure to rise with age in some individuals may simply be a reflection of selective survival in those individuals. Cassel[66] has suggested, though, that we not overlook the relationship of increased blood pressure among the elderly and the societal pressures placed on older persons in modern technological culture. Childhood, adolescence and early adult life is the time in which our society inculcates its value systems. Stress may develop when the aging individual finds himself or herself in a social milieu in which it is hard to adapt because these values are not being supported. The elderly are also at risk for the occurrence of a blockage of aspirations, a decrease of meaningful human intercourse and an uncertainty about future events.

Alexander[61] viewed the central emotional problem in asthma as a fear of separation from the mother and concluded that the asthmatic attack is equivalent to a repressed cry for the lost mother. The elderly individual (at risk for a loss of important emotional ties and decreasing self-sufficiency) may undergo an increased need for dependency upon others. In fact, Leigh suggests that an emotional factor may be more important in the etiological complex of late onset asthma than of asthma which originates earlier in life.[70] Leigh also suggests that a substantial number of patients develop asthma in the middle years (16% to 34% of asthmatics first experience symptoms after about 35 years of age). In one series, emotional factors were seen to be of importance as a precipitating factor in 47% of the patients 35 and over. Yet the psychological symptoms showed considerable variation with anxiety and depression being the most common. Other writers suggest that bronchial asthma is infrequent in the elderly.[68] Recent evidence has indicated that emotional factors are only one of a number of factors including immunologic predisposition, which contributes to the development of an asthmatic attack.[3] The data on the prevalence of asthma in late life is uncertain. Therefore it is difficult to draw any firm conclusions concerning the contribution of psychic factors to the development of bronchial asthma in late life. Many questions arise in consideration of asthma as a condition where psychic factors play a significant role in the etiology. If psychic factors are of importance, why doesn't the condition present earlier in life when the individual must negotiate developmental crises? Is the psychic stress secondary to a specific etiologic conflict (i.e., specific to the disease) or is generalized stress the most important factor? To what extent does social support, a loving and effective caretaker, modify the response to the psychic stress?, etc.

Rebellion against restrictive influences leading to anxiety and subsequent repression of rebellious tendencies are thought to be elements of the dynamic constellation in patients with rheumatoid arthritis.[61] A number of investigators have agreed that rheumatoid arthritics are more likely to be "self-sacrificing, masochistic, conforming, self conscious, shy, inhibited, perfectionistic and interested in sports and games. They also tend to overreact to their illness."[69] Again one could make a case for the elderly being specifically at risk for the development of arthritic symptoms given the restrictions (both physical and psychosocial) experienced during the later years in our society. Rheumatoid arthritis does have its onset after the age of 65 (2% of the patients in one series).[70] Another study revealed a 15% prevalence of rheumatoid arthritis among women in the 65 and over age group.[71] The discrepancy in prevalence studies of rheumatoid arthritis in late life coupled with the problems of differential diagnosis in separating this condition from osteoarthritis has limited the psychosomatic studies of rheumatoid arthritis in late life. A review of the literature does not reveal any information concerning the psychosocial characteristics of individuals who have rheumatoid arthritis in late life. Given the prevalence of arthritic conditions, such studies would seem to be warranted. The pathophysiology of this condition also raises some intriguing prospects. Though normal immune functions decline with aging, infections and autoimmunity increase.[71] Rheumatoid arthritis is an autoimmune disease, though the antigen primarily responsible for this immunologic activity is unknown.

Thyrotoxicosis (Graves' disease) has been claimed to be the health outcome of some individuals who had frustrated dependent longings and a persistent threat to their security (either exposure to death or other threatening experiences) in early life which in turn led to premature attempts to identify with the objects of dependent cravings. The failure of these strivings for self-sufficiency and the caring of others was seen as the precipitant of the condition.[61] Again the dependency needs and security that accompany late life might be considered risk factors for the development of thyrotoxicosis in the elderly. Yet careful studies do not substantiate previously held views regarding the role of personality factors in the etiology of the condition.[3] This condition has increasingly been thought of as another of the autoimmune conditions. Those 60 and over account for 10% to 17% of the thyrotoxic population.[73] The typical symptomatology of nervousness, sweating, etc. may be inconspicuous or absent in the elderly. These symptoms are likely to be replaced by other symptomatology, such as angina, atrial fibrillation and congestive heart failure. A review of the literature sheds no light on the contribution of psychosocial factors to the development of thyrotoxicosis in late life.

The development of gastrointestinal symptoms in late life has been described previously. Ulcerative colitis is rare among the elderly and there is no evidence that psychosocial factors play a significant role in the etiology of the condition. Active peptic ulcer disease is seen in about the same prevalence among the elderly as in a younger population, but there is much greater likelihood that the ulcer will be gastric (1 in 3 as opposed to 1 in 10 for a younger individual.[53]) There is no evidence that psychological factors play an etiologic role in late life. We are therefore left with little if any information concerning the contribution of psychosocial factors to the classical psychophysiological illnesses. Yet clinical intuition leads to the assumption that psy-

chosocial factors indeed play some role in illness onset and progression. The study of the psychobiology of human disease in late life is an important but relatively untouched field. The absence of simple etiologic models coupled with the countless extraneous factors that must be considered over the life span have certainly contributed to the vacuum of studies in this area. Medical treatment for these conditions in the elderly is basically similar to that for individuals throughout the life span. Psychosocial intervention in the elderly (save in the area of hypertension) has received few if any comments in the literature.

DRUG USE DISORDERS

Alcohol continues to be the most common drug used by the adult elderly for its central nervous system effects. The use of alcohol as a therapeutic agent in the social setting has been advocated by Chien, et al.[74] A simulated pub milieu was developed in two nursing homes. Alcohol was appreciated in the settings but did not appear to offer significant therapeutic effects. However, other clinicians have suggested from their own experience that alcohol is of value in enhancing the social atmosphere of the long-term care facility. Alcohol has also been used as an appetite stimulant. A small glass of wine before the evening meal may be of both physiologic and psychologic value in increasing the appetite of the anorexic elderly patient both in the home and in institutional setting. Older people may use alcohol as a sedative to help relieve tension. The immediate effects may be the induction of sleep but the ensuing sleep is often fragmented. Other agents are thought to be of more value as sedatives (e.g., chloral hydrate). The tranquilizing effects of alcohol are also somewhat difficult to control and, if alcohol is being given solely for its tranquilizing effect, other agents (such as diazapam) may be substituted. Depending on the situation and the effects desired, alcohol can be used therapeutically among older patients, but the relative advantages and disadvantages must be weighed in each situation. More studies are needed in this area.

Schmidt[75] has indicated that alcohol intake decreases in late life. Drinking problems are less common and one sees a smaller percentage of heavy drinkers, a smaller percentage of problem drinkers and a smaller percentage of alcoholics. The reasons for this decrease in alcohol consumption are many. First, among men over the age of 60, more than one-half have reduced their drinking from a previous high level of intake with only 10% reporting a recent increase in alcohol consumption. Among women over 60, only 4% reported an increase use in alcohol in the later years. The majority of the abstainers in late life stopped drinking after the age of 45. Those individuals in early and midlife who consume alcohol heavily may not survive to the later years. Individuals over the age of 65 may therefore represent a select group of individuals who, on the average, have mild to moderate alcohol intake. In addition, individuals presently over the age of 65 may represent a cohort who have never demonstrated the heavy alcohol intake of earlier age groups.

The above findings are substantiated in another study by Rathbone-McCuan, et al.[76] in Baltimore. Among individuals 55 and over, the rate of problem drinking was 12%. The ratio of males to females was 5 to 1 among the 695 persons surveyed in community, high rise apartment, nursing home and domiciliary settings. The highest proportion of those "at risk" lived in community and domiciliary type settings and the lowest proportion lived in high rise complexes or nursing homes. Among the 55 to 69 age group (the young old) the rate of problem drinking was 22%. Among individuals 70 years and older (the old old), 4% were problem drinkers. The older problem drinker was typically single, divorced or separated, socially inactive, underemployed, Protestant, and male. All income levels were represented. The problem drinkers generally reported poorer health states and evidence of a greater number of physical problems.

They did not make frequent use of community services or individual service providers and 85% did not receive any type of service directly related to their drinking problem. They typically viewed themselves as being alienated from society.

Two studies appear to contradict the above findings. Zinsberg[77] found that in San Francisco, 2.2% of individuals 65 to 74 were alcoholics compared to 1.7% in the age range of 55 to 64. Of 722 individuals age 60 or more arrested, 82.2% were charged with drunkenness, a much higher proportion than in any other age group. Gaitz[78] found that among 100 patients 60 and over who were screened in a psychiatric ward, 36 had a primary diagnosis of alcoholism and 44 had some type of alcoholism. The discrepancy is more apparent than real, however. Though the rate of drinking probably decreases in the later years, the risk of the problem drinker being incarcerated and/or admitted to a psychiatric ward may in fact increase. The likelihood of individuals with problem drinking developing an acute or chronic brain syndrome may increase in late life, thus further placing these individuals at risk for incarceration or psychiatric hospitalization.

Individuals who develop problem drinking in late life generally fall into two categories.[79] The first are the delayed problem drinkers. These are individuals who consume alcohol heavily prior to the age of 50 but only become problem drinkers between the age of 50 and 60 (a decade later than usual). The second are the decompensated social drinkers. These are individuals who were moderate drinkers over many years and who developed excessive drinking in the sixties. Problem drinking in late life may in part be due to a decrease in energy level, restriction in social activities or reflection of mental and/or physical impairment.[80]

The treatment of the severely intoxicated or problem drinker should first begin within an institutional setting. The initial step of treatment is directed toward withdrawal of alcohol and restoration of fluid and electrolyte balance. Chlordiazepoxide is the drug of choice for withdrawal because of its relatively long half-life and cross-tolerance with alcohol. Between 50 and 200 mg. of the drug every 6 to 12 hours for sedation until delirium has cleared, and then a gradual reduction (usually 20% per day) to effect withdrawal has usually been found effective. If delirium tremens with seizures develop, diazapam may be a more active anticonvulsant because of its more rapid onset. The general guidelines of drug usage in the elderly (lower dosage over a longer period of time) continue to apply in treatment of the alcoholic. It is most important to restore fluid and electrolyte balance. Yet clinicians must avoid overhydration. It has been found that chronic alcoholics often suffer from a deficiency in magnesium and the addition of magnesium parentally is therefore an important adjunct to therapy.[81] Multivitamin therapy, especially with the B complex vitamins, is also very important. Once the individual has been successfully withdrawn from alcohol, a contract with the patient and family members is essential for future treatment. Psychotherapy may be indicated if alcoholism is secondary to a recognized emotional conflict which the patient is willing to explore. Family therapy is the intervention of choice when family dynamics appear to play the major role in the development of alcoholism.[82] The patient-therapist contract may include the use of disulfurim. However, some clinicians feel that the use of disulfurim in the elderly is contraindicated. In summary, once the acute effects of alcohol have been alleviated and the drug has been physiologically withdrawn, further treatment is contingent upon the active cooperation of patient and family members if it is to be successful.

The elderly also are subject to the abuse of prescribed psychotropic agents (and over-the-counter preparations). The minor tranquilizers, especially the benzodiazepines, and the sedative hypnotic agents, especially, the barbiturates, are the most frequently abused. Medications, such as methylphenidate, are also abused. 98.7% of the elderly who use psychotropic drugs obtain

them through physicians' prescriptions. One study in Ohio showed that 35% to 40% of all prescriptions for elderly consumers under Medicaid were tranquilizers and sedatives.[83] An NIDA study[50] revealed that 50% of those using psychotropic drugs indicate they could not perform their daily activities without these agents (indicating psychological dependency). 39% of those taking psychotropic drugs indicate they took several kinds of drugs both prescription and over-the-counter. Therefore the potential for drug drug interaction among the elderly is high. Sedatives and tranquilizers were used by 14% of the population studied (cardiovascular drugs being used by 39%). 1% were using antidepressants. An additional HEW study[84] revealed that the average number of drugs prescribed in skilled nursing facilities was 6.1%. 10% of all prescriptions were for tranquilizers and 47% of the patients in such facilities were receiving tranquilizers. 35% received sedative hypnotic agents and 8.5% received antidepressants. 25% were taking more than one tranquilizer and 6% were taking more than one sedative. The high rate of use of tranquilizers and sedative hypnotic agents in long-term care facilities is particularly alarming and points to the need of the physician to be aware of the potential for drug abuse in this population.

Treatment of the abuse of the minor tranquilizers and sedative hypnotic agents involves the gradual withdrawal of these agents over a period of time. The barbiturate containing sedative hypnotics cannot be withdrawn at a rate greater than 10% per day. The benzodiazepines (especially diazapam and chlordiazepoxide) may be withdrawn at a faster rate. Withdrawal over a 1- to 2-week period is generally optimal for both of these agents and should take place in the hospital or long-term care facility. The need for withdrawal and the plan of withdrawal should be explained clearly to the older patient and the cooperation of the patient should be obtained, if possible. Again, the real test is the period of time following withdrawal. Cooperation of patient and family along with primary care physicians interacting with the patient is essential. These patients are particularly at risk for "doctor hopping" and may be receiving prescriptions for tranquilizers and sedative hypnotics from a number of different sources. One physician should coordinate the use of all psychotropic medications in the older patient, thus avoiding the potential for multiple drug use and abuse. As a rule of thumb, any patient suffering from chronic insomnia, persistent anxiety or chronic organic mental disease should be withdrawn from all medications possible as a first step in therapy. Clinicians who have taken this step in the management of the elderly are often surprised at the prevalence of the abuse of tranquilizers and sedative hypnotics plus the dramatic improvement of these patients upon withdrawal.

REFERENCES

1. *Diagnostic and Statistical Manual-III.* Draft of April 15, 1977, American Psychiatric Association, 1977.
2. *Diagnostic and Statistical Manual of Mental Disorders* (Second Edition). Washington, D.C.: American Psychiatric Association, 1968.
3. Weiner, H. *Psychobiology and Human Disease.* New York: Elsevier, 1977.
4. Raffway, H. P., Muzio, J. N. and Dement, W. C. Ontogenic development of the human sleep-dream cycle. *Science,* **152:** 604 (1966).
5. Feinberg, I., Koreska, R. L. and Heller, N. EEG sleep patterns as a function of normal and pathological aging in man. *J. Psychiatric Res.,* **5 (2):** 107, June (1967).
6. Pfeiffer, E. and Busse, E. W. Affective disorders; paranoid, neurotic, and situational reactions, In E. W. Busse and E. Pfeiffer (eds.) *Mental Illness in Later Life.* Washington, D.C.: American Psychiatric Association, 1973.
7. Pfeiffer, E. Psychopathology and social behavior, In J. E. Gruen and K. W. Schaie (eds.) *Handbook of the Psychology of Aging.* New York: Van Nostrand and Reinhold, 1977.
8. Ginsberg, R. Sleep and sleep disturbances in geriatric psychiatry. *J. American Geriatric Soc.,* **3:** 493 (1955).
9. Prinz, P. N., Marsh, G. R., Thompson, L. W. Normal human aging: relationship of sleep variables to longitudinal changes in intellectual function. *Gerontologist,* **14:** 41 (1974).
10. Feinberg, I. Sleep in OBS, In A. Kales, (ed.) *Sleep: Physiology and Pathology.* Philadelphia: Lippincott, 1969.
11. Mendels, J., Hawkins, D. R. Sleep and depression: further considerations. *Arch. Gen. Psychiat.,* **19:** 445 (1968).
12. Cameron, D. E. Studies in senile nocturnal delirium. *Psychiatric Quart.,* **15:** 47 (1941).
13. Nowlin, J. B. *et al.* The associations of nocturnal angina pectoris with dreaming. *Ann. Intern. Med.,* **63:** 1040 (1965).
14. Kales, A. *et al.* All night sleep patterns in hypothyroid patients, before and after treatment. *J. Clin. Endoc.,* **27:** 1593 (1967).
15. Adams, R. D. Sleep and its abnormalities, In G. W. Thorn, R. D. Adams, E. Braunwald, *et al. Harrison's Principles of Internal Medicine.* New York: McGraw Hill, 1977.
16. Rechtschaffen, A. and Dement, W. C. Narcolepsy and hypersomnia, In A. M. Kales (ed.) *Sleep: Physiology and Pathology.* Philadelphia: Lippincott, 1969.
17. Schmidt-Kessen, W. and Kendel, K. Einfluss der Raumtem peratur alif den Nachlschlaf. *Res. Exp. Med.* (Berlin), **160:** 220 (1973).
18. Harris, P. *The Sleep Disorders.* Kalamazoo, Michigan: Upjohn Company, 1977.
19. Reeves, R. L. Comparison of triazolam, flurazepam and placebo as hypnotics in geriatric patients with insomnia. *Journal of Clinical Pharmacology.* p. 319, May—June (1977).
20. Hartmann, E. L-triptophan: a rational hypnotic with clinical potential. *American Journal of Psychiatry,* **134:** 366 (1977).
21. Flernenbaum, A. Pavornocturniss: A complication of single daily tricyclic or neuroleptic dosage. *American Journal of Psychiatry,* **133:** 570 (1976).
22. MacArthur, J. W. Diseases of the ovary, In G. W. Thorn, R. D. Adams, E. Braunwald, *et al., Harrison's Principles of Internal Medicine.* New York: McGraw-Hill, 1977.
23. Master, W. H. and Johnson, V. E. *Human Sexual Response.* Boston: Little Brown and Company, 1966.
24. Pfeiffer, E., Verwoerdt, A. and Wang, H. S. Sexual behavior in aged men and women. I. Observations on 254 community volunteers. *Arch. Gen. Psychiatry,* **19:** 753 (1968).
25. Pfeiffer, E., Verwoerdt, A. and Wang, H. S. The natural history of sexual behavior in a biologically advantaged group of aged individuals. *Journal of Gerontology,* **24:** 193 (1969).
26. Verwoerdt, A., Pfeiffer, E. and Wang, H. S. Sexual behavior in senescence. I. Changes in sexual activity and interest of aging men and women. *Journal of Geriatric Psychiatry,* **24:** 163 (1969).
27. Verwoerdt, A., Pfeiffer, E. and Wang, H. S. Sexual behavior in senescence. II. Patterns of sexual activity and interest. *Geriatrics,* **24:** 137 (1969).
28. Nieschlag, E., Kley, H. K., Wiegelmann, W.,

Solback, H. G., and Krüshemper, H. L. Lebensalter und endokrine function der testes des erwachsenan mannes. *Deut. Med. Wochscher,* **98:** 1281 (1973).

29. Masters, W. H. and Johnson, V. E. *Human Sexual Inadequacy.* New York: Little Brown, 1970.

30. Anderson, W. F. *Practical Management of the Elderly.* London: Blackwell, 1976.

31. Kinsey, A. C., Pomeroy, W. B. and Martin, C. E. *Sexual Behavior in the Human Male.* Philadelphia: W. B. Saunders, 1948.

32. Goy, R. W. and Jakway, J. S. Role of inheritance in determination of sexual behavior patterns, In E. L. Bliss, (ed.) *Roots of Behavior.* New York: Harper, 1962.

33. Woods, J. S. Drug effects on human sexual behavior, In N. F. Woods, (ed.) *Human Sexuality in Health and Illness.* St. Louis: Mosby, 1975.

34. Green, L. F., Kelalis, P. P. and Weeks, R. E. Retrograde ejaculation of semen due to diabetic neuropathy. *Fertility and Sterility,* **14:** 617 (1963).

35. Rubin, I. Climax without ejaculation. *Sexology,* **30:** 694 (1964).

36. Bors, E., Coman, A. E. and Haycock, C. Effects of rectal surgery. *Sexology,* **27:** 478 (1961).

37. Heller, C. T. and Maddock, W. O. The clinical use of testosterone in the male. *Vitamins and Hormones,* **5:** 393 (1947).

38. Kelly, J. The aging male homosexual. *Gerontologist,* **17:** 329 (1977).

39. Clark, W. C. and Mehl, L. Thermal pain: A sensory decision theory analysis of the effect of age and sex on d; various response criteria and 50 percent pain threshold. *J. Abnormal Psychol.,* **78:** 202 (1971).

40. Lasagna, L. Influence of age on analgesic pain relief. *J. American Medical Association,* **218:** 1831 (1971).

41. Fordyce, W. E., Fowler, R. S. and Lehmann, J. F. Some implications of learning in problems of chronic pain. *J. Chron. Dis.,* **21:** 179 (1968).

42. Ziegler, D. K., Hassanein, R. S. and Couch, J. R. Characteristics of life headache histories in a nonclinic population. *Neurology,* **27:** 265 (1977).

43. Hauser, W. A., Ferguson, R. H. and Holley, K. E., *et al.* Temporal arterites in Rochester, Minnesota, 1951 to 1967. *Mayo Clin. Proc.,* **46:** 597 (1971).

44. Medina, J. L., Diamond, S. and Rubino, F. A. Headaches in patients with transient ischemic attacks. *Headache,* **15:** 182 (1975).

45. Busse, E. W., Barnes, R. H. and Dovenmuehle, R. H. The incidence and origin of hypochondriacal patterns and psychophysiological reaction in elderly persons. *First Pan American Congress on Gerontology,* Mexico City, September 1956.

46. Strain, J. J. and Grossman, S. *Psychological Care for the Medically Ill.* New York: Appleton Century Crofts, 1975.

47. Verwoerdt, A. *Clinical Geropsychiatry.* Baltimore: Williams and Wilkins, pp. 107–118, 1976.

48. Alarcon, R. Hypochondriasis and depression in the aged. *Geront. Clin.,* **6:** 266 (1964).

49. Blazer, D. G. and Houpt, J. Perception of poor health in the healthy elderly. *J. of the American Geriatrics Society* (in press).

50. NIDA Services Research Report: A Study of Legal Drug Use by Older Americans. USDHEW, Publications #77–495, 1977.

51. Maddox, G. L. and Douglas, E. D. Self-assessment of health: A longitudinal study of elderly subjects. *Journal of Health and Social Behavior,* **14:** 87 (1973).

52. Busse, E. W. The treatment of hypochondriasis. *Tri-State Medical Journal,* **2:** 7 (1954).

53. Sklar, M. Functional bowel distress and constipation in the aged. *Geriatrics,* **27:** 79 (1972).

54. Brockelhurst, J. C. *Textbook of Geriatric Medicine and Gerontology.* New York: Churchill Livingston, 1973.

55. Gebves, K. and Bossaert, H. Gastrointestinal disorders in old age. *Ageing,* **6:** 197 (1977).

56. Welton, D. G. and Greenberg, B. G. Trends in office practice of dermatology, part III. *Arch. Derm.,* **90:** 296 (1964).

57. Tindall, J. P. Geriatric dermatology, In W. Reichel (ed.) *Clinical Aspects of Aging.* Baltimore: Williams and Wilkins, 1978.

58. Brockelhurst, J. C. Personal correspondence.

59. Issacs, B. and Walkey, F. A. A survey of incontinence in the elderly. *Geront. Clin.,* **6:** 37 (1964).

60. Brockelhurst, J. C. Recent advances in incontinence, In W. F. Anderson and T. G. Judge, (eds.) *Geriatric Medicine.* New York: Academic Press, 1974.

61. Alexander, F. *Psychosomatic Medicine.* New York: Norton, 1950.

62. Harris. R. E., Soholow, M., Carpenter, L. G., Freedman, M. and Hunt, S. P. Response to psychologic stress in persons who are potentially hypertensive. *Circulation,* **7:** 874 (1953).

63. Moses, L., Daniels, G. E. and Nickerson, J. L. Psychogenic factors in essential hypertension: Methodology and preliminary report. *Psychosomatic Medicine,* **18:** 471 (1956).

64. Donnison, C. P. *Civilization and Disease.* Baltimore: William Wood and Company, 1938.

65. Cruz-Coke, R. Environmental influences and arterial blood pressure. *Lancet,* **2:** 885 (1960).

66. Henry, J. P. and Cassel, J. C. Psychosocial factors in essential hypertension. Recent epidemiologic and animal experimental evidence. *American J. Epidemiol.,* **90:** 171 (1969).

67. Leigh, D., Rawnsky, K. Bronchial asthma of late onset. *Int. Arch. Allergy Appl. Immunol.,* **9:6,** 305 (1956).

68. Lee, H. Y. and Stretton, T. B. Asthma in the elderly. *Brit. Med. J.,* **2:** 93 (1972).

69. Moos, R. H. Personality factors associated with rheumatoid arthritis: A review. *J. Chronic Dis.,* **17:** 41 (1964).

70. Grob, D. Prevalent joint diseases in older persons, In W. Reichel, (ed.) *Clinical Aspects of Aging.* Baltimore: Williams and Wilkins, 1978.

71. Brewerton, D. A. Rheumatic disorders, In I. Rossman, (ed.) *Clinical Geriatrics.* Philadelphia: Lippincott, 1971.

72. Walford, R. L. *The Immunologic Theory of Aging.* Copenhagen, Munksgaard, 1969.

73. Davis, P. J., and Davis, F. B. Hyperthyroidism in patients over the age of 60. *Medicine,* **53:** 161 (1974).

74. Chien, C., Stolsky, B. A. and Cole, J. O. Psychiatric treatment for nursing home patients: drug, alcohol, milieu. *Am. J. Psychiat.,* **130:** 543 (1973).

75. Schmidt, W. and Lint, J. Causes of death of alcoholics. *Quart. J. Struct. Alc.,* **33:** 171 (1972).

76. Rathbone-McCuan, E., *et al. Community Survey of Aged Alcoholics and Problem Drinkers.* Baltimore: Levindale Geriatrics Research Center, 1976.

77. Zinberg, S. Studies showing seriousness of alcoholism in the elderly. *Addiction Research Foundation Journal,* February, 1974.

78. Gaitz, C. M., Baer, P. E. Characteristics of elderly patients patients with alcoholism. *Arch. Gen. Psychiatry,* **23:** 372 (1971).

79. Hyde, R. W. Alcohol and geriatrics. Read at G.W.A.N. Conference. Sugarbash, October, 1971.

80. Mayfield, D. Alcohol problems in the aging, In Fann and Maddox, *Drug Issues in Geropsychiatry.*

81. Beard, J. D., Knott, D. H. Fluid and electrolyte balance during acute withdrawal in chronic alcoholic patients. *JAMA,* **204:** 133 (1968).

82. Beresen, D. Alcohol and the family system, In P. J. Guerin, (ed.) *Family Therapy.* New York: Gardner Press, 1976.

83. United States Senate Special Committee on Aging, 1971.

84. *Physician's Drug Prescribing Patterns in Skilled Nursing Facilities.* Long Term Care Facility Improvement Campaign Monograph No. 2, USDHEW, Publication No. (OS) 76-50050, 1976.

Chapter 19
Grief, Death, and Dying

James Spikes, M.D.

Montefiore Hospital and Medical Center

INTRODUCTION

Although the issues of personal death and object loss are extremely important psychological matters from the age of five or six onward,[1] they become areas of more immediate and conscious concern in the elderly. The presence of physical illness, reduction in cognitive capacity, and the deaths of peers are only a few of the factors that serve to remind the older person of the finiteness of the existence of himself and his loved ones. It is not known how profoundly the fact of death influences the adaptation to late life, but psychological studies have documented the supposition that thoughts of death are both more frequent and more easily tolerated in the elderly.[2]

This is not to imply, however, that the elderly differ in any significant way from younger people in the manner in which they react to and deal with the ending of life. In fact, the immediacy of this concern in the elderly may serve to highlight the psychological mechanisms that are employed to adapt to the fact of death.

Clinical studies and observations suggest that the ability to tolerate emotional and conscious awareness of mortality of the self and the object is dependent on two rather broadly conceived capacities: (1) the capacity to develop a fantasy or belief of immortality, and (2) the capacity to mourn. The term fantasy is not used as whimsical imagination but as a psychic mechanism by which harsh reality is changed into an imaginary experience that satisfies a specific human need.[3] That these capacities, fantasy and mourning, are quite closely related will become apparent below. There is no evidence to suggest that these characteristics are any less important in the elderly than in the younger population.

The most obvious examples of this fantasy are seen in the widely held religious beliefs of both Eastern and Western cultures—specifically, the ideas of reincarnation and of life after death. This fantasy is less obvious in persons who are more intellectually inclined, and the specific religious character of the fantasy has lost much of its impact on Western culture due to the decline of the influence of religion on everyday life. Nevertheless, the conviction of some sort of immortality persists and can be seen in such ideas as living on through children or though creations or possessions that are left behind.

In stressing the importance of this fantasy, Eissler[4] goes so far as to suggest that the psychiatrist who is working with the dying patient must maintain a paradoxical attitude: "on the one hand he must fully recognize the magnitude and gravity of the situation . . . and on the other he must [imply] a belief in the patient's indestructibility." He adds that the necessity for such an archaic, animistic belief indicates a lack of integration of the idea that "death is the matrix of life and that in dying [one] fulfills life's primary law." Other writers[5,6] are inclined to the view that his tendency is an innate characteristic of human beings and not (as Eissler seems to suggest) a generalized neurosis. Freud proposed that the necessity for the formation of the fantasy lies in the supposition that in the id the idea of nonexistence is inconceivable. These remarks apply specifically to the nonexistence of the self. With regard to object loss, it is tempting to speculate that a similar phenomenon occurs in identification. By means of this mechanism the loss is managed by preserving the dead person within the self. Practical considerations must intervene at this point. Although these questions remain unanswered theoretically, clinical observations indicate over and over that the idea of death does not appear to be tolerated without the simultaneous generation of a fantasy of immortality. Stated another way, the process of mourning does not appear to be possible unless the self or the object can be viewed, in some important way, as possessing permanence.

The clinical implications of this are apparent: if the optimal psychological integration of death is to be achieved through successful mourning, then the erection of a fantasy of immortality would seem to be a crucial determinant in being able to manage this task. If the patient cannot erect such a fantasy himself, it falls upon the clinician to aid him in doing so.[7]

The psychology of death appears to be virtually synonymous with the psychology of loss. Coming to terms with death means integrating the idea of the eventual loss of the self or the object into one's conscious experience. The ability to achieve this integration is dependent upon the person's capacity to tolerate loss—that is, the capacity to mourn. Although the process of mourning has been described more than amply by a number of writers, a few brief remarks are in order here. It involves the conscious awareness of an actual or anticipated loss and the simultaneous discharge of painful affect. These affects are usually a combination of sadness and rage. The mourner almost always feels a sense of relief after such a discharge and then is able to turn his attention to other matters. One can observe this phenomenon in people who are dying and in people who have lost, or who anticipate the loss of, a loved one. When it does not occur, the person either ignores the fact of death or becomes symptomatic in one way or another. Some frequently observed symptom complexes are depression, regression with anxiety, social withdrawal, and compulsive, driven behavior that seeks to avoid the awareness of the loss. These complexes may occur along or in combination, or they may alternate with each other. They are always an attempt to maintain a defense of denial that has been severely shaken.

The progression of mourning has been amply described by a number of writers, most notably Freud[5] and Lindemann.[8] At the completion of the process the person has integrated the loss into his current state of being and is then free to pursue other tasks. Lindemann identified several stages that he thought were characteristic of this process: (1) denial, (2) depression, and (3) readjustment. One is immediately struck by the similarity between these stages and the stages of dying, as described by Kubler-Ross:[6] (1) denial, (2) anger, (3) bargaining, (4) depression, and (5) acceptance. This observation strengthens the notion that personal death and death of the object have remarkably similar psychological consequences and meanings. (It is important to note that the orderly progression of the mourning process that is suggested by this enumeration is a fiction. These stages are meant to serve only as guidelines. In actuality, patients may alternate rapidly between and among the stages. Kubler-Ross, herself, has expressed concern about some of the compulsive pigeon-holing that has resulted from her work.)

This chapter will explore and describe what is known about the older person's adaptation to death. An attempt will be made to achieve consistent clinical reliance. As detailed above, this task involves evaluating the capacities of the aged to mourn and to form fantasies of immortality. It is possible to identify several factors that are crucial in determining these capacities: (1) personality factors; (2) the general state of physical health; (3) the state of cognitive function; (4) the cause and the course of death; (5) the sociocultural climate in which the person lives; and (6) the age of the person.

PERSONALITY FACTORS

In the absence of severe cognitive dysfunction, personality factors are clearly the most important determinants of a person's approach to death. In general, older persons tend to have reached a stage in development that is characterized by a rigidification of character structure, so that one may observe some inflexibility in handling stress. If the stress is severe, one encounters more disorganization and anxiety since it is so difficult to replace failing defenses with others that are more effective. The result can be an extreme solution, such as a mutual suicide pact or the development of paranoid, depressive, or hypochondriacal ideation. (It is well known that the rate of suicide increases sharply with advancing age).[9] Although these reactions may be related to social conditions or illness and pain, they are still determined to a large extent by the intrapsychic equipment of the individual. Psychological studies have succeeded in positively relating the fear of death to the presence of character pathology (Magni, 1972).[9a] Wahl (1958)[9b] suggests that the well-loved child is more likely to retain an unconscious conviction of omnipotence which he is able to use to handle death anxiety, as he has had the confidence to face new situations in the past.

With these considerations as a background, personality characteristics can be more specifically viewed from two standpoints: (1) the meaning of death for the individual, and (2) object relations.

Personality determines the way in which death is viewed symbolically. To the narcissistic person, death and old age are seen simply as weakness. Thus, the realization of death produces strong reactions of humiliation and rage. Younger persons are viewed with envy. If denial cannot be maintained by counterphobic or other measures, serious depression, even suicide, may be the result. Suicide is often an attempt to regain the lost power by dictating the time and circumstances of death.

Case Example

A 63-year-old woman developed an inoperable cancer. She had already suspected the diagnosis and requested complete honesty from her physician. Her major personality characteristic was her pride in being able to exert power and control over both herself and others. She was given the diagnosis and after a brief period of shock became suicidally depressed. Thinly veiled reaction formations cloaked a seething rage at her physicians. When she was interviewed by the psychiatrist, it became clear that she felt devastated by the idea that her cancer had power over her. She seemed particularly preoccupied with the idea that there was *no chance* of survival. When informed by the psychiatrist that no matter how bleak the prognosis there is always a chance, she immediately began to feel better. By the next day she was determined to fight the illness and left the hospital in good spirits. She recalled that the psychiatrist had "said something that made me feel better," but could not remember what it was. She anxiously declined further interviews and "died fighting" two months later.

It is clear from this example that the patient could not tolerate the loss of strength that she associated with death. Thus, recognition of the loss would have been too painful for her and she could not grieve. Since she could not entertain the idea of death without becoming severely depressed, it was impossible for her to develop a comforting fantasy of immortality. Instead, she behaved as if she were immortal in reality. Since it is more difficult for older people to erect such defensive structures, they may be more prone to intractable depressive reactions.

Compulsive personalities generally associate death with guilt and loss of control of aggression. They view their own deaths as punishment, and death of the object as something for which they can be blamed. In the former case they will be preoccupied with ruminations about possible sins or wrongdoings committed in the past, and in the latter, by possible ways in which they could have contributed to the death of the object. The depressions they suffer are more of the superego (conscience) type, as opposed to those of the narcissistic personality, which are more likely to be of the ego ideal (failure of aspiration) variety.

Case Example

A 68-year-old diabetic woman came to consultation shortly after the death of her husband, because she had been unable to control her blood sugar properly. The interview revealed that she had been careless with her insulin because she was preoccupied with thoughts that she had contributed in some way to her husband's death. She described classical vegetative signs of depression. From the history it was clear that the husband had been both

domineering and unkind in his treatment of her. Her reaction to this had been to submit to his demands and to comfort herself with meticulous housework. When asked if she ever thought of pleasurable experiences she had had with him, she replied that whenever such thoughts came to her she would become anxious and immediately dismiss them.

This patient could not mourn the death of her husband, because to allow full emotional awareness of it would have touched her ambivalence (death wishes) too closely. Instead, she behaved as if he were still alive and tortured herself as he had.

If compulsive preoccupations are unable to control the awareness of aggression, the patient can develop projective defenses that may lead to paranoid reactions. Clinical experience suggests that the inflexibility in the character structures of older persons makes them more prone to these solutions, and one often finds them looking for ways to blame others.

An 84-year-old man who was dying of intractable heart failure refused to see his physician, stating that the doctor was there only to get his money.

Hysterical personalities often view death as a kind of ugliness that robs them of the opportunity to enjoy the admiration and concern of others. They are more likely to feel cheated by death. The death of the object frequently stimulates the search for a new object, and depression may result if the search is unrewarded.

Dependent and infantile personalities tend to ignore death altogether and, instead, anxiously attempt to attach themselves regressively to some powerful object. This is more likely to happen in old age, as the limitation of power makes the dependency even more acceptable to the patient.

Depressive and masochistic personalities are quite different in their approach to death in the sense that they often appear to welcome it. For masochists, the process of dying may become an almost idyllic experience as they glow with the admiration that others express for their ability to tolerate suffering. Chronic depressives sometimes see death as a welcome relief from their suffering. Weisman[10] reported a striking example of a woman who actually felt better when informed of a fatal prognosis.

It should be emphasized that most of these reactions to death are common, even in people whose characters are not formed along the lines that have been described. Only in persons who exaggerate these reactions can any conclusion about this basic personality be drawn.

OBJECT RELATIONS

Although this category clearly overlaps with the one above, it is necessary to point out that the particular quality of a person's relations with others strongly influences the way he handles death. This is true regardless of the way that he had fared in other aspects of his life. Jeffers and Verwoerdt[9] state that "One of the most satisfying adaptations to ending of life is a close [and] nonambivalent relationship with children and grandchildren. This satisfies not only the mutual affectional needs but bestowed on the older person the reminder of continuity of life and tangible evidence of his ongoing contribution to mankind." Thus a relationship with children and grandchildren makes it easier for the person to partially satisfy a need for immortality. Further, the process of mourning is greater facilitated by the presence of interested listeners.[11,12]

GENERAL STATE OF PHYSICAL HEALTH

It might be supposed that the presence of chronic illness could be an important determinant in the person's capacity to deal with the idea of death. On the one hand, the presence of illness could heighten the fear of and awareness of death. On the other, it could limit the ability to handle death itself, because the pain or other discomfort caused by the illness would take up the patient's coping energies. He would therefore be too concerned about life to contemplate death; or, if the discomfort were quite severe, he might even wish for death as a relief. Jeffers and Verwoerdt[9] conclude that "from the expressions of older persons it appears that death is feared much less than prolonged illness, dependency or pain . . ." Further, Feifel and Jones[13] found that the chronically ill did not show any more concern about death than did the healthy or the mentally ill, while the terminally ill revealed much more anxiety and depression over futurity than did the other three groups. Clearly, this issue is much more complicated than it would appear, and it is therefore difficult to make any meaningful statement that would have general validity. Nevertheless, the author's clinical impression is that chronic illness and disability increase one's concern about death and decrease the capacity to handle this concern in an effective way.

STATE OF COGNITIVE FUNCTION

It is clear from the foregoing chapters that late life is often accompanied by significant alterations on cognitive functioning. The usual effect of these changes, particularly in the early stages, is a reduction in the patient's capacity to cope with any stress. As a result, mature defenses may be replaced by more archaic ones such as projection and denial. The patient is no longer as able to process information, both from without and from within, so that distortions occur as anxiety is mobilized. Concern about personal death or about object loss may then be transformed into terrifying ideas or delusions.

Case Example

An 84-year-old woman was admitted for treatment of advanced carcinoma of the breast. On the second hospital day she was found mumbling to herself and seemed irritated. When asked what the trouble was, she replied that her physicians had injected her with dangerous drugs that were creating bumps on her skin (these lesions were metastatic nodules). Examination revealed a mild dementia. Except for her delusions about her physicians and her illness, the patient's reality testing was intact.

As dementia becomes more severe, there is a reduction in the patient's ability to think, to develop fantasies, and to have meaningful relationships. At this point, ideas about death and object loss begin to pale into insignificance as they are replaced by more simple concerns, such as physical comforts.

THE CAUSE AND THE COURSE OF DEATH

The vagueness that attended the category of the general state of physical health is not apparent here. There is no question that the particular illness that causes death will have a profound influence on how death is perceived and handled. This influence is exerted from two sources: (1) the effect of the illness on the central nervous system and on the general state of well-being; and (2) the psychological meaning of the illness itself.

It has been pointed out that the compromise of cognitive function that is so common in old age can have a pronounced effect on the patient's view of his situation. Any illness can aggravate this dysfunction by either a direct or an indirect impact on the central nervous system. The timing, course, and degree of the effects are dependent on two variables: (1) the severity of the insult; and (2) the rapidity with which it occurs.[14]

Thus, a slow rise in blood urea nitrogen due to arteriosclerosis may not exert such a profound influence until the patient is near death, because the central nervous system will have had time to adjust. In general, the older the patient is, the more rapid and profound the disturbance will be. That this factor has not been given sufficient consideration is attested to by the work of Massie,

Glass and Holland.[15] They showed that 15 of 20 patients on an oncology ward, who appeared to be in a state of quiet acceptance (as defined by Kübler-Ross),[6] were actually suffering from organic brain syndromes of varying severity.

The general state of well-being may be so severely affected by an illness that errors can be made in psychological evaluation. This is particularly true in cases where the medical staff judges the patient to be suffering from a depresseive response to a potentially fatal illness. Closer examination reveals that the patient's apparent mood alteration is due to the debilitation of the illness itself.

Although is it usually less profound, the psychological meaning of an illness to the persons afflicted or to the object can strongly influence their reactions. First, the psychological effect may proceed through identification with a loved one who had a similar illness.

Case Example

A 68-year-old woman developed a carcinoma of the sigmoid: It was considered operable by her internist and surgeon and she was told she had an 80% chance for a cure. She refused the surgery at first, stating that it would be useless because she was doomed. When questioned further, she related that she had watched her older brother die of cancer of the larynx. He had had several operations and after each of them he had seemed worse.

Since the character structures and coping styles of older people are more rigid, such identificatory tendencies may not yield easily to reality testing. The patient described above was able to have the surgery only after she was made to feel that she was doing it only for her friends and relatives.

The impact of the specific meaning of the illness is nowhere more apparent than it is with cancer. The mere mention of this word strikes terror into the hearts of most hospitalized patients. In an unreported consecutive sampling of 20 hospitalized patients, the author and a medical colleague found that 15 were afraid that they had cancer (none of them did). Clinical impressions indicate that the fantasies evoked by this illness all have to do with violence and sadism. This is clearly shown in the title of the book *Stay of Execution* by Stewart Alsop, who had leukemia. Thus, patients and their families usually have the conscious or unconscious idea that the patient is forced to submit passively to a merciless killer. This idea is very likely to tap ambivalence, particularly in the object.

Case Example

A 70-year-old woman was visiting her 75-year-old husband, who was hospitalized for treatment of prostatic carcinoma. Upon observing that his physician was relaxing in the conference room, she bitterly attacked him for relaxing his vigil. Interview revealed that she had been tortured by thoughts that her husband's cancer could have been cured if she had gotten him to the doctor sooner. Since the plot of this drama revolves around contributing to a fatal illness, the question must arise as to who is the culprit.

The course of the illness has yet another kind of significance. Obviously, a rapid course does not allow time for mourning and reflection, while a slower course may involve more pain and suffering. Kalish and Reynolds[2] showed that most people preferred a sudden and unexpected death, although the elderly considered sudden death and slow death as equally tragic. In a more detailed exploration, Holland[16] charted several possible courses for the patient following the diagnosis of a malignancy: (1) treatment leading to a cure; (2) no treatment, leading to progressive illness and death; and (3) treatment leading to one or more remissions followed finally by progressive illness and death. She showed how the psychological task for the patient may be

quite different with each of these courses. For courses (1) and (2), the task is more direct and simple. The patient who has remissions, however, may have to go through several episodes of preparation. The uncertainty of the outcome may then become the crucial variable, thereby heightening anxiety and further stressing the coping capacities of the patient and his family.

SOCIOCULTURAL ENVIRONMENT

The views that a society holds toward death obviously have a significant effect on the dying patient. With the decline in the power of religion, Western culture has sought a strange kind of immortality through the development of medical technology. Patients, families, and physicians all view the physician as possessing a power over the forces of disease that is reminiscent of the religious man's expectations of God.[17] The evidence for this is the depression the physician feels when he cannot cure his patient, and the rage the patient feels when he cannot be cured. Often patients and physicians avoid recognition of the doctor's helplessness by simply agreeing to ignore it. Families frequently play a similar game, and the result of it all is abandonment of the patient. Eissler,[4] Kübler-Ross,[6] and Norton[12] speak eloquently of the consequences of this abandonment. Norton specifically shows how the availability of objects prevents the severe regressions that are seen so commonly in the dying. Kübler-Ross expresses the view that depressions occur in the dying because they have no one with whom to share the experience. It appears that this abandonment is caused by the dying person's reminding the object of his own mortality. In a society that is geared up for fighting illness and death, the dying person is often not welcome. Since the patient, himself, often holds similar views, he fears that he will not be tolerated. He cannot express his rage at this abandonment for fear that the situation will only worsen. He then turns the rage against himself and a depression ensues. Too frequently this depression is viewed by family and medical staff as a simple reaction to the illness. (In narcissistic personalities, as shown above, this may, indeed, be the case.)

Case Example

A psychiatry resident was asked to see a 68-year-old man, who was dying of lung cancer, because he had mentioned thoughts of suicide. In his interview the resident was struck by the man's despair and hopelessness and wondered if he shouldn't be allowed to kill himself. The supervisor encouraged the resident to take a closer look, with the result that the patient revealed that he wanted to go home to die but was concerned that his wife would be too burdened with his care. He was afraid to ask her, anticipating becoming devastated at her refusal.

This constellation of dynamics is compounded for the elderly person because in old age there is a diminished social value of life, i.e., the elderly person places less value on his own life, while others in his environment tend to share his evaluation, (Glaser, 1966).[17a] Kalish[18] comments, "At the same time our future-oriented value system emphasizes the need to expend its energies on the producers of tomorrow rather than on those of yesterday. As is sometimes said of the elderly, their future is behind them."

Clearly, under these circumstances the opportunity to mourn and to develop fantasies of immortality may be severely hindered. The isolation of the elderly can lessen the availability of objects to share and promote these processes.

Closely knit, religious communities appear to deal with the problem much more effectively. Support systems are available and the religion provides a fantasy of immortality that is shared by everyone. The studies of Feifel and Branscomb,[19] Kalish and Reynolds,[2] and Swenson,[20] to name only a few, amply confirm this view. This offers a challenge to the nonreligious sectors of society to develop a similarly effective support system.

A similar phenomenon may be observed with the elderly who are bereaved. In a recent essay, Engel[21] provocatively expounds on the proposition that grief could be considered a disease. He raises this question in the context of developing a "biopsychosocial" model of illness to replace the reductionist concepts of a "biomedicine" which would confine itself to biochemical observations and neglect the social implications of illness. One of his major points is that grief is a discrete syndrome that usually mobilizes forces within the society that provide for the mourner. It is clear from what has been said above that the isolated elderly, who are usually in such dire need of these forces, are the ones to whom they are often denied. The result can be that grief, instead of running its course discretely, will become a chronic depression that is superimposed on another "illness," old age. Perhaps the responsibility for developing a viable support system for the elderly has come to lie with a modern medicine that is designed along biopsychosocial lines. Katz and Gardner[22] clearly lean in this direction through their suggestion to medical caregivers that one of the important aspects of the autopsy consent interview can be the doctor's aiding the bereaved to begin the mourning process.

AGE

There is data that suggests that the older a person is the less fearful he is of dying. Kalish and Reynolds[2] and Feifel and Branscomb[19] showed that the elderly both think and talk more about death and are less fearful of it than younger persons. Kalish suggests that several factors may be responsible for this. First, the diminished social value of life makes life easier to contemplate giving up. (This may be a depressive response, as outlined above.) Second, once a person has lived to his life expectancy or more, he may feel that he has received his entitlement. And third, as people become older they are socialized to their own death and the deaths of spouses and peers. The rehearsal for widowhood begins at a fairly early age (Kalish, 1971)[22a] and runs concurrently with thoughts about one's own death. By the time the elderly person faces his own death (or that of his spouse), he has dealt with death often enough to be socialized to it.[18]

On the other hand, as a person grows older, social isolation occurs and illness intervenes, so that the person may become closer to, and more dependent on, the spouse. Such a strong libidinal tie may develop, along with the inability to find new objects, that the old person becomes even more threatened by the idea of object loss. It is well known that conversations between elderly spouses concerning "who will go first" are frequent. A pathological result of such conversations is the mutual suicide pact. The author has observed several elderly patients who, even after as long as 15 years, had not fully mourned the loss of a husband or wife. A typical tearful statement was, "How do you ever get over the death of a person you spent over 50 years with?"

That this question remains problematic is attested to by the work of Cartwright, *et al.*,[23] who showed that the proportion of the bereaved who visited doctors and required medicine for mental symptoms decreased with age. Further, although psychosomatic studies[24,25] have shown a significant increase in morbidity and mortality among the bereaved, Wiener, *et al.*,[26] in studying an older population, showed no difference in mortality between the grieving population and matched controls, although there was a significant increase in morbidity, as shown by more frequent visits to physicians. These findings are more in support of the hypothesis that the elderly handle death better, both mentally and physically.

A clinical example in more detail and depth will serve to illustrate the complex manner in which these variables may interact to produce a dysfunctional result.

Case Example

A psychiatry resident was called to see a hospitalized 75-year-old woman because she appeared withdrawn and depressed. She had been admitted to the hospital from a nursing home 2 weeks before in a comatose state and was found to have lobar pneumonia. She had responded well to treatment and was quite alert, but the house staff and nurses found her withdrawn and somewhat uncommunicative, and assumed that she was depressed.

In the interview she presented as anxious and angry rather than depressed. All of her responses to questions were given in a clipped, irritated tone of voice. She fidgeted nervously, and often glanced around the room. She stated that she did not know what was going on. She had been feeling somewhat ill in the nursing home, went to bed one night, and woke up in the hospital. She was told she had pneumonia. (Her affect indicated that she wasn't sure that this was the truth.) She had been "manhandled" the previous day by a "gorilla-doctor," and she often woke up at night and thought that she had been moved to another part of the hospital. She wanted to get out of the hospital as soon as possible in order to care for her husband, who was a resident of the same nursing home. Her husband was sick with periarteritis nodosa, was partially blind, and had trouble walking. They had "given up everything" two years ago to move to the nursing home because of his illness. (She indicated some sadness at this point and her voice also betrayed possible irritation at her husband). When asked how sick she felt she had been, she became quite nervous, and irritably stated, "Not as sick as they (the doctors) seem to think I was!" How sick did they think? "Pretty sick, but I'm feeling good now and want to get out of here." When asked further about the curious experiences at night, she stated that she knew she wasn't being moved but it seemed that way. She added that she observed movements in the room and had the feeling that someone was coming to get her. Further questioning revealed that she had always been a somewhat "crabby" and irritable person and that this had increased over the past few years because of discomfort from arthritis. She and her husband were alone in the world and needed each other. She couldn't wait to return to him.

A cognitive examination revealed a mild organic mental syndrome (patient could remember one or two out of three objects after three minutes) that appeared to be chronic, since she reported having had some difficulty with her memory for the past two years.

The resident and supervisor tentatively formulated the case as follows. The severe and sudden illness (*course of this illness*) that she had suffered had awakened fears in the patient of death and object loss. The sudden transfer to the hospital had exacerbated these fears, as had the previously existing *social situation* in which she and her husband felt isolated, with only each other on whom to depend. The *mild organicity* and the *personality trait* of irritability (exacerbated by *chronic illness*) had clearly affected her capacity to cope with a new *social situation,* the hospital. The organicity had made it more difficult for her to process new information in a meaningful way, and the irritability (of which she was aware) further threatened her relationships with hospital staff. Her intrapsychic solution for all this was mainly to externalize the problem. It was not that she had been seriously ill but that misinformed physicians had attempted to force their views on her. Thus, she now had two reasons to fear the doctors: (1) they signified death, illness, and separation from her husband; and (2) they could retaliate against her because of her anger. The result was anxiety and withdrawal, accompanied by fearful fantasies (and perhaps hallucinations) of being harmed by the "gorilla-doctor."

The supervisor thought that the most therapeutic approach to the patient would be to help her to explore her anger. He noted that the resident had not pointed out to the patient that she seemed angry with him. If she could see that someone could tolerate her rage and frustration without retaliating, then she might be able to relieve her sense of isolation and deal with her experience more adaptively.

The resident returned to see the patient the following day. She appeared even more reluctant and irritable. When he gently confronted her with her anger, she at first denied it and then admitted that she had felt insulted by the recommendation of psychiatric intervention. She had been afraid to reveal this because her doctors "might not like it." Her nervousness decreased noticeably at this point, and she revealed that she was afraid that if she stayed any longer in the hospital she might get sick again and that she would lose her bed in the nursing home. The resident reassured her that she would not get sick and offered to speak to the social worker to insure that she would not lose her nursing home bed. He recommended trifluperazine 2 mg. P.O. hs to relieve her frightening nocturnal symptoms. Her remaining three days in the hospital was uneventful.

It is important to re-emphasize how this patient's defenses had continued to isolate her and to prevent her from obtaining the help that she needed. The resident's successful intervention began at the intrapsychic and interpersonal level but also extended to the involvement of the social milieu and to the use of a pharmacologic agent to counteract the effects of the organicity.

PSYCHOTHERAPY

An exhaustive treatment of this subject is beyond the scope of this chapter. The remarks offered here will be confined to some of the more salient features encountered in psychotherapy.

The major therapeutic task with the dying and the bereaved is to help the patient to mourn and to develop some sense of immortality.[4]

(The difficulties of this task with the elderly have been outlined above.) However, it is important that the therapist (or consultant) be acutely aware of the unique capacities of the patient to engage in the mourning process. For example, the first patient who was reported above was clearly unable to mourn and needed to act out a conviction of immortality.

Jeffers and Verwoerdt[9] caution against encouraging the life review in certain patients. They point out that "there are those tragic instances when the review and the stock-taking lead to the discovery that one 'missed the boat' and that it is now too late to repair previous mistakes." Becker[7] similarly suggests that new insights may be seen as having arrived too late. He adds that the dying patient may not have the time to explore and handle resistances and defenses. On the other hand, Jung[27] reports on a fascinating case of an older woman who was totally unable to gain insight into herself until she knew that she had a serious illness and that the end was near. In this case the patient was motivated to "take stock" before it was too late. Although the cautionary comments described above must be taken seriously, it is clear that generalizations are insufficient, and that the therapist must carefully evaluate the specific characteristics of each patient.

The profound effect of available objects on the mourning process has been emphasized above. Kübler-Ross[6] and Eissler[4] have espoused some interesting views on this subject. They appear to contend that the modern psychotherapist may come to occupy a more pivotal position with the dying patient than might be expected. This is because family members and friends may be too overcome with despair and grief to offer the pity and understanding that the dying person needs. (This statement may apply just as well to the person who is grieving.) Although this idea appears to have some validity, a word of caution is in order. The author has observed a number of older couples mourning together quite effectively when one of the couple was afflicted with a fatal illness. Perhaps the major task of the psychotherapist will be to facilitate the process of mutual mourning when it has gone awry. Of course, when psychopathology is the major determinant of the difficulty, individual work with a therapist is indicated.

CONCLUSION

This chapter has attempted to elucidate some of the psychological aspects of the phenomena of death and grief in the elderly. Although much of what has been said appears valid from a clinical point of view, it must be apparent that some of the more theoretical questions remain unanswered. It may be that the answers to these theoretical questions will have profound clinical relevance. Of particular note is the question of whether or not a transcendent (death and immortality) attitude toward death is a necessary accompaniment to the human condition. This question is closely related to another question which is even more intriguing. What is the place of denial in the reaction to death? Is the transcendent attitude merely an altered, albeit less intense, form of denial, by which the person allows some tolerance of death awareness but largely avoids the terror of the idea of nonexistence? Kalish[18] provocatively comments on the studies of Magni (1972) that showed a negative correlation between conscious death fear (as measured by attitude scales) and psychophysical measurements of unconscious death fear. He interprets this data as suggesting that "denial intensified as fear of death increased." The logical conclusion of this is that "a lower conscious death fear masks a greater actual (unconscious) fear through a more powerful form of denial!

The elderly form a population that is ripe for the study of these issues. The recent development of more sophisticated psychological and psychophysical research methods make this endeavor more possible than it ever was before.[18]

But perhaps the most important, and most socially relevant, question for humanistic medicine concerns the increased death-readiness of the elderly. Is this primarily an increased tolerance for the idea of death or a kind of depressive response to the prospects of a life that has become unbearable? The furtherance of a biopsychosocial model of medicine, as proposed by Engel, may well produce the climate that generates the answer.

REFERENCES

1. Nagy, M. H. The child's view of death. *Journal of Genetic Psychology* 73: 3–27 (1948).
2. Kalish, R. A. and Reynolds, D. K. 1976. *Death and Ethnicity: A Psychocultural Study.* Los Angeles: University of Southern California Press.
3. *Dorland's Medical Dictionary,* 23rd Edition, 1961. Philadelphia and London: W. B. Saunders and Company.
4. Eissler, K. R. 1955. *The Psychiatrist and the Dying Patient.* New York: International Universities Press, Inc.
5. Freud, S. (1915) On transience. In *Collected Papers IV.* London: The Hogarth Press (1953).
6. Kübler-Ross, E. 1969. *On Death and Dying.* New York: Macmillan.
7. Becker, E. 1973. *The Denial of Death.* New York: The Free Press.
8. Lindemann, E. Symptomatology and management of acute grief. *American Journal of Psychiatry* 101: 141–148 (1944).
9. Jeffers, F. C. and Verwoerdt, A. 1968. How the old face death. In E. W. Busse & E. Pfeiffer (eds.) *Behavior and Adaptation in Late Life.* Boston: Little, Brown and Co., pp. 163–181.
9a. Magni, K. G. The fear of death, In A. Godin (ed.), *Death in Perspective,* Brussels: Leumen Ditae Press, 1972.
9b. Wahl, C. W. The fear of death. *Bulletin of the Menniger Clinic,* 22: 214, (1958).
10. Weisman, A. D. 1972. *On Dying and Denying.* New York: Behavioral Publications.
11. Shands, H. An outline of the process of recovery from severe trauma. *AMA Archives of Neurology and Psychiatry* 13: 403–409 (1955).
12. Norton, J. The treatment of a dying patient. *Psychoanalytic Study of the Child* 18: 541–560 (1963).
13. Feifel, H., and Jones, R. Perception of death as related to nearness of death. Proceedings of the 76th Annual Convention of the American Psychological Association 3: 545–546 (1968).
14. Lipowski, Z. J. Delirium, clouding of consciousness, and confusion. *Journal of Nervous and Mental Disease* 9: 260–267 (1967).
15. Massie, M. J., Glass, E. and Holland, J. C. B. 1977 Personal communication of unpublished work.
16. Holland, J. C. B. 1973. Psychologic aspects of cancer. In J. Holland and E. Frei, III (eds.) *Cancer Medicine,* pp. 991–1021. Philadelphia: Lea and Febiger.
17. Spikes, J. and Holland, J. C. B. The physician's response to the dying patient. In J. Strain and S. Grossman (eds.) *The Psychological Care of the Medically Ill—A Primer of Liaison Psychiatry,* pp. 138–148. New York: Appleton-Century-Crofts (1975).
17a. Glaser, B. G. The social loss of aged dying patients. *Gerontologist,* 6: 77 (1966).
18. Kalish, R. A. 1976. Death and dying in a social context. In R. Binstock and E. Shanas (eds.), *Handbook of Aging and the Social Sciences.* New York: Van Nostrand Reinhold.
19. Feifel, H. and Branscomb, A. B. Who's afraid of death? *Journal of Abnormal Psychology* 81: 282–288 (1973).
20. Swenson, W. M. Attitudes toward death in an aged population. *Journal of Gerontology* 16: 49–52 (1961).
21. Engel, G. L. The need for a new medical model: A challenge for biomedicine. *Science* 196: 129–134 (1977).
22. Katz, J. L. and Gardner, R. The intern's dilemma: The request for autopsy consent. *Psychiatry in Medicine* 3: 197–203 (1972).
22a. Kalish, R. A. Sex and marital role differences in anticipation of age produced dependency. *Journal of Geriatric Psychology,* 119: 53, (1971).
23. Cartwright, A., Hockey, L. and Anderson, J. L. 1973. *Life Before Death.* London: Routledge & Kegan Paul.
24. Parkes, C. M. and Brown, R. J. Health after bereavement: a controlled study of young Boston widows and widowers. *Psychosomatic Medicine* 34: 449–461 (1972).
25. Rees, W. D. and Lutkins, S. G. Mortality of bereavement. *British Journal of Medicine* 4: 13–16 (1967).
26. Wiener, A., Gerber, I., Battan, D. and Arkin, A. The process and phenomenology of bereavement. In, B. Schoenberg, I. Gerber, A. Wiener, A. Kutscher, D. Peretz, and A. Carr (eds.), *Bereavement, Its Psychosocial Aspects,* pp. 53–65. New York and London: Columbia University Press (1975).
27. Jung, C. G. 1959. (Originally published 1934) The soul and death. In H. Feifel (ed.), *The Meaning of Death,* pp. 3–15. New York: McGraw-Hill.

Chapter 20
Treatment in the Ambulatory Care Setting

Lawrence W. Lazarus, M.D.
Illinois State Psychiatric Institute

Jack Weinberg, M.D.
University of Illinois

In this chapter, we will discuss the psychiatric treatment of the elderly in the ambulatory care setting. The hesitation of elderly patients, their families and physicians to utilize psychiatric services, the reluctance of psychiatrists to treat the elderly, and ways in which to overcome these obstacles will be reviewed. Discussion of the developmental tasks and challenges which face the elderly and their families will provide the background for an elucidation of individual, group, family, and psychopharmacological treatment approaches.

DEVELOPMENTAL TASKS OF THE ELDERLY

The developmental tasks of the last phase of the life cycle can be divided into three main areas—intrapsychic, familial, and societal.

Intrapsychic

The aging person attempts to maintain his current functioning, self-esteem, and sense of purpose in life at the phase in the life cycle characterized by diminishing ego resources, increasing self-doubt, and the onslaught of narcissistic traumas.[1] Narcissistic traumas refer to those events which erode one's self-esteem, confidence, and positive self-image. Constantly threatened with extinction are those activities responsible for the maintenance of a person's positive self-image and self-esteem. Retirement, separation from family and friends, failing health, economic uncertainty, and approaching death—these are the potential traumas one faces during this phase of the life cycle.

For Erickson,[2] achievements and satisfactions during this developmental phase include a lifetime's accumulated knowledge, mature judgment, and a state of ego integrity. The opposite, a state of despair and disgust, is characterized by the fear of death and represents the failure to achieve a state of integrity. Cath[3] characterizes the middle and later years as a period in which there exists a balance between factors which lead to emotional depletion and factors which promote a person's sense of self and self-

427

esteem. Among the latter are the wisdom derived from life-long experience, the attainment of a satisfying philosophical and religious world view, past accomplishments within the family and at work, and the continuing opportunity for satisfaction of instinctual drives. Cath[3] believes that given adequate ego resources and a supportive, sustaining environment, most elderly people achieve a sense of integrity, a final integration of an altered body-image, and a mastery of the challenges characteristic of the last stage of the life cycle.

Post[4] believes that if old age is viewed in relation to the evolution and preservation of the human species, the inevitabe changes accompanying the aging process can be shown to be conducive to optimal adaptation. What to young people may be losses, such as diminishing sexual prowess or interest in others, may have adaptive value for older people and not be a cause of subjective dissatisfaction. For example, a decline in physical mobility may protect the elderly individual from the dangers of over exertion.

The disengagement theory, formulated by Cumming and Henry,[5] postulates that under normal circumstances the aging individual withdraws gradually from life in preparation for his diminished role and for the inevitable isolation and aloneness that is death. Most elderly accept comfortably their autumn years and adjust satisfactorily to diminishing physical, economic, and social capacities. Some elderly persons, as a means of denying their diminished abilities, engage in bouts of frantic activity, dress in the style of the young, or search for medicines to recapture their youth.

Butler[6] notes the universal tendency of the aging person to reflect upon and to reminisce about the past—a process which helps him to conceptualize his life over time and to give it significance and meaning. The life review process is stimulated by the realization of approaching death.

The Family

Contrary to the widespread belief that the stabilizing influence of the nuclear and ex-
tended family was eroded by America's change from an agricultural to an industrialized society and the increased mobility of family members, empirical studies have shown that family life continues to be a vitally important stabilizing influence in today's society. It is estimated that in 8% of families in the United States three generations live in the same household. About 80% of all older people have living children. Shanas[7] notes that 82% of all currently unmarried old persons in the United States who have children are less than 30 minutes distance from at least one of these children. Sussman[8] emphasizes the importance for the elderly of the "extended" family, which consists of a complex and integrated network of social relationships that operates along bilateral kin lines and vertically over several generations. Butler and Lewis believe that:

".... when families do not offer to help their older members a whole range of personal, social, and economic forces are usually at work rather than an attitude of neglect and abandonment."[9]

Some of the developmental tasks for the elderly person with regard to his family include accommodation—to the role of grandparent, to changing relationships with children, adjustment to a spouse's increasing debility, to the possibility or fact of widowhood, and to the inevitability of death.

The elderly derive self-esteem and enjoyment by contributing to the welfare of the family. For example, a grandparent may be called upon to be a temporary or permanent parent surrogate. Grandparents are sometimes the repository of family myths and secrets and the reservoir of wisdom derived from life-long experiences. Benedek views grandparenthood as a time which permits the elderly to:

". . . project the hope of the fulfillment of their narcissistic self-image to their grandchildren. Since they do not have the responsibility for raising the child toward that unconscious goal, their love is not as burdened by doubts and anxieties as it was when their own children were young."[10]

A life-long marriage may supply a bedrock of support and companionship during a period in life characterized by multiple losses. Divorce is uncommon late in life because the marriage has survived and perhaps been strengthened by mutual support during previous life stresses. In addition, the elderly were raised in an era when religious and societal pressures served as deterrents to divorce. Children, grandchildren, and mutual friendships strengthen the bonds between the elderly couple. However, progressive physical or mental debility of one spouse may impose tremendous emotional, physical, or financial hardship on the healthy, care-giving spouse. This may lead to marital conflict. The healthier spouse, because of his or her own unfulfilled dependency needs, may become angry and withdraw from the impaired partner.

Widowhood can be an exceedingly difficult period. The incidence of mortality and illness in the surviving spouse is far greater than the general geriatric population.[11] Remarriage of a widow or widower may cause conflict among the children of both sides of the family over such issues as family alliance and inheritance, and allegiance to the deceased parent.

Middle-aged children of aging parents face several developmental tasks of their own. As a result of their parents' increasing dependency and debility, the adult children realize that they may be called upon for emotional and financial support. Blenkner[12] believes that one indication that the adult children of aging parents have achieved maturity with regard to their filial responsibility is their ability to help their parents, both emotionally and financially. Adult children may have difficulty responding helpfully to their parent's diminishing capacities, especially if they need to preserve a childhood image of their parent as being all-powerful and omnipotent. Sometimes

they require counseling to help them resolve their ambivalent feelings and to accept some responsibility for their parents. With regard to a dying parent, the adult child faces the developmental task of resolving feelings of ambivalence toward the parent, beginning the mourning process, and realizing that he, too, faces the inevitability of death.

The decision as to who will accept responsibility for an aging parent may stimulate unresolved sibling rivalry and other family conflicts. This may take the form of family indecision and disagreement about placement in a long-term care facility, resentment toward the sibling with whom the parent decides to live, and disagreements about division of the family estate and debts. Psychotherapeutic approaches to these problems will be discussed later in this chapter.

Societal

Butler[13] and others[14,15] have written extensively about society's prejudices toward, and stereotypes of, the elderly. They are often portrayed in movies, television, and novels as meddling in the lives of their children, as emotional and financial drains on family and society, and as asexual, senile, depreciated objects of scorn and pity. Mandatory retirement together with America's preoccupation with youth and economic productivity, tend to reinforce this image. These stereotypes and prejudices are internalized and then passed on to successive generations.

Physicians are not immune to these myths and misconceptions. Exposed during their training primarily to hospitalized elderly patients with serious illnesses, physicians may continue to view all elderly people as debilitated and incapacitated. Most psychiatrists have had limited training and experience in geropsychiatry.[16] They are sometimes discouraged from working therapeutically with the elderly because of difficulty in sorting out the relative contribution of psychological and organic factors, the increased time and energy required to consult with family, health professionals and agencies, and inadequate third-party reimbursement.[17] Young psychiatrists may find it emotionally draining and anxiety producing to work with patients who are preoccupied with loss, death, and dying. Karasu and Waltzman, discussing work with the chronically ill, believe that: "To be impotent in the face of rampant disease is a blow to the physician's self-esteem and strikes at the heart of his narcissism."[18]

THE ROLE OF PRIMARY PHYSICIAN AND PSYCHIATRIST

Ambulatory geriatric patients with organic and/or emotional impairments are generally under the care of their primary physician (internist, family or general practitioner). He assumes a crucial role in coordinating his patient's treatment. It is not uncommon for an elderly patient to visit several different physicians which makes coordination of treatment quite difficult. The elderly patient may not inform one physician about medication and other treatments prescribed by his other physicians. The primary physician must therefore work closely with other health professionals and the patient's family in order to orchestrate his patient's treatment.

Depending on the setting in which he works, the psychiatrist may function in various capacities—as consultant to assist the primary physician in diagnostic and treatment issues, as psychotherapist, as consultant to a team of health professionals involved in patient care, and as consultant to the administration of an institution which sets policy ultimately effecting all patient care.

REFERRAL FOR PSYCHIATRIC EVALUATION

Referral of the geriatric patient for psychiatric consultation requires time, tact, and patience on the part of the primary physician. Raised in an era before medical specialization, the elderly patient expects his primary physician to be solely responsible for all his medical care. Since he is sometimes emotionally dependent on his primary physician, referral to another physician may be perceived by him, either consciously or unconsciously, as a rejection. The elderly patient is more apt than the younger patient to attribute feelings of anxiety, depression, and other feeling states to physical causes. He therefore expects physical remedies. The idea that he may obtain relief for his problems by talking about them may seem foreign to him. He may even perceive psychiatric referral as an accusation that he is crazy and is therefore destined for incarceration in a mental institution.

Having experienced economic and other hardships earlier in life, the elderly patient, in contrast to the younger patient, may be more accepting of physical and emotional discomfort. He may have accepted society's myth that unhappiness and discomfort is to be expected during the latter years. Older people tend to attribute their physical symptoms to being old. Osfelt[19] studied a sample of elderly people in Chicago and found that although 50% were clearly in need of medical care, only 25% recognized this need and identified themselves as being ill. The remainder believed that their condition was due to being old.

The older patient's family may, in a like manner, be resistant to considering psychiatric evaluation for their aging family member. The family may erroneously attribute his disordered behavior to "growing old" in order to preserve their previous image of him or to compensate for feelings of guilt and shame regarding their possible contribution to his problem.

The primary physician may have difficulty deciding which family member requires psychiatric evaluation because emotional disturbance of other family members or disturbance of the family's homeostasis may precipitate psychiatric symptomatology in one of its elderly members. For example, a family's ambivalence about where its elderly member should live may contribute to the elderly person's depression.

These considerations lead to the following suggestions regarding psychiatric referral of the elderly patient. The success of the referral process will depend largely upon the nature and quality of the primary physician's relationship with his patient and the manner in which the referral is effected. A trusting, positive relationship with his primary physician increases the likelihood that the elderly patient will follow through with the referral. The primary physician reassures his patient that he will continue to assume responsibility for his overall management. The patient's family can be useful allies to support the referral. If the primary physician anticipates that his patient will respond negatively to the suggestion, he may wish to contact the psychiatrist beforehand for suggestions about ways to best facilitate the process. Referral should be considered soon after the onset of psychiatric symptoms. Zinberg,[20] Butler,[21] Oberleider,[22] and Feigenbaum[23] note that the elderly person is usually not referred for psychiatric evaluation until an emergency exists. This is unfortunate because the longer the time that elapses between the onset of psychiatric symptoms until treatment is instituted the less likely treatment will be effective.

The primary physician is faced with the decisions as to when and how to refer for psychiatric evaluation. Referral should be considered in the following situations: for assistance in diagnosis and treatment; when emotional factors interfere with patient cooperation regarding medical treatment; and for ongoing psychiatric treatment. The reasons for the referral should be presented in a positive, constructive manner in language the patient and his family can understand. The physician allows time to answer his patient's questions, responds empathically to his ambivalence, and reassures him about its potential usefulness in his treatment. The physician explains, particularly to those whose depression or cognitive impairment may interfere with communication, that more than one psychiatric interview may be required. It is preferable for the primary physician to talk directly with the psychiatrist about the pa-

tient rather than by a written request. More information can be exchanged in this way and the psychiatrist can sometimes discover problems within the patient-physician relationship which may be causing difficulties.

Unless it is apparent that the entire family is having emotional difficulties, it is usually best first to interview the elderly patient alone. It is informative, after obtaining the patient's permission, also to interview his family for the purpose of obtaining collaborative information, evaluating the quality of the affective ties and relationships and establishing a working alliance with the family. Throughout the assessment process, the psychiatrist maintains a high index of suspicion for undetected medical illnesses which may be contributing to the patient's condition.

The psychiatrist discusses his findings and recommendations with the referring physician. He may continue to be accessible to assist the primary physician or, when indicated, may see the patient regularly for psychiatric treatment. All physicians and health professionals involved in the patient's care should clearly understand which physician will be responsible for coordinating the efforts of all.

OUTPATIENT PSYCHOTHERAPY—SOME PROBLEMS AND SOLUTIONS

Although U. S. citizens age 65 and older comprise about 10% of the population and are a population especially at risk for developing psychiatric illness, they comprise only about 2 to 4% of cases in psychiatric outpatient clinics[24] and even less in most private psychiatric practices.[16] The reason for this low utilization of psychiatric outpatient services can be understood from four perspectives: the patient, his family, the primary physician, and the psychiatrist. Having discussed the first two in the preceding section, we will now discuss the primary physician and the psychiatrist.

The primary physician may be reluctant to refer the elderly patient for outpatient evaluation and psychotherapy because of doubts about its value, a tendency to attribute all disordered behavior in the elderly to physical causes and "senility," lack of family cooperation, and the unavailability of a psychiatrist with special interest and training. Some physicians, having accepted society's devaluation of, and prejudices about, the elderly, are reluctant to invest time and energy in exploring other modalities of treatment.

Psychiatrists have, in general, been resistant to work therapeutically with the elderly. A 1970 study[25] found that 56% of psychiatrists surveyed spent no time with patients over age 65. More than 86% of the psychiatrists spent less than 10% of their working time with the elderly. An American Psychiatric Association report in 1973 indicates that only 50% of the psychiatric residency programs surveyed offered an opportunity for clinical experiences with the elderly. It therefore may be the psychiatrist's inadequate training that accounts for his reluctance to treat the elderly.

Psychotherapists erroneously believe that elderly patients with psychiatric disorders have a poorer prognosis than younger patients. Some feel that because the elderly have less time to live they are less deserving of the psychiatrist's time. Also, inadequate family and community resources make it difficult for some elderly patients to attend therapy sessions regularly.

Young psychiatrists may have difficulty empathizing with the problems of older patients and older psychiatrists may, because of overidentification, experience anxiety. The therapist's unresolved conflicts with parents and grandparents may be reactivated and lead to countertransference difficulties. A physician whose self-image and self-esteem is overly dependent upon the success of his therapeutic efforts may experience frustration and disappointment when confronted by a patient with serious physical as well as psychiatric disorders.

Several ways have been demonstrated to overcome these obstacles to outpatient psychotherapy with the elderly. At the Langley Porter Neuropsychiatric Institute[25] a special psychiatric outpatient program was developed for geriatric patients and the availability of these services was then publicized. Before the initiation of this special program, the elderly comprised 2% of the psychiatric outpatient population. After 3 years, the proportion of elderly patients rose to over 5%. The improvement rates of different age groups was fairly similar. The San Francisco Geriatric Screening Project[27] demonstrated that early detection, evaluation, and treatment of emotionally impaired elderly in the community reduced the admission rate of elderly patients to state mental hospitals. A myriad of both public and private community-based health care programs which provide supportive health services to the elderly have been developed in recent years to help maintain mentally and physically impaired elderly people in the community.[28]

If today's young citizens are more psychologically sophisticated than the elderly about utilizing psychiatric services, we may anticipate greater utilization of these services by successive generations of senior citizens. Increasing knowledge about psychiatric disorders of the elderly will hopefully lead to more preventive measures as well as more effective therapies. Preventive measures and early detection would require more effective use of outpatient diagnostic services which may lead ultimately to a decrease in the need for psychiatric hospitalization.

INDIVIDUAL PSYCHOTHERAPY AND COUNSELING

Following a brief historical review of psychotherapy and counseling with the elderly, we will discuss the clinical application of recent psychoanalytic theory about self psychology and narcissism, the major themes, strategies, and nuances of psychotherapy, and typical transference-countertransference reactions that occur during treatment. Clinical vignettes will be used to illustrate the main concepts.

Historical Review

Psychotherapeutic approaches to the elderly have been influenced by the period in history in which they developed, the theoretical orientation and personality of the therapist, and the ego strength and social support systems of the patients with whom he worked.

Psychologist Lillian J. Martin, the founder in 1929 of the San Francisco Old Age Counseling Center, described in three books[29-31] a supportive, educational, and inspirational approach to the elderly. The elderly were advised, during a series of highly structured interviews, about ways to enrich their lives. Although this approach has been criticized as being superficial, she was nevertheless one of the first to advocate psychotherapy for the emotionally impaired aged.

Freud was pessimistic about the elderly's suitability for traditional psychoanalysis. He believed that:

" . . . near or above the fifties the elasticity of the mental processes, on which the treatment depends, is as a rule lacking—old people are no longer educable. . . . "[32]

The mass of material from accumulated life experiences would prolong the duration of treatment indefinitely and a cure would be reached at such a late period in life that its influence on the remaining years would be of little value.[33] Despite Freud's pessimism, psychoanalysts Abraham,[34] Kaufman,[35] Jellifee[36] and others[37,38] reported successful analyses of elderly patients. Alexander and French[39] proposed modifications of traditional analytic techniques. Grotjahn,[40] Meerlo,[41] Weinberg,[42] Hollender,[43] and Wayne[44] advocated supportive therapeutic techniques in which the therapist is active, supportive, and involved with the patient in a real and meaningful way. Weinberg[42] believes that allowances be made for the possibility of unduly disturbing those patients who have severe psychosomatic conditions and for the reduced vigor, agility, and learning capacity of the aged. Hollender cautions:

"When a person has turned to the past or developed fixed ways of doing things to derive narcissistic gratifications or to protect injuries to self-esteem, we should not tamper with these defenses unless we are sure that we can provide adequate substitutes for them."[43]

Goldfarb[45] describes a brief therapeutic technique for institutionalized, brain damaged elderly patients. Using the patient's dependency to therapeutic advantage, he encourages the patient to feel as if he controls the therapist, who is perceived as an omnipotent, parental figure. The patient's dependency needs are thereby gratified and his sense of mastery, security, and self-esteem is enhanced. Although this technique has been criticized for being partly based on the creation of an illusion, this approach may have great value in institutional settings because of limitations on the therapist's time. Linden[46] advocates an optimistic approach to the brain damaged elderly which includes environmental manipulation, physical activity, resocialization, group therapy, and careful medical management.

The therapist understands that the elderly patient's propensity to reminisce about his past serves several purposes—to maintain ego integrity and self-esteem, to avoid depression, and to cope with an unstable life situation. The therapist is therefore attentive to, and encouraging of, this normal process.

Despite the numerous encouraging reports about the value of individual therapy, Rechtschaffen's conclusion in his excellent review article about geriatric psychotherapy is, unfortunately, as pertinent today as it was in 1959.

"As is true for psychotherapy as a whole, systematic, controlled studies of the effectiveness of various treatments of older people are still lacking. Ultimately, there must be empirical grounds for predicting which type of treatment will work best for which type of patient."[47]

In recent years, more attention has been focused on the elderly person in the context of his entire biopsychosocial milieu than primarily on his intrapsychic processes. Attempts have been made to avoid protracted institutionalization for the elderly by providing the necessary support systems to help maintain them in the community.

NARCISSISM AND AGING — THEORY AND CLINICAL APPLICATION

Recent psychoanalytic theory about normal and pathological narcissism has lent itself to important clinical applications in psychotherapeutic work with the elderly. Psychoanalyst Heinz Kohut, extending the work of Freud,[48,49] Mahler,[50] Bibring,[51] and Reich[52] has proposed that there is a distinct line of development for the narcissistic sector of the personality, just as there is a distinct developmental line with regard to object relationships.

Narcissism is defined by Kohut and others as the emotional investment in the self. Narcissism has to do with the integration and cohesiveness of the self. It's antithesis, object love, is an emotional investment in others. According to Goldberg:

"The self as a psychological construct is an enduring experience of an individual's uniqueness with a correlated and coherent developmental line."[53]

There are healthy as well as pathological forms and expressions of narcissism. Psychopathological parent-child interactions during critical stages in the development of the narcissistic sector of the personality can lead to later defects in the adult's estimation of himself, self-esteem regulation and interpersonal relationships, and a propensity to shame, depression, and rage.

The following summary of Kohut's[54-57] theory regarding the normal and psychopathological development of the narcissistic sector of the personality will then be applied to the theory and practice of psychotherapy with the elderly. Infantile narcissism refers to the psychological state of the infant in whom differentiation between self and object has not yet taken place. Kohut identifies two principal forms of infantile narcissism. The first, the grandiose self, occurs during the stage of undifferentiated symbosis with the mother. The infant feels omnipotent and perfect and has an accompanying fantasy of greatness. This primitive form of narcissism, under normal circumstances, gradually undergoes transformation into healthy expressions of pride, enjoyment, and satisfaction in one's activities and successes. Failure to achieve one's ambitions results in transitory feelings of shame and disappointment. The second form of infantile narcissism, the idealized parental imago, results from the projection of the child's original feelings of perfection (the grandiose self) onto the parent, leading to idealization of the parent. Normally, there is a gradual, phase-specific discovery by the child of the parent's real, as opposed to idealized, qualities. The child reacts to this loss and disappointment by internalizing the idealized qualities, a process which contributes to the formation of values and ideals (the ego ideal) to which he aspires. The idealizing aspect of the superego is the final developmental maturation of the idealized parental imago. The final developmental achievement by the mature adult is the transformation and integration within the personality of such healthy expressions of the self as creativity, humor, empathy, acceptance of one's impermanence, and wisdom. The extent to which these achievements are realized varies with each individual and accounts, in part, for one's individuality and identity. The touchstone of each person's individuality and identity stems from the intricate interplay between the narcissistic self, the ego, and the superego. Kohut believes[58] that experiences during the formation of the self become the prototype of our security and vulnerability in the narcissistic realm. These early life experiences account for the variability in our self-esteem, need for praise, wish for merger into idealized figures, and for other forms of narcissistic sustenance. They influence the degree of cohesion of the self during stressful periods of transition, such as the transition to adolescence, maturity, or old age.

The disturbances of narcissistic balance which Kohut refers to as narcissistic injury,

"are usually easily recognized by the painful affect of embarrassment or shame which accompanies them and by their ideational elaboration which is known as inferiority feeling or hurt pride."[59]

The ego ideal and the goal structure of the ego are the personality's best protection against narcissistic vulnerability and shame propensity. Emotional responses to narcissistic injury may range from unbridled anger and rage toward those he believes have inflicted the insult, to the massive inhibition of feeling which may manifest itself as withdrawal or depression.

Narcissistic psychopathology in the adult or elderly patient may manifest itself in recurring depressions or defensive grandiosity in response to minor slights or disappointments, self-consciousness, overdependence on approval from others for maintenance of self-esteem, and transitory periods of fragmentation and discohesiveness of the self. He searches for a person to idealize and from whom he can obtain approval, protection, and stabilization of his brittle sense of self and self-esteem. Self-centered and egocentric, he views others not as separate objects but as extensions of himself to be used for self-serving purposes and for enhancement and stabilization of his self-esteem. Goldberg[60] and Horowitz[61] believe that psychotherapy of most neurotic and character types should consider narcissistic aspects of the personality. As patients with narcissistic pathology grow older, one observes an increase in hypochondriasis, an overconcern with physical appearance and possessions, and past accomplishments. They continually seek approval and reassurance from others. Narcissistic indivi-

duals are especially vulnerable and easily devastated by the biopsychosocial losses associated with aging. With diminishing physical attractiveness, health, and productivity to feed a previously unstable sense of self, they resort to primitive defenses to guard against further loss of self-esteem. Especially sensitive to slights and insults from relatives and friends, they are liable to withdraw into a fantasy world in which memories or fantasies of real or imagined past accomplishments take on great importance. They are prone to depression and paranoid reactions.

Cath,[3] Meissner,[1] and Muslin and Epstein[62] believe that a major developmental task of the aging individual is to find restitution for the inevitable biopsychosocial losses associated with this stage of the life cycle. The basic problem of aging, according to Meissner, is that of narcissistic loss. Referring to Rochin's discussion of the issue, Meissner[63] notes that the greatest test of narcissism is old age. The attributes which contribute to man's self-esteem and narcissism, such as his skills and powers, which provided gratifications as they functioned to effect adaptation, wane in this phase of the life cycle. Man's energies, resources, and the intimate relationships upon which he depended are continually being depleted and lost. Aging is not unlike gambling in that the longer one lives, the more regularly one loses.

It is not surprising then that anger, rage, despair, and withdrawal are frequent emotional reactions of the elderly to these losses. Kohut cites the example of the aging person who, due to brain injury, is unable to solve simple problems. Failing in this, he becomes enraged "due to the fact that he's not in control of his own thought processes, of a function which people consider to be most intimately their own—i.e. as a part of the self."[64]

How do the elderly attempt to cope when they fail to find restitution for the innumerable losses associated with aging and fail to maintain a sense of self and self-esteem? One psychological reaction is regression along narcissistic, as well as object libidinal, developmental lines. As developmentally more mature mechanisms of defense become impaired because of brain deterioration and/or emotional illness, there is regression to more primitive defenses such as denial, projection, and withdrawal. If these defenses fail to defend against self-esteem diminishment and overwhelming anxiety, the elderly person may experience transitory feelings of fragmentation and discohesiveness of the self.

For example, a 64-year-old woman recovering from a life-threatening stroke which paralyzed her left side told her psychotherapist: "It feels as if parts of my body are in different places. I no longer have control over them." In the advanced stages of senile dementia, one observes regression to very primitive forms of narcissism manifested by autoerotic sexual activity, grandiose, wish-fulfilling fantasies and delusions, and infantlike behavior.

Defending against the recognition of increasing incapacity and debility, the elderly person may have brief flurries of frantic activity in which he makes unrealistic, grandiose plans for the future. It is as if the aging person were insisting: "It cannot be! I am as capable, lovable, and competent as I always was."

Case Example

An elderly architect who had derived lifelong enjoyment from playing golf with cronies every weekend became significantly depressed following a life-threatening heart ailment which forced him to consider retirement and cessation of all sports activities. In a desperate attempt to deny his increasing disability in order to preserve his self-image as a healthy and competent sportsman, he made an elaborate plan to join a group of sports enthusiasts on a European golf tour. Before leaving, he finally agreed to his physician's insistence that he see a psychiatrist. It was apparent during his first inter view

that his self-esteem had always been nourished by achievements in work and athletics. The threatened loss of these sources of narcissistic gratification and the threat of the ultimate of narcissistic traumas, death, accounted for his anxiety, depression, and grandiose plans. When this was interpreted to him, he agreed to cancel his trip, but then insisted on having psychiatric appointments on days other than those he usually played golf because he could not bear the humiliation of having a psychiatric visit on the same day he formerly enjoyed the cameraderie of his golf friends.

Paranoid ideas may surface as a defense against further loss of self-esteem and to defend against the recognition of increased dependency on others. The paranoid defense is not only a projection of unacceptable aggressive and hostile impulses, but also serves to attribute responsibility to others for the loss of competency and bodily intactness. It is as if the paranoid were saying: "It is not I who has lost my abilities, it is they who have stolen them from me." When the elderly paranoid woman accuses her daughter, who has assumed responsibility for her mother's financial affairs, of stealing from her, the symbolic meaning of the accusation may be: "You have taken from me that function which I have always valued and cherished and which contributed to my feelings of competency and self-esteem."

These theories about narcissistic development and psychopathology have a number of important clinical applications. If one developmental task of the elderly person is to find restitution for narcissistic and other losses associated with aging, the therapist first helps his patient work through the grief and mourning over the losses and then gradually encourages him to find realistic substitute sources of gratification. If a second developmental task for the elderly person is to modify the cherished aspirations and goals of his ego ideal to which he aspired when younger, the therapist helps him to revise former goals in accordance with his diminished capabilities. Modifying former aspirations may protect him from recurrent feelings of defeat, humiliation, and shame. The therapist understands that his patient's denial of diminishing abilities may symbolize the continued insistence of the ego to live up to its former ego ideals. Considerable time may be required for the patient to modify these cherished aspirations. For example, even a year after her life-threatening stroke, the 64-year-old woman previously discussed admitted to her psychotherapist that she could not accept her disability. She described her continuing disappointment upon awakening each morning to discover that her fantasy of a return of bodily intactness and wholeness had not been realized.

The therapist conveys his understanding of these developmental tasks and challenges and indicates, by word and by gesture, his willingness to assist his patient to work through the losses, to find new sources of satisfaction and gratification, and to modify the goals to which he formerly aspired. As well, the therapist needs to accept his elderly patient's limitations and to modify repeatedly the goals of therapy in keeping with the patient's true capabilities. If treatment goals are unrealistically ambitious, both he and the patient will experience frustration and disappointment.

The therapist is sensitive to his patient's tendency to attribute his own feelings of hopelessness and inferiority to the therapist, thus believing him to be rejecting and critical. The elderly patient, especially if he has narcissistic psychopathology, is exquisitely sensitive to subtle behavior indicating the therapist's annoyance or indifference. The therapist's careful listening, empathizing, and interpreting, gradually enable the patient to begin feeling that he is a valuable worthwhile person. The therapist may also serve as a replacement for those important friends and relatives he has lost. An elderly patient with impoverished self-esteem and without meaningful relationships may tend to idealize the therapist, believing his therapist to be perfect, all-knowing, and of immeasurable value to him. He feels secure and protected by this parentlike figure. Some therapists misidentify the patient's idealization as a defense against hostility toward the therapist, or attempt to discourage the idealization under the assumption that they are improving the patient's reality testing. In many instances, the patient's idealization serves an important intrapsychic function and in these instances it may be therapeutically best not to interpret it.

Case Example

A 76-year-old retired college professor had a series of attractive women as companions throughout his life to whom he related not as separate objects to be loved and cherished, but rather as extensions of himself. These women served to bolster his insecure sense of self and his self-esteem. He felt flattered whenever his colleagues saw him with one of his attractive women. When chronic illness made it impossible for him to continue this lifestyle, he became profoundly depressed and finally sought psychiatric treatment. He was referred to a woman therapist with whom he quickly established a narcissistic transference. He believed that his wit and charm won her acceptance and interest. The therapist's acceptance of his implicit need to be admired led to his rapid improvement. The transference was never interpreted and periodic appointments over the ensuing years maintained his improvement.

In summary, the numerous narcissistic trauma which the elderly person experiences poses identifiable developmental tasks for him to master—to modify former goals and ideals, to mourn and find restitution for narcissistic and other losses, and to maintain self-esteem and a sense of integrity in the wake of biopsychosocial losses. The therapist helps the patient to master these developmental tasks. The treatment plan is carefully and realistically tailored to the patient's needs and strengths. The therapist communicates, both verbally and nonverbally, his respect, acceptance, and involvement. At times the therapist is a replacement object for those important persons whom the patient has lost. At other times, the therapist may be a narcissistic object whose protection and positive regard enable the patient to re-establish feelings of self-worth and self-esteem.

Individual Psychotherapy — Other Themes and Issues

Because of concern about approaching death, the elderly's sense of time is focused on the present, the here and now. His concern with death, although often denied or rationalized, is often revealed in dreams or when describing his reactions to the death of friends and relatives. A patient who is mourning the death of his wife will sometimes describe a pact he has made with death so that he can reunite with his spouse.[65]

Another important issue in psychotherapy with the elderly is that of termination. Many patients, particularly those who are in supportive forms of psychotherapy, do not formally terminate psychotherapy. Even during the final stages of therapy, the therapist will usually indicate his continued availability should the patient require psychotherapy in the future. The therapist continues to be available because he recognizes that the stresses of advancing years and its associated losses may precipitate a recurrence of emotional conflict and decompensation. The knowledge of the therapist's continued availability should help be needed is very reassuring to the elderly patient.

In reminiscing about the past, some elderly patients have a tendency to experience guilt and despair about past behavior. The therapist tries to distinguish between realistic guilt and that which is irrational and imposed by the patient's punitive superego. Butler and Lewis state:

"Facing genuine guilt as well as the attrition of the person's physical and emotional world is what makes psychotherapy with the aging an intellectually and emotionally powerful experience."[66]

Other recurring themes in psychotherapy include fear about increasing dependency on the family, physical and mental deterioration, and the continued wish to resolve old and new conflicts.

TRANSFERENCE — COUNTER-TRANSFERENCE

The elderly patient develops parental or filial transference reactions to his therapist; the latter especially occurs when the therapist is similar in age to the patient's children. The patient may idealize the therapist. This may derive partly from belief in the physician's healing powers, projection onto the therapist of the patient's grandiosity, or from inner feelings of emptiness and despair associated with an overvaluation of a perceived helper. The trust and security which the patient feels toward the therapist can be used to encourage him to regain old, and establish new social relationships.

Negative transference reactions also occur fairly often. If the patient is angry and humiliated about having been coerced by his family and physician into seeing a psychiatrist, and has little understanding of the purpose of the interviews, he at first may be understandably suspicious and uncooperative. Coping already with numerous losses and disappointments, he anticipates and fears that the therapist will likewise reject him. His initial hostility may also serve to test the therapist's sincerity. He may express paranoid ideas regarding his family which may be difficult to distinguish from realistic reactions to slights and disappointments. To establish a therapeutic alliance with the paranoid patient, the therapist initially accepts and tries to understand the patient's point of view. Understanding that the patient's anger and hostility, which may also be directed at the therapist, is a natural outcome of past disappointments with significant friends and family will enable the therapist to be tolerant, understanding, and accepting.

Psychotherapy with the elderly may rekindle unresolved conflicts with the therapist's parents and grandparents. The frequent omission of a sexual history from psychiatric case reports of elderly patients may represent unconscious prohibitions against discussing sexual issues with one's elders (i.e. one's parents). Psychotherapy with the elderly may stimulate the therapist's own fears about aging and death. The inevitability and nearness of the older patient's death may make both patient and therapist shun a close, meaningful relationship. Meerlo believes that:

"Treating a declining life hurts our medical narcissism and our expectations of magical cure."[67]

THE THERAPIST'S BASIC STANCE

In reviewing the work of noted geropsychiatrists, several guiding principles emerge concerning the psychotherapist's basic stance and attitude when working with the elderly. One principle is that of therapeutic flexibility. The ever-changing and intricate interplay of organic and functional factors requires that the therapist have a good medical background as well as experience with a variety of therapeutic techniques. For example, the elderly person's adult children may require therapy to help them adjust to a parent's deterioration from organic brain impairment. The family's expectations that their elder member "be as he was before" may contribute to the elderly patient's depression. Individual therapy may be indicated for some elderly patients and family therapy may be indicated for others. During one phase of the patient's treatment, the therapist may function in the traditional role of individual therapist, but at another time he may be called upon to function as family

therapist, pharmacotherapist, social planner, or as a member of a team of health professionals.

Secondly, the psychotherapist, by gesture and by touch,[68] by his genuine acceptance and regard, and by his respect and interest, helps the patient to regain a sense of self and self-esteem. The therapist encourages the patient to become interested in relationships with others and with meaningful activities. As Meerlo stated:

"Psychotherapy has to reconstitute the contact with the outer world, it has to replace the delusion of the need for money and for more material needs with the impact of human contact and sympathy."[69]

Thirdly, the psychotherapist understands that in some treatment situations he is only one member of a multidisciplinary team of health professionals. The psychiatrist, with the patient's permission, shares certain information about him and assists other members of the health care team. Mutual exchange of information between physicians and other health care providers minimizes the likelihood of mismanagement and duplication of services. One physician is identified as the primary physician. Other physicians and health professionals should confer with the primary physician about proposed changes in the patient's treatment plan.

FAMILY THERAPY

The medical model has traditionally regarded the individual patient as the primary focus for diagnosis and treatment. Family therapists believe that the correct therapeutic focus is not the single individual but rather two or more people within the nuclear or extended family. The family member who demonstrates psychiatric symptoms is, according to most family therapists, expressing the disequilibrium within the family.

The early family theoreticians applied principles of individual therapy to the whole family, encouraged family members to express their feelings, and later began to interpret the interactions between family members. With the development of communication theory, family therapists clarified the meaning of the family member's communications.[70] Bowen,[71] working with families with a schizophrenic member, advocated a therapeutic approach which supported each family member's autonomy and independence. System's theory[72,73] views family interactions as occurring in a repetitive fashion which strives to maintain stability and uniformity. Change or deviation in one member of a family affects others in the family system.

Another theoretical model of family therapy is based on the concept of family structure. A hierarchy exists within the family with rules that are similar, in some respect, to most organizations. Psychopathology becomes manifest in a family member when there is confusion or a violation of rules in the family organization. Haley[74] cites, as an example, the family distress which occurs when a grandmother consistently forms a coalition with a child against the child's mother.

Families have a life history. The roles of family members, the hierarchial structure, and family coalitions undergo change over time.[75] The family and each of its members have specific developmental tasks to accomplish at different stages in its life cycle. Children shift from being taken care of, to being peers of their parents, to taking care of their parents in their old age. Developmental crises and family disequilibrium can occur because of failure to accomplish a stage-specific task. For example, failure of an adult child to assume some responsibility for the emotional and financial support of an aging parent can lead to guilt and depression amongst the family members.

These three major theories of family therapy—systems theory, the theory of hierarchial structure, and the family life cycle—have important applications with families of the elderly. The primary physician and psychiatrist enhances his understanding of the elderly patient by familiarizing himself with the family. Evaluation of the elderly patient alone without collateral assessment of the family's style of communication and interaction may result in a restricted view of the presenting problems. Just as in individual psychotherapy with the elderly, working with the family requires the therapist to be flexible, active, and sometimes directive. The therapist usually avoids taking sides with family members despite their attempts to win his alliance. At other times, the therapist may find it necessary to be the advocate of the elderly family member and to help other family members understand the older person's behavior and communication.

It is often an emergency which brings the family and its elderly member to the physician's office. In a crisis, the family is sometimes most amenable to intervention and change. Early detection and treatment of psychiatric disorders in the elderly helps to prevent chronicity. The following section includes a discussion of therapeutic strategies for common family problems facing the primary physician and psychiatrist.

The Family's Reaction to its Aging Parent

The elderly person living in the home of children and grandchildren (the three generation family) may provide assistance to, and derive gratification from, the family. Weinberg notes that:

> "The multigeneration family provides the aged the meaningful and repeated contacts needed to stave off deterioration."[76]

Despite these reciprocal benefits, some degree of psychological stress is commonplace.[77]

Difficulties may occur because of the adult children's inability to accept age-related physical and mental changes in the parent, their frustration and annoyance with his deterioration, and guilt and ambivalence over the wish to be freed of the emotional and financial burden of caring for the parent. The elderly person's caretakers may become angry, depressed, and develop physical illness because of the burden of taking care of the elderly parent at home.

Inability of the family to cope at home with the elderly's problems may result in his hospital admission. Sanford,[78] in a study conducted in England, estimated that 12% of all geriatric hospital admissions are for patients whose relatives can no longer cope with them at home. Interviews with the principal family member from 50 such families revealed that 92% could identify which problems would have to be alleviated to facilitate the return to home of the elderly member. Sleep disturbance was tolerated by only 16% of the 50 principal family members, while fecal incontinence was tolerated by 43%, and urinary incontinence by 81%. Sanford concluded that medical attention to these and other problems as well as community aid and support to the families of the elderly would reduce the need for hospitalization.

The adult children of aging parents may have difficulty accepting their parent's deterioration, especially if they need to preserve a childhood image of him as being omnipotent. The adult child's own ego is threatened since the parent's approaching demise is a harbinger of his own fate.[79] The family may react by withdrawing, as evidenced by decreasing visits to the nursing home where he is residing. Misidentifying the withdrawal as abandonment, the staff of the long-term facility may criticize the family, thus provoking guilt and remorse. In such situations the primary physician, psychiatrist, or social worker may help the family to understand the reasons for their withdrawal. The family may be gradually helped to accept their parent as he now is and to prepare for eventual mourning of the loss. Cath believes that grief and mourning, if these occur, represent a step in growth since the capacity to tolerate and work through this is an essential step toward human maturity.[79]

Although most families accept and will-ingly fulfill their filial obligations, some families do reject their elderly. The rejection is more comprehensible if viewed within the total perspective of the family's life cycle. If the aging parent did not, in former years, evoke a loving response from his children, it may now be difficult to evoke these emotions. Working with families who are struggling with ambivalence and guilt about their responsibility to aging parents requires that the therapist be comfortable with regard to his feelings toward his own parents. Otherwise, the therapist's bias about these moral and ethical issues may make him intolerant of the families of the elderly.

In the clinical situations described above, the therapist helps the family to understand the underlying reasons for their ambivalence and conflict. The therapist may offer advice about how the family can relate better to their aging parents. For example, teaching the adult child about the therapeutic value of listening, "really" listening, to what their elderly parent says, can often benefit both parent and child.[80] By assuming the role of interested listener on the one hand, and knowledgeable teacher on the other, the therapist can help the family through its conflict and grief and help them to master the developmental challenges of this stage of the family's life cycle.

Institutionalization of an Aging Parent

Despite the increasing proportion of citizens over age 65 in the U.S., in 1970 only 4% were living in institutions. It is usually a combination of increasing debility of the elderly person and decreasing emotional and financial resources of the caretaking family members which raises the emotionally charged question of institutionalization.

The prospect of any change, particularly a move from familiar to unknown surroundings, is usually experienced by the elderly person as a threat to his security. According to Sussman,[81] for some elderly institutionalization may be seen as a final surrender to the recognition that they can no longer care for themselves and that the hope of regaining the activity lost due to illness or natural aging processes is permanent. To other elderly people, the term "nursing home" may connote safety and security. The elderly person may become increasingly aware of his need for more comprehensive care and the burden that his failing health imposes on his family. Nevertheless, this recognition may conflict with his wish to remain in the family home. Although ostensibly agreeable about the move to a nursing home, he may nevertheless covertly sabotage it by provoking guilt and ambivalence in other family members. The family's guilt about institutionalizing its elderly may lead to procrastination and indecision. Having to consider a long-term care facility for their aging parent may force the family to recognize their parent's increasing debility, the eventual task of mourning the image of the parent as he once was, and their own eventual aging and death.

Following the elderly parent's admission to a long-term care facility, the family's guilt over having abandoned their elderly member may lead to difficulty in the family's adjustment to this new situation. The family may accuse staff of not caring adequately for their parent's needs. The family may behave toward their parent in an overprotective, solicitous, manner. Rather than working cooperatively with one another, the family and nursing home staff may find themselves on opposing sides. The elderly patient may instigate these disagreements about his care, only to find himself confused and anxious about the disputes. The physician or psychiatrist can help minimize such reactions in the following ways. He helps the family to arrive at a realistic decision concerning institutionalization. He helps the family to understand and work through conflicts which interfere with effecting a realistic treatment plan and encourages the elderly patient to participate, whenever possible, in all decisions regarding his future. Whenever possible, trial visits should precede the transfer to a long-term care facility so that the elderly person is less subject to the trauma which so frequently accompanies relocation.[82,83] Personal possessions, such as photographs, books, and valued objects, should accompany him to his new home. These objects provide a sense of continuity with the past and help to preserve his sense of identity. The family is encouraged to develop a close working relationship with the staff at the facility. Frequent family visits, particularly if they are constructive, are usually encouraged, particularly during the ofttimes difficult period of adjustment. Some families may need counseling before and after their elderly member's admission to a facility in order to understand their feelings and behavior toward the parent and the nursing home staff.

The Surviving Spouse and Family

The death of a family member can place a tremendous stress on the survivors. The suicide rate is highest after divorce or separation, and next highest after widowhood. The risk of suicide is highest during the first year of widowhood and it remains higher than average for at least 5 years.[84] The surviving spouse has to cope not only with the loss, but also with a changed financial and social status. A widow who was dependent on her husband may require assistance in managing financial and other matters. If attractive, she may find herself avoided by her married women friends, and if depressed, she may be avoided by all. Yet a woman may adjust better than a man to the death of a spouse because widowhood usually occurs at a younger age when coping mechanisms are more readily available. A woman is more likely to anticipate widowhood because she has observed the reactions of her widowed women friends and has experienced, perhaps in a more emotional way, the departure of her children from the family home. The surviving widower, whose wife formerly managed all household tasks, may have to learn new skills. The opportunities for remarriage are better for men because of the greater proportion of available women.

The physician helps to educate the surviving family members about what to anticipate with regard to the mourning process. Major decisions, such as a move to a new location, are best deferred until part of the mourning process is completed and the mourners can make realistic plans about the future. The family is reassured that the mourning period is usually time-limited. The family is informed about the availability of voluntary organizations, various self-help groups,[85] and health professionals who can help those requiring further assistance.

GROUP PSYCHOTHERAPY

Group psychotherapy provides the elderly patient with a setting of acceptance and trust to re-establish feelings of worth and self-esteem and become interested, once again, in becoming involved with others. The goals of group therapy vary with the setting in which it takes place, the patients composing the group, and the theoretical orientation and personality of the therapists.

The early workers in the 1950s such as Silver,[86] Linden,[87] Rechtschaffen,[88] and Wolff[89] reported the therapeutic value of group psychotherapy with elderly, regressed institutionalized patients. Linden,[87] utilizing group psychotherapy for 51 institutionalized senile women over a 2-year period, found that 45% were able to be discharged or awaited placement, whereas only 13% of those who did not receive group therapy were able to leave the hospital. Linden concluded, and others[90,91] working in hospital settings have concurred that:

"in a setting of acceptance, interested care, and creative participation, old values regain their importance, hunger for social relationships returns, regression is halted, and an urge to contribute to group cohesion emerges."[92]

There have been fewer reports about group psychotherapy with elderly outpatients, probably because of the practical difficulties involved in assembling six to eight elderly patients at one time. Schwartz and Goodman,[93] conducting outpatient group therapy with 19 obese elderly diabetics, found that 13 were able to lose considerable weight and two were able to discontinue insulin. Butler and Lewis[94] have conducted "age-integrated, life crisis" group therapy. Their groups are composed of patients of different ages who are experiencing a life crisis. Elderly members made unique contributions to other group members by serving as role models for growing older, for dealing with loss and grief, and for their creative use of reminiscing. They believe that psychotherapy groups should be composed of patients of varied ages because heterogeneity minimizes the elderly's sense of isolation and encourages discussion of issues pertinent to the whole range of the life cycle.

Despite these encouraging reports about the value of group therapy for elderly patients, there is a paucity of carefully performed control studies to substantiate its efficacy. After a careful review of the group therapy literature, Eisdorfer and Stotsky concluded:

"It is hard to sort out the more from the less successful programs and to determine the importance of therapist skill and type and mix of patients in achieving successful group experiences."[95]

Group psychotherapy appears to benefit the elderly in at least 10 ways. Group psychotherapy may serve to (1) enhance self-esteem and self-worth; (2) provide information and suggestions for problem solving; (3) encourage socialization; (4) provide contact with therapists who serve also as role models for identification; (5) encourage reality testing and orientation; (6) increase motivation to renew former interests and relationships; (7) supplement the goals of individual and other forms of psychotherapy; (8) provide an opportunity for patients to share and help one another; (9) clarify the patient's diagnosis and prognosis; (10)

clarify and resolve intrapsychic and interpersonal conflicts.

Principal Themes and Issues

The principal issues discussed by elderly patients in outpatient group therapy include: concerns about somatic illness; coping with loss; memories about the past; family conflict; death and dying; and fear and ambivalence about increasing emotional and physical dependency. The universality of these themes enhances group cohesion and sharing.

Case Example

Mr. S., a retired businessman, lamented the recent death of his son. Mrs. R., a depressed widow remarked empathically, "I know what you are going through. I lost my son a few years ago." This was followed by a revival of memories about their sons which provided them and other group members the opportunity to further work through feelings about these and other losses.

Less experienced therapists may tend to view the elderly as more impaired than they really are, resulting in attempts to gratify patients' inappropriate demands for gratification of dependency wishes. This overprotectiveness serves only to reinforce feelings of helplessness, dependency, and impotency. It is usually more therapeutic to support the patients' own ability and resourcefulness to solve his problems.

Case Example

Mrs. H., a 70-year-old dependent, depressed woman with hemiplegia, concluded each session by asking the cotherapists to assist her into her walker. After complying with her request several times, the therapist began encouraging her to try this on her own. She responded angrily at first but her

later accomplishment of this act led to eventual mastery of other more independent behavior.

A major problem in conducting group psychotherapy in an ambulatory care setting is inconsistent attendance because of patients' physical illness, depression, lack of interest, withdrawal, or social uneasiness. Group members may turn to the therapists to solve this problem or they may welcome the increased attention. There are several ways to address this problem. During the preparatory interview before members are selected for the group, the patient's resistances to group therapy are explored and worked through. The importance of regular attendance is emphasized and the patient is encouraged to discuss ambivalent feelings he may have about the group as they arise. If concurrently involved in individual psychotherapy, his individual therapist can support regular attendance and the working through of these resistances. Group pressure also serves as a deterrent to absenteeism. In addition to realistic, unavoidable factors, poor attendance may arise because of interpersonal problems between group members, individual resistances, conflicts between the cotherapists, and other factors. Discontinuity of patient membership is compensated for by the permanency of the therapists.

Transference—Countertransference Issues

The types of transference reactions which develop to the group therapists depend upon patient and group psychodynamics, and the personality of the therapists. In general, elderly patients transfer idealized or ambivalent feelings felt toward their own parents or children. The group setting acts as a catalyst which reactivates issues and conflicts pertinent to each patient's family life. For example, if sibling rivalry had been a problem for a patient in his own family, this may be expressed in the group as competition with other patients for the therapists' attention.

Case Example

Mrs. D., a cantankerous paranoid 70-year-old woman, constantly tried to leave the group when the cotherapists' attention was not on her. She was able to modify her behavior into more socially acceptable means for gaining attention after she understood how rivalrous feelings toward her siblings were reactivated in the group therapy setting.

The manner in which transference distortions are handled is dependent on many factors, including the patient's ego strength, his capacity for insight, the goals of treatment, and group dynamics. Sometimes the patient's idealization of the therapist is best left uninterpreted, because he may derive considerable support by feeling protected by someone he believes to be a protective parental figure.

Typical reactions on the part of the group therapists include overprotectiveness, competition between cotherapists for patients' affection, therapeutic overzealousness, and premature closure of discussion of such issues as death, dying, and sexuality. The therapists' unresolved feelings and conflicts toward parents or grandparents may resurface. The therapists' anxiety when the elderly discuss such issues as death, dying, and sexuality may lead the therapists to covertly discourage these discussions. Reduction of the therapists' anxiety about these issues will facilitate adequate discussion.

Linden[96] reported the many benefits to be derived from cotherapy group leadership. The cotherapy relationship facilitates sharing and clarification of each therapist's observations and interventions, promotes parental transference reactions, and provides the therapist with the support and assistance of a trusted colleague. In an outpatient setting, it is especially helpful if one cotherapist is a social worker who is knowledgeable about community resources for the elderly because coordination of medical, psychological, social and other services ensures continuity of patient care.

In summary, group psychotherapy is a valuable addition to the therapist's armamentarium. It provides both a social and therapeutic setting for elderly patients to re-establish feelings of worth and self-esteem, to share and discover ways to cope with and find restitution for losses, and to find assistance and encouragement to seek new, and re-establish old, relationships. The problem of irregular attendance is countered by careful patient selection and preparation, group pressures, and confrontation of patient resistances. Cotherapy leadership helps to diffuse patients' dependency needs and to share and clarify the therapists' observations and interventions.

OUTPATIENT PHARMACOTHERAPY

Principles and strategies regarding the use of psychopharmacological agents for the geropsychiatric outpatient will be discussed in this section. For a detailed review of specific drugs, the reader is referred to the chapter on the Neuropharmacology of Aging.

The physician is faced with several dilemmas when he considers the use of a psychotropic drug for an elderly patient. The elderly patient often has several chronic illnesses for which he visits different physicians, each of whom may prescribe various medications. Also, he may secretly abuse over-the-counter medication, alcohol, or other drugs. These, in combination with prescribed medication, may contribute to his confusion and anxiety. For example, chronic ingestion of over-the-counter bromides may precipitate an organic brain syndrome. In addition, some elderly patients exert considerable pressure on the physician to prescribe a favored drug. The intricate interplay of medical, psychological, and sociocultural variables make it difficult for the physician to determine the degree that each variable contributes to the patient's symptomatology. The manufacture of new psychotropic agents not only increases the physician's options, but also his uncertainty about which drug to select. The following principles are useful guidelines regarding the use of psychotropic drugs for the elderly.

Before prescribing a psychotropic drug, the physician performs a comprehensive evaluation which includes a review of medical and psychiatric history, current stress factors and use of prescribed and over-the-counter medication, mental status and physical examination, and other tests as indicated. It is especially useful to have the elderly patient or his family bring to the physician all currently used medications because multiple drug usage may be contributing to his symptoms. If the patient is taking psychotropic drugs at the time of this comprehensive evaluation, it is helpful, whenever possible, to discontinue these medications and to reevaluate him during a drug-free baseline period. The psychotropic drugs, alone or in combination with other drugs, may be contributing to his symptoms. Learoyd et al.[97] found that the abnormal behavior of 16% of 236 patients who were receiving psychotropic drugs before admission to a psychogeriatric hospital unit was directly attributable to the drug's deleterious effects.

The comprehensive evaluation may reveal a recent stress, such as a death in the family, which may account for a change in the patient's behavior. The patient's symptoms may therefore respond better to environmental support or psychotherapy than to a major tranquilizer.

Drug selection and dosage is sometimes determined more by the presenting signs and symptoms than by the specific psychiatric syndrome. One psychotropic drug, rather than a combination of such drugs, should be used to minimize side effects and to evaluate its effectiveness. It is best to select a psychotropic drug which has withstood the test of time and with which the physician has the most knowledge and experience. The dosage should be individualized. In general, with most psychotropic drugs, one begins usually with a quarter to one-third of the initial dose prescribed to healthy adults, with gradual increments based on the clinical response and the development of side effects. For debilitated patients, the initial dose may be even less. When prescribing drugs to an elderly patient, both he and his family should be instructed about their use and side effects.

Most psychotropic drugs should be given in equally divided doses three or four times over a 24-hour period because elderly patients may be intolerant of a sudden rise in drug blood level resulting from one large daily dose. There should be careful monitoring for changes in blood pressure, pulse, and other side effects. For patients with insomnia, however, giving the major portion of a tranquilizer or antidepressant at bedtime takes advantage of its sedating and soporific effect. Liquid preparations are useful for elderly patients who cannot swallow tablets, or who refuse to do so.

The patient should be reassessed at frequent intervals to determine the need for maintenance medication, changes in dosage, and development of side effects. An antiparkinsonian drug to counteract extrapyramidal side effects of a major tranquilizer should be used only as needed and not prophylactically. It may further aggravate the anticholinergic side effects of the major tranquilizer and other medications. If an antiparkinsonian drug is used, Fann and Lake[98] recommend that it be discontinued on a trial basis after 4 to 6 weeks since only 18 to 20% of patients whose antiparkinsonian drug is discontinued will have a recurrence of extrapyramidal side effects. If extrapyramidal side effects are mild, decreasing the dosage of the neuroleptic may circumvent the need for an antiparkinsonian drug.

If a major tranquilizer is indicated for such symptoms as agitation, delusions or hallucinations, it is best to choose a drug which is least likely to further aggravate concurrent medical problems. For example, an elderly psychotic patient whose cardiovascular system is impaired may be particularly sensitive to the hypotensive side effect of a phenothiazine drug such as chlorpromazine. Haloperidol, because it produces less hypotension and sedation, may be preferable for this patient. A phenothiazine, rather than haloperidol, is preferable for the elderly patient who has difficulty in motor coordination because haloperidol produces more extrapyramidal side effects.[99] Most of the major tranquilizers, particularly when used in high dosages, can exacerbate psychotic symptoms and confusion, leading the physician erroneously to prescribe still higher doses of the offending medication. When in doubt, a trial discontinuation of the medication in question may not only clarify, but may also ameliorate, the problem.

The elderly person, particularly if he has organic brain disease, is especially susceptible to the side effects of the major tranquilizers. Although discussed in the chapter on the Neuropharmacology of Aging, two particularly distressing side effects merit discussion here. The first, tardive dyskinesia, is characterized by disfiguring, involuntary buccal and lingual maticatory movements. Akathesia, choreaform body movements, and rhythmic extension and flexion movements of the fingers may also be present. Examination of the patient's protruded tongue for fine tremors and vermicular movements is a useful diagnostic procedure. More common in elderly women than men, tardive dyskinesia occurs most typically in patients who have taken high doses of neurotropics over a long period of time, but it can also occur soon after such drugs are initiated. The condition may persist or even worsen after discontinuation of the offending drug and continued treatment may mask or reduce the symptoms.[100] At present, there is no definitive treatment. Preventive measures include the use of minimum dosages of neuroleptics, frequent reevaluation of the need for maintenance treatment, drug holidays, immediate withdrawal of the offending medication after the appearance of this side effect, and avoidance of the injudicious use of antiparkinsonian agents.

A second distressing side effect of psychotropic drugs is a toxic confusional state resulting from the anticholinergic properties of a single or a combination of psychotropic drugs with an antiparkinsonian drug or a tricyclic antidepressant.[101] Also referred to as the "central anticholinergic syndrome" or atropine psychosis, it is characterized by a marked disturbance in short-term memory, impaired attention, disorientation, anxiety, visual and auditory hallucinations, increased psychotic thinking, and peripheral anticholinergic side effects. The syndrome is sometimes difficult to recognize, particularly in patients who are psychotic, confused, and agitated before they develop this side effect. Its onset may be signaled by a worsening of the preexisting psychosis or by the addition of toxic symptoms to the existing psychotic symptomatology. The syndrome may be attributed incorrectly to a worsening of the psychosis, which leads the physician to increase the medication, resulting in a predictable increase of the symptoms. The anticholinergic properties of the antiparkinsonian agent may be a major causative factor. Since many elderly patients receiving a neuroleptic and an antiparkinsonian drug may no longer require the latter, the most efficacious treatment may be to discontinue the antiparkinsonian drug and/or to reduce or discontinue the neuroleptic. The confusional state will usually clear within one or two days after discontinuation of the offending drug(s).

The elderly patient with mild to moderate anxiety may be a candidate for a mild tranquilizer. The effective dosage is usually less than in adult patients. Chlordiazepoxide or diazepam, in doses of 5 to 10 mg bid or t.i.d., is often effective. A mild tranquilizer can also be used at bedtime for its hypnotic effect. Compared to the barbituates, the minor tranquilizers have a higher ratio of therapeutic effectiveness to side effects and are considered safer. However, the minor tranquilizers, although to a lesser extent than the barbituates, can also be addictive and can produce paradoxical reactions characterized by confusion, disorientation, excitement, and exacerbation of psychiatric symptoms.

Depression is the most common psychiatric disorder of the elderly. Elderly white men have the highest suicide rate of any age group. Reactive depressions are fairly common among the elderly and are generally responsive to psychotherapy. Depression is a frequent concomitant of dementia and may cause the patient to appear more cognitively impaired than he actually is. Treatment of the concomitant depression may result in a significant improvement in the patient's cognitive deficit and overall clinical state, particularly if the apparent cognitive deficit was aggravated by the depression.[102] As with the use of other psychotropic drugs in the elderly, it is best to begin with lower doses of an antidepressant and then gradually increase the dose to therapeutic levels. The tricyclic antidepressants, such as amitriptyline and imipramine, can be used in initial doses of 20 to 50 mg/day and gradually increased according to patient response and the development of side effects. Doxepin is believed by some to be the safest tricyclic antidepressant to use in patients with heart disease because it is least cardiotoxic. However, careful cardiac monitoring is nevertheless mandatory. The tricyclic antidepressants, like other psychotropic drugs, have more side effects in older than in younger patients. These include anticholinergic side effects, exacerbation of psychotic symptoms, parkinsonism and tremors, the central anticholinergic syndrome, cardiotoxicity, and others. There is considerable variability among elderly patients with regard to the optimal dosage and the development of side effects. Patients unresponsive to one tricyclic antidepressant may respond to another. If a patient is still significantly depressed despite psychotherapy and a trial with antidepressants, hospitalization should be considered. In the hospital, a monoamine oxidase inhibitor such as phenelzine or electroconvulsive therapy may be considered.

In summary, psychotropic drugs are an important addition to the physician's armamentarium in the treatment of psychiatric disorders of the elderly. However, the advent of any new and successful mode of treatment sometimes results in its overutilization and its use as a substitute for other modalities of treatment. These drugs should be viewed as only one component of a comprehensive, multi-dimensional approach to the elderly patient. A comprehensive evaluation should precede their use followed by frequent evaluations for detection of side effects and dosage regulation. Drug selection and use should be based on the physician's understanding of concurrent medical problems, the etiology and psychodynamics of the presenting symptomatology, the drug's side effects and pharmacokinetics, and knowledge of the special way in which the elderly respond to these drugs. The physician's ability to develop a trusting therapeutic relationship with the patient and his family will augment patient cooperation and possibly improve his responsiveness to these drugs.

CONCLUSION

Psychiatric treatment of the elderly patient and his family in the ambulatory care setting is a challenging and rewarding task for the primary physician and the psychiatrist. The carefully performed, comprehensive clinical evaluation serves as the cornerstone of this process.

Early detection of psychiatric and medical disorders may prevent chronicity and refractoriness to treatment. The physician's diagnostic skill and acumen is challenged as he attempts to unravel the delicate and intricate interplay of biological, psychological, and sociocultural variables which contribute to the patient's symptomatology. To accomplish this comprehensive evaluation, the physician gathers information from various sources—the patient, his family, other physicians and health professionals, and agencies. With the patient's permission, the physician's findings and treatment recommendations are shared with other health professionals who are involved in the patient's care. All health professionals should understand who is primarily responsible for coordinating the efforts of all. Proper coordination of care reduces the possibility of mismanagement resulting from overmedication and other problems associated with miscommunication among health professionals.

The psychotherapist who works with the elderly patient must be knowledgeable about the developmental tasks and challenges of the last phase of the life cycle. The therapist conveys to the patient, both verbally and nonverbally, his respect, interest, and availability. The therapist understands that his patient's varying, uneven course may necessitate different forms of therapeutic intervention at different stages of treatment. The therapist may function at one point as an individual therapist, and as family therapist or pharmacotherapist at another time. The treatment goals are carefully and realistically tailored to the patient's current capabilities and deficits so that both patient and therapist avoid the frustration and disappointment resulting from unrealistic goals.

Most elderly patients require more supportive forms of psychotherapy which require the therapist to be active, directive, and involved with the patient in a real and meaningful way. The patient's tendency to idealize the therapist should not be mistaken for defended hostility. Some patients may need to feel secure and protected by having some control over someone perceived to be an omnipotent, parentlike figure. As treatment comes to a close, the elderly patient is reassured that the therapist continues to be available should he require further assistance in the future. Psychotherapy with the elderly patient provides the therapist with the opportunity to learn about different adaptations and maladaptations to the aging process, the joys and sorrows associated with this stage of the life cycle and the opportunities for continued growth. The elderly have a lifetime of experience and knowledge to teach us. Our interest and curiosity about what they have to say provides patient and therapist alike with a mutually rewarding relationship.

REFERENCES

1. Meissner, W. W. Normal psychology of the aging process, revisited—I, Discussion, Presented at the 15th anniversary annual scientific meeting of the Boston Society of Gerontologic Psychiatry, Nov. 1, 1975.

2. Erickson, E. H. The human life cycle, In *International Encyclopedia of the Social Sciences,* New York: Macmillan, 1968.

3. Cath, S. H. Functional disorders: An organismic view and attempt at reclassification, In L. Bellak and T. B. Karasu, (eds.) *Geriatric Psychiatry—A Handbook for the Psychiatry and Primary Care Physician,* New York: Grune and Stratton, 1976.

4. Post, F. *The Clinical Psychiatry of Late Life,* Pergamon Press, London, 1965.

5. Cumming, E. and Henry, W. E. *Growing Old—The Process of Disengagement,* New York: Basic Books, 1961.

6. Butler, R. The life review: An interpretation of reminiscense in the aged, *Psychiat.* 26: 65-76 (1963).

7. Shanas, E. The unmarried old person in the United States: Living arrangements and care in illness, myth and fact. Presented at the International Social Science Research Seminar in Gerontology, Markaryd, Sweden, August, 1963.

8. Sussman, M. B. Relationships of adult children with their parents in the United States, In E. Shanas, G. F. Streib, (eds.) *Social Structure and the Family: Generational Relationships,* Englewood Cliffs, N. J.: Prentice-Hall, 1965.

9. Butler, R. N. and Lewis, M. I. *Aging and Mental Health, Positive Psychosocial Approaches,* St. Louis: C. V. Mosby, p. 107, 1973.

10. Benedek, T., Parenthood during the life cycle, In E. J. Antony, (ed.) *Parenthood,* Boston: Little Brown, p. 201, 1970.

11. Karasu, T. B. and Waltzman, S. A. Death and dying in the aged, In L. Bellak and T. B. Karasu, (eds.) *Geriatric Psychiatry—A Handbook for Psychiatrist and Primary Care Physician,* New York: Grune and Stratton, 1972.

12. Blenkner M. Social work and family relationships in later life with some thoughts on filial maturity, In E. Shanas, and G. F. Streib, (eds.), *Social Structure and the Family: Generational Relations,* Englewood Cliffs, N. J.: Prentice-Hall, 1965.

13. Butler, R. N. The effects of medical and health progress on the social and economic aspects of the life cycle, *Industrial Geront.* 1: 1-9 (1969).

14. Palmore, E. Gerontophobia versus ageism. *The Gerontologist,* 12: 213 (1972).

15. Gallagher, E. B., Sharaf, M. R. and Levinson, D. J. The influence of patient and therapist in determining the use of psychotherapy in a hospital setting, *Psychiat.,* 28: 297-310 (1965).

16. Finkel, S. Geriatric psychiatry training for the general psychiatric resident, *Am. J. Psychiat.* 135: 101-103 (1978).

17. Gibson, R. W. Insurance coverage for treatment of mental illness in later life, In E. W. Busse, and E. Pfeiffer, (eds.), Mental Illness in Later Life,

American Psychiatric Association, Washington, D.C., 1973.

18. Karasu, T. B. and Waltzman, S. A. Death and dying in the aged, *Geriatric Psychiatry—A Handbook for Psychiatrist and Primary Care Physician, op. cit.,* p. 252.

19. Osfelt, A. Frequency and nature of problems of retired persons, In F. M. Corp, (ed.) *Retirement Process,* Wash., D.C., U.S. Public Health Service Publication, No. 1778, 1968.

20. Zinberg, N. E., Special problems of gerontologic psychiatry, In M. A. Berezin, and S. H. Cath, (eds.) *Geriatric Psychiatry,* New York: International University Press, 1965.

21. Butler, R. N. Psychiatric evaluation of the aged, *Geriatrics,* **18:** 220–232 (1963).

22. Oberleider, M. Psychotherapy with the aging: An art of the possible, *Psychotherapy: Theory, Research, and Practice,* **3:** 139–142 (1966).

23. Feigenbaum, E. Ambulatory treatment of the elderly, In E. W. Busse, and E. Pfeiffer, (eds.) *Mental Illness in Later Life,* American Psychiatric Association, Washington, D. C., 1973.

24. Eisdorfer, C. and Stotsky, B. A. Intervention, treatment, and rehabilitation of psychiatric disorders, In J. E. Birren, and K. W. Schaie, (eds.), *The Handbook of the Psychology of Aging,* New York: Van Nostrand Reinhold, pp. 724–748, 1977.

25. Arnhoff, F. and Kumbar, A. The nation's psychiatrists—1970 survey, Washington, D. C.: American Psychiatric Association, 1970.

26. Gurel, L. A survey of academic resources in psychiatric residency training, Washington, D. C.: American Psychiatric Association, 1973.

27. Simon, A. and Lowenthal, M. F. *Crisis and Intervention: The Fate of the Elderly Mental Patient,* San Francisco: Jossey-Bass, 1970.

28. Butler, R. N. and Lewis, M. I. How to keep people at home, In R. N. Butler, and M. I. Lewis (eds.) *Aging and Mental Health, Positive Psychosocial Approaches,* St. Louis: C. V. Mosby pp. 186–207, 1973.

29. Martin, L. J. and deGrunchy, C. *Salvaging Old Age,* New York: Macmillan, 1930.

30. Martin, L. J. and deGrunchy, C. *Sweeping the Cobwebs,* New York: Macmillan, 1933.

31. Martin, L. J. A Handbook for Old Age Counsellors, San Francisco: Geertz Printing, 1944.

32. Freud, S. On psychotherapy, *Collected Papers,* Vol. I, London: Hogarth Press, pp. 249–261, 1924.

33. Freud, S. Sexuality in the aetiology of the neuroses, *Collected Papers,* Vol. I, London: Hogarth Press, pp. 220–248, 1924.

34. Abraham, K. The applicability of psychoanalytic treatment to patients at an advanced age, *Selected Papers on Psychoanalysis,* London: Hogarth Press, pp. 312–317, 1949.

35. Kaufman, M. R. Psychoanalyses in late life depressions, *Psychanal. Quart.,* **6:** 308–335 (1937).

36. Jellifee, S. E. The old age factor in psychoanalytic therapy, *Med. J. Rec.,* **121:** 7–12 (1925).

37. Grotjahn, M. Psychoanalytic investigation of a seventy-one-year-old man with senile dementia, *Psychoanal. Quart.,* **9:** 80–97 (1940).

38. Wayne, G. J. Modified psychoanalytic therapy in senescence, *Psychoanal. Rev.,* **40:** 99–116 (1953).

39. Alexander, F. G. and French, T. M. *Psychoanalytic Therapy: Principles and Applications,* New York: Ronald Press, 1946.

40. Grotjahn M., Analytic psychotherapy with the elderly, *Psychoanal. Rev.,* **42:** 419–427 (1955).

41. Meerlo, J. A. M. Psychotherapy with elderly people, *Geriatrics,* **10:** 583–587 (1955).

42. Weinberg, J. Psychiatric techniques in the treatment of older people, In W. Donahue, and C. Tibbits, (eds.), *Growing in the Later Years,* Ann Arbor: University of Michigan Press, 1951.

43. Hollender, M. H. Individualizing the aged, *Soc. Casework,* **33:** 337–342 (1952).

44. Wayne, G. J. Modified psychoanalytic therapy in senescence, *Psychoanal. Rev.,* **40:** 99–116 (1953).

45. Goldfarb, A. I. and Turner, H. Psychotherapy of aged persons. Utilization and effectiveness of brief therapy, *Am. J. Psychiat.,* **109:** 916–921 (1953).

46. Linden, M. E. Group psychotherapy with institutionalized senile women: Study in gerontologic human relations, *Int. J. Group Psychother.,* **3:** 150–170 (1953).

47. Rechtschaffen, A. Psychotherapy with geriatric patients: A review of the literature, *J. of Gerontology,* **14:** 73–84 (1959).

48. Freud, S. On narcissism: An introduction, *The Standard Edition,* Vol. 14, London: Hogarth Press, pp. 67–105 (1914).

49. Freud, S. Mourning and melancholia, *The Standard Edition,* Vol. 14, London: Hogarth Press, pp. 237–259, 1917.

50. Mahler, M. S., On child psychosis and schizophrenia: Autistic and symbiotic infantile psychosis, *Am. J. Psychoanal. Assoc.,* **7:** 286, (1952).

51. Bibring, E. The mechanism of depression, In P. Greenacre, (ed.) *Affective Disorders,* New York: International Universities Press, 1953.

52. Reich, A. Pathological forms of self-esteem regulation, *Am. J. Psychoanal. Assoc.* **15:** 215–232 (1960).

53. Goldberg, A. Narcissism and the readiness for psychotherapy termination, *Arch. Gen. Psychiat.,* **32:** 695–699 (1975).

54. Kohut, H., Forms and transformations of narcissism, *Amer. J. Psychoanal. Assoc.,* **14:** 243–272 (1966).

55. Kohut, H. The psychoanalytic treatment of nar-

cissistic personality disturbances, *Psychoanal. Study of the Child,* **23:** 86–113 (1968).

56. Kohut, H. Thoughts on narcissism and narcissistic rage, *Psychoanal. Study of the Child,* **27:** 360–400 (1972).

57. Kohut, H. *The Analysis of the Self,* New York: International Universities Press, 1971.

58. Kohut, H. Forms and transformations of narcissism, *op. cit.,* pp. 368–369.

59. *Ibid,* p. 244.

60. Goldberg, A. Psychotherapy of narcissistic injuries, *Arch. Gen. Psychiat.,* **28:** 722–726 (1973).

61. Horowitz, M. Stress Response Syndromes, New York: Jason Aronson, pp. 170–185, 1976.

62. Muslin, H. and Epstein, L. J. Personal communication.

63. Meissner, W. W. Normal psychology of the aging process, revisited—I, Discussion, *op. cit.,* pp. 156–157.

64. Kohut, H. Thoughts on narcissism and narcissistic rage, *op. cit.,* p. 383.

65. Meerlo, J. A. M. Modes of psychotherapy in the aged, *J. Amer. Geriat. Society,* **9:** 225–234, 1961.

66. Butler, R. N. and Lewis, M. I. *Aging and Mental Health—Positive Psychosocial Approaches, op. cit.,* p. 233.

67. Meerlo, J. A. M. Modes of psychotherapy in the aged, *op. cit.* p. 227.

68. Pearson, L. Opportunities for psychotherapy with the aging, Presented at the American Psychological Association, Chicago, September, 1955.

69. Meerlo, J. A. M. Modes of psychotherapy in the elderly, *op. cit.,* p. 233.

70. Satir, V., *Conjoint Family Therapy,* Palo Alto: Science and Behavior Books, 1964.

71. Bowen, M., The use of family theory in clinical practice, *Compr. Psychiatry* **7:** 345 (1966).

72. Weiner, N. *Cybernetics,* New York: John Wiley, 1948.

73. Jackson, D. D. The question of family homeostasis, *Psychiatry,* **31:** 79 (1957).

74. Haley, J. The perverse triangle, In G. Zuk, and Boszormenyi-Nagy, (eds.) *Family Therapy and Disturbed Families,* Palo Alto: Science and Behavior Books, 1967.

75. Haley, J. *Uncommon Therapy,* New York: W. W. Norton, 1973.

76. Weinberg, J. Interpersonal relations in multigeneration families, In W. Donahue, J. L. Kornbluh, and L. Power, (eds.) *Living in the Multigeneration Family,* Ann Arbor: The University of Michigan—Wayne State University, pp. 52–59, 1969.

77. La Barre, M. B., Jessner, L. and Ussery, L. The significance of grandmothers in the psychopathology of children, *Am. J. Orthopsychiatry,* **30:** 175–185 (1960).

78. Sanford, J. R. A. Tolerance of debility in elderly dependents by supporters at home: its significance for hospital practice, *Brit. Med. J.,* **3:** 471–473 (1975).

79. Cath, S. H. The geriatric patient and his family. The institutionalization of a parent—a nadir of life. *J. Geriat. Psych.* **5:** 1 (1972).

80. Weinberg, J. What do I say to my mother when I have nothing to say? *Geriatrics,* **29:** 11 (1974).

81. Sussman, M. B. The family life of old people, In R. H. Binstock, and E. Shanas, (eds.) *Handbook of Aging and the Social Sciences,* New York: Van Nostrand Reinhold, pp. 218–243, 1976.

82. Aldrich, C. K. and Mendkoff, E. Relocation of the aged and disabled: a mortality study, *J. Am. Geriatr. Soc.,* **11:** 185–194 (1963).

83. Lieberman, M. A. Relationship of mortality rates to entrance to a home for the aged, *Geriatrics,* **16:** 575–579 (1961).

84. Bunch, J., Recent bereavement and suicide, *J. Psychosom. Res.,* **163:** 361 (1972).

85. Silverman, P. R. The widow-to-widow program, *Arch. of the Foundation of Thanatology,* **2:** 133–135 (1970).

86. Silver, A. Group psychotherapy with senile psychotic patients, *Geriatrics,* **5:** 147–150 (1950).

87. Linden, M. Group psychotherapy with institutionalized senile women: studies in gerontologic human relations, *Inter. J. Group Psychother.,* **3:** 150–170 (1953).

88. Rechtschaffen, A. Intensive treatment program for state hospital geriatric patients, *Geriatrics,* **9:** 28–34 (1954).

89. Wolff, K., Group psychotherapy with geriatric patients in a mental hospital. *J. Am. Geriatrics Soc.,* **5:** 13–19 (1957).

90. Lazarus, L. W. A program for the elderly in a private psychiatric hospital, *The Gerontologist,* **16:** 125–131 (1976).

91. Oradei, D. and Waite, N. Group psychotherapy with stroke patients during the immediate recovery phase, *Am. J. Orthopsychiat.,* **44:** 386–395 (1974).

92. Linden, M. Group psychotherapy with institutionalized senile women: studies in gerontologic human relations, *op. cit.,* p. 169.

93. Schwartz, E. and Goodman, J., Group therapy of obesity in elderly diabetics, Geriatrics, **7:** 280–283 (1952).

94. Butler, R. N. and Lewis, M. I. *Aging and Mental Health—Positive Psychosocial Approaches, op. cit.,* pp. 238–239.

95. Eisdorfer, C. and Stotsky, B. A. Intervention, treatment, and rehabilitation of psychiatric disorders, *The Handbook of the Psychology of Aging, op. cit.,* p. 734.

96. Linden, M. The significance of dual leadership in gerontological group psychotherapy. Studies in gerontologic human relations. *Int. J. of Group Psychother.,* **4:** 262–273 (1954).

97. Learoyd, B. M. Psychotropic drugs in the aging patient, *Med. J. Aust.,* **1:** 1131–1133 (1972).

98. Fann, F. E. and Lake, C. R. Drug-induced movement disorders in the elderly: an appraisal of treatment, In W. E. Fann, and G. L. Maddox, (eds.) *Drug Issues in Geropsychiatry,* Baltimore: Williams and Wilkins, pp. 41–48, 1974.

99. Salzman, C., Kolk, B. V. and Shader, R. I., Psychopharmacology and the geriatric patient, In R. I. Shader, (ed.) *Manual of Psychiatric Therapeutics,* Boston: Little, Brown, pp. 171–184, 1975.

100. Fann, W. E., Davis, J. M., Wilson, I. C. and Lake, C. R. Attempts of pharmacological management of tardive dyskinesia, In *Psychopharmacology and Aging, Advances in Behavioral Biology,* London: Plenum Press, pp. 89–96, 1973.

101. Davis, J. M., Fann, W. E., El-Yousef, M. K. and Janowsky, D., Clinical problems in treating the aged with psychotropic drugs. *Psychopharmacology and Aging, Advances in Behavioral Biology,* London: Plenum Press, pp. 111–125, 1973.

102. Folstein, M. P., Folstein, S. E., and McHugh, P. R., Mini-mental state. A practical method for grading the cognitive state of patients for the clinician, *J. Psychiat. Res.,* **12:** 189–198 (1975).

Chapter 21
Treatment Within The Institution

Alan D. Whanger, M.D.

Duke University Medical Center

INTRODUCTION

Utilization of the Institution for the treatment of Mental Illness

Until recently institutionalization, usually in a state mental hospital, was virtually the only alternative for the aged patient with psychiatric problems who could not be cared for at home. Philosophical and economic considerations have led to a greater emphasis on community services for mental health care, and to a transfer of patients out of state mental hospitals to the community and to other institutions such as nursing homes. Between 1969 and 1973, the population of elderly patients in state mental hospitals declined by 40%.[1] Although mental illness can be treated in settings other than institutions, and the mere fact of institutionalization certainly does not guarantee that treatment is taking place, it is important that neither the state mental hospital, its newer community alternatives, nor nursing homes, be utilized without careful and continuing attention to the needs of the patient population. Elderly patients

with mental disorders are not uncommonly placed in a particular type of institution as a matter of convenience rather than as a therapeutic measure,[2] and it is increasingly true that those who once would have had no viable alternative to the state mental hospital now have no viable alternative to the nursing home.[3] The treatment of mental illness is not a generally recognized function of the nursing home as an institution, however. Stotsky found diagnosable psychoses in over half of nursing home patients without a psychiatric history.[4] Our own studies confirmed the impression of others that over 80% of those elderly in nursing care facilities have diagnosable psychiatric problems.[5] This finding may be interpreted either as an indication of the suitability of nursing home care for psychiatric patients or more likely as an index to the need for increased mental health services. Sherr and Goffi found that preventive and therapeutic psychiatric care within a nursing home setting was an effective and economical approach for both the patients and the home.[6] Kahn notes that the modern trends in development of community psychiatric services have led to many elderly patients "dropping out" of the psychiatric system altogether rather than receiving improved care.[7]

A continuing increase in the quality and quantity of community facilities and services for elderly persons is desirable, but even with ideal community programs, institutions could still appropriately provide useful and important services. Butler recommends the use of general and psychiatric hospitals for emergency and short-term psychiatric care.[1] State and county mental hospitals could provide active therapeutic programs for those patients requiring long-term care.

History of Institutional Care

Prior to the seventeenth century, families or religious institutions assumed primary responsibility for the care of the physically or mentally infirm elderly. Governmental and secular involvement in caring for the elderly began with King Henry VIII in England when he, for his own personal reasons, demolished the monasteries and the systems of care in the churches.[8] The Poor Relief Act, which was passed in England in 1601, imposed a tax to establish almshouses and workhouses for custodial care of the poor, including the elderly.[9,10,11] The Salpêtrière in France, originally established for elderly indigents, was admitting increasing numbers of psychiatric patients by 1790 under the direction of Pinel. Treatment was based on environmental manipulation, exercise, and nursing care.[12] During the early 1800s several small, humane, and quite effective mental hospitals were established in Britain and the United States.[13] In later years, the great numbers of immigrants to the United States led to an increase in the population of mentally ill poor beyond the capacity of small town hospitals. Large state hospitals proliferated, becoming convenient but overcrowded, understaffed, and hardly therapeutic warehouses for the mentally ill. These hospitals were often used for permanent and terminal care of the elderly, and

many persons still perceive them as places to die.[14] In Great Britain, the workhouses adopted the principle of "lesser eligibility" in making the conditions therein worse and therefore less appealing than any outside, and this system prevailed until 1948 when the development of the National Health Service occurred, and the specialty of Geriatrics was begun as described by Brocklehurst.[8] The state mental hospital population in the United States peaked in 1955, at 558,922, and has been declining steadily since.[15] Between 1963 and 1969 the resident population in American nursing care homes increased from 505,000 to 895,000. Mental hospitals are again becoming treatment centers for psychiatric disorders, and pessimism about the possibility of effective therapeutic intervention for aged psychiatric patients is less prevalent.

Types of Facilities Available

The types of institutions in which elderly patients with psychiatric problems are commonly placed include general hospitals, psychiatric hospitals, nursing homes, and boarding care facilities. General hospitals may contain psychiatric units, suitable for the treatment of active mental illness and problems correctable within a brief period; private mental hospitals may serve similar functions.[16] Public psychiatric hospitals care for many patients, both those with long-standing illness who have grown old in the hospitals and those whose psychiatric disturbance began late in life.[17] Feder and Junod describe a geriatric hospital in Switzerland which integrates physical and psychiatric care in its basic treatment concepts,[18] but such facilities are generally unavailable in the United States. Nursing homes, both skilled care and intermediate care, contain increasing numbers of psychiatric patients. Although specialized psychiatric care is infrequently provided in nursing homes, Colthart outlines the functioning of a mental health unit in a skilled nursing home, and reports that one-third of the patients are able to function more independently as a result of treatment.[19]

Day hospitals and day care centers, which are more widely available in Britain than in the United States, provide semiinstitutional care for patients not requiring continuous care in a hospital. Day hospitals furnish diagnostic and minor treatment services, and therapeutic, social, and recreational activities.[20,21] Psychogeriatric day care may be included as an aspect of a psychiatric hospital, or may be privately managed.[22,23] Psychiatric day hospital care may ease the transition from hospital to community for some patients and may provide a short-term alternative to other forms of treatment for some; however, most participants have chronic psychiatric disabilities requiring long-term supportive care. This form of care is useful particularly for those with behavioral problems induced by organic brain impairment and for those with chronic or intermittent functional disorders.[24]

Other facilities accepting persons with psychiatric problems include board-and-care facilities, foster care homes, and congregate housing facilities. These are most appropriate for patients whose illness is stabilized or in remission.[3,16]

Admission Factors

Predisposing and Precipitating Factors. If the findings of Kay, Beamish, and Roth apply to the United States as well as to Britain, a minority of elderly persons with organic or functional psychiatric disorders are receiving institutional care.[25] In general terms, combined physical and mental disabilities and lack of access to personal or community supportive services predispose to institutionalization.[26] Among the aged factors associated with increased chance of admission to an institution include living alone, singleness or separation from spouse, and few or no living children; blacks, and the poor have lower rates of institutionalization than those in higher economic groups.[27]

In most cases, identifiable events precede and precipitate admission. Potentially harmful behavior such as self-neglect or wandering precipitates admission in about one-third of the cases; about one-fifth display actually harmful behavior such as heavy drinking, fire setting, violence, or refusing medical care. Environmental factors such as depletion of funds, loss of a caretaker, or a physician's recommendation lead to about 23% of admissions. Depression, delusion, incoherence, and other disturbances of thought or feeling precipitate about 13% of admissions, and about a tenth result from physical factors such as strokes, falls, malnutrition, or feebleness.[28,29]

Criteria for Institutionalization. For maximum benefit to the individual and most effective use of the institution it is helpful to utilize general criteria to distinguish between appropriate and inappropriate admissions. Patients with the following characteristics might appropriately receive treatment at a state mental hospital or other institution providing psychiatric care for the aged.[30,16,31]

1. Those who are dangerous to themselves or others, and are actually capable of carrying out destructive behavior.

2. Those with organic brain disease whose usual behavior such as fire setting, escaping, or attacking others is intractable to medication and is too disturbing to be managed at home or in a less restrictive facility.

3. Those with chronic brain syndrome during periods of restlessness and agitation caused by stress.

4. Those with moderate organic brain syndrome who are likely to improve with active treatment in a controlled environment.

5. Those with functional psychoses for whom out-patient care is not feasible.

6. Those with chronic psychoses who require periodic medication readjustments not possible or practical on an out-patient basis.

7. Alcoholics and drug abusers needing in-patient detoxification and subsequent rehabilitation.

8. Medically ill persons with significant reversible psychiatric disorders who do not

have access to psychiatric services within a general hospital.

Those who are comatose, moribund, or acutely ill physically; those with minor mental symptoms related to medical problems; those with mild organic mental impairment; and those who need only adequate living arrangements with some support services would be clearly inappropriate admissions to psychiatric institutions.

Diagnostic Categories. Psychiatric diagnosis of the elderly patient is frequently complicated by coexisting physical disease, multiple psychiatric disorders, family and socioeconomic difficulties, and the tendency to attribute all problems to senility. Some apparent psychiatric disorders result from unrecognized major medical illness.[32] While figures vary, among aged patients in public psychiatric hospitals, about 50% have been diagnosed as having organic brain syndrome, 42% have functional psychoses, 2% have neuroses, and 4% have various other diagnoses. Organic brain syndromes are more frequent among the new admissions, where they represent 72% of the patients, than among patients who have grown old in the hospital, where they represent 45%.[33,34,35] Among the aged in psychiatric wards of general hospitals and in private psychiatric hospitals, about 46% have organic brain syndrome, 18% have functional psychoses and 26% have neurotic disorders.

These averaged percentages have applied to the United States, but different prevalence rates have been noted elsewhere, as in Britain. It is not certain to what extent this represents differences in actual prevalence, differences in diagnostic criteria, differences in utilization of institutions, or other factors.[36,37]

Preadmission Screening Programs. Prehospitalization screening teams evaluate the need for psychiatric hospital care, and may also assist patient and family to find alternate arrangements when this seems more suitable.[38,39] Such teams, most effective when composed of a psychiatric nurse, a social worker, and a psychiatrist, should evaluate the prospective patient at home when possible. The home environment provides a valuable opportunity for realistic assessment of physical and social conditions and family interaction patterns. Wolff studied 105 elderly persons proposed for state mental hospital admission, and found after screening that only 47% required such hospitalization, while 23% were sent to nursing care facilities and 30% were returned to their family, often with outpatient treatment.[40] The preadmission screening visit can be a time to help ease the transition by informing the patient what to expect in the way of surroundings and treatment. This may help reduce the shock of hospitalization or institutionalization, and enhance the effectiveness of the treatment program.[31]

Matching Patient and Facility. Lack of clear admitting criteria, inaccurate diagnoses, lack of prescreening programs, and patterns of availability of beds contribute to the frequent placement of aged patients in less than optimal surroundings. The decision between a psychiatric and a medical ward present particular difficulties. Various studies have shown mixed illness to be quite common among the elderly, with as much as 65% of the psychiatric patients having physical illness and 63% of the physically ill patients having psychiatric disorders.[41] Kidd classified elderly patients according to their predominant problem, and found that 24% of those in a psychiatric setting had predominantly medical problems and 34% of those in a medical service had mainly psychiatric problems. Those who were over 75 years of age, the single or widowed patients, and those of a low socioeconomic status were most likely to be inappropriately placed. Consequences of misplacement included prolonged hospitalization, increased mortality rate, increased incontinence, restlessness, disorientation, immobility, and reduced staff efficiency.[42,43]

Geropsychiatric patients who are assaultive, threatening, noisy, destructive, negativistic, and prone to wandering are generally not suitable for nursing home placement,[15] although some nursing home facilities satisfactorily manage very disturbed patients.

TREATMENT MODALITIES FOR THE INSTITUTIONALIZED ELDERLY PSYCHIATRIC PATIENT

Milieu Therapy and the Therapeutic Community

In recent years increasing attention has been focused on the impact of the social milieu on the patient. The concept of the therapeutic community was developed by Maxwell Jones, and numerous programs applying this conceptual framework have been implemented.[44] The most extensive research in the United States on the effects of the therapeutic community on the geropsychiatric patient probably comes from Gottesman, Coons, and their group at the University of Michigan. Traditional care is seen as detrimental in that patients are expected to be sick and to fulfill a passive role. The lack of demands on the patient often leads to deterioration of ego skills and regression, and does not provide for the learning of new skills.[45] Milieu therapy is a treatment mode based on the principle that all elements of the environment, including the staff, the patients, the treatment program, and the physical environment, should be used as therapeutic agents. The therapeutic community is the setting in which milieu therapy takes place. Staff relate to patients as therapists and teachers, and patients are provided opportunities to assume the normal social roles of friend, consumer, worker, and citizen. They participate in ward planning, operate ward stores, and perform contract work for pay in workshops. Activities are broken down into a structured series of steps allowing the patient to advance to progressively more difficult or complex tasks as he succeeds at initial levels. The sexes are mixed on the wards and patients wear their own clothes. The physical environment is designed to encourage socialization and self-management, and to provide for privacy.[46,47,48]

Investigators such as Risdorfer, Goldstein, and Grauer have applied milieu therapy techniques with good results, although difficulties were encountered.[49,50,51] Steer and Boger found that milieu therapy was more effective in the treatment of patients who had been very regressed and socially deprived than in less regressed individuals.[52]

Bok studied the problems of milieu therapy for aged psychiatric patients.[53] The major sources of difficulty were lack of patient potential for change; rigid attitudes of staff members; chronic shortage of funds and personnel; and lack of desirable community alternatives to hospital care.

Behavior Modifications and Habit Training

Behavior modification techniques are based on the premise that behaviors are learned response patterns, and that therefore maladaptive behaviors can be altered by manipulating stimulus variables or reinforcements. Techniques to modify disturbed behavior may include counter-conditioning, extinction procedures, desensitization, or negative reinforcement. Lindsley suggested outlines for the development of behavioral "prosthetic environments" for geriatric patients by the application of operant conditioning techniques, to give maximal support to the behavior of aged persons and compensate for behavioral deficits in a sense analogous to the use of physical prostheses.[54] Many of the treatment modalities for geropsychiatric patients involve behavior modification principles, but there have been few studies of the specific use of behavior modification techniques in these patients. Ankus and Quarrington found that individually appropriate reinforcements, such as money, could modify behavior even in patients with severe organic mental impairment.[55] Birjandi and Sclafani described the use of positive reinforcement techniques in small groups of aged patients.[56]

Geriatric mental patients frequently exhibit deterioration of personal hygiene, particularly of toilet habits. Incontinence has multiple physiological causes, among which are neurologic disease, prostatic disease, uterine prolapse, urinary tract infection, and severe confusion from organic impairment; however, it may also be an active expression of hostility and rejection, resulting from feelings of neglect and insufficient attention.[57] Urinary urgency is common among the elderly, and some episodes of incontinence may be avoided by having toilets near all patient areas with the doors clearly marked by bright colors, by name, and by a silhouette for more rapid location of the facility. Bladder and bowel training programs are successful or at least helpful in some cases. Taking the patient to the toilet after meals and every 2 hours during the day, and every 3 hours at night, greatly reduces the problem with some patients. Adequate exercise, adequate fluid intake, and foods such as prune juice and bran cereal are also helpful in establishing bowel regularity and predictability. However, there are still patients who wet or soil themselves on the way back from the toilet.

Attitude Therapy

In attitude therapy, as developed by James Folsom, one of five basic attitudes is prescribed for the patient, according to his problems. These attitudes are termed kind firmness, for depressed patients; no demand, for destructive patients; active friendliness, for withdrawn and apathetic patients; passive friendliness, for suspicious and paranoid patients; and matter of fact, for alcoholic and sociopathic patients. Consistency of approach and involvement of all staff in the treatment process are critical to the success of this therapy. The attitude adopted toward a patient may be changed during the course of treatment if his needs change.[58]

Reality Orientation

Reality orientation techniques, also developed by Folsom, are helpful in reducing confusion and disorientation among organically impaired patients, and those who have been institutionalized for long periods of time.[16] One aspect of this is a continual reality orientation. Staff address patients by name and remind them of their location, present or upcoming events, time of day, and so on. Rambling or unrealistic conversation is directed back to reality. Prominent sign boards provide a reference source for information about the date, place, weather, and activities. Another aspect is reality orientation classes. These are carried out daily, usually by a nursing assistant, for small groups of patients. The instructor, in a calm, friendly manner, goes over basic information with each patient, such as his name, the date, the weather, the menu, and upcoming holidays. Positive feedback such as "good" or "that's fine" are given immediately for correct responses; the correct information is supplied in an encouraging, noncritical manner when an incorrect response is given. More complex information is added as the patient progresses, and advanced classes may be held for the less severely confused.[59,60] In a study of geriatric mental patients in a state hospital, Harris and Ivory found that patients who received reality orientation displayed significantly more verbal orientation than a control group who received only the routine hospital care.[61]

Remotivation

Remotivation is a structured program intended to reawaken the interest of regressed and apathetic patients in their surroundings through an effort to reach the healthy, normal aspects of patients' personalities. Remotivation groups, usually led by a nursing assistant, consist of 10 to 15 patients. Meetings are held once or twice weekly. The five steps involved in group meetings are creating a climate of acceptance; building a bridge to reality, as by reading and discussing objective poetry or newspaper items; sharing the experiences of the world, through discussions of objective topics selected to be of interest to the patients; an appreciation of the work of the world, to prompt the patient into thinking about work in relation to himself; and a climate of appreciation.[62]

Remotivation is intended to be adjunctive to other means of therapy and should be followed by rehabilitative activities, such as occupational and recreational therapy.[16]

Individual Psychotherapy

Contrary to widespread attitudes that individual psychotherapy is beneficial only to the relatively young, which spring partly from Sigmund Freud's belief that psychoanalysis of the elderly would be pointless,[62a] numerous therapists have found individual psychotherapeutic techniques helpful in their aged patients. Rechtschaffer summarized some suggested modifications for the psychotherapeutic approach to elderly patients, including: the therapist must be more active, environmental manipulation may be desirable, some educational techniques may be used, resistance and transference are handled gently, and therapy is tapered but rarely terminated.[63] Some of the complexities of transference and countertransference that may arise in relationships of an aged patient and a younger therapist are described by Hiatt.[64]

Meerloo and others have used psychoanalytic techniques with the elderly, but these appear more applicable to patients not requiring institutional care.[65] A technique developed by Goldfarb and Turner has proved useful for hospitalized geropsychiatric patients, especially those with organic brain impairment.[66] These patients have low self-esteem due to their mental deterioration, and are looking for a strong parent figure. The therapist fills this role, allowing expression of hostile and dependent feelings. Two short sessions of this therapy are held the first week to establish this relationship, and then the patient is seen briefly at infrequent intervals for an indefinite period of time. Even patients with less organic impairment frequently have low self-esteem, and Wolff found ego supportive individual therapy to be helpful.[40]

Among the common themes found in psychotherapy with the elderly, Butler and Lewis list desire for new starts and second chances; disguised fears of death; awareness of, and concern with, time; grief and restitution; guilt and atonement; and concerns related to autonomy and identity.[16]

Group Therapies

Man is by nature a social creature, and much of his life takes place in formal or informal groups. The use of the group as a deliberate therapeutic tool has become increasingly popular in recent years. A therapy group differs from others in that it is planned; group members share identifiable problems, diseases, or concerns; there is at least one therapist or leader; the group has a formal or informal understanding or contract. Although specific goals of group therapy are dependent on the particular group, some general goals for geropsychiatric groups may include alleviation of psychiatric symptoms, ability to live successfully in a group, increased self-esteem of group members, and ability to make decisions and function more independently. Groups can help patients achieve these goals through the variety of role models they provide; through reality contact and opportunities for reality testing with peers in a structured situation; through alleviation of isolation and loneliness; through contact with others who face similar problems; and through social contacts and opportunities to help one another.[67,68]

Desirable group characteristics include relative homogeneity of problems, needs, and mental status; sexual integration; and regular times and places for meeting. It is preferable to have at least two therapists, a male and a female, who should be warm, positive, and fairly active. Group size may be variable, depending upon the type of group and the needs and characteristics of its members. It should be large enough to provide variation and protection, and small enough to facilitate personal involvement and interaction by all members. Six to twelve members is frequently a good size.

Groups in institutional settings are usually open because of the practical difficulties of maintaining a closed group, stable in membership. This decreases group cohesion and intensity of interaction, but the changes in membership can be used to help patients learn to cope with loss and change. Klein, Leshan, and Furman have described helpful techniques and goals in group therapy.[69]

After 3 months of group therapy with the elderly, Wolff found better verbalization and controlled feelings, better ward adjustment, increased communication and activity, better orientation, better grooming, more appropriate sex role adjustment, lessened anxiety and feelings of isolation, favorable group identification, and sustained improvement which facilitated adjustment after discharge from the hospital.[40] Lazarus noted improvement both in disordered affect and in regressive hostile behavior, and found that patients with organic brain syndrome as well as those with functional impairment can benefit from group therapy.[70]

Socialization Groups. Patients who are reasonably alert may benefit from the opportunity to discuss matters of interest. Content of discussions may range from practical situations of finances, health, and relationships with children, to more abstract concepts such as religion or happiness.

Coping Groups. Groups may be formed to help persons find ways of coping with shared problems, such as adjustment to widowhood and the subsequent alterations in life style. Groups can also provide opportunities to regain valued but deteriorated or neglected skills, such as cooking or grooming.

Conjoint and Family Therapy Groups. Family and marital disorders frequently accompany mental illness among geriatric patients, and resolution of these difficulties is important for successful rehabilitation. Spark and Brody; Grauer, Betts and Birnbom describe some family interventions.[71,72] Family therapy groups usually consist only of the immediate family, but unrelated families with similar problems may also meet together.

Inspirational Groups. Groups such as Alcoholics Anonymous and religious groups, by providing support, enhancement of values, and inspiration, may be of great benefit to some geropsychiatric patients.

Predischarge Groups. Adjustment to the transition from hospital life to community life may be facilitated by groups organized to deal with problems and anxieties created by this transition. Group activities include not only discussion of these problems but also practical experiences such as shopping or visiting various community agencies.

Occupational Therapy

Occupational therapy is loosely defined, and may include such varied activities as arts and crafts, gardening, cooking, and working in sheltered workshops. General goals are increased self-esteem, increased self-confidence, the development of friendships, and acceptable expressions of aggressive drives, through constructive activity suitable to the individual's interests and capacities.[40] Physical disabilities such as poor vision or arthritis may limit the geriatric patient, and short attention span may also be a problem. Pincus noted that supposed learning deficits in the elderly often stem, to a considerable extent, from performance factors such as increased response time, lack of motivation, and sensory and psychomotor deficits.[73] Motivation to participate can be improved by encouraging patient participation in the selection of the activities that will become a part of his rehabilitation program.[74] Wolk and his group mention a bedside occupational therapy program for the benefit of patients who are physically or emotionally unable to come to the activity area.[75]

Sheltered workshops where contract work is performed for compensation can provide opportunities for meaningful activity, particularly to those persons who place high value upon work roles and productivity.

Nathanson and Reingold found that even patients with moderate to severe chronic organic brain syndrome could participate successfully in a sheltered workshop.[76]

Recreational Therapy

Relaxation and enjoyment remain as important for mental and physical health in old age as in the younger years. Recreational activities for the geropsychiatric patient should involve more than merely entertainment or diversion; they should be genuinely "recreational," reviving, stimulating, or maintaining creative functions. Reading, ceramics, card games, sewing, drawing, picnics, cooking, woodwork, and parties are among the numerous activities than can be therapeutic as well as entertaining. Less sedentary activities, such as walking, dancing, gardening, and exercising, are beneficial physically and psychologically provided that they are undertaken within the patient's actual physical capabilities. A handbook on dramatic activities for elderly persons was written by Harbin and adapted by Metzelaar, incorporating milieu therapy concepts.[77]

It will be noted that the line of demarcation between recreational therapy and occupational therapy is not sharp, suggesting the value of broadly trained rehabilitation therapists.

Music Therapy

Music, according to Congreue, has charms to soothe a savage beast; music therapy, according to Boxberger and Cotter, leads to reduction in aggressiveness, more appropriate behavior, reduction of incontinence, less physical and verbal reaction to hallucinations, a decrease in the level of undesirable patient noise, and improvements in personal appearance of geriatric patients.[78] Certainly music can provide pleasure, facilitate socialization, and revive happy memories. Bright describes the use of music as an aid to speech therapy and physical therapy, as well as in psychological rehabilitation.[79] Rhythmic movement is a natural accompaniment to music, and can provide a pleasant means of getting exercise.

Dance Therapy

Dance, both creative and social, can provide a means for increasing self-awareness, expressing thoughts and feelings, and socialization. Regular participation by the elderly in dance activities leads to increased communication and socialization and to improved physical endurance.[80]

Physical Therapy

Physical disabilities are common among elderly psychiatric patients. Strokes or fractures may cause or compound emotional disturbances. The prolonged immobility of bedridden or restrained patients rapidly leads to weakness and atrophy without preventive physical therapy.

Rodstein reports that mild daily exercise increases the cognitive abilities and orientation of elderly mental patients.[81] Hydrotherapy and massage may be beneficial in malaise, weakness, and withdrawal; warm baths may calm the agitated or restless patient; pain may be alleviated by heat and massage.[40] Illness and infected wounds may be treated with whirlpool baths. Although motivation level is generally considered crucial in rehabilitation following a disability such as a stroke or hip fracture, Steinberg cautions that depression from the emotional impact of the disability is to be expected, resulting in low initial motivation.[82] Physical improvement also improves enthusiasm and motivation.

The attention and human contact provided by the physical therapist are significant benefits, in addition to the specific physical benefit provided through therapy.

Physical Aids and Sensory Stimulation

Sensory deprivation may contribute to psychopathology, and sensory limitations may restrict participation in rehabilitative programs. Glasses will often enable a person to participate in crafts and activities or to lip read; magnifying glasses and large print books make reading possible for some persons with declining vision. Provision of a hearing aid or removal of impacted ear wax will reduce suspiciousness and hostility among many patients who are unable to perceive clearly what is going on around them.

Sensory stimulation is a structured therapeutic modality used with extremely regressed or organically impaired patients. Bower believes that part of the confusion seen in such patients results from sensory deprivation and cerebral "disuse atrophy."[83] The goal of sensory training is to increase sensitivity and discrimination of feelings. This is carried out in a small group, to provide feedback and consensual validation. The following sensory modalities are stimulated independently: kinesthetic and proprioceptive, tactile, olfactory, auditory, and visual. Group singing and playing of rhythm instruments at the end of the sessions stimulates social and cognitive functions.[84]

Power and McCarron found that bodily contact and social interaction is a helpful approach in the alleviation of depressive symptoms.[85]

Nutritional Therapy

The significance of nutritional deficiencies in the development of psychiatric disorders, and of nutritional therapy in the treatment of psychiatric disorders, is uncertain, and opinions vary widely. The reader is referred to the chapter in this volume on "Nutrition, Diet, and Exercise." Classical deficiency syndromes are relatively uncommon among elderly psychiatric patients, but milder deficiency states appear more frequently. In one study, over 70% of geropsychiatric patients admitted to a state hospital had doubtfully adequate or inadequate diets; borderline or low levels of folic acid were found in 50% and borderline or low levels of Vitamin B_{12} were found in 12%. Both of these vitamins may be associated with psychiatric disorders.[86,87] When vitamin deficiencies occur in the elderly, they are generally multiple deficiencies.

When nutritional deficiencies are found in association with psychiatric disorders, the direction of causation may be difficult to ascertain. Probably a vicious circle of mental illness, self-neglect, nutritional deficiency, physical illness, and further mental deterioration is operative in many of these cases. Institutional care does not ensure prevention or alleviation of nutritional deficiencies. Geropsychiatric patients waste about 30% of the food they are served.[88] Poor food habits may be longstanding and not amenable to change. Vitamins, particularly folic acid and vitamin C, may be lost in significant amounts during food preparation and service.

Eating has social as well as physiological importance. Attractively prepared food served in pleasant surroundings may have beneficial tonic effects. A daily glass of beer or wine in a pub situation among geropsychiatric patients has been found to increase social interaction, decrease incontinence, and reduce the need for other medications.[89]

Drug and Somatic Therapies

Most of the institutionalized elderly who are mentally ill (and some who are not) are on various psychotropic drugs, and will be more likely to need treatment such as ECT. These subjects are covered in other chapters of this volume and elsewhere.[90]

ENVIRONMENTAL FACTORS IN TREATMENT

Ward Types and Placement

For the most effective treatment of the elderly psychiatric patient, several types of wards should be available, although not necessarily at the same location. A planned program for each of these and periodic reassessments of the patient's current status and needs are essential for adequate care.[91]

Admission and Diagnostic Wards. Comprehensive assessment of a patient before admission is frequently impractical, and admission may be precipitated by a medical or social emergency, increasing the difficulty of assigning the patient to the most appropriate service.[92] Admission and diagnostic wards allow for thorough medical, social, and psychiatric assessment, and subsequent placement in the most suitable facility.[93,94,95,96] Andrews notes that problems hindering the functioning of such units may include lack of resources for patients needing long-term care, inadequate staffing, and difficulties in transferring patients to the appropriate services.[97] Facilities must be available for guaranteed discharge of patients admitted for assessment.[98] Some diagnostic units have specific time limits that a patient may be maintained on that ward.[99]

In addition to assessment, intensive treatment of problems amenable to correction within 2 or 3 months may be conducted on these wards.

Rehabilitation Wards. These wards are suitable for patients needing institutionalization of intermediate duration, and for chronically psychotic patients who have grown old in the hospital.

Chronic Care Wards. These should provide a supportive, humane, and protective environment for patients with progressive mental deterioration.

Minimal or Self-Care Wards. Similar in function to a half-way house, these are for individuals awaiting community placement, and for those capable of working outside the hospital during the day.

Ambulatory Senile Wards. Severe degrees of organic brain impairment can occur without marked physical impairment or psychotic disturbance;[100] such individuals need protection from wandering and getting lost.

Nursing Care Facilities. Nursing care wards are needed in mental hospitals when significant physical deterioration is accom-

panied by behavioral or other problems hampering placement in nursing homes.

Medical Wards. Similarly, wards for elderly psychiatric patients requiring medical care are needed especially in large psychiatric hospitals. Attempts to treat major medical illness in psychiatric wards often result in much less than optimal care, and is a heavy drain on the staff as well.

Age Distribution

The desirability of age segregation is a debatable topic. Proponents of age segregation cite research findings indicating beneficial effects of age-segregated housing for normal elderly persons, and feel that the elderly on age-mixed wards receive disproportionately little staff attention and risk harm from young violent patients. Furthermore, age segregation is thought to provide more appropriate role models and expectations. However, studies have shown age-homogenous custodial wards to be significantly less helpful than age-integrated custodial wards, and even detrimental to the behavioral and functional status of their occupants, regardless of patient diagnosis. Actively therapeutic wards are the most effective.[101,102]

Sex Distribution

It is common for wards of state mental hospitals and their facilities for elderly patients to rigidly segregate the sexes. However, acceptance and practice of a realistic and appropriate sex role is facilitated by sexually integrated wards.[103] Socialization, grooming, and manners tend to improve on mixed wards, and problems of annoying or improper behavior toward members of the opposite sex are rare.

Transfer Difficulties

The sudden transfer of an aged person to unfamiliar surroundings may result in confusion, disorientation, depression, withdrawal, or anger; and there is a real concern about the phenomena of "transfer mortality."

Rodstein and his group documented that indeed admission to an institution for the aged is stressful, with two-thirds of his patients showing problems in either the physical or emotional areas within the first month.[104] This was related not only to the acute environmental change, but also to the "process of institutionalization" involving a major change in life style. The majority of those initially stressed had made good adjustments by 6 months afterward. A detailed study of the effects of transfer on the elderly was carried out by Zweig and Csank who observed distinct phases in patient adjustment before and after the move, some of them associated with significantly increased mortality.[105] In their experience the most stressful times (and those associated with a higher mortality) were the time before the move when anticipation anxiety was high, and then between 4 and 6 months following the move, for less clear reasons. They advocated a stress-prevention program to help ease such transitions. Staff who are unaware of this will give little assistance to help the patient adjust, and their assessments of the patient's behavioral capacities may be inaccurate.[106] One study found results of transfer to be variable, with approximately equal numbers showing deterioration, improvement, and no change.[107] Mortality rate does not seem to increase with interinstitutional transfer.[108]

Physical and Architectural Factors

Too few of the facilities caring for elderly mental patients have incorporated physical, architectural, and environmental features designed for the convenience, pleasure, and maximum independence of the residents. Landscaping, gardening areas, sheltered walkways, and terraces provide pleasant atmosphere and the opportunity to be outdoors. Wheelchair ramps, wide corridors, handrails, absence of doorsteps or thresholds, nonslip flooring, doors which open automatically, pedestal-type tables, fairly short corridors, a lack of glass doors, and windows which open out rather than in are among features which can minimize the dangers and activity restrictions resulting from physical disabilities or limitations. Toilets should be located near dining and activity areas, as well as near rooms, and clearly marked. Space should be provided for physical therapy, occupational therapy, a library, hair dressing facilities, lounges, examination and treatment rooms, laundry machines, and other services. Carpeting reduces noise and breaks falls, but is impractical around incontinent patients. Furniture should be arranged to allow adequate room for patients with walkers or wheelchairs and to facilitate socialization. Tablecloths, flowers, lamps, upholstered furniture, books, magazines, and a television set create a more homelike atmosphere.[109,15]

Although excessive noise levels are irritating and can be confusing to the person with hearing loss, excessive silence can deprive the patients of important orienting background noise and also reduce the ability to hear.[110]

Mental function and vision appear to be related, and it is probable that at least part of this correlation stems from the effect of declining vision on behavior.[111] Vision testing and provision for glasses are certainly important; the appropriate use of color and lighting is another useful approach to limiting the disabilities caused by poor vision. Glare is a greater problem for older people than young ones; however, lighting must be bright enough to allow discrimination of color and detail, and to help in lip reading. Night lights help prevent falls and getting lost.[112] Color coding of wards and doors with contrasting wall paints and bright floor tiles are stimulating, provide a more cheerful atmosphere and help orient the confused and the visually impaired patients.[113]

Air temperature should be held fairly constant, and should be between 68° and 83°F. Air conditioning, heating, and humidity control are important, as ability to adjust to temperature extremes is much reduced with age.[16] Excessive heat is particularly dangerous to patients on phenothiazines or anticholinergic drugs, as dehydration or fatal hyperpyrexia may develop very rapidly.

SPECIAL PROBLEMS OF THE INSTITUTIONALIZED ELDERLY PATIENT

Regression and "Institutionalism"

Institutional care can increase the risk of regression and social breakdown, and impede the improvement of patients already exhibiting such behaviors. Rigid routines, loss of responsibility for decisions relating to personal activities, lack of privacy, unavailability of affectionate and supportive relationships, lack of intellectual stimulation, and spiritual deprivation may lead to loss of self-respect, narrowed interests and emotional responses, and behavior similar to that found in organic brain syndrome.[114] Butler and Lewis list the symptoms of "institutional neuroses" as erosion of personality, overdependence, expressionless faces, automatic behavior, and loss of interest in the outside world.[16] Staff attitudes may foster infantilization and desexualization. It is often easier and quicker to do things for a patient than to encourage or assist him to care for himself, and understaffing or misconceptions among staff regarding appropriate nursing care foster dependency and regression.[115]

Some evidence, however, suggests that the effects of institutional life may be less deleterious than commonly supposed. Preadmission characteristics, which are frequently related to the reasons for institutionalization, and the impact of the changes caused by entry into the institution appear partially responsible for the observed physical and psychological disadvantages of the institutionalized elderly.[116] Personality characteristics associated with successful adaptation to institutional life are high activity, high aggression, and narcissistic body image.[117] The impact of institutionalization upon the amount of social interaction appears to be a more important influence on self-esteem than institutionalization in itself; thus, institutionalization could be beneficial to self-esteem by increasing opportunities for interaction and age-appropriate social roles.[118] This research has largely focused on nursing homes, retirement homes, and homes for the aged. The possible influences of the stigmatization attached to psychiatric hospitalization and the varying totality of these institutions is uncertain.

Many of the therapeutic modalities previously discussed are applicable to the prevention or amelioration of the ill effects of institutionalism as well as to the treatment of the problems leading to institutionalization.

Adverse Drug Reactions

The high incidence of multiple system pathology among the elderly predisposes to multiple medication. The problems of drug interactions inherent in this are compounded when the patient is attended by two or more physicians, who are not necessarily aware of each other's prescriptions. In addition, physiologic changes of aging may alter the rate of drug absorption, distribution, metabolism, and excretion.[119] Some admissions to psychiatric institutions are related to drug toxicity and complications of overmedication; some adverse drug reactions occur following institutionalization. Acutely agitated patients may initially need high doses of antipsychotic medication. A much lesser maintenance dose may then suffice, but without careful review of the pharmacotherapy the initial dosages may be continued unnecessarily.

Side effects and manifestations of adverse reactions may be mistaken for worsening psychiatric or physiological conditions, and may be erroneously treated by adding further medications rather than withdrawing or reducing the responsible agent.[90]

Incontinence

As noted earlier, incontinence may stem from many causes, including physiological, psychological, and environmental (lack of rapid access, or sufficient assistance to toilet facilities). Success in controlling incontinence is highly variable and is often dependent on the accurate diagnosis of the cause of the condition. Incontinence may contribute to social isolation, limit participation in therapeutic activities, and predispose to skin irritation and breakdown, particularly in patients who are debilitated, obese, inactive, or bedridden.

Fecal Impactions

Relative inactivity, patterns of food and fluid intake, and the anticholinergic effects of many drugs all contribute to the great frequency of fecal impactions among elderly institutionalized mental patients. Fever, agitation, diarrhea, walking or sitting bent to one side, vomiting, lethargy, and increased confusion are among the possible manifestations of an impaction, and a rectal examination should be included in the investigation of any of these conditions.

Sleep Problems

Wakefulness at night may have several causes, and sedation is not always the most appropriate intervention. Excessive napping during the day may be reduced by providing interesting activities. Arthritic pains and other discomforts sometimes inhibit sleep, and an analgesic at bedtime may promote better rest. Although older people often need more sleep than younger ones, patients who are put to bed very early in the evening naturally awaken very early in the morning or in the middle of the night, having had sufficient sleep for their needs.[16] Deep sleep decreases with increasing age, with the result that some patients believe that they sleep less than they actually do. It is wise to ascertain the actual extent and pattern of sleeplessness, and for the nursing staff to try such measures as back rubs, snacks, or warm milk before prescribing hypnotic drugs.

OUTCOMES OF INSTITUTIONAL TREATMENT OF THE ELDERLY MENTALLY ILL

Factors Influencing Outcome

The outcome of institutional care of geropsychiatric patients is affected by several factors, the most important ones being the nature of the initial problem and the nature of the therapy. Patients with affective disorders are very likely to be released, but those with chronic organic brain syndrome or physical disease are less likely to be released. The admission of physically ill persons to psychiatric hospitals results in an excessive morbidity and mortality rate.

The average geriatric mental patient on a traditional custodial ward a number of years ago would probably have had no more than a 5 to 10% chance of getting out alive. In an active milieu program, well over half of the new admissions can be discharged within 6 months. Intensive therapy upon admission is desirable, as those who improve sufficiently to be discharged within 3 months have a much better chance of successful return to the community than those who are hospitalized longer.

An interested family and previous good adjustment increase the likelihood of release from the hospital. Differences in staff attitudes regarding rehabilitation potential of aged patients have been noted, with professional nurses, social workers, secretarial staff, administrative staff, and relatives displaying significantly more positive views than nonprofessional nursing staff, housekeepers, and the institutionalized elderly themselves. The influence of these attitudes upon quality and outcome of care is undetermined, however.[120]

Goals of Institutionalization

The goals of institutional care are not always stated, although it would perhaps be beneficial for the patient and for the most appropriate use of the various institutions if this were done. Naturally the goals, whether explicit or implied, will vary both with the type of institution and with the particular patient. The functions of nursing homes, mental hospitals, and other institutions providing care to aged patients may overlap, but they are not identical. In the unfortunate but not uncommon situation of utilizing a particular type of institution for lack of adequate alternatives, the goals of institutionalization may be unclear or difficult to fulfill effectively. Basic goals of the mental hospital are provision of the most effective treatment possible for the patient's disorders, and rehabilitation to the individual's maximum potential. Many patients experience cure or remission of their psychiatric disorder. Goals for others may be a slowing of the rate of disability, or humane comfort and support. Dying with dignity may be the best achievement possible with some patients. Physician goals my appropriately focus more on disability management than disease identification.[121]

Mortality

Urinary or fecal incontinence is consistently related to high mortality rates among aged psychiatric patients; other important factors are marked physical dependency and severe organic brain disease, as noted by Goldfarb and Neiditch.[122,39] Significant organic impairment from cerebral arteriosclerosis leads to death in an average of 3.8 years. When the cause is senile dementia the patient lives an average of 5.1 years after onset, as Wang and Whanger noted.[123]

Alternating Hospitalization and Respite Care

Planned intermittent hospital care is a possible approach when an individual does not require continuous institutional care but cannot be maintained indefinitely in the community without undue stress on his family or other support systems. Lear describes an arrangement in which geropsychiatric patients spent alternate months in the hospital and in the community, which allowed each hospital bed to be used for two patients.[124] Respite care, in which an ailing person is admitted for a temporary, planned interval of institutional care, may provide sufficient relief to the patient's family to enable the patient to live at home most of the time without disrupting family integrity and equilibrium.

Deinstitutionalization

The two crucial variables in planning for deinstitutionalization are the patient himself and the community to which he is returning. Leaving an institution, particularly after an extended stay, may be a stressful event in itself. Predischarge groups as noted earlier can ease this transition. May describes a halfway house for elderly mental patients.[125] Through increased sharing of tasks, increased responsibility for environmental maintenance, and replacement of a highly structured therapeutic community with a less structured situation, these patients are prepared for the realities of life in the community. Bykowski mentions the utilization of a placement and aftercare team consisting of a nurse, a social worker, and a group worker to minimize problems associated with deinstitutionalization. Facilities and services available vary considerably, but ideally should include community mental health clinics, day hospitals, day care centers, general practitioners, other medical facilities, home nursing services, home help services, meals services, laundry services, social welfare services, provisions for transportation, telephone directory services, physical therapy, occupational therapy, sheltered workshops, and residential facilities, including nursing care, homes for the aged, facilities for the confused, foster homes, and hotel type rooming. Furthermore, provisions should be made for elderly couples to be housed and cared for together, to prevent breakdown of longstanding supportive relationships.[127] In practice, all the services desirable for a particular patient may not be readily available, and placement must be made according to the realities of the situation. Eighty percent of state mental hospitals surveyed indicated that it is difficult to obtain sufficient placements, with the major problem cited as simple unavailability of community resources.[128] Helpful manuals for deinstitutionalization have been prepared by Grant and Folsom and her group.[129,130]

Results of Placement

In a study of geriatric patients discharged from a state hospital to various types of facilities, including apartments for independent living, family dwellings, boarding homes, and skilled nursing homes, Bourestom found significant differences in morale and in descrepancy levels between desired and actual participation in instrumental, social, and leisure activities.[131] The nursing home patients reported the lowest morale and life satisfaction, and those living in apartments the highest; similarly, levels of participation in relation to initial desire were lowest among nursing home residents and highest among apartment dwellers, with residents located in other types of facilities displaying intermediate levels.

The early stages of adjustment following placement in a nursing home are the most critical, as crises or psychiatric symptoms which develop during this initial period tend to lead to rehospitalization or physical illness unless treated.[15] Successful adjustment to nursing home placement depends most strongly upon presence or absence of psychiatric symptoms and behavioral disturbances.[132] Psychiatric patients show greater incidence of psychopathology and mental impairment than those without psychiatric histories; however, these differences are more apparent in psychiatric interviews and tests than in behavior, and nursing homes seem able to manage these patients.[133] Dobson and Patterson found that schizophrenic patients adjusted as well in nursing homes as in hospitals, but that those with organic brain disease experienced a greater decrease in physical and self-care activities in the nursing home than in the hospital.[134]

Determination, motivation, and ability to manipulate a familiar environment contribute to successful adjustment to noninstitutional placement, as observed by MacLeod in a series of case histories.[135] Persons may be willing and able to adapt to living situations which, in the value system of the therapist, are inadequate and undesirable.

Coordination with Community Programs

The existence of a broad spectrum of community facilities, programs, and services is of little benefit without adequate means to ensure coordination of patient needs with available services. A patient being discharged should be assigned a coordinator, usually a nurse or social worker, to provide for mobilization and integration of community resources.[136] Common obstacles impeding delivery of effective follow-up services include rigidity and territoriality of professionals and agencies; poverty, stubbornness and suspiciousness in the patient, overburdening with forms and red tape, unwillingness of physicians to treat aged clients, communication difficulties, impairment of mobility, tendencies to stop medications prematurely, resistance from families, difficulties in following diets, trouble in getting to more than one medical clinic in a day, the tendency of some nursing homes to oversedate and unnecessarily immobilize patients, and the sheer lack of facilities.[137]

CONCLUSION

At last the active treatment of the mental disorders of the elderly is becoming a national issue, if not a priority, and increasingly professionals are seeking skills and knowledge about how to accomplish it. The role of various institutions in the treatment spectrum is still often uncertain, suffering from a mixture of tradition, neglect, underfunding, expediency, and hope. The almshouse mentality is being abandoned, and many innovations and creative programs are being developed and tried, some of which will help to make our institutions more effectively responsive to the needs of our mentally ill older citizens.

ACKNOWLEDGEMENT

The author would like to thank Elizabeth A. Whanger, R. N., of the Health Care Center of the Durham Methodist Retirement Home for her valuable assistance in reviewing the literature, and her helpful comments on institutional care from a nurse's standpoint.

REFERENCES

1. Butler, R. N. They are only senile. Chap. 8 in *Why Survive? Being Old in America.* New York: Harper & Row, 1975.
2. Eisdorfer, C. and Stotsky, B. A. Intervention, treatment, and rehabilitation of psychiatric disorders. In J. E. Birren and K. W. Schaie, (eds.) *Handbook of the Psychology of Aging.* New York: Van Nostrand Reinhold Co., 1977.
3. Glasscote, R., Gudeman, J. E. and Miles, D. *Creative Mental Health Services for the Elderly.* Washington, D. C.: American Psychiatric Association and the Mental Health Association, 1977.
4. Stotsky, B. A. Psychiatric disorders common to psychiatric and nonpsychiatric patients in nursing homes. *J. Amer. Geriat. Soc.* 15(7): 664–673 (1967).
5. Whanger, A. D. and Lewis, P. Survey of institutionalized elderly In E. Pfeiffer, (ed.) *Multidimensional Functional Assessment: The OARS Methodology* Durham, N. C.: Duke University, 1975.
6. Sherr, V. T. and Goffi, M. T. Sr., On-site geropsychiatric services to guests of residential homes. *J. Amer. Geriat. Soc.* 25(6): 269–272 (1977).
7. Kahn, R. L. The mental health system and the future aged. *Gerontologist* 15: 24–31 (1975).
8. Brocklehurst, J. Personal Communication, 1978.
9. Gold, J. G. Development of care of the elderly: Tracing the history of institutional facilities. *Gerontologist* 10: 262–274 (1970).
10. Hawker, M. *Geriatrics for Physiotherapists and the Allied Professions.* London: Faber & Faber, 1974.
11. Whanger, A. D. The history and development of geriatric psychiatry. *Career Directions* 5(3): 2–11 (1977).
12. Hader, M. and Seltzer, H. A. La Salpétrière: An early home for elderly psychiatric patients. *Gerontologist* 7: 113–135 (1967).
13. Busse, E. W. and Pfeiffer, E. (eds.) *Behavior and Adaptation in Late Life.* Boston: Little, Brown and Company, 1969.
14. Markson, E. A hiding place to die. *Transactions,* Dec. 1971. pp. 48–54.
15. Stotsky, B. A. *The Nursing Home and the Aged Psychiatric Patient* T. F. Dwyer, F. H. Frankel and M. T. McGuire, (eds.) New York: Meredith, 1970.
16. Butler, R. N. and Lewis, M. I. *Aging and Mental Health,* 2nd Edition. St. Louis: C. V. Mosby, 1977.
17. Kahana, E. and Kahana, B. Health care facilities. Chap. 31 In Cowdry's—*The Care of the Geriatric Patient,* 5th Edition. St. Louis: C. V. Mosby, 1976.
18. Feder, M. and Junod, J. P. Psychiatry in the geriatric hospital: Its goals and limitations. *Geront. Clin.* 17: 58–60 (1975).
19. Colthart, S. M. A mental health unit in a skilled nursing facility. *J. Amer. Geriat. Soc.* 22(10): 453–456 (1974).
20. Lorenze, E. J., Hamill, C. M. and Oliver, R. C. The day hospital: An alternative to institutional care. *J. Amer. Geriat. Soc.* 22: 316–320 (1974).
21. Matlack, D. R. The case for geriatric day hospitals. *The Gerontologist* 15: 109–113 (1975).
22. Wilson, J. W. Starting a geriatric day care center within a state hospital. *J. Amer. Geriat. Soc.* 21(4): 175–179 (1973).
23. Berger, M. M. and Berger, L. F. An innovative program for a private psychogeriatric day center. *J. Amer. Geriat. Soc.* 19(4): 332–336 (1971).
24. Arie, T. Day care in geriatric psychiatry. *Geront. Clin.* 17: 31–39 (1975).
25. Kay, D. W. K., Beamish, P. and Roth, M. Old age mental disorders in Newcastle upon Tyne. *Brit. J. Psychiat.* 110: 146–158 (1964).
26. Grauer, H. and Birnbom, F. A geriatric functional rating scale to determine the need for institutional care. *J. Amer. Geriat. Soc.* 23(10): 472–476 (1975).
27. Palmore, E. Total chance of institutionalization among the aged. *Gerontologist* 16(6): 504–507 (1976).
28. Lowenthal, M. F. *Lives in Distress.* New York: Basic Books, 1964.
29. Lowenthal, M. F., Berkman, P. L. and Associates. *Aging and Mental Disorder in San Francisco.* San Francisco: Jossey-Bass, 1967.
30. Whanger, A. D. and Busse, E. W. Care in hospital In J. A. Howells, (ed.) *Modern Perspectives in the Psychiatry of Old Age.* New York: Brunner/Mazel, 1975.
31. Whanger, A. D. When should a mentally ill older person be sent to the hospital? In E. W. Busse and E. Pfeiffer, (eds.) *Mental Illness in Later Life.*

Washington, D. C.: American Psychiatric Association, 1973.

32. Weinberg, J. Mental health in the aged. Chap. 15 In M. M. Dacso, (ed.) *Restorative Medicine in Geriatrics* Springfield: Charles C Thomas, 1963.

33. U. S. Department of Health, Education, and Welfare, 1968. *Patients in Mental Institutions, 1966, Part II: State and County Mental Hospitals.* Public Health Service Publication No. 1818, Part II. Washington, D.C.

34. Whanger, A. D. Geriatric mental health in North Carolina. *N. C. Journal of Ment. Health* 5: 43–49 (1971).

35. Redick, R. W., Kramer, M. and Taube, C. A. Epidemiology of mental illness and utilization of psychiatric facilities among older persons. In E. W. Busse and E. Pfeiffer (eds.) *Mental Illness in Later Life* Washington, D.C.: American Psychiatric Association, 1973.

36. Scottish Health Services Council, 1970. *Services for the Elderly with Mental Disorder.* Edinburgh: Scottish Home and Health Department, 1970.

37. Burvill, P. W. Elderly patients in mental hospitals, geriatric hospitals and nursing homes in Perth, Western Australia. *Acta. Psychiatr. Scand.* 46: 258–272 (1970).

38. Kobrynski, B. and Miller, A. D. The role of the state hospital in the care of the elderly. *J. Amer. Geriat. Soc.* 18: 210–219 (1970).

39. Neiditch, J. A. and White, L. Prediction of short-term outcome in newly admitted psychogeriatric patients. *J. Amer. Geriat. Soc.* 24(2): 72–78 (1976).

40. Wolff, K. *The Emotional Rehabilitation of the Geriatric Patient.* Springfield: Charles C Thomas, 1970.

41. Langley, G. E. and Simpson, J. H. Misplacement of the elderly in geriatric and psychiatric hospitals. *Gerontologia Clinica* 12: 149–163 (1970).

42. Kidd, C. B. Criteria for admission of the elderly to geriatric and psychiatric units. *J. Ment. Science* 108: 68–74 (1962).

43. Kidd, C. B. Misplacement of the elderly in hospital. *Brit. Med. Journal* 2: 1491–1495 (1962).

44. Jones, M. *The Therapeutic Community.* New York: Basic Books, 1953.

45. Gottesman, L. E. The response of long-hospitalized aged psychiatric patients to milieu treatment. *Gerontologist* 7: 47–48 (1967).

46. Bykowski, J. and Harrison, S. *Research and Reality: Development of an Empirical Model and Training Program in Milieu Therapy.* Institute of Gerontology, Ann Arbor, Mich., 1975.

47. Coons, D. H. *Designing A Therapeutic Community.* Institute of Gerontology, Ann Arbor, Mich., 1973.

48. Maney, H. *A Self-care Program for a Group of Elderly Men Living in a Therapeutic Community.* Institute of Gerontology, Ann Arbor, Mich., 1975.

49. Risdorfer, E. N. Review of Results in a Geriatric Intensive Treatment Unit: Some Prospects. *J. Amer, Geriat. Soc.* 18: 47–55 (1970).

50. Goldstein, S. A critical appraisal of milieu therapy in a geriatric day hospital. *J. Amer. Geriat. Soc.* 19(8): 693–699 (1971).

51. Grauer, H. Institutions for the Aged— Therapeutic Communities. *J. Amer. Geriat. Soc.* 19(8): 687–692 (1971).

52. Steer, R. A. and Boger, W. P. Milieu therapy with psychiatric-medically infirm patients. *Gerontologist* 15: 138–141 (1975).

53. Bok, M. Some problems in milieu treatment of the chronic older mental patient. *Gerontologist* 11: 141–147 (1971).

54. Lindsley, O. R. Geriatric behavioral prosthetics. In R. Kastenbaum, (ed.). *New Thoughts on Old Age.* New York: Springer Publishing Company, 1964.

55. Ankus, M. and Quarrington, B. Operant behavior in the memory-disordered. *J. Gerontol.* 27: 500–510 (1972).

56. Birjandi, P. F. and Sclafani, M. J. An interdisciplinary team approach to geriatric patient care. *Hosp. & Commun. Psychiat.* 24(11): 777–778 (1973).

57. Macmillan, D. and Shaw, P. Senile breakdown in standards of personal and environmental cleanliness. *Brit. Med. J.* 2: 1032–1037 (1966).

58. Folsom, J. C. Attitude therapy and the team approach. Tuscaloosa: Veterans Administration Hospital, 1966.

59. Folsom, J. C. Reality orientation for the elderly mental patient. *J. Geriat. Psychiat.* 1: 291–307 (1968).

60. Anonymous author. Tips on teaching classroom R. O. *The Rope* 5(2): Winter (1977–1978).

61. Harris, C. S. and Ivory, P. B. C. B. An outcome evaluation of reality orientation therapy with geriatric patients in a state mental hospital. *Gerontologist* 16(6): 496–503 (1976).

62. American Psychiatric Association: *Remotivation Kit.* Washington, D. C.: American Psychiatric Association, 1965.

62a. Freud, S. On psychotherapy, *Collected Papers,* Volume I. London: Hogarth Press, pp. 249–262, 1924.

63. Rechtschaffen, A. Psychotherapy with geriatric patients: A review of the literature. *Gerontology* 14: 73–84 (1959).

64. Hiatt, H. Dynamic psychotherapy of the aged. In J. H. Masserman, (ed.) *Handbook of Psychiatric Therapies* New York: Aronsen, 1973.

65. Meerloo, J. A. M. Modes of psychotherapy in the aged. *J. Amer. Geriat. Soc.* 9: 225–234 (1961).

66. Goldfarb, A. I. and Turner, H. Psychotherapy of aged persons, II. Utilization and effectiveness of "Brief" therapy. *Amer. J. Psychiat.* 109: 916–921 (1953).

67. Koslofsky, L. Group work with the aged, 1973. An unpublished manuscript.

68. Linden, M. E. Group psychotherapy with institutionalized senile women, II. Study in gerontologic human relations. *Int. J. Group Psychother.* **3:** 150–170 (1953).

69. Klein, W. H., Leshan, E. J. and Furman, S. S. *Promoting Mental Health of Older People Through Group Methods.* New York: Manhattan Society for Mental Health, 1965.

70. Lazarus, L. W. A program for the elderly at a private psychiatric hospital. *Gerontologist* **16**(2): 125–131 (1976).

71. Spark, G. M. and Brody, E. M. The aged are family members. *Family Process* **9**(2): 195–210 (1970).

72. Grauer, H., Betts, D. and Birnbom, F. Welfare emotions and family therapy in geriatrics. *J. Amer. Geriat. Soc.* **21**(1): 21–24 (1973).

73. Pincus, A. New findings on learning in old age: Implications for occupational therapy. *Amer. J. Occupational Therapy* **22**(4): 300–303 (1968).

74. Lewis, S. A patient-determined approach to geriatric activity programming within a state hospital. *Gerontologist* **15:** 146–149 (1975).

75. Wolk, R. L., Seiden, R. B. and Wolverton, B. Unique influences and goals of an occupational therapy program in a home for the aged. *J. Amer. Geriat. Soc.* **13**(11): 989–997 (1965).

76. Nathanson, B. F. and Reingold, J. A workshop for mentally impaired aged. *Gerontologist* **9:** 293–295 (1969).

77. Harbin, S. *Dramatic Activities for the Elderly.* Institute of Gerontology, Ann Arbor, Mich., 1976.

78. Boxberger, R. and Cotter, V. W. Music therapy for geriatric patients. In E. T. Gaston, (ed.) *Music in Therapy* New York: Macmillan, 1968.

79. Bright, R. *Music in Geriatric Care.* Sydney, Australia: Halstead Press, 1972.

80. Maney, J. A class in creative movement for residents of an in-hospital halfway house within a geriatric therapeutic community. Institute of Gerontology, Ann Arbor, Mich., 1975.

81. Rodstein, M. Challenging residents to assume maximal responsibilities in homes for the aged. *J. Amer. Geriat. Soc.* **23**(7): 317–321 (1975).

82. Steinberg, F. U. Rehabilitation medicine. In Cowdry's—*The Care of the Geriatric Patient,* 5th Edition. St. Louis: C. V. Mosby Company, 1976.

83. Bower, H. M. Sensory stimulation and the treatment of senile dementia. *Med. J. of Australia* **1**(22): 1113–1119 (1967).

84. Richman, L. Sensory training for geriatric Patients. *Amer. J. Occupational Therapy* **23:** 254–257 (1969).

85. Power, C. A. and McCarron, L. T. Treatment of depression in persons residing in homes for the aged. *Gerontologist* **15:** 132–135 (1975).

86. Whanger, A. D. and Wang, H. S. Vitamin B_{12} deficiency in normal aged and elderly psychiatric patients. In E. Palmore, (ed.) *Normal Aging, II* Durham, N. C.: Duke University Press, 1974.

87. Whanger, A. D. Vitamins and vigor at 65 plus. *Postgrad. Med.* **53:** 167–172 (1973).

88. Gericke, O. L., Lobb, L. G. and Allenger, D. E. Nutritional supplementation for elderly patients in a state mental hospital: Effect on appetite and weight gain. *J. Amer. Geriat. Soc.* **9:** 381–387 (1961).

89. Chien, C. P. Psychiatric treatment for geriatric patients: "Pub" or Drug?'' *Amer. J. Psychiat.* **127:** 1070–1075 (1971).

90. Whanger, A. D. Drug management of the elderly in state hospitals. In W. E. Fann and G. L. Maddox, (eds.) *Drug Issues in Geropsychiatry.* Baltimore: Williams and Wilkins, 1974.

91. World Health Organization. *Psychogeriatrics.* World Health Organization Technical Representatives Series No. 507. Geneva: World Health Organization, 1972.

92. Kay, D. W. K., Roth, M. and Hall, M. R. P. Special problems of the aged and the organization of hospital services. *Brit. Med. J.* **2:** 967–972 (1966).

93. MacMillan, D. Problems of a geriatric mental health service. *Brit. J. Psychiat.* **113:** 175–181 (1967).

94. Exton-Smith, A. N. and Robinson, K. V. Psychogeriatric assessment units. *Lancet* **1:** 1292 (1970).

95. Burrows, H. P. Psychogeriatric assessment units. *Lancet* **1:** 1121 (1970).

96. Anonymous author. Mental disorder in the elderly. *Lancet* **2:** 867 (1970).

97. Andrews, J. Psychogeriatric assessment units. *Lancet* **1:** 1004 (1970).

98. Hurst, L. and Morton, E. V. B. Psychogeriatric assessment units. *Lancet* **2:** 47–48 (1970).

99. Morton, E. V. B., Barker, M. E. and MacMillan, D. The joint assessment and early treatment unit in psychogeriatric care. *Gerontol. Clin.* **10:** 65–73 (1968).

100. Anonymous author: Psychogeriatric care. *Brit. Med. J.* **3:** 202–203 (1971).

101. Kahana, B. Changes in mental status of elderly patients in age-integrated and age-segregated hospital milieus. *J. Abnormal Psychol.* **75:** 177–181 (1970).

102. Kahana, E. and Kahana, B. Therapeutic potential of age integration. Effects of age-integrated hospital environment on elderly psychiatric patients. *Arch. Gen. Psychiat.* **23:** 20–29 (1970).

103. Ciarlo, J. A. and Gottesman, L. E. The effects of differing treatment milieus upon the ward behavior of geriatric mental patients. A paper given at the American Psychological Association meetings, Sept. 1–6, 1966, New York City.

104. Rodstein, M., Savitsky, E. and Starkman, R. Initial adjustment to a long-term care institution: Medical and behavioral aspects. *J. Amer. Geriat. Soc.* **24**(2): 65–71 (1976).

105. Zweig, J. P. and Csank, J. Z. Mortality fluctuations among chronically ill medical geriatric pa-

tients as an indicator of stress before and after relocation. *J. Amer. Geriat. Soc.* **24**(6): 264–277 (1976).

106. Shaughnessy, M. E. Emotional problems of patients in nursing homes. *J. Geriat. Psychiat.* **1**: 159–166 (1967–68).

107. Raasoch, J., Willmuth, R., Thomson, L. and Hyde, R. Intrahospital transfer: Effects on chronically ill psychogeriatric patients. *J. Amer. Geriat. Soc.* **25**(6): 281–284 (1977).

108. Markson, E. W. and Cumming, J. H. The post-transfer fate of relocated mental patients in New York. *Gerontologist* **15**: 104–113 (1975).

109. McClannahan, L. E. Therapeutic and prosthetic living environments for nursing home residents. *Gerontologist* **13**: 424–429 (1973).

110. Busse, E. W. Problems affecting psychiatric care of the aging. *Geriatrics* **15**: 97–105 (1960).

111. Snyder, L. H., Pyrek, J. and Smith, K. C. Vision and mental function of the elderly. *Gerontologist* **16**(6): 491–495, (1976).

112. Maxwell, J. M. *Centers for Older People.* New York: National Council on Aging, 1962.

113. Agate, J. N. *The Practice of Geriatrics,* 2nd Edition. Springfield: Charles C. Thomas, 1970.

114. Stotsky, B. A. and Dominick, J. R. Mental patients in nursing homes, I. Social deprivation and regression. *J. Amer. Geriat. Soc.* **17**(1): 33–44 (1969).

115. Lieberman, M. A. Crises of the last decade of life: Reactions and adaptations. In A. G. Feldman, (ed.) *Community Mental Health and Aging: An Overview* Los Angeles: University of Southern California, 1973.

116. Lieberman, M. A. Institutionalization of the aged: Effects on behavior. *J. Gerontol.* **24**: 330–340 (1969).

117. Turner, B. F., Tobin, S. S. and Lieberman, M. A. Personality traits as predictors of institutional adaption among the aged. *J. Gerontol.* **27**(1): 61–68 (1972).

118. Anderson, N. N. Effects of institutionalization on self-esteem. *J. Gerontol.* **22**: 313–317 (1967).

119. Ingman, S. R., Lawson, I. R., Pierpaoli, P. G. and Blake, P. A survey of the prescribing and administration of drugs in a long-term care institution for the elderly. *J. Amer. Geriat. Soc.* **23**(7): 309–316 (1975).

120. Kosberg, J. I. and Gorman, J. F. Perceptions toward the rehabilitation potential of institutionalized aged. *Gerontologist* **15**: 398–403 (1975).

121. Miller, M. B. Restructuring medical education for management of the chronically ill aged. *J. Amer. Geriat. Soc.* **22**(11): 501–510 (1974).

122. Goldfarb, A. I. Predictors of mortality in the institutionalized aged. In E. Palmore and F. C. Jeffers, (eds.) *Prediction of Life Span.* Lexington: Heath Lexington Books, 1971.

123. Wang, H. S. and Whanger, A. D. Brain impairment and longevity. In E. Palmore and F. C. Jef-

fers, (eds.) *Prediction of Life Span.* Lexington: Heath Lexington Books, 1971.

124. Lear, J. E. Sharing the care of the elderly between community and hospital. *Lancet* **2**: 1349–1353 (1969).

125. May, W. W. A halfway house for geriatric patients at Ypsilanti State Hospital—An experience in de-institutionalizing. A paper presented to the Michigan Association of Neuropsychiatric Hospital and Clinic Physicians, June, 1973, Northville, Michigan.

126. Bykowski, J. The institution goes one step beyond. American Psychological Association, New Orleans, La., 1974.

127. Poliquin, N. and Straker, M. A clinical psychogeriatric unit: Organization and function. *J. Amer. Geriat. Soc.* **25**(4): 132–137 (1977).

128. Glasscote, R. M., Beigel, A., Butterfield, A., Jr., Clark, E., Cox, B. A., Elpers, J. R., Gudeman, J. E., Gurel, L., Lewis, R. V., Miles, D. G., Raybin, J. B., Reifler, C. B. and Vito, E. H., Jr. *Old Folks at Homes.* The Joint Information Service of the American Psychiatric Association and the National Association for Mental Health, Washington, D. C., 1976.

129. Grant, F. E. Rehabilitation and placement programs for psycho-geriatric treatment. *Catawba Hospital Handbook for Facilitators.* Institute of Gerontology, Ann Arbor, Mich., 1976.

130. Folsom, G. S. *Life Skills for the Developmentally Disabled: An Approach to Accountability in Deinstitutionalization,* Vols. 1, 2, & 3. Washington, D. C.: George Washington University, 1975.

131. Bourestom, N. Reactions of elderly mental patients to different community facilities. Institute of Gerontology, Ann Arbor, Michigan. A paper given at the Gerontological Society meetings in Denver, Colorado, November 1968.

132. Stotsky, B. A. A controlled study of factors in the successful adjustment of mental patients to nursing homes. *Amer. J. Psychiat.* **123**: 1243–1251 (1967).

133. Stotsky, B. A. and Frye, S. Comparison of psychiatric and nonpsychiatric patients in nursing homes. *J. Amer. Geriat. Soc.* **15**(4): 355–363 (1967).

134. Dobson, W. R. and Patterson, T. W. A behavioral evaluation of geriatric patients living in nursing homes as compared to a hospitalized group. *Gerontologist* **1**: 135–139 (1961).

135. MacLeod, R. D. Unrealistic discharges. *Geront. Clin.* **12**: 31–39 (1970).

136. Gaitz, C. M. The coordinator: An essential member of a multidisciplinary team delivering health services to aged persons. *Gerontologist* **10**: 217–220 (1970).

137. Gaitz, C. M. and Hacker, S. Obstacles in coordinating services for the care of the psychiatrically ill aged. *J. Amer. Geriat. Soc.* **18**: 172–182 (1970).

Chapter 22
Nutrition, Diet, and Exercise

Alan D. Whanger, M. D.
Duke University Medical Center

INTRODUCTION

In this chapter we will consider aspects of nutrition and exercise as they relate to the mental health and the mental disorders of the elderly. Perhaps the rationale for considering these together is that there are relatively few "hard facts" and well-controlled studies, but there are an abundance of programs and regimens claiming remarkable results for a wide spectrum of human ills, especially in the aged. Both nutrition and exercise are fertile fields for the faddists. A short article in a recent nationally circulated weekly newspaper supplement quoted a somewhat aging and controversial tennis professional on his nutritional practices as follows: "I am a great believer in vitamins. I know over 400 (vitamins and supplement pills) seems like a lot to be taking in one day, but actually it isn't, because I take them three times a day, and package them ahead of time. It seems like very little to be doing for all the benefit I derive from them."[1] The nutritional radicals clash with the dietary reactionaries. The health food

store bookracks bulge with such books as *Supernutrition Megavitamin Revolution* which promises on the cover that "In just 10 weeks you can have the kind of energy and vibrant health you never dreamed possible,"[2] and *Mental health Through Nutrition* by a state judge who feels he shows that "regardless of what the medical and legal books say about senility and old age, senility is not a result of age, but of starvation of the body and the brain. With proper nutrition one will never be old mentally, provided, of course, he observes certain fundamental rules of health with which we are all familiar."[3] The Foundation for Infinite Survival, Inc., offers a mineral evaluation by hair analysis and computerized nutritional analysis as part of their life-extension and control of aging program.[4]

The opposition replies in such articles as "The Perfect Environment for Nonsense" in which the author feels that out of the fury of the ecology movement and the anti-establishment mood of the young people "fanned by immature faculty members, emerged a great distrust of the establishment—big business, the government, medicine, and academia itself. All of which played right into the hands of the nutrition fanatic. Health food people capitalized on the whole mess by featuring the organic bit while themselves smearing food science, the food industry, and the medical profession."[5] In an article entitled "Americans Love Hogwash," Rynearson details the background of a number of the popular nutrition writers and cites their many fallacious and poorly documented statements.[6] Using psychoanalytic dynamic terms, Bruch explains how those concerned with pure foods may have had early unwholesome experiences causing failure of the development of basic trust, and that the fear of being poisoned is one of the commonest delusions of those becoming manifestly mentally ill.[7] The Food and Drug Administration (FDA) defended its position that there is little wrong with the American food production and distribution system in their Fact Sheet of 1967 stating that it is a "modern marvel" that the natural value of foods is not lost in processing, and that foods can even get better in the processing. The FDA further assured us that scientific knowledge, working through laws to protect consumers, would assure the "safety and wholesomeness of every component of our food supply."[8] In their attempt to clamp down on false nutritional claims, the FDA proposed that all vitamin and mineral preparations state on the label: "Vitamins and minerals are supplied in abundance by the foods that we eat. The Food and Nutrition Board of the National Research Council recommends that dietary needs by satisfied by foods. Except for persons with special medical needs, there is no scientific basis for recommending routine use of dietary supplements."[9]

Counterattacks have come from various sources, such as Ralph Nader's study group report *The Chemical Feast,*[10] which deals with the Food and Drug Administration and the poorly checked practices of additives, adulterants, and deceptive practices of the food industry. Schroeder points out that food processing usually separates the various micronutrients, vitamins, and minerals present in the food and necessary for its metabolism into the various component parts, leaving each product deficient in some way. For instance the processing of wheat results in the loss of 50% to 86% of seven vitamins in the white flour. The flour is then "enriched" by adding back three of the eight known vitamins and one of the thirteen minerals removed. I 1973, the FDA moved to force any preparation containing Dietary Allowances (RDA) of any vitamin or mineral to be treated as a drug rather than a diet supplement, and to bar substances of unproved nutritional value from supplements.[11] These actions raised a storm of protest, well documented in the Hearings before the House Subcommittee of Public Health and Environment[12] and in the reported 26,000 pages of testimony produced in the FDA's decade long vitamin hearings.[13] The director of the FDA's Bureau of Foods stated that "those people who need more than the RDA need medical supervision because there is something wrong with them."[11]

Actually the RDA vitamin values have fluctuated nine times since 1941, and there is wide international variation.[9] Those who go to their doctors for clarification of this nutritional confusion may be disappointed, as Dr. Jean Mayer observed after a study of the knowledge of Harvard physicians that the average doctor knew a little more about nutrition than his secretary, unless his secretary had a weight problem, in which case the average secretary knew a little more about nutrition than the average doctor. Nutrition is still a severely neglected subject in most medical school curricula.[14] It is obvious that all of the data are not in, and that this chapter will not be able to give the answers to these complex and emotionally charged subjects. The reader is invited to separate the wheat from the chaff in general references on geriatric nutrition such as those by Weg,[15] Schroeder,[9] Barrows and Roeder,[16] Howell and Loeb,[17] Watkin,[18] Williams,[19] Anderson,[20] Burton,[21] Exton-Smith and Scott,[22] Caster,[23] and Winick.[24]

NUTRITIONAL NEEDS OF THE ELDERLY

Introduction and Factors in Nutritional Variability

According to the pronouncements of the Food and Nutrition Board, the nutritional requirements of older people are little different from those of the young adult, excepting that the caloric intake should decrease as the person ages. The recommended dietary allowances are designed for the maintenance of good nutrition of practically all healthy people in the U.S.A., and the allowances are intended to provide for individual variations among most normal persons as they live in the United States under usual environmental conditions.[25] (see Table 22-1). Theoretically, one might think that the need for many nutrients should be lower in the elderly because of the decreased calories and diminished number of active cells in the body. Actually, Michelsen[27] feels there is little experimental evidence to support these contentions, and Watkin[18] states that in man aging is so modified by disease that its uncomplicated course is unknown, so that nutritional recommendations directed at the aged as a class must be couched

in terms so general as to be meaningless. Williams[19] advocates an individual approach to geriatric nutrition, pointing out that no individual's body ages uniformly in all its functions, and that no individual, aging or not, possesses a nutrition that is typical in every way. Most of the signs of old age are probably connected with failure of cells and tissues somewhere in the body to perform their functions properly, and one major cause of these failures is cell and tissue malnutrition. While there are aging processes in the cells that cannot be modified nor overcome, it is o bvious that the longer they will continue to remain in good working order. Different cells in the body have different nutritional requirements, and there is some intercellular symbiosis wherein certain cells depand on the functioning of other cells for their own nutrition. Because of these factors, Williams[19] feels that some "non-essential" nutrients, i.e., those that the body itself can manufacture or are not proven to be required for metabolism, may become more "essential" during the aging process because of various cellular and metabolic features. He found, for instance, a 4.5-fold range of calcium and a 6.5-fold

Table 22-1.   The RDA for persons over age 51, as revised in 1974 by the National Research Council is adapted as follows.[26]

NUTRIENT	MEN	WOMEN
Calories	2,400	1,800
Protein	56 gm	46 gm
Vitamin A	5,000 IU	4,000 IU
B₁ (Thiamine)	1.2 mg	1.0 mg
B₂ (Riboflavin)	1.5 mg	1.1 mg
B₆ (Pyridoxine)	2.0 mg	2.0 mg
B₁₂	3.0 mcg	3.0 mcg
Folacin	400 mcg	400 mcg
Niacin	16 mg	12 mg
C (Ascorbic Acid)	45 mg	45 mg
D	400 IU	400 IU
	(not determined)	(not determined)
E	15 IU	12 IU
Calcium	800 mg	800 mg
Phosphorus	800 mg	800 mg
Iodine	110 mcg	80mcg
Iron	10 mg	10 mg
Magnesium	350 mg	300 mg
Zinc	15 mg	15 mg

range of leucine minimal requirements in humans, and a 25-fold variation in needs for vitamin A in rats and a 32-fold variation in vitamin C requirements in guinea pigs. There are about 35 nutrients that are known to be individually essential in human nutrition, and about a half dozen more that may at times be necessary. Obviously our knowledge about these complex interactions, as well as out ability to apply them clinically, is still quite limited, especially in the elderly.

Not only do variations exist on a cellular level, but there are other factors which, as Howell and Loeb detail,[17] may cause nutritional imbalance even if the presented diet is well-balanced. These are interference with intake; interference with absorption by such things as salivary enzyme loss, gastric atrophy and achlorhydria, decrease in the digestive enzymes of the stomach, pancreas, and small intestine, decreased quantity of bile, hypermotility of the stomach, decreased motility of the intestines, and altered intestinal flora; interference with storage and utilization by such things as altered endocrine function,[28] loss of storage cells, decreased vascular efficiency,[29] and increased fibrous tissue in vessels and tissues; and increased excretion and loss rates, such as that associated with intestinal malabsorption, loss of muscle (and protein) mass, urinary protein excretion, and loss of cellular potassium and intracellular water.

Calories

The energy-producing content of foods is measured in units of heat, the kilocalorie. A person needs energy both to provide for the basal body needs, and to supply the additional demands of various activities. The basal metabolism declines with aging, but Bierman[30] states this is due to the altered body composition of lean mass, and does not in reality represent a decline. Energy expenditure for lying, standing, and walking changes little with age, but as work efficiency declines from 37% in the young to 28% in the elderly, the older person uses more energy to perform the same amount of work.[15] Factors which may cause variation in the caloric needs of individuals are age, sex, basal metabolism, size, occupation, environment, temperature, hormonal balance, and physical activity patterns and habits.[17]

Carbohydrates

The plant carbohydrates, such as the grains and root vegetables, serve as the major human energy supply. An increasing amount of energy in the American diet is derived from refined sugar, now averaging about 120 pounds of sugar per person per year.[14] Milling renders the grains, such as wheat, rice, and corn, partially deficient; and processing renders sugar totally deficient in micronutrients. Man's ability to metabolize carbohydrate is reduced with advancing age, reflected in the impaired glucose tolerance curves.[29] Infrequent ingestion of large quantities of carbohydrate, i.e., three meals a day, results in greater insulin demands on the pancreas and causes an accumulation of triglycerides synthesized endogenously from carbohydrate, as well as a lessened nitrogen retention.[18]

Fats

Fats serve as a source of the essential fatty acids, as a carrier of the fat-soluble vitamins (A, D, E, K), and as a major energy source. Up to 43% of the calories in the American diet is derived from fat, 66% from animal and 34% from vegetable sources.[9] There has been an enormous interest in the relationship between dietary fat and atherosclerosis, a major cause of morbidity and mortality in the aged. There is strong circumstantial evidence that lowering the total fat intake and substituting unsaturated fats for the saturated ones will reduce atherosclerotic problems, but the evidence is still controversial.[18,23,29] Hazzard[31] reports on an 8-year prospective study showing that a substitution of vegetable oils for saturated fats results in a significant reduction of myocardial infarction, sudden death, and cerebrovascular accidents, but the overall death rate in the experimental and control groups was similar because of a significantly increased rate of neoplasm in the unsaturated fat group. From animal studies, Caster[23] reported that caproic acid esters (saturated fatty acids, present in butter fat, coconut oil, corn grits, and chicken skin) were probably more important in raising blood cholesterol levels than was dietary cholesterol itself. In addition he found a significant increase in systolic blood pressure when the amount of fat in the diet was increased from 10% to 25%.

Proteins

The function of protein is to supply the eight essential amino acids, and to provide the nitrogen for the synthesis of the others. The requirement for protein in relation to age is uncertain because of vast individual variations.[18,32] There is a frequent age-related decrease in the serum albumin and increase in globulins, but the albumin drop may be related to chronic protein undernutrition. Not only is it necessary for the essential amino acids to be present in the diet, but they must be available to the tissues at the same time and in proper proportions for the body to use. The diets of older people must continue to supply the quantity of amino acids necessary for tissue maintenance daily.[17] While the RDA is 56 gm. per day for the 70 kg. ideal man, others recommend up to 1 gm. per kg. of body weight of good quality protein, such as that in meat, milk products, or eggs.[9]

EATING HABITS OF THE ELDERLY

Introduction and General Surveys

There are two principal ways to study the eating habits and the nutritional status of the elderly; namely, cross-sectional surveys on groups at various ages and longitudinal studies on the same individuals over a long period of time. While the latter is much more informative, relatively few longitudinal studies have been initiated, according to Exton-Smith.[33] Some of the results of those studies conducted in Western countries will be reported. Again there are wide differences of results, interpretations, and opinions.

Shock reported, in 1970, that there was little experimental evidence to indicate substantial age differences in nutritional requirements or for the incidence of widespread nutritional deficiencies of the elderly living in their own homes.[34] One of the largest surveys undertaken was the Ten-State Nutrition Survey by the U. S. Center for Disease Control reported in 1972. This study collected data from 24-hour recall of food consumed, as well as information about food purchasing, preparation, and usage. They especially studied groups at nutritional risk.[35] Among their findings were that persons 60 years old and older consumed far less food than needed to meet the nutrient standards for their age, sex, and weight. While no subgroup met the caloric adequacy standards, blacks and Spanish-Americans in general had the poorer diets. Over half of the male population had caloric intakes below 2000 calories, and over half of the females had less than 1500 calories. From a practical standpoint, it is difficult to maintain adequate micronutritional intakes at these levels. While the mean intakes of most nutrients met or closely approximated the standards except for iron and protein intakes in women, there was a wide range of intakes for most nutrients so that a "high percentage" of individuals consumed specific nutrient intakes below the standards. The most frequently reported deficiencies were of protein, iron and vitamin A. The median intakes for iron were less than the 10 mgm. standard for black males and all females. Cumulative frequency distribution showed large numbers of black and Spanish-American males and all females had low intakes of vitamin A. With the exception of vitamin A, the quality of the diets of older persons in the survey were not much different among the various subgroups, and the differences were more influenced by the total food consumption than by the nutrient density. Generally people in the low-income-ratio states had lower dietary intakes than persons in the high-income-ratio states, but it was not strongly related to income on a per 1000 calorie basis. Certain nutrients were mildly related to income, with increased amounts of calories, protein, calcium, and vitamins A anç C in the wealthier groups. No consistent relationship between body weight and nutrient intake was observed. Females tended to have lesser intakes than males, and blacks had the lowest values for most nutrients, except that Spanish-Americans had the lowest intake of vitamin A. Biochemical tests indicated that intakes of protein, iron, and vitamin A were dependent of total food intake, while differences in riboflavin and vitamin C reflected selection of foods high in these substances. Comparison of the mean nutrient intake per 1000 calories of the older age group with adolescents indicated that the foods selected by the elderly tended to have a generally higher nutritional content. Comparison of the mean nutrient intakes of those over age 60 in this survey with the corresponding age group in a previous U.S.D.A. survey in 1965 revealed minor differences, but a definite trend toward lower intakes in the later study.

Barrows and Roeder[16] summarize a number of different nutritional surveys and feel that, taken as a whole, the studies do not indicate consistent evidence of poor nutritional status or of marked deficiencies in nutrient intake among older members of most population groups. Todhunter[36] reported a survey conducted in a community group in 1973, looking especially at how life styles affected nutrient intakes in the elderly. Those who lived alone did not differ significantly in dietary adequacy from those who lived with others. Neither various health problems nor lack of teeth had much effect on food practices. More blacks than whites tended to economize on food, and meat was the first food to be limited. Most subjects indicated a willingness to try new foods, and ate three meals a day. Better education was correlated with a better diet, and economic factors strongly influenced the dietary adequacy, both in the choices and the serving size. Black females were the most disadvantaged group. In this study, two-thirds of the RDA was considered "satisfactory." In summary, about one-half of the dietary intake for the whole group met the RDA for protein; two-thirds were satisfactory for calcium; less than half of the women were satisfactory for iron; less than half of the total group were satisfactory for vitamin A and thiamine; only 37% of the group was satisfactory for riboflavin; and two-thirds were satisfactory for vitamin C.

Some recent studies of the elderly at home have been done in the United Kingdom by Macleod and her group.[37,38,39] Some of the RDA's are different, and some regional differences were noted as well. The problem of the realistic assessment of data because of lack of precise criteria was noted, but it was observed that 13% of the men and 25% of the women took less than the recommended RDA of protein. The intake of most nutrients except sucrose declined with age. Calcium intake was below the national average, and potassium and magnesium were felt to be below optimal levels. About 45% took less than 50 mgm. of ascorbic acid daily, and about one-third of the men and over half of the women took less than the recommended dose of thiamine. Mean intakes of nicotinic acid declined with age, and only 31% of the men and 11% of the women reached the recommended intakes. The mean intakes for all ages and groups were below the recommended levels for riboflavin. In spite of these problems, comparatively little overt clinical malnutrition was seen. Caird, Judge, and Macleod[40] analyzed this Glasgow data, and noted that those variables most likely to predict malnutrition in the elderly at home were the amount spent on food per week, taking seven or less hot meals per week, and physical disability. The uncertainty as to the extent of malnutrition present in the community-living elderly was addressed by Berry and Darke.[41] They could not find significant overt malnutrition, and felt those at greatest risk were those with various debilitating diseases, or mental or physical conditions which interfere with their ability to obtain, prepare, and eat an adequate diet. A recent study by E. A. Whanger[42] among older lower-middle-class women attending a day care center showed that none of them had adequate intakes when measured by the frequency of intake of the four basic food groups and caloric intake. The most common group of inadequate intake was in dairy foods. One-half of the subjects were taking vitamin supplements, two-thirds of these on the recommendations of their doctors. Most did not know the name nor the ingredients of their vitamin or mineral supplement, and one thought her antihypertensive medicine was a vitamin. Investigation of the subjects' nutritional knowledge and beliefs showed no significant correlation with their dietary practice.

Within various institutions, studies have been done on nutritional status. In a general hospital in 1965, Leevy and his group[43] studied eleven vitamin levels, and found that in 88% of the patients there was a reduction in the blood levels of one or more vitamins, and that in 10% there was a decrease in the levels of at least five vitamins. The more frequent deficiencies were folacin in 45% of the patients, thiamine in 31%, niacin in 29%, vitamin B_6 in 27%, vitamin C in 12%, and vitamin B_{12} in 10%. Only 40% of the patients with hypovitaminosis had a history of abnormal dietary habits, and objective evidence of vitamin deficiency was present in only 38% of this group. The causes for reduced dietary intake in a long-stay hospital were studied by MacLennan, Martin, and Mason[44] who noted that subjects requiring help with feeding because of physical problems were likely to have low levels of nicotinic acid and iron. In contrast, those with severe mental disorders were more likely to have reduced intake of riboflavin, nicotinic acid, ascorbic acid, potassium and iron. Intake of different types of food was related to physical and mental impairment, such as inability to communicate needs and loss of appetite. A survey by Basu and his group[45] of blood values of vitamins in long-stay psychogeriatric patients showed that 83% had evidence of thiamine deficiency, 50% had low ascorbic acid levels, and 44% had low vitamin A levels. Morgan and his group[46] studied blood and urine vitamin levels in acute geriatric admissions to a hospital, and found that none of them had a normal nutritional profile. About 35% had over 50% of their various tests abnormal; vitamin C, vitamin E, carotene and nicotinic acid were low in over 50% of the patients.

Taste and Smell as Dietary Determinants

The elderly commonly complain about the taste and smell of food, especially its sourness, bitterness, and dryness. Schiffman documents the marked loss of smell in the elderly, as well as variations in taste so that older persons are often unable to distinguish one food from another when blindfolded and thus lose important hedonic stimuli.[47,48,49] These losses undoubtedly are related to the shift in many elderly away from such foods as vegetables, which have a pleasant odor but a bitter taste, to sweet tasting but often nutritionally inadequate foods. Flavor and odor enhancement increase the desirability and palatability of foods for the elderly, but the market in geriatric foods has been virtually undeveloped. Perhaps the complaints of some elderly about the flatness or bitterness of life may have some physiologic as well as psychologic basis.

Psychologic Implications of Eating Patterns of the Elderly

The older person's search is for a nourishment that transcends the nutritional factors. As Weinberg[50] notes, food is utilized as a symbol for the maintenance of the psychologic life of the person, as feeding is one of the basic determinants of personality patterning and socialization. Thus eating becomes a medium of social interchange; an expression of, or a substitute for, love; and a source of basic pleasure. For the older person, with whom he eats is often more important than what he eats. As losses of other gratifications and relationships occur, eating patterns assume a greater positive or negative role in the person's psychologic environment.

RELATIONSHIP BETWEEN NUTRITION, HEALTH AND AGING

Patterns of Nutrition, Disease, Mortality, and Aging

A number of the relationships between nutritional factors and disease have already been explored, and obviously a great deal more research needs to be done.

A circular pattern of interaction between aging and nutrition is postulated by Rao,[51] who speculates that the aging process leads to reduced energy, causing retirement, which entails a low earning capacity resulting in poverty. This results in poor housing conditions, causing relative food and improper food habits. The resulting poor state of nutrition predisposes to chronic diseases, which gives impetus in turn to the aging process.

Two older studies showed a relationship between nutrient intake and physical well-being. Kelley and her group[52] found that, in older women, with one or more nutrients below 80% of the RDA, 40% reported unexplained tiredness, joint pains, and shortness of breath. The mortality rate over the next 7 years was higher among women who had at least one nutrient below 40% of the RDA. In 1954, Chope[53] observed low intakes of vitamin A, niacin and ascorbic acid in the 4 years prior to death in 49 of 50 individuals. He noted that low vitamin A intake was correlated with increased incidence of nervous, circulatory and respiratory disorders, and low thiamine intake was associated with subsequent diseases of the nervous and circulatory systems. In a more recent study, Schlenker and his associates[54] did a follow-up on a group of older women showing a high correlation between an increased fat intake and a shortened life span, independent of the caloric effect and resul-

tant obesity. Those women ingesting a diet with large amounts of thiamine had a lower incidence of death from cardiovascular disease, and those with diets high in ascorbic acid lived longer.

Frequency of Classical Deficiency Syndromes

Perhaps a complicating factor in clinical nutrition is that the classical deficiency syndromes are infrequently seen today. A useful guide to these is the volume by Goldsmith.[55] A survey of patients admitted to Duke University Medical Center, a referral and teaching facility, from 1951 through 1971, showed only 7 cases of vitamin A deficiency, 5 cases of beriberi (thiamine), 9 cases of pellagra (niacin), 17 cases of scurvy (ascorbic acid), and 38 cases of rickets (vitamin D) among 411,000 patients, for a prevalence of 18 deficiency diseases per 100,000 admissions. There were 326 cases of pernicious anemia (vitamin B_{12}) during this time, however.

Subclinical Malnutrition

In view of the infrequent states of clinical deficiency syndromes, the question arises of subclinical malnutrition. Anderson[56] addresses this issue, pointing out the deficiencies of our methods of analysis as well as our clinical correlations. While overt deficiencies are described as the tip of the iceberg of malnutrition, it is not at all certain how large the rest of the iceberg is. He felt that, in general, malnutrition arose sporadically and characteristically in situations of specific stress such as an illness or loss of spouse impinging on otherwise borderline nutritional states. Watkin alludes to this problem in two of his observations. In 1968 he observed the reports of low nutritional intakes and serum values of various nutrients in the aged, but felt these parameters were cause for little concern about the nutritional status of this population, for although physical examinations revealed many conditions not found in younger people, none of these could be attributed to nutrient deficiencies *per se.*[57] By 1976, however, Watkin[58] felt that nutrition is the most impressive environmental key to good health in man, but he lamented the very slow progress in researching the area of nutrition, health, and aging, feeling even that the investigations have been equipped with the wrong tools.

Some important observations were made by Brin[59] on the stages of development of vitamin deficiency disease, based on the experimental development of thiamine deficiency in young men. He observed a sequence of five stages: (1) a preliminary stage of decreased urinary vitamin excretion within 5 days; (2) a biochemical stage within 10 days of alterations in blood chemistry; (3) a physiological stage within 21–30 days with loss of body weight and appetite, general malaise, insomnia, and increased irritability; (4) a clinical phase within 30–300 days with increased malaise, weight loss, polyneuritis, and cardiovascular symptoms; and (5) the anatomical phase after 200 days with cardiovascular changes and neurologic changes including degeneration of the granular layer of the cerebellum, perivascular cerebral hemorrhages with neuronal degeneration, swelling of microglia, proliferation of astrocytes, and mammillary body pathology. How these observations might fit with various clinical conditions seen in the elderly is not known, but the diffuse signs seen in the subclinical phases are certainly common complaints of the elderly.

Obesity

Obesity is rarely considered a form of malnutrition, although it is a major health hazard in the United States. It is of course the result of an excess of calories as compared with the expenditure of energy in both body maintenance and exercise. The obese individual is more prone to conditions such as dyspnea, diabetes, hypertension, and generalized atherosclerosis, as well as a greater tendency to falls and accidents. Thus obesity significantly reduces life expectancy.

Rockstein and Sussman point out[60] that the life expectancy of an obese 45-year-old male is reduced by about 25%. They speculate that if all cancer could be eliminated the average life span would increase by 2 years, whereas if obesity and its associated problems could be controlled, the average life span would increase by 4 years or more. Andrus, in a recent review of the literature, concludes that mild to moderate obesity in middle and late life does not decrease expectancy.[60a] However, one must question if this is a cohort effect. Other nutritional deficiencies are common among the overweight since much of the obesity comes from the consumption of "empty calorie" foods such as sugar, cooking fats, and alcohol, which also decrease the appetite for other foods of higher nutritive value.[17] The difficulties of achieving weight loss are described by Stunkard,[61] who also cites an interesting 3-year controlled study on diet restriction in an old age home. The death rate for the restricted group was less than half of the control groups, and the restricted spent only a little over half of the time in the infirmary as did the controls.

VITAMINS AND THEIR ROLE IN GERIATRIC MENTAL ILLNESS

Introduction

The term "vitamine" was introduced in 1912 by Funk, who believed that there were four indispensable dietary factors.[62] In describing the role of vitamins in metabolic function, Roe[63] said "Each step of the chain of reactions through which a nutrient passes, as it follows in appropriate metabolic pathways, is mediated by at least one enzyme system, and the function of every enzyme system calls for the combined action of an apoenzyme (composed for the most part of amino acids) and a coenzyme which usually includes a vitamin and/or mineral element." Since the body cannot synthesize vitamins, it must get them from external sources either in an active form or as an inactive precursor (provitamin). Every vitamin may take part in multiple metabolic reactions, often interrelating with other vitamins; hence, a deficiency of one may affect the metabolism of several others. The individual vitamins and related compounds have been designated in approximate order of discovery by letters of the alphabet and numerical subscripts. The studies of vitamin metabolism in animals are not always relevant to man because of considerable species specificity. The vitamins are divided into the fat-soluble (A, D, E, and K) and the water-soluble groups. The latter generally are stored to a limited degree in the body, and the amount that is maintained is probably related to the saturation capacity of an apoenzyme.[15] The B-complex group are chemically different, but are generally bound together in nature and function somewhat similarly. The classical deficiency syndromes are seen only in advanced stages of deficiency, and the symptoms of early malnutrition of any one of the B-complex vitamins tend to be similar. Considerable uncertainty still exists about the vitamin requirements and interactions in old age, and about the significance of marginal or subclinical deficiencies. In this chapter only those vitamins having some known or likely role in geriatric mental illness will be discussed.

Vitamin A (Retinol)

The term vitamin A now designates several active compounds; namely, the retinols and their esters, retinal and retinoic acid, and the carotinoids with provitamin activity as listed by Roels and Lui.[64] The preformed compounds are found mainly in liver, meat, fats, eggs, and dairy products, and the provitamin in yellow and green vegetables and fruits. Deficiencies may arise from inability to store the vitamins because of liver disease, difficulty in converting the provitamin as in diabetes or hypothyroidism, or impaired absorption because of such things as lack of dietary fat, inadequate bile secretion, use of mineral oil, pancreatic insuffi-

ciency, or use of antibiotics. In chronic illness the liver stores may be depleted or the metabolism of vitamin A interfered with. Low levels of vitamin A in older people were noted to be correlated with a heightened incidence of unspecified nervous diseases by Chope.[53] Studies with rats reported by Bertolini[29] indicated that by quadrupling the minimal necessary amount of vitamin A, the length of the useful segment of maturity, i.e., nonsenile, could be extended about 10%. Doubling the amount again caused a reduction in life span and caused other problems, however.

Vitamin B$_1$ (Thiamine)

Thiamine serves as a coenzyme in oxidative decarboxylation and according to Neal and Sauberlich is important in the phosphogluconate pathway of the interconversion of various sugars.[65] It is found in meat, whole grains, yeast, green vegetables, and beans. Deficiencies may occur when thiamine requirements increase because of a febrile condition, malignant disease, or a high carbohydrate intake. Diuretics increase the rate of excretion. Some experimental evidence indicates that the gastric secretions of the aged may inactivate thiamine, especially if hydrochloric acid is absent, and that altered intestinal flora may bind ingested thiamine. Tolerance tests indicate there may be altered metabolism of thiamine in the aged.[29] The classical deficiency syndrome is beriberi, usually manifested in the elderly in the "dry" form with an ascending symmetric polyneuritis, fatigue, decreased attention span, and impaired capacity to work. In more severe or acute situations there may be the "wet" form with associated cardiac symptoms, or Wernicke's encephalopathy with ophthalmoplegia, cerebellar ataxia, confusion, and coma.[66] Other mental symptoms in milder forms of thiamine deficiency are listed by Cheraskin[14] as loss of appetite, depression, irritability, confusion, memory loss, inability to concentrate, and sensitivity to noise.

Vitamin B₂ (Riboflavin)

Riboflavin acts as the prosthetic group of the flavo-protein enzymes involved in a number of oxidative enzyme systems essential to cell growth and repair.[67] Its best sources are milk, eggs, and meat. A deficiency of this vitamin alone is unusual, and is characterized by glossitis, cheilosis, and seborrheic dermatitis, as well as depression.

Vitamin B₃ (Niacin, Nicotinic Acid Amide, Niacinamide, Vitamin PP)

The active form of this vitamin is nicotinic acid amide, forming parts of a number of enzymes such as codehydrogenase and respiratory enzymes, and is involved in carbohydrate, fat, protein, and cytochrome metabolism.[68] Niacin is especially found in liver, meat, yeast, and legumes, and dietary tryptophan can be converted to niacin. Pellagra is the classic deficiency disease, with its "three D's" (dermatitis, diarrhea, and dementia). Common signs early in the deficiency include headaches, irritability, apprehension, sleeplessness, emotional instability, and loss of recent memory; while in advanced cases a confusional psychosis with delirium and catatonia may be seen.[69] There is a great controversy about the use of niacin in large doses to treat mental illness. This is discussed in the section on megavitamin therapy. Nicotinic acid in doses of 3 to 6 gms. per day have been used to lower levels of cholesterol and glycerides in the blood as a treatment for atherosclerosis.[15]

Vitamin B₆ (Pyridoxine)

There are three forms of vitamin B₆, which are incorporated in a large number of enzymes concerned with nitrogen metabolism.[70] Since it is widely distributed in many foodstuffs, clearcut deficiencies are infrequent, but lesser deficiency manifestations include irritability, weakness, nervousness, insomnia, apathy, depression, and a loss of the sense of responsibility. There is a gradual drop in serum levels with age, and the administration of pyridoxine to aged subjects is reported to produce a hypotensive effect, and a lowering of cholesterol levels.[29]

Pantothenic Acid

This vitamin forms coenzyme-A, and is active in a large number of metabolic reactions. Like pyridoxine, it is widely distributed in nature and hence obvious deficiencies are infrequent. Williams[71] reports that mice fed on a pantothenic acid supplement all of their lives lived about 20% longer than controls. He points out that pantothenic acid is essential to brain functioning and that profound depression may result from its deficiency. It is also reported that this vitamin may give relief in nutritional neuropathy and Korsakoff's psychosis, as well as improving the ability to withstand stress.[72]

Folacin (Folic Acid, Pteroylglutamic Acid, Vitamins B₉, B₁₀, B₁₁, and M).

The generic term folacin includes several compounds involved in a variety of metabolic actions such as single carbon metabolism and nucleic acid structure, norepinephrine and serotonin biosynthesis, and a close interrelation with vitamin B₁₂ as described by Herbert.[73] It is found in liver and other organ meats, yeast, fresh green vegetables, and some fruits. In geriatric mental illness folacin is important both because it is probably the most common vitamin deficiency, and because early mental symptoms of deficiency include apathy, weakness, lassitude, irritability, forgetfulness, lack of motivation, hostility, paranoid behavior, and depression, and later of dementia (as described by Kane and Lipton,[74] Strachan and Henderson,[75] Hallstrome,[76] Carney and Sheffield,[77] and Sneath,[78] among others). Several factors may play a role both in folate and vitamin B₁₂ utilization: (1) inadequate ingestion, such as from a poor diet; (2) inadequate absorption because of drug interference or specific malabsorption from the gut; (3) a metabolic block such as folic acid antagonists or liver disease; (4) increased requirement as in anemia, carcinomas, or hyperthyroidism; and (5) increased excretion, such as found in vitamin B_{12} deficiency or liver disease.[73] A recent study by Baker, Jaslow, and Frank[79] demonstrated a rather marked impairment in the ability to utilize dietary falocin because of a diminished supply of intestinal folate conjugase enzyme which converts the dietary folylpolyglutamates to an absorbable form. There is a active absorption process, apparently by a carrier-protein similar to vitamin B_{12}, as well as a very limited passive diffusion. A low intake of iron may also decrease the absorption of folacin and vitamin B_{12}. A vicious cycle may develop in thatr a persistent folacin deficiency causes enzyme and morphologic changes in the intestinal epithelial cells, further compromising the ability to absorb dietary folacin and other nutrients.[79] this situation requires vitamin supplementation, sometimes parenterally.

Vitamin B_{12} (Cobalamin, Cyanocobalamin)

Cobalamin is a generic term for several related compounds functioning as coenzymes in the synthesis of nucleic acid and nucleoprotein, in red cell formation, in the metabolic pathways of nervous tissue, in energy cycles, and as a reducing agent (as described by Herbert[73] and Weg[15]). It is found almost entirely in animal tissues such as liver and kidney, but is synthesized by some bacteria.

The clinical deficiency disease is pernicious anemia, although megaloblastosis is the end product of deranged DNA synthesis of any cause. Since both folic acid and vitamin B_{12} are required for DNA formation, deficiency of either may lead to megaloblastosis which affects not only the blood cells, but other body cells as well. For a yet unclear reason, there is inadequate myelin synthesis in vitamin B_{12} deficiency, but not in folacin deficiency. Thus various neurologic signs and symptoms may occur in vitamin B_{12} deficiency including loss of vibratory and position sense, paresthesias, poor muscle coordination, ataxia, confusion, memory loss, moodiness, agitation, depression, delusions, hallucinations, and psychosis, often with paranoid features, as described by Herbert,[73] Kallstrom and Nylof,[80] Smith[81] and MacCallum.[82] There is still uncertainty about what the normal levels of vitamin B_{12} are in the elderly, and what effects low levels may have, especially regarding psychiatric illness, as described by Buxton and his group,[83] Shulman,[84] and Whanger and Wang.[85] Our surveys among 164 older psychiatric patients and controls revealed no levels in the low pernicious anemia range, but a 5% incidence of levels in the questionably deficient range (i.e., 100–149 picograms/ml) and a 13% incidence in the "indeterminant" range of 150–199 pg/ml, with a significantly higher mean level in black subjects. The absorption of vitamin B_{12} is complex, beginning with the attachment of the vitamin to the gastric intrinsic factor glycoprotein which then adheres to the ileal wall. Under optimal conditions, the vitamin is passed across the ileal wall into the portal blood stream where it is attached to another glycoprotein. In high concentrations, there is some direct diffusion of vitamin B_{12} from the entire small intestine into the bloodstream. The body stores of vitamin B_{12} will usually last over 3 years. More than 60 different conditions in which vitamin B_{12} deficiency may arise are listed by Herbert,[73] with common ones in old age being inadequate intake and gastric atrophy. There are high concentrations of vitamin B_{12} in human brain tissue, and especially high levels have been noted in the pituitary in animals. Ordonez[86] reports that these concentrations decrease by up to 80% during dietary deficiency.

Vitamin B_{15} (Pangamic Acid, Calcium Pangamate)

This substance was discovered in 1951 by E. T. Krebs, and is a water-soluble compound found with other B-complex vitamins in fruit kernels, seeds, rice bran and whole grain cereals, yeast, and liver. The vitamin is scantily discussed in the standard English literature, as it is felt that vitamin B_{15} activity has not been demonstrated in man.[87] The East Europeans have used it extensively and enthusiastically for a number of years, feeling that it contributes, along with other micronutrients, to "a decrease in the inertness of the cerebral rhythms, an improvement of protein, lipid, vitamin, and electrolyte metabolism and the stimulation of oxidative processes in tissues" in the aging, according to Chebotarev.[88] The Russians in particular advocate its use in cardiovascular and arteriosclerotic disorders, elevated cholesterol, emphysema, mental retardation, premature aging, and senility, and they ply their athletes with it to stimulate energy in muscular activity. Professor Yakov Shpirt of the Moscow Clinical Hospital feels that the effects of vitamin B_{15} on improving cerebral oxygen utilization and avoiding atherosclerotic problems are so substantial that he foresees calcium pangamate "next to the saltcellar on the table of every family with people past forty."[89] The tablets have recently shown up in health food stores, and the recommended dosage is 50 mg three times daily for about 30 days, with a 2- or 3-month rest period before its next course.[90] It is reportedly virtually nontoxic, but, obviously, further research is a necessity.

Vitamin C (Ascorbic Acid)

Vitamin C is a rather simple compound, although it has several derivatives and analogs which play a number of metabolic roles including that of an intracellular oxidation-reduction potential regulator, an antioxidant, an aid in conversion of folic acid to folinic acid, a facilitator of iron absorption, an essential for collagen formation and blood vessel integrity, a factor in the utilization of vitamin B_{12}, a detoxifying agent, and a somewhat uncertain role in adrenal cortical function and cholesterol metabolism as mentioned by Hodges and Baker[91] and Weg.[15] Its best sources are rapidly growing fruits and vegetables, but it is quite vulnerable to heating and processing. Levels in tissue, and possibly even the ability of the tissue to retain vitamin C, may decline with age.[92] The classical deficiency syndrome is scurvy, which includes a profound fatigue and lethargy. Psychologic changes are common and have been characterized by Kinsman and Hood[93] as a neurotic triad of hysteria, depression, and hypochondriasis.

Riccitelli[94] reports malaise, irritability, and emotional disturbances in the hypovitaminosis state. Surveys of the elderly ill show a high incidence of vitamin C deficiency, such as 68% mentioned by Morgan and his group.[46] They showed a significantly increased mortality rate among the elderly with low leucocyte ascorbic acid levels. The controversy over the use of high doses of ascorbic acid in colds and other conditions is still unsettled.

Vitamin E (Tocopherols)

Vitamin E comprises a group of at least seven related compounds, the most active of which is alpha-tocopherol. The richest sources are vegetable and seed oils, but it is found rather widely in leafy vegetables, whole grains, egg yolk, liver, and milk. Its metabolic functions are not completely clear, but it has an antioxidant action which tends to protect tissue and various compounds such as membrane phospholipids, coenzyme Q, vitamin A, and polyunsaturated fatty acids (PUFA) from breakdown by peroxidation or free radical reactions, according to Horwitt.[95] Some feel that it may have some enzymatic functions, and a role in protein synthesis.[18] Clear cut deficiency states are very rare in humans except in malabsorption syndromes. Among geriatric admissions to an acute hospital, however, Morgan and his group[46] noted low plasma levels in 67% of the subjects. Of major concern to the older age group are the reported effects of increased vitamin E on cardiovascular disease, on sexual function, and on the aging process itself. Many are using a diet with an increased amount of

PUFA, with some reduction in cardiovascular disease, but a possible attendant rise in neoplastic disease. The need for vitamin E increases with the amount of PUFA taken in as the vitamin E generally present in the PUFA vehicle is often destroyed in the processing.[95] There is some documentation that vitamin E in a dosage of 300 IU nightly may reduce idiopathic leg cramps, and 1200 IU daily may help intermittent claudication with a femoropopliteal block or poor distal arteries.[96] The effect of vitamin E on impotence in sexual functioning is probably a placebo effect, but often a happy one, and its role in the aging process in humans remains to be elucidated.

Results of Supplementation of Vitamins in the Elderly

As was mentioned previously, there is enormous controversy on the use of vitamin supplements. Where there is a rare case of a classical deficiency disease, then of course the appropriate action would be to supply the missing vitamin, although this would usually be inadequate in the elderly since deficiencies tend to be multiple. The pill purveyors promise panaceas while the FDA reports in the *Myths of Vitamins*[97] that foods can and do supply most Americans with adequate nutrients, and that consumers should not expect any major physical benefits from multivitamin pills, "contrary to the myth." One of the most striking deficiencies is the lack of studies of the effects of long-term nutritional supplements on physical and mental well-being, especially in the elderly. One of the few long-term studies is by Chebotarev[88] from Russia. Multiple vitamin supplements were given for years to large numbers of elderly. He reported improved functioning of the cardiovascular and central nervous system in over half of the elderly, with EEG improvement in 26%. One of the best controlled studies was that reported by Taylor[98] of 80 chronically ill, hospitalized elderly patients, of whom 95% showed some sign of nutritional deficiency and 90% had low levels of thiamine and/or ascorbic acid. Those who received a vitamin B complex and vitamin C supplement showed highly significant improvement in physical and mental functioning, although the positive effects were not manifest before a year or more. When the vitamin supplement was stopped, signs of deficiency reappeared in many of the subjects in about 6 months' time, even though they were eating the regular hospital diet. The biochemical levels returned to normal rapidly, but it was obvious that even 1 year was not adequate for full clinical restitution. Incidentally, at the end of the year 30% of the controls had bedsores, while only 6% of those receiving supplements had bedsores. Most of the control group demonstrated significant deterioration during the study period, as noted by Brocklehurst.[99] In a similar study reported in 1972, MacLeod[100] did not find significant change in the physical signs, but did not comment on mental changes. The preparation used was only a partial supplement.

Other studies include one by Kral and his group[101] in which 63 elderly patients with organic brain syndrome were studied for vitamin B_{12} levels (28% were clinically deficient) and folic acid levels (36% clinically deficient). 11% were deficient in both. There was not a clear correlation between the degree of dementia and the B_{12} level, and 3 months of vitamin B_{12} injection did not change the picture significantly. In a similar study Carney and Sheffield[77] found that those treated with folate had significant improvement in functional and organic psychoses, and were discharged from the hospital earlier, although those treated with B_{12} showed only minor improvement in the same 40 days of the observations. In a controlled trial of chronically hospitalized psychiatric patients, Milner[102] noted that 3 weeks of vitamin C supplementation produced significant improvement in depressive, manic, and paranoid symptomatology. A later study by Dymock and Brocklehurst,[103] using individual vitamin supplements to try to treat physical signs of deficiency, did not yield significant results. Hughes and his group[104] gave vitamin B_{12} to a group of community elderly with low vitamin B_{12} levels over a 4-week period and did not notice significant change. Altman *et al.*[105] gave a vitamin B complex and C preparation to psychogeriatric inpatients for 6 weeks, and noted a significant reduction in the level of excitement. An interesting finding reported by Pennington[106] in an uncontrolled study was that a multiple vitamin preparation plus glutamic acid significantly enhanced the speed and effectiveness of a variety of psychotropic drugs.

An issue arises of how often the elderly take vitamin supplements and under what circumstances. We conducted a survey among several different groups, finding that 20% of the elderly being admitted to a state hospital were taking supplements, while 48% of those who had been there 6 months or more were taking supplements on doctor's orders. A comparable but elite outpatient volunteer group from the first Longitudinal Study of the Duke University Center for the Study of Aging and Human Development showed that 42% were taking supplements, mostly on their own. A random sample of the community living elderly showed that 30% were using supplements. There was a steady increase with age, so that usage below age 65 was 14%, increasing to 25% at age 65 and to 50% of those over age 90. Whites tended to take supplements in a significantly higher percentage than blacks, and women significantly more than men. The use of vitamin supplements was only slightly higher in the economically well off as compared to the destitute. There was a steady rise in vitamin supplement usage with increasing levels of education in both blacks and whites. Among occupational groups, only 21% of unskilled workers were using supplements, while 48% of the professional people were using them. Of course, it is difficult to draw etiologic conclusions from these observations.

Another factor mentioned by the opponents of vitamin supplementation is the "damage to the budget" of buying supplements rather than food.[97] It is often tempting to buy exotic and extremely expensive vitamin supplements, depending on one's taste and gullibility. Most elderly do not tend to be faddish, however. A major brand name vitamin and mineral supplement costs 4¢ a day, while the generic equivalent is less than 2¢ a day. A "natural vitamin and mineral capsule" would cost about 9¢ per day at present.

Toxicity of Vitamins

Toxic effects may develop when large doses of certain vitamins are ingested, yet vitamins are quite safe when one considers how often they are taken in extreme or irrational ways. Those with major toxic potential are the fat soluble vitamins A and D, but they are much more a hazard to children than to adults. Vitamin A, when taken in doses of 20 to 30 times the RDA over a period of time may produce fatigue, malaise, abdominal and joint pains, severe headaches, insomnia, and restlessness. High doses of carotene produce an orange cast to the skin, but no other toxic symptoms.[64] Hypervitaminosis D causes hypercalcemia, which may lead to nausea, weight loss, anorexia, abnormal calcification, head pain, and possibly atherosclerosis.[107,108] In adults symptoms may occur after 50,000 units of vitamin D is taken for several weeks. Vitamin E is virtually nontoxic, although some increase in clotting time and rare depression have been reported.[108] In high doses, vitamin K may damage red blood cell membranes. The water soluble vitamins generally have a lower toxicity. Rare cases of anaphylactic shock have been reported following injections of thiamine in a person previously sensitized to it.[65] Toxicity with ribroflavin, pantothenic acid, pyridoxine, and vitamin B_{12} are almost unknown, except for a rare allergic type reaction after B_{12} injections. Niacin is a significant risk at high pharmacologic doses, i.e., over 3 gms. daily, producing occasional arrythmias, gastrointestinal problems such as peptic ulcers, and liver toxicity.[68,108] Folic acid has a very low toxicity, but may produce some diarrhea above 15 mg. daily; and, at enormous dosage, can precipitate in the kidneys.[73] A real danger is the use of folic acid in the presence of an undiagnosed vitamin B_{12} deficiency or pernicious anemia, as the hematologic picture will improve, but the neurologic symptoms may progress dangerously.[73] In high doses (5 to 15 gms daily) ascorbic acid may cause diarrhea. Theoretically there might be an increase in urinary tract stones, and this may interfere with the absorption of some trace minerals.[91] A survey of vitamin toxicity among patients admitted to the Duke University Medical Center from 1952 to 1971 revealed a rate of hypervitaminosis of 4 per 100,000 patients; about one-fifth the rate of classical vitamin deficiency during the same period. Not one case of hypervitaminosis in the Boston Drug Surveillance Project has been identified to date among the elderly.[109]

Megavitamin Therapy

There have been great interest and debate over the use of huge doses of various vitamins to treat various psychiatric disorders, as mentioned by Hawkins and his group[110] and Osmond.[111] This has been adressed by Lipton and Kane[112] and others, and since as far as is known, it has no particular relevance to the elderly, it will not be pursued here.

To B or Not To B

A major question comes as to whether or not to use vitamin supplements rather liberally in the elderly. Of course many elderly solve the issue by taking supplements on their own, either deliberately or unwittingly, in the increasing number of food preparations containing substantial amounts of supplemental vitamins and minerals. Many physicians, when faced with the multiple nonspecific complaints of the elderly, may out of frustration prescribe vitamins as a placebo, or in hopes of accomplishing something. Certainly subclinical deficiencies are often hard and expensive to prove or disprove. To suggest that vitamin deficiencies cause most depletion states in the elderly is unscientific, but to ignore the fact that they do cause some is unwise.

My own approach is to use balanced multivitamins and mineral supplements almost regularly in impaired older persons on the basis that the probable value considerably offsets the minor and theoretical hazards, and the expense is minor. It is important to first do a thorough work-up, and make sure that pernicious anemia is ruled out. If the person is obviously malnourished, I may give a parenteral injection of multivitamins on each of two successive days on the basis of frequent alimentary upset and impaired absorption.[113] If the folic acid is low, I give folic acid supplement, one mg. twice daily for a month. I rarely use single vitamin preparations only, as the deficiencies are almost always multiple. In addition there is some evidence, including some from our study on the vibratory sense in the elderly, that single or incomplete vitamins may make the metabolic and neurologic state worse by further upsetting the nutritional balance.[114]

One does not like adding unnecessary medications or fixing an older person's attention further on body functions, but I think that this concern is a counsel of perfection in our society. Discussing nutrition with a patient may well keep him from using faddish, irrational, or excessively expensive products, and may contribute significantly to his wellbeing.

MINERALS AND THEIR POSSIBLE ROLE IN GERIATRIC MENTAL ILLNESS

Introduction

Minerals make up about 3.5% of the total body weight, and of the 90 naturally occurring elements, 26 are presently known to be essential for animal life. According to Underwood[115] these can be divided into 11 major (or bulk or macrominerals) and 15 trace elements or microminerals. The daily requirements for the major minerals are above 100 mg. per day, and they consist of carbon, hydrogen, oxygen, nitrogen, sulfur, calcium, phosphorus, potassium, sodium, chlorine and magnesium. The requirements for the trace elements are several milligrams per day or less[116] and these microminerals consist of iron, zinc, copper, manganese, nickel, cobalt, molybdenum, selenium, chromium, iodine, fluorine, tin, silicon, vanadium, and arsenic. In addition, there are some 20 to 30 minerals not meeting the criteria for being essential to proper cellular function which are present in variable concentrations in living tissue, and these include aluminum, cadmium, mercury, lead, silver, and gold. These latter elements probably represent environmental contaminants, and may increase with age and exposure. The essential elements have a dose range of biological action, determined in part by the homeostatic capacities of the animal. At high levels all minerals may have a pharmacological action, independent of any deficiency states, and at even higher and prolonged dosages, all may produce various toxic effects. Of course, the elements cannot be synthesized and must come ultimately from the soil. There are obligatory losses in urine, feces, sweat, skin, hair, and nails; and in the elderly the sweat losses may be substantial. The elements are widespread in animal and vegetable substances, but substantial loses of them may occur in food processing and cooking. As Schroeder[9] points out, from 50% to 90% of the minerals are removed in producing white flour, and refined sugar is virtually depleted of minerals necessary for its metabolism.

Much of the knowledge of the trace elements has become known in the past decade, and much remains to be clarified. They generally either form parts of various enzymes or serve as activators. There are many complex reactions and interactions and the reader is referred to some of the basic works such as those by Underwood,[115] Davies,[117] Schroeder[118] and Hine.[116] Perhaps the most useful is the report on the biomedical role of trace elements in aging by Hsu, Davis, and Neithamer.[119] Only those

minerals with some likely relevance to mental illness will be discussed here. These may be of special importance to the elderly, as they tend to have a reduced mineral intake because of both decreased caloric and/or protein intake, and poor food selection.[120] In addition, there are alterations in absorption and in enzyme concentrations and interactions that occur during the aging process, as mentioned by Lawton.[121]

Calcium

Calcium is the most abundant mineral, with most of it being found in the bones and teeth. In addition, it serves in its circulating form at least seven other functions, including the release of neurotransmitters from nerve endings.[122] The serum level is maintained at relatively constant levels, but at the expense of the skeletal system which is related in a complex way to osteoporosis. Substantial numbers of the elderly have inadequate intake of calcium, and Cheraskin[14] reports that anxiety, tension, and irritability may be related to inadequate calcium. Dairy products are the major food source of calcium, but in the face of deficiencies, generally a supplement such as calcium lactate or gluconate is needed, as the interrelated phosphorus intake is usually quite high in adults.

Phosphorus

Phosphorus, the second most abundant mineral, is vital in many roles in cellular functioning, such as formation of RNA and DNA, energy transfer in ADP, and formation of B vitamin coenzymes. Its deficiency in the elderly is unusual except as a result of prolonged use of nonabsorbable antacids. Clinically it may be manifested by weakness, anorexia, and malaise. The RDA of both calcium and phosphorus is 800 mg.[26]

Potassium

Potassium is the fourth most common mineral in the body, being found primarily intracellularly. This pool serves to keep the serum level relatively constant, so that a low serum level reflects a significant body depletion. It functions in the propagation of nervous impulse and muscle contraction as well as in intellectual and emotional tasks. Deficiencies increase with age, and can be related to diuretics, diarrhea, and restricted diets. A community study by Judge[123] showed that 56% of the elderly had inadequate dietary intake of potassium. These deficiencies lead to depressive states, weakness, inability to concentrate, incontinence, and disorientation. A minimal daily intake of 2.7 gm. is recommended by Schroeder.[9]

Magnesium

The body magnesium is found mainly intracellularly in bone and muscle tissue, and is involved in many metabolic functions including protein synthesis, and neuromuscular transmission. The mineral is found rather widely in vegetables and in milk, but its deficiency can be produced in the elderly by diabetes, diarrhea, congestive heart failure, diuretic therapy, alcoholism, hypertension, and renal disease, as observed by Martin,[124] and Flink and Jones.[125] Symptoms occurring with magnesium deficiency have been reported as weakness, lethargy, anorexia, and personality changes by Shils,[126] as well as hallucinations, being easily startled, and mental confusion.[14] Hypocalcemia and hypokalemia are often associated. The RDA is 350 mg., and treatment is usually by IM or IV magnesium sulfate.

PROTEINS AND THEIR POSSIBLE ROLE IN GERIATRIC MENTAL ILLNESS

Early Protein Deprivation and the Nervous System

Studies have shown that prolonged deficiencies of protein intake retard the development and affect the composition of the brain.[127] Pollitt and Thompson[128] cite evidence that severe protein deficiency in the first 12 months of life results in severe permanent deficits in intellectual function, while that occurring in the second year of life may, but generally does not, leave measurable retardation in intellectual function. In the adult, the brain takes up about 20 gm. of amino acids daily from the plasma, but Nowak and Munro[129] indicate that the brain draws preferentially on proteins from other body tissues to maintain its own protein synthesis. There is no clear evidence of how variable degrees of brain damage, early in life, might affect mental functioning late in life when the normal neuronal drop-out infringes on the early damage, but Howell and Loeb[17] feel that the ability of an older person to deal with complex problems and to adjust to changing circumstances can be permanently impaired by early protein deficit. The psychologic effects of protein-calorie undernutrition in adults include reduction in voluntary intellectual activity, depression, irritability, apathy, sensitivity to noise, reduced ambitions, poor concentration and comprehension. However, no permanent neurologic or psychiatric syndromes have been ascribed to simple protein-calorie undernutrition in the adult in the absence of an associated vitamin deficiency, as described by Dodge, Prensky, Feigin, and Holmes.[130]

Effects of Late Life Protein Deficiency on Mental Function

Protein undernutrition is associated with impairment of psychological performance, as proteins are necessary in the transmission of nerve impulses.[17] Recently it has been found that rapid and specific changes in brain composition normally occur after each meal. Wurtman and Fernstrom[131] report that particular brain constituents such as the neurotransmitter serotonin and its amino acid precursor tryptophan vary with the foods consumed. It is felt that protein deficits in the adult relax both excitation and inhibition in the nervous system, with both the alertness and selectivity of nerve cells to stimulation becoming defective.[132] The definitive studies of the effects of protein undernutrition in the elderly remain to be done.

Protein Supplementation

Tests a number of years ago suggested that the administration of the amino acid glutamic acid could increase the performance of animals in experimental behavior situations. Glutamic acid is found in high concentration in the brain and plays an important role in the formation of gamma a-minobutyric acid in the nervous system.[133,134] While recommendations have been made for its use in the mentally impaired elderly, there is no present proof that such supplementation beyond the normal diet can enhance the mental state of a senile older person.[135]

DENTAL FACTORS IN GERIATRIC NUTRITION

Dental status can significantly influence nutritional status, and this is a particularly relevant concern in the geriatric patient. Changes in the tissues of the oral cavity are very common in elderly persons, some of which result from normal aging processes, although others are consequences of disease or malnutrition. Gingival tissues atrophy and become dehydrated and bleed easily. Connective tissues and muscles shrink and lose elasticity. Taste acuity diminishes as the number of taste buds decline. Teeth yellow and become more brittle. Saliva production diminishes greatly, and the saliva becomes thick and ropy. This gummy, mucinous saliva is conducive to caries formation, and often leads to dental decay, even in individuals whose teeth have been resistant to caries for many years. Increasing age is associated with decreasing numbers of teeth, which are lost due to peridontal disease, receding gums, decay, and other factors. Stomatitis, ulceration, and necrosis are common findings among aged patients, as is glossodynia, a painful burning tongue which is frequently associated with nutritional

deficiencies, anemia, hormonal imbalances, and emotional disturbances.[136,137]

Dental problems frequently lead to ingestion of a diet consisting primarily of soft foods and liquids. Such a diet is likely to be nutritionally inadequate.[136] Dentures can ameliorate this situation; however, satisfactory dentures cannot always be obtained. Resorption of the mandibular and maxillary bones, and dryness and fragility of the soft tissues, lead to ill-fitting dentures which are difficult to manage effectively. A study conducted by Soremark and Nilson found that about 50% of the men and 35% of the women reported difficulties in chewing such foods as fruits, vegetables, and meat due to poor dentures. This underscores the potential etiological significance of dental factors in nutritional deficiencies of geriatric patients. A study by Todhunter[36] indicated that patients with dental problems would still be likely to get adequate food intake, however.

EXERCISE AND ITS ROLE IN GERIATRIC MENTAL ILLNESS

Effects of Activity on Body and Brain

Physical activity is commonly reduced greatly in the elderly. Cardiac, respiratory, neurologic, musculoskeletal, and other conditions may impose some activity limitations; additional contributary factors include reduction of the kinesthetic pleasure derived by younger persons from motor activity and societal expectations of appropriate behavior in the aged. Physical inactivity leads to perception of the body as broader and heavier than it actually is, resulting in clumsiness and further activity restriction.[138] Physical inactivity aggravates changes associated with normal aging, and often has deleterious effects mistakenly assumed to result from the aging process. Decreased physical fitness may contribute to increased reaction time. Flexor muscles shorten; antigravity muscles which support the head, body, and joints weaken; back and shoulder muscles weaken. These muscular changes cause poor posture and a humpback appearance, and contribute to restriction of breathing, which restricts capacity for physical activity and may impair blood supply to the brain, according to Harris.[139] Cardiac degeneration may also be an effect of physical inactivity.[138]

Physical activity can delay or retard many age-related changes, and lead to some improvement when deterioration has already occurred. The musculoskeletal, respiratory, cardiovascular, and central nervous systems all benefit from appropriate exercise. Physical activity stimulates metabolism, respiration, circulation, digestion, and glands of external secretion. Stimulation of nerve cells inhibits involution and atrophy. Patients who suffer from emphysema or cardiovascular disease can improve respiratory efficiency, circulation, and exercise tolerance through physical exercise. Activity promotes relaxation, and some forms of exercise reduce electrical activity of muscles as well as the tranquilizer Meprobamate.[139] There are definite limits on what exercise can do, as detailed by Niinimaa and Shepard in their recent articles on physical endurance training in the elderly which showed no difference in pulmonary diffusing capacity nor increase in the stroke volume after conditioning.[140,141] Of course the amount and rate of exercise must be determined by the general condition of the older person, and useful guidelines for this are given by de Vries[142] and Rodstein[143] in the excellent volume edited by Harris and Frankel.[144] The stress of inactivity has been pointed out by Wenger,[145] who showed orthostatic hypotension, a decrease in maximal oxygen uptake of up to 25%, and a loss of muscle contractile strength up to 45% of an otherwise healthy person put in bed for three weeks.

Therapeutic Exercise and its Results

Exercise can be a useful therapeutic modality in geriatric patients with physical, mental, or mixed problems. In addition to the physiological benefits, activity can improve motivation, independence, and self-image; provide new interests, abilities, and goals; and relieve psychological tension.[139] Regression of basic skill patterns can be delayed, thus contributing to enjoyment of life.[146] Maddox has shown a positive relationship between the level of activity in the elderly and the degree of life satisfaction and morale.[147]

Planned activity programs for the aged should provide relaxation, endurance exercises, muscle strengthening exercises, and stretching exercises. Relaxation techniques, rhythmic movements, and deep breathing exercises reduce tension, fatigue, anxiety, and dependency. Patients who regularly practice relaxation sleep better and demonstrate increased attention and concentration. Walking is generally the best endurance exercise, although other activities requiring use of the major muscles are also suitable, as tolerated. Endurance exercises enhance neuromuscular coordination, improve joint flexibility, stimulate metabolism, aid digestion, and reduce constipation and fatigue, as well as increase cardiovascular fitness. Muscle strengthening calisthenics aid posture. By increasing joint mobility and flexibility, stretching exercises contribute to greater independence and capacity for self-care. Such exercises may also alleviate muscular and joint aches and pains.[139]

Favorable results have been reported from a variety of exercise programs. Liberty[148] initiated a physical fitness program for aged members of a religious community consisting of exercises, suitable for wheelchair patients and modifiable for bedfast patients, which could be done to music. Participants reported better balance, increased joint flexibility, increased energy, and decreased pain; in addition, social interaction and participation in other activities also increased. Mogilevsky[149] describes a physical education class in Argentina for retired persons. General goals of the class include mobility, strength, coordination, endurance, relaxation, and recreation. These objectives are achieved through activities such as rhythmic movement, lifting small weights, walking, dance steps, balance exercises, various calisthenics, relaxation techniques, and ball games. It is desirable to alternately exercise various parts of the body, to precede mobility exercises with strength exercises, to avoid movements which would induce the Valsalva maneuver, and to vary the order of the exercises. Bardone[150] developed a Yoga program for older people. Yoga exercise involves maintaining physical postures for periods of time ranging from 30 seconds to 5 minutes. These are said to increase strength, balance, and flexibility; to strengthen muscles, spine, ligaments, and arteries; and to stimulate the brain, internal organs, and nerves. Deep breathing and relaxation also are taught as part of Yoga. Class participants reported that they felt better, gained more control over muscles and joints, experienced increased energy, were more relaxed, worried less, and slept better at night.

Physical activity may be used, in conjunction with other therapies, for the treatment of psychiatric disorders. The aged patient with neurotic depression accepts physical contact readily, and this may facilitate psychotherapy. Gradual physical activity for the patient with endogenous depression may be a prelude and a preparation for overcoming psychomotor retardation sufficiently to participate in the usual daily tasks. The manic patient can benefit from regulated physical activity such as gymnastics or dancing to control overactivity and constant goal changing.[151]

It is appropriate to close this chapter by citing the late Dr. Paul Dudley White, who gave a prominent example of vigorous physical activity until late in life, and felt that brisk walking to the point of fatigue and also other exercises are ideal antidotes against emotional stress.[152] He said, "Exercise is the best tranquilizer in the world."

REFERENCES

1. Riggs, B. *Family Weekly,* October 28, 1973.
2. Passwater, R. A. *Supernutrition: Megavitamin Revolution.* New York: Pocket Books. August, 1976.
3. Blaine, T. R. *Mental Health Through Nutrition.* New York: The Citadel Press, 1969.
4. Everone, C. A. A systematic approach to life extension and control of ageing. In press: *J. Applied Nutrition,* 1978.
5. White, P. L. The perfect environment for nonsense. *Nutrition News* 36(3): 9-12 (1973).
6. Rynearson, E. H. Americans love hogwash. *Nutrition Reviews/Supplement* 32: 1-14 (1974).
7. Bruch, H. The Allure of Food Cults and Nutrition Quackery. *Nutrition Reviews/Supplement* 32: 62-66 (1974).
8. FDA Fact Sheet, May 1967. Reprinted in McGovern Hearings, *Senate Select Committee on Nutrition and Human Needs, Part13-A,* Pg. 2956.
9. Schroeder, H. A. Nutrition. *Cowdry's—The Care of the Geriatric Patient* F. V. Steinberg (ed.), Fifth Edition. St. Louis: C. V. Mosby Company, 1976.
10. Turner, J. S. *The Nader Report: The Chemical Feast.* New York: Grossman Publishers, 1970.
11. Prohibition set on OTC sale of high-dose vitamins A, D. *Hospital Tribune,* September 24, 1973.
12. Hearings before the subcommittee on public health and environment. House of Representatives, Ninety-third Congress. *Parts 1 and 2. Serial No. 93-58 and 93-59.* Washington, D.C.: U.S. Government Printing Office, 1974.
13. Rosenberg, H. and Feldzamen, A. N. *The Doctor's Book of Vitamin Therapy.* New York: G. P. Putnam's Sons, 1974.
14. Cheraskin, E. and Ringsdorf, W. M., Jr. *Psychodietetics.* New York: Stein and Day, 1974.
15. Weg, R. B. *Nutrition and The Later Years.* Los Angeles: University of Southern California Press, 1978.
16. Barrows, C. H., Jr. and Roeder, L. M. Nutrition. In C. E. Finch and L. Hayflick, (eds.) *Handbook of the Biology of Aging.* New York: Van Nostrand Reinhold Co., 1977.
17. Howell, S. C. and Loeb, M. B. "Nutritional Needs of the Older Adult." *Gerontologist* 9: 17-30 (1969).
18. Watkin, D. M. Nutrition for the aging and the aged. In R. S. Goodhart and M. E. Shils, (eds.) *Modern Nutrition in Health and Disease.* Fifth Edition. Philadelphia: Lea & Febiger, 1973.
19. Williams, R. J. The individual approach to geriatric nutrition. In *Duke University Council on Aging and Human Development: Proceedings of Seminars* F. Jeffers (ed.). Durham, N. C.: Duke University Press, 1965-1969.
20. Anderson, W. F. Nutrition of the elderly. In *Practical Management of the Elderly,* Third Edition. Oxford: Blackwell Scientific Publications, 1976.
21. Burton, B. T. Geriatric Nutrition. In *Human Nutrition,* Third Edition. New York: McGraw-Hill Book Co., 1976.
22. Exton-Smith, A. N. and Scott, D. L. *Vitamins in the Elderly.* Bristol: John Wright & Sons, 1968.

23. Caster, W. O. The role of nutrition in human aging. In M. Rockstein and M. Sussman, (eds.) *Nutrition, Longevity, and Aging*. New York: Academic Press Inc., 1976.

24. Winick, M. *Nutrition and Aging*. New York: John Wiley & Sons, 1976.

25. Mayer, J. *A Diet for Living*. New York: David McKay, 1975.

26. National Research Council. *Recommended Dietary Allowances*, Eighth Revised Edition. Washington, D.C.: National Academy of Sciences, 1974.

27. Michelsen, O. The possible role of vitamins in the aging process. In M. Rockstein and M. Sussman, (eds.) *Nutrition, Longevity, and Aging*. New York: Academic Press, 1976.

28. Shank, R. E. Nutritional characteristics of the elderly—An overview. In M. Rockstein and M. Sussman, (eds.) *Nutrition, Longevity, and Aging*. New York: Academic Press, Inc., 1976.

29. Bertolini, A. M. *Gerontologic metabolism*. Springfield, Ill.: Charles C Thomas, 1969.

30. Bierman, E. L. Obesity, carbohydrate, and lipid interactions in the elderly. In M. Winick, (ed.) *Nutrition and Aging*. New York: John Wiley & Sons, 1976.

31. Hazzard, W. R. Aging and atherosclerosis: Interactions with diet, heredity, and associated risk factors. In M. Rockstein and M. Sussman, (eds.) *Nutrition, Longevity, and Aging*. New York: Academic Press, 1976.

32. Munro, H. N. Protein requirements and metabolism in aging. In *Symposia of the Swedish Nutrition Foundation X: Nutrition and Old Age*. Sweden: Almqvist & Wiksell, 1972.

33. Exton-Smith, A. N. Nutrition of the elderly. In *Reports of 9th International Congress of Gerontology 1*, 1972.

34. Shock, N. W. Physiologic aspects of aging. *J. Amer. Dietetic Assoc.* **56**: 494–495 (1970).

35. U.S. Center for Disease Control. *Ten-State Nutrition Survey*. DHEW Publication No. (HSM) 72-8130. Washington, D.C.: DHEW, 1972.

36. Todhunter, E. N. Life style and nutrient intake in the elderly. In M. Winick, (ed.) *Nutrition and Aging*. New York: John Wiley & Sons, 1976.

37. Macleod, C. C., Judge, T. G. and Caird, F. I. Nutrition of the elderly at home, I. Intakes of energy, protein, carbohydrates and fat. *Age and Ageing* **3**: 158–166 (1974).

38. Macleod, C. C., Judge, T. G. and Caird, F. I. Nutrition of the elderly at home, II. Intakes of vitamins. *Age and Ageing* **3**: 209–220 (1974).

39. Macleod, C. C., Judge, T. G. and Caird, F. I. Nutrition of the elderly at home, III. Intakes of minerals. *Age and Ageing* **4**: 49–57 (1975).

40. Caird, F. I., Judge, T. G. and Macleod, C. Pointers to possible malnutrition in the elderly at home. *Geront. Clin.* **17**: 47–54 (1975).

41. Berry, W. T. C. and Darke, S. J. Nutrition of the

elderly living at home. *Age and Ageing* **1**: 177–181 (1972).

42. Whanger, E. A. Nutritional needs and dietary intake of non-institutionalized aged persons. Unpublished manuscript, 1977.

43. Leevy, C. M., Cardi, L., Frank, O., Gellene, R. and Baker, H. Incidence and significance of hypovitaminemia in a randomly selected municipal hospital population. *Amer. J. Clin. Nutr.* **17**: 259–271 (1965).

44. MacLennan, W. J., Martin, P. and Mason, B. J. Causes for reduced dietary intake in a long-stay hospital. *Age and Ageing* **4**: 175–180 (1975).

45. Basu, T. K., Jordan, S. J., Jenner, M. and Williams, D. C. Blood values of some vitamins in long-stay psycho-geriatric patients. *Int. J. Vit. Nutr. Res.* **46**: 61–65 (1976).

46. Morgan, A. G., Kelleher, J., Walker, B. E., Losowsky, M. S., Droller, H. and Middleton, R. S. W. A nutritional survey in the elderly: Blood and urine vitamin levels. *Int. J. Vit. Nutr. Res.* **45**: 448–462 (1975).

47. Schiffman, S. S. Food recognition by the elderly. *J. Gerontol.* **32**(5): 586–592 (1977).

48. Schiffman, S. S., Moss, J. and Erickson, R. P. Thresholds of food odors in the elderly. *Experimental Aging Res.* **2**(5): 389–398 (1976).

49. Schiffman, S. S. Changes in taste and smell with age: Psychophysical aspects. In J. M. Ordy, (ed.) *Sensory Systems and Aging in Man*. In press. New York: Raven Press.

50. Weinberg, J. Psychologic implications of the nutritional needs of the elderly. *J. Amer. Dietetic Assoc.* **60**: 293–296 (1972).

51. Rao, D. B. Problems of nutrition in the aged. *J. Amer. Geriat. Soc.* **21**: 362–367 (1973).

52. Kelley, L., Ohlson, M. and Harper, L. Food selection and well-being of aging women. *J. Amer. Dietetic Assoc.* **33**: 466–470 (1957).

53. Chope, H. D. Relation of nutrition to health in aging persons. *California Med.* **81**(5): 335–338 (1954).

54. Schlenker, E. D., Feurig, J. S., Stone, L. H., Ohlson, M. A. and Mickelsen, O. Nutrition and health of older people. *Amer. J. Clin. Nutr.* **26**: 1111–1119 (1973).

55. Goldsmith, G. A. *Nutritional Diagnosis*. Springfield: Charles C Thomas, 1959.

56. Anderson, W. F., Cohen, C., Hyams, D. E., Millard, P. H., Plowright, N. M., Woodford-Williams, E. and Berry, W. T. C. Clinical and subclinical malnutrition in old age. *Symposia of the Swedish Nutrition Foundation X: Nutrition in Old Age*. Sweden: Almqvist & Wiksell, 1972.

57. Watkin, D. M. Nutritional problems today in the elderly in the United States. In A. W. Exton-Smith and D. L. Scott, (eds.) *Vitamins in the Elderly*. Bristol: John Wright & Sons, 1968.

58. Watkin, D. M. Biochemical impact of nutrition of the aging process. In M. Rockstein and M. I.

Sussman, (eds.) *Nutrition, Longevity, and Aging.* New York: Academic Press, 1976.

59. Brin, M. Biochemical methods and findings in U.S.A. surveys. In A. N. Exton-Smith and D. L. Scott, (eds.) *Vitamins in the Elderly.* Bristol: John Wright & Sons, 1968.

60. Rockstein, M. and Sussman, M. L. Introduction: Food for thought. In M. Rockstein and M. I. Sussman, (eds.) *Nutrition, Longevity, and Aging.* New York: Academic Press, 1976.

60a. Andrus, R. Paper presented at the International Congress of Gerontology, Tokyo, Japan, 1978.

61. Stunkard, A. J. Nutrition, aging and obesity. In M. Rockstein and M. I. Sussman, (eds.) *Nutrition, Longevity, and Aging* New York: Academic Press, Inc., 1976.

62. Whanger, A. D. Vitamins and vigor at 65 plus. *Postgrad. Med.* **53**(2): 167–172 (1973).

63. Roe, D. A. Dietary interrelationships. In M. G. Wohl and R. S. Goodhart, (eds.) *Modern Nutrition in Health and Disease* Fourth Edition. Philadelphia: Lea & Febiger, 1968.

64. Roels, O. A. and Lui, N. S. T. Vitamin A and carotene. In R. S. Goodhart and M. E. Shils, (eds.) *Modern Nutrition in Health and Disease: Dietotherapy* Fifth Edition. Philadelphia: Lea & Febiger, 1973.

65. Neal, R. A. and Sauberlich, H. E. Thiamine. In R. S. Goodhart and M. E. Shils, (eds.) *Modern Nutrition in Health and Disease: Dietotherapy* Fifth Edition. Philadelphia: Lea & Febiger, 1973.

66. Sandstead, H. H. Clinical manifestations of certain vitamin deficiencies. In R. S. Goodhart and M. E. Shils, (eds.) *Modern Nutrition in Health and Disease: Dietotherapy* Fifth Edition. Philadelphia: Lea & Febiger, 1973.

67. Horwitt, M. K. Riboflavin. In R. S. Goodhart and M. E. Shils, (eds.) *Modern Nutrition in Health and Disease: Dietotherapy* Fifth Edition. Philadelphia: Lea & Febiger, 1973.

68. Horwitt, M. K. Niacin. In R. S. Goodhart and M. E. Shils, (eds.) *Modern Nutrition in Health and Disease: Dietotherapy,* Fifth Edition. Philadelphia: Lea & Febiger, 1973.

69. Dakshinamurti, K. B vitamins and nervous system function. In R. J. Wurtman and J. J. Wurtman, (eds.) *Nutrition and the Brain, Vol. 1* New York: Raven Press, 1977.

70. Sauberlich, H. E. and Canham, J. E. Vitamin B-6. In R. S. Goodhart and M. E. Shils, (eds.) *Modern Nutrition in Health and Disease: Dietotherapy,* Fifth Edition. Philadelphia: Lea & Febiger, 1973.

71. Williams, R. J. *Nutrition Against Disease.* New York: Bantam Books, 1973.

72. Sauberlich, H. E. Pantothenic acid. In R. S. Goodhart and M. E. Shils, (eds.) *Modern Nutrition in Health and Disease: Dietotherapy* Fifth Edition. Philadelphia: Lea & Febiger, 1973.

73. Herbert, V. Folic acid and vitamin B_{12}. In R. S.

Goodhart and M. E. Shils (eds.), *Modern Nutrition in Health and Disease: Dietotherapy* Fifth Edition. Philadelphia: Lea & Febiger, 1973.

74. Kane, F. J., Jr. and Lipton, M. Folic acid and mental illness. *So. Med. J.* **63**: 603–607 (1970).

75. Strachan, R. W. and Henderson, J. G. Dementia and folate deficiency. *Qtrly, J. Med.* **36**(142): 191–204 (1967).

76. Hallstrom, T. Serum B_{12} and folate concentrations in mental patients. *Acta Psychiat. Scand.* **45**: 19–36 (1969).

77. Carney, M. W. P. and Sheffield, B. F. Associations of subnormal serum folate and vitamin B_{12} values and effects of replacement therapy. *J. Nerv. & Ment. Dis.* **150**(5): 404–412 (1970).

78. Sneath, P., Chanarin, I., Hodkinson, H. M., McPherson, C. K. and Reynolds, E. H. Folate status in a geriatric population and its relation to dementia. *Age and Ageing* **2**: 177–182 (1973).

79. Baker, H., Jaslow, S. P. and Frank, O. Severe impairment of dietary folate utilization in the elderly. *J. Amer. Geriat. Soc.* **26**(5): 218–221 (1978).

80. Kallstrom, B. and Nyloff, R. Vitamin B_{12} and folic acid in psychiatric disorders. *Acta Psychiat. Scand.* **45**(2): 137–152 (1969).

81. Smith, A. D. M. Megaloblastic madness. *Brit. Med. J.* **2**: 1840–1845, December 24, 1960.

82. MacCallum, W. A. G. Recoverable psychiatric illness occurring with low serum vitamin B_{12} levels. *J. Irish Med. Assoc.* **57**: 187–192 (1965).

83. Buxton, P. K., Davison, W., Hyams, D. E. and Irvine, W. J. Vitamin B_{12} status in mentally disturbed elderly patients. *Geront. Clin.* **11**: 22–35 (1969).

84. Shulman, R. A survey of vitamin B_{12} deficiency in an elderly psychiatric population. *Brit. J. Psychiat.* **113**: 241–251 (1967).

85. Whanger, A. D. and Wang, H. S. Vitamin B_{12} deficiency. In E. Palmore, (ed.) *Normal Aging II.* Durham, N. C.: Duke University Press, 1974.

86. Ordõñez, L. A. Control of the availability to the brain of folic acid, vitamin B_{12} and choline. In R. J. Wurtman and J. J. Wurtman, (eds.) *Nutrition and the Brain, Vol. 1.* New York: Raven Press, 1977.

87. Goodhart, R. S. Criteria of an adequate diet. In R. S. Goodhart and M. E. Shils (eds.) *Modern Nutrition in Health and Disease: Dietotherapy* Philadelphia: Lea & Febiger, 1973.

88. Chebotarev, D. F. Biological active agents ("Geriatrics") in prevention and treatment of premature aging. In D. F. Chebotarev, (ed.) *The Main Problems of Soviet Gerontology.* Material for the IX International Congress of Gerontology. Kiev, 1972.

89. Clark, L. A. *Know Your Nutrition.* New Canaan, Conn.: Keats Publishing, 1973.

90. Newbold, H. L. *Mega-Nutrients for Your Nerves.* New York: Peter H. Wyden, 1975.

91. Hodges, R. E. and Baker, E. M. Ascorbic acid. In R. S. Goodhart and M. E. Shils, (eds.), *Modern Nutrition in Health and Disease: Dietotherapy* Fifth Edition. Philadelphia: Lea & Febiger, 1973.

92. Spittle, C. R. Atherosclerosis and vitamin C. *Lancet* 1(7737): 1280–1281 (1971).

93. Kinsman, R. A. and Hood, J. Some behavioral effects of ascorbic acid deficiency. *Amer. J. Clin. Nutr.* 24(1): 455–464, 1971.

94. Riccitelli, M. L. Vitamin C therapy in geriatric practice. *J. Amer. Geriat. Soc.* 20: 34–42 (1972).

95. Horwitt, M. K. Vitamin E. In R. S. Goodhart and M. E. Shils, (eds.) *Modern Nutrition in Health and Disease: Dietotherapy,* Fifth Edition. Philadelphia: Lea & Febiger, 1973.

96. Williams, H. T., Fenna, D. and Macbeth, R. A. Alpha tocopherol in the treatment of intermittent claudication. *Surg. Gynecol. Obstet.* 132: 662 (1971).

97. Health Education and Welfare. *Myths of Vitamins.* Publication No. (FDA) 78–2047, U. S. Government Printing Office. February, 1978.

98. Taylor, G. F. A clinical survey of elderly people from a nutritional standpoint. In A. N. Exton-Smith and D. L. Scott, (eds.). *Vitamins in the Elderly* Bristol: John Wright & Sons, 1968.

99. Brocklehurst, J. C., Griffiths, L. L., Taylor, G. F., Marks, J., Scott, D. L. and Blackley, J. The clinical features of chronic vitamin deficiency: A therapeutic trial in geriatric hospital patients. *Geront. Clin.* 10: 309–320 (1968).

100. MacLeod, R. D. M. Abnormal tongue appearances and vitamin status of the elderly—A double blind trial. *Age and Ageing* 1: 99–102 (1972).

101. Kral, V. A., Solyom, L. and Ledwidge, B. Relationship of vitamin B_{12} and folic acid to memory function. *Biol. Psychiat.* 2: 19–26 (1970).

102. Milner, G. Ascorbic acid in chronic psychiatric patients—A controlled trial. *Brit. J. Psychiat.* 109: 294–299 (1963).

103. Dymock, S. M. and Brocklehurst, J. C. Clinical effects of water soluble vitamin supplementation in geriatric patients. *Age and Ageing* 2: 172–176 (1973).

104. Hughes, D., Elwood, P. C., Shinton, N. K. and Wrighton, R. J. Clinical trial of the effect of vitamin B_{12} in elderly subjects with low serum B_{12} levels. *Brit. Med. J.* 2: 458–460 (1970).

105. Altman, H., Mehta, D., Evenson, R. C. and Sletten, I. W. Behavioral effects of drug therapy on psychogeriatric inpatients II. Multivitamin supplement. *J. Amer. Geriat. Soc.* 21(6): 249–252 (1973).

106. Pennington, V. M. Enhancement of psychotropic drugs by a vitamin supplement. *Psychosom.* 7: 115–120 (1966).

107. Omdahl, J. L. and DeLuca, H. F. Vitamin D. In R. S. Goodhart and M. E. Shils, (eds.), *Modern Nutrition in Health and Disease: Dietotherapy* Fifth Edition. Philadelphia: Lea & Febiger, 1973.

108. Kreutler, P. A. Vitamins. In R. B. Howard and N. H. Herbold, (eds.) *Nutrition in Clinical Care.* Boston: McGraw-Hill Book Company, 1978.

109. Jick, H. *Personal Communication,* April 1978.

110. Hawkins, D. R.; Bortin, A. W. and Runyon, R. P.: Orthomolecular psychiatry: Niacin and megavitamin therapy. *Psychosom.* 11: 517–521 (1970).

111. Osmond, H. Reply to 'Nutrition and psychiatric illness'. In G. Serban, (ed.) *Nutrition and Mental Functions.* New York: Plenum Press, 1975.

112. Lipton, M. A. and Kane, F. J., Jr. The use of vitamins as therapeutic agents in psychiatry. In R. I. Shader, (ed.) *Psychiatric Complications of Medical Drugs.* New York: Raven Press, 1972.

113. Chow, B. R. and Yeh, S. D. Vitamin and mineral supplements in the diet of the elderly. In J. T. Freeman, (ed.) *Clinical Principles and Drugs in the Aging.* Springfield: Charles C Thomas, 1963.

114. Whanger, A. D. and Wang, H. S. Clinical correlates of the vibratory sense in elderly psychiatric patients. *J. Gerontol.* 29(1): 39–45 (1974).

115. Underwood, E. J. *Trace Elements in Human and Animal Nutrition,* Fourth Edition. New York: Academic Press, 1977.

116. Hine, J. Minerals. In R. B. Howard and N. H. Herbold, (eds.) *Nutrition in Clinical Care.* New York: McGraw-Hill Book Company, 1978.

117. Davies, I. J. T. *The Clinical Significance of Essential Biological Metals.* London: William Heinemann Medical Books, 1972.

118. Schroeder, H. A. *The Trace Elements and Man, Some Positive and Negative Aspects.* Old Greenwich, Conn.: Devin-Adair Company, 1973.

119. J. M. Hsu; R. L. Davis and R. W. Neithamer, (eds.) *Biomedical Role of Trace Elements in Aging.* St. Petersburg, Fla.: Eckerd College Gerontology Center, 1976.

120. Smith, J. C., Jr. Golden ages and trace elements. In J. M. Hsu, R. L. Davis and R. W. Neithamer, (eds.) *Conference on the Biomedical Role of Trace Elements in Aging.* St. Petersburg, Fla.: Eckerd College Gerontology Center, 1976.

121. Lawton, A. H. Introductory remarks: Trace elements in aging. In J. M. Hsu; R. L. Davis and R. W. Neithamer, (eds.) *Conference on the Biomedical Role of Trace Elements in Aging* St. Petersburg, Fla.: Eckerd College Gerontology Center, 1976.

122. Hegsted, D. M. Calcium and phosphorus. In R. S. Goodhart and M. E. Shils, (eds.) *Modern Nutrition in Health and Disease: Dietotherapy* Fifth Edition. Philadelphia: Lea & Febiger, 1973.

123. Judge, T. G. Potassium metabolism in the elderly. In *Symposia of the Swedish Nutrition Foundation X: Nutrition in Old Age.* Sweden: Almqvist & Wiksell, 1972.

124. Martin, H. E. Clinical magnesium deficiency. *Annals of the New York Academy of Sciences* **162**(2): 891–900 (1969).

125. Flink, E. B. and Jones, J. E. The pathogenesis and clinical significance of magnesium deficiency. *Annals of the New York Academy of Sciences* **162**(2): 705–984 (1969).

126. Shils, M. E. Magnesium. In R. S. Goodhart and M. E. Shils, (eds.) *Modern Nutrition in Health and Disease: Dietotherapy* Fifth Edition. Philadelphia: Lea & Febiger, 1973.

127. Shoemaker, W. J. and Bloom, F. E. Effect of undernutrition on brain morphology. In R. J. Wurtman and J. J. Wurtman, (eds.) *Nutrition and the Brain, Vol. 2.* New York: Raven Press, 1977.

128. Pollitt, E. and Thomson, C. Protein-calorie malnutrition and behavior: A view from psychology. In R. J. Wurtman and J. J. Wurtman, (eds.) *Nutrition and the Brain, Vol. 2* New York: Raven Press, 1977.

129. Nowak, T. S. and Munro, H. N. Effects of protein-calorie malnutrition on biochemical aspects of brain development. In R. J. Wurtman and J. J. Wurtman, (eds.) *Nutrition and the Brain, Vol. 2.* New York: Raven Press, 1977.

130. P. R. Dodge, A. L. Prensky, R. D. Feigin and S. J. Holmes, (eds.) *Nutrition and the Developing Nervous System.* St. Louis: C. V. Mosby Company, 1975.

131. Wurtman, R. J. and Fernstrom, J. D. Effects of the diet on brain neurotransmitters. *Nutrition Reviews* **32**(7): 193–200 (1974).

132. N. S. Scrimshaw and J. E. Gordon (eds.) *Malnutrition, Learning, and Behavior.* Cambridge, Mass: M. I. T. Press, 1968.

133. S. Davidson, R. Passmore, J. F. Brock and A. S. Truswell, (eds.) *Human Nutrition and Dietetics.* Edinburgh: Churchill Livingstone, 1975.

134. Albanese, A. A. and Orto, L. A. The proteins and amino acids. In R. S. Goodhart and M. E. Shils, (eds.) *Modern Nutrition in Health and Disease: Dietotherapy,* Fifth Edition. Philadelphia: Lea & Febiger, 1973.

135. Rockstein, M.: Questions and responses. In E. W. Busse, and E. Pfeiffer, (eds.) *Mental Illness in Later Life.* Washington, D. C.: American Psychiatric Association, 1973.

136. Elfenbaum, A. Oral care for the elderly. In F. Jeffers, (ed.) *Duke University Council on Aging and Human Development: Proceedings of Seminars.* Duke University, Durham, N. C.: Duke University Press, 1965–1969.

137. Söremark, R. and Nilsson, B. Dental status and nutrition in old age. *Symposia of the Swedish Nutrition Foundation X: Nutrition in Old Age.* Sweden: Almqvist & Wiksell, 1972.

138. Kreitler, H. and Kreitler, S. H. Movement and aging: A psychological approach, In D. Brunner and E. Jokl, (eds.) *Medicine and Sport 4: Physical Activity and Aging.* Basel: S. Karger, 1970.

139. Harris, R. Physical activity and mental health in the aged. In U. Simki, (ed.) *Physical Exercise & Activity for the Aging: Proceedings of an International Seminar.* Jerusalem: Wingate Institute, 1975.

140. Niinimaa, V. and Shephard, R. J. Training and oxygen conductance in the elderly, I. The respiratory system. *J. Gerontol.* **33**(3): 354–361 (1978).

141. Niinimaa, V. and Shephard, R. J. Training and oxygen conductance in the elderly, II. The cardiovascular system. *J. Gerontol.* **33**(3): 362–367 (1978).

142. de Vries, H. A. Physiology of physical conditioning for the elderly. In R. Harris and L. J. Frankel, (eds.) *Guide to Fitness After Fifty.* New York: Plenum Press, 1977.

143. Rodstein, M. Changing the habits and thought patterns of the aged to promote better health through activity programs in institutions. In R. Harris and L. J. Frankel, (eds.) *Guide to Fitness After Fifty.* New York: Plenum Press, 1977.

144. R. Harris and L. J. Frankel, (eds.) *Guide to Fitness After Fifty.* New York: Plenum Press, 1977.

145. Wenger, N. K. The early ambulation of patients after myocardial infarction. *Cardiol.* **58**: 1–6 (1973).

146. Eckert, H. M. Physical activity and developmental aspects of aging. In U. Simri (ed.) *Physical Exercise & Activity for the Aging: Proceedings of an International Seminar,* pp. 226–228 Jerusalem: Wingate Institute, 1975.

147. Maddox, G. L. Activity and morale: A longitudinal study of selected elderly subjects. *Social Forces* **42**: 195–204, (1963–1964).

148. Liberty, S. J. Adventures with a modified physical fitness program. Institute of Gerontology, University of Michigan-Wayne State University, Ann Arbor, Michigan, 1975.

149. Mogilevsky, A. Gymnastics is for everybody. In U. Simri, (ed.) *Physical Exercise & Activity for the Aging: Proceedings of an International Seminar,* pp. 111–116. Jerusalem: Wingate Institute, 1975.

150. Bardone, M. Yoga and the older person. In U. Simri, (ed.) *Physical Exercise & Activity for the Aging: Proceedings of an International Seminar,* pp. 95–110. Jerusalem: Wingate Institute, 1975.

151. Kral, V. A. Motivation and activity. In U. Simri, (ed.) *Physical Exercise and Activity for the Aging: Proceedings of an International Seminar,* pp. 110–124. Jerusalem: Wingate Institute, 1975.

152. White, P. D. Preface. In D. Brunner and E. Jokl, (eds.) *Medicine and Sport 4: Physical Activity and Aging.* Basel: S. Karger, 1970.

Part III
Future Directions

Chapter 23
The Continuum of Care:
Movement Toward the Community

George L. Maddox
Duke University Medical Center

OVERVIEW

In recent decades public discussion of care for older persons has continually concentrated on what has come to be called "the alternative issue." The attention of congressional committees initially focused on this issue because older persons consume public health and related welfare resources at a rate that is higher than adults generally. Older persons therefore provide a very visible illustration of a general problem of securing quality care at bearable cost. What has clearly concerned the Congress about care of older people was and is the very high cost of services that appear to be poorly distributed, and inappropriate care of debatable quality.[1] Public discussion of efficient and effective alternative forms of care for older people, however, has generated a great deal of rhetoric but little definitive evidence which would inform choices among a bewildering array of competing options. At the beginning of the 1970s discussion focused on alternatives to institutionalization. A consensus among both professionals and laity did emerge that too many older people

were inappropriately and unnecessarily institutionalized in mental hospitals and nursing homes. This consensus unquestionably had some basis in fact; but since no definitive consensual procedures existed for determining appropriate levels and locales for care, estimates of the number of older people inappropriately institutionalized or receiving too much care varied widely from as little as 6% to as much as 40% or more. The confidence that too many people were receiving care, and perhaps too much care, in the wrong care settings, was matched by confident assertions that care in the community and, if possible at home, provided obviously preferable alternatives at obviously lower cost. The obviousness of these conclusions has repeatedly been confronted by a troublesome fact: The efficiency and effectiveness of alternatives to the current organization of services continues to be asserted rather than systematically demonstrated. Relevant evidence is beginning to accumulate, however, options are becoming more clearly defined, and systematic evaluation is increasingly possible. With clearer conceptualization of issues and more definitive research than has been evident in the past decade, definitive discussion of alternative forms of care for older persons is increasingly probable as relevant evidence accumulates.

STRUCTURING THE ISSUES

The development of scientific knowledge, the transfer of that knowledge to professionals through training, and the translation of knowledge into professional practice takes place in the context of organizations. Understanding the delivery of care to a population therefore benefits from a sociological understanding both of how organizations define the roles and rules which organize the interactions of the professional helpers and those they help, and of how societies and communities allocate resources among organizations.

Over a decade ago Charles Perrow[2] wrote a very insightful sociological analysis of key factors which influence the behavior of organizations whose product is personal care. His analysis provides a conceptual structure for thinking about some basic issues in the organization of helping resources. Perrow concentrated on three interactive societal factors: (1) the *cultural system* of a society embodying values and beliefs which influence the setting of legitimate organization goals; (2) the available *technology* that determines the means for goal attainment; and (3) the *social structure* of organizations in which specific techniques are embedded in ways that facilitate or inhibit goal attainment. Perrow's illustration of these three factors was care in mental hospitals. His basic argument, however, is broadly applicable to an understanding, organized response to impairment generally.

Culture is a shared, socially transmitted construction of reality. The concept refers broadly to the goals members of a society value and pursue; to the rules and roles which structure social life; to the technologies, and to the material and symbolic products of group life. Through processes of socialization and social control, most individuals' cultural expectations are transmitted from generation to generation. Consequently, conformity to social expectations is the common experience of everyday life; most members of most social groups want to become and be what they are expected to become and be. Nonconformity does occur, and when it does, cultural belief systems provide plausible explanations and suggest corrective measures. Illness is a case in point. Illness has social as well as personal significance in all societies. This is so because illness typically impairs the performance of social roles. There are, therefore, social as well as personal reasons for limiting the impact of illness. Illness typically evokes temporary exemption from usual role obligations and helpful social response but usually with the expectation that the sick individual wants to limit the debilitating effects of illness as much as possible. Modern societies attach considerable importance to controlling the effects of illness. In our own society, for example, one of our largest industries, to which we devote over 8% of our annual Gross National Product (GNP), is health care. Scientific medicine and its related technologies, manpower, and organization are integral parts of our culture. This is so much the case that some observers refer to belief in the "Great Equation," that is, Medical Care Equals Health.[3] Others refer to the "medicalization" of western societies and the necessity of "demedicalization."[4]

There is no question that, in the last half century, advances in medical technology have raised public expectations regarding the conquest of disease. Average life expectancy has increased dramatically.[5] Sick people, for the most part, expect to receive care and expect to be cured. Unfortunately, very high expectations encounter substantial obstacles. Health resources, particularly primary health care, are not equally distributed geographically and, hence, not equally accessible. Moreover, as Wildavsky contends, the "Great Equation" is probably wrong; medical care does not equal health.[6,7] The medical system—doctors, other health professionals, hospitals, drugs—may account for and deal with only a small proportion of the factors affecting health. A much larger proportion appears to be determined by factors over which the medical system has little or no control—factors such as lifestyle (smoking, eating, drinking, worrying, inactivity); social conditions (income, inheritance); and social environment (air, water, noise, safety). This is why Wildavsky[5] and others[6,7] feel that the medical system cannot insure health at any cost, much less at a bearable cost. Even in a society becoming accustomed to high inflation generally, the total cost of health care is escalating more rapidly than other services.[8,9] The result is a widespread sense of concern which reflects, according to public opinion polls, less a crisis in confidence in the value of medical care than the belief that appropriate care will not be received at a bearable cost.[10] Or, in terms of the three interacting factors stressed by Perrow, cultural beliefs and expectations about health care are mismatched with both the available technology and the organization of care for achieving shared goals for insuring health care. Medical technology available for diagnosis and treatment is impressive, although it is directed primarily toward acute illness. The organization for health care delivery concentrates on medical care dependent on high technology controlled by highly specialized personnel centralized in or near hospitals. Financing of health care is directed primarily to medical care and to care which must be certified by medical practitioners. There is a growing body of opinion that Wildavsky's extreme conclusion regarding the important but modest contribution which medicine can make in insuring health is more right than wrong.[6,7] Hence, increasing amounts of resources poured into health services as they are currently organized are likely to produce a decreasing marginal return on investment and less satisfaction with the outcome. In regard to health services, doing better in many ways but feeling worse[11] has been the outcome. Problems related to the health care of older persons are specific and instructive illustrations of why there is a sense of crisis regarding our capacity to achieve adequate health care at a bearable cost and a continuing interest in "alternatives to institutionalization."[12,5]

HEALTH CARE FOR OLDER PERSONS

The cultural beliefs and values regarding the care of older persons in the United States is most accurately described as complex, ambiguous, and contradictory. All citizens, including older ones, have a right to the best available care. What is *best* tends to be associated with high technology i.e., sophisticated equipment manned by specialized personnel, centralized in hospitals and medical centers. The short-stay hospital in recent decades has come to be associated with curative therapies and tends to evoke, with the exception of misgivings about costs, a very positive image. Long-stay institutions, on the other hand, evoke a very negative image as indicated by public attitudes toward mental hospitals and nursing homes. Such institutions have been the focus of social concern and have provided the illustrations of unnecessary and inappropriate custodial, as distinct from curative, service. Nursing homes as they have developed extensively in this country since the advent of Medicare and Medicaid programs are clearly extensions of a medical model of care. Access to and continuation in nursing homes is contingent on medical certification. And, critics of the very extensive development of nursing homes (almost 22,000 homes, 1¼ million beds, and a $12.5 billion annual cost in 1977) usually comment that the care provided does not emphasize the social components of care enough; nursing homes suffer from the appearance of being second rate, understaffed, and underfunded hospitals.[12]

Deinstitutionalization of the mentally ill, including many older persons, has been the intention of public policy as well as cultural preference in this country for over a decade.[13,14] Both public policy and cultural preference regarding deinstitutionalization reflect evidence as well as emotion. Media coverage of dramatic events involving older persons in long-term care institutions— events such as deaths resulting from fires, incidents involving abuse and inadequate care, and evidence of fiscal mismanagement—provide fuel for strong emotional response. But there is also evidence of what appears to be unnecessary institutionalization, dependency-producing overcare, and questionable effectiveness of high cost services.[12,14] A large number of persons, including many older persons, have been removed from mental institutions. Hospital censuses and length of stay have been reduced. There is little definitive evidence, however, with regard to the selection procedure used to determine who will be placed in the community, the fate of older individuals who have been so placed, or the impact of this placement on neighborhoods and communities. The best evidence indicates that many of the "deinstitutionalized" are reinstitutionalized in less publicly visible long-term care facilities in the community.[12] Occasionally those who rally under the banner of deinstitutionalization make rather extravagant claims about the proportion of older individuals who are inappropriately institutionalized, with estimates running as high as 40%. In fact, we do not have definitive evidence on this point, although there is some evidence indicating that the great majority of individuals in, for example, nursing homes are significantly impaired, that 13–14% might be cared for appropriately in a situation providing less intensive care, and that perhaps another 10% who probably benefit from institutionalization overall, receive more care than their functional impairments require.[5,15]

In the absence of a definitive technology in long-stay institutions which gives reasonable assurance of achieving the restoration of functioning, the inference is invited that such institutions are not only primarily custodial, i.e., focusing on maintenance rather than rehabilitation, but also that the organization of life within them unnecessarily increases the dependence of residents. Unlike hospitals and medical centers, where high cost at least is associated with the hope for restoration of function, high cost in long-stay institutions has come to be associated with the expectation of increased dependence in a custodial environment. The organization of long-term care in the United States continues to be dominated by and to suffer from comparison with what has been called "a medical model" of care, a model symbolized by a specialized physician in a hospital supported by technicians and technology. While the continuing dominance of a medical model of long-term care might be interpreted as additional evidence of medicine's control of health care, this dominance does reflect continuing hope that current medical technology and organization of care can effect cures for the chronically ill in the face of discouraging evidence to the contrary. The current search for alternatives to institutionalization and a preference for deinstitutionalization of health care for older persons is therefore hampered by the lack of demonstrably effective, efficient and adequately distributed organizations for care in communities whose performance is superior to the overall performance of medical institutions. Nevertheless, both professional and public opinion increasingly reflect a belief in the desirability as well as the feasibility of more long-term care in the community rather than institutional settings. This opinion is buttressed with increasing experience of satisfactory care outside institutions which is, at least, no more expensive than institutional care and possibly less expensive.[5,16] The United States is, consequently, entering an era in which experimenting with alternative organization and financing of care will increase. The actual transformation of the care system to emphasize community-based rather than hospital-based care will probably move slowly, at least in the near future. This is the case, in part, because reliable and valid procedures for determining the proper level and locale for care and for measuring outcome are inadequately developed and neither routinely available nor consistently applied even when available.[14,17,18] The implications of a substantial reorientation of care to emphasize community-based services for professional training and manpower development are also not yet well understood. It is not at all clear that public preference for high-technology medicine will be significantly reduced by the addition of opportunities for care in the community or that the total cost of care will be reduced by additional forms of care unless the alternative forms are a substitute for existing forms. And, finally we currently understand very little about the impact on kin and friendship networks of placing more responsibility for care in the community.[13,15] But these constraints notwithstanding, extensive development of community based care for older persons is appropriately in the nation's future.

THE CASE FOR COMMUNITY-BASED CARE

The case for increasing the probability that the locale for care will be outside institutions and that the care offered will stress social and psychological as well as medical components is outlined briefly here and developed in the sections which follow. In brief, first, community and home care for impaired older persons are commonsense responses to common problems of dependency in late life. Historically, these forms of care preceded institutionalization and continue today to provide most of services required; community and home care are old ideas that are currently being rediscovered.[5,13] Public attitudes and public policy regarding appropriate sources and location of care have, at least until recently, reflected high regard for professional expertise and limited confidence in the competence and responsibilities of families to deal with impaired members. The transfer of presumed responsibility for impaired members of families from families to professional family-surrogates has been pro-

nounced.[4] Nevertheless, a substantial majority of the care provided to impaired older persons is provided not by public agencies, but by a network of kin and friends.[13,15,19] Community and home care is hardly a novel idea or an unusual experience.

Second, a wide array of community and home services e.g., home health and home help in the public and private sector already exist.[19,20,21,22,23] The feasibility of establishing a wide variety of community-based services is not at issue. Services for community and home care, like health and social services generally are, however, typically fragmented, uncoordinated, and not routinely accessible to a majority of the impaired elderly.

Third, discussions of the economics of community and home services continue to be inconclusive. Intuitively, offering services outside institutions where high technology is concentrated ought to achieve economies. This has not, however, been demonstrated to be the case, particularly when the quality and quantity of professionally prescribed services are controlled. In any case, the crucial economic issue is the total cost of all services to the care system of acceptable levels and quality of care, not the cost of a discrete set of services. The reduction of total service system cost attributable to community and home services has not been demonstrated.[5,16,24]

Fourth, concentration of public discussion on the cost-effectiveness of community and home services probably is an interesting diversion from a more basic issue. The basic issue is the fragmented, unsystematic organization of care and of the public financing of care. Only comprehensive, integrated care delivery systems at local levels offer any prospect for achieving cost-effectiveness for community and home care. And the most significant contribution of community and home care to the achievement of economy, according to some economic analysts, may be the removal of patients from exposure to high-technology, high-cost health care centers.[25,26]

Fifth, achieving an appropriately comprehensive, integrated system of care delivery at the local level will probably take the form of current proposals for a type of care system illustrated by health maintenance organizations (HMOs).[27,10] This type of care system may continue to emphasize the medical as distinct from social and psychological aspects of care for older persons. Yet the emerging tradition of the HMO may offer a significant opportunity for melding the strengths of medical and social-psychological components of care in a way which is publicly and politically appealing and viable. The HMO offers an opportunity for local variations in the specific organization of a care system while providing both for prepayment and for a relatively comprehensive, integrated, and controllable system of care. Manpower development and training, financing and procedures for assignment to alternative types of care within any care system are critical problems whose solution will determine how adequate, effective, and efficient that system of care will be.

REDISCOVERING COMMUNITY AND HOME CARE

Scientific medicine in the United States and optimism about the beneficial effects of exposure to physicians and hospitals date only from the second decade of this century.[6] Care of impaired individuals in general and of elderly individuals in particular tended to be a family, a neighborhood, or a community responsibility. Until World War II, federal spending for health care was largely confined to investment in traditional public health activities such as immunization. In the postwar era, a change in public attitudes and policy occurred, resulting in federal programs of increasing variety and scale. Prior to 1965, the federal investment in health care for the aged and poor was $4.4 billion. By 1977 that investment was $49.6 billion, of which Medicare and Medicaid accounted for $35.7 billion and the Department of Defense and the Veterans Administration for another $6 billion.[9] The financing of

long-term care by Medicare and Medicaid was a prime factor in promoting the development of a nursing home industry, which, by the mid-1970s, included some 22,000 nursing homes with 1.25 million beds at a cost of over $12 billion annually. These beds are occupied by very elderly impaired persons—75% of them are over the age of 75, most having multiple impairments, and and over half with significant mental impairment. In the same period, persons 65 years of age and older accounted for an average of 64 million hospital days annually and, on average, each visited a physician almost seven times annually, and the total health cost to older persons was about three times higher than that of adults generally.[28,29] About 5% of persons 65 years of age and older are institutionalized at any point in time in the United States, and the estimated probability of a period of long-term institutionalization in late life is about 25%.

These widely quoted statistics are impressive and invite the incorrect inference that institutional care has supplanted traditional community and home care. This is far from the case. Epidemiological surveys provide evidence that about 60% of older persons are not significantly impaired in five important dimensions of functioning—social support networks, economic security, physical health, mental health, and the capacity for performing basic activities of daily living.[20,18] Over 9 out of 10 will live most of their later years in the community. And for the approximately 12–15% of older persons in the community who are seriously impaired, approximately 80% of the services they receive are provided by kin and friends, not by a public agency.[21,19]

The fact that currently an estimated 20% of health and social services provided to seriously impaired older persons have a public source surely constitutes a change and a historical trend. This change challenges a cultural preference for asserting familial responsibility for older persons and activates anxieties about the weakening of family ties and related social obligations. Social theorists have accentuated this concern with discussions of what may be called "the consequences of modernization" thesis, which contends the inevitable price of industrialization, urbanization, and rapid social change is the weakening of familial and communities ties. The dependent old, in turn, would obviously be vulnerable to isolation, social irrelevance, and neglect. There is evidence that family structure and function has changed in recent decades. The divorce rate is high, single parent families are now common; alternative family lifestyles are more visible than formerly; and families have access to and use an increasing array of experts to help in solving personal and familial problems. Yet the fact remains that most older people are not isolated from kin and friends; and impressive majorities of adult children indicate a continuing willingness to care for an older adult family member.[30,13,12] In sum, community and home care of dependent, impaired older persons have been and continue to be the rule, not the exception. Therefore, current discussions of community and home care most appropriately stress a long-established pattern which may be in need of rediscovery and revitalization but which is certainly not a daring new adventure.

PROLIFERATION OF COMMUNITY SERVICES

Community and home services, both public and voluntary, have been widely available and widely used in Western European countries for many years. In European settings, particularly those with comprehensive care systems, public debate focuses not on whether community and home services are feasible and desirable, but on how to increase their availability to underserved and unserved populations. Based on such experience, a considerable body of documentation and expertise exists regarding the organization, training, staffing, and performance of noninstitutional services for older persons. In general such services have high social visibility, are integrated into comprehensive care systems, and are reasonably

well financed. Experience in Europe suggests that one community or home care worker to help with household maintenance and personal care is required for every 100 older persons, a rate that is currently approximated in the Nordic countries. The United Kingdom has achieved a rate of 1/750. In the United States the current rate is about 1/5000.[5]

Contemporary health care in the United States is characterized by a high degree of specialization of information, personnel, therapeutic procedures, and locales for delivering services. This specialization includes community and home care, but to a minimal degree. The permutations and combinations of specialized people, activities, and locales has no known limits and therefore generates acute problems of fragmentation, requires organizational coordination, and tends to have gaps in coverage. The proliferation of specialized components in health care illustrates one logical outcome of disaggregating health care into its specialized components. Early in this century health care was considerably less specialized in terms of knowledge, personnel, techniques, and locale of service. Hence, one encountered general practitioners and general nurses offering services primarily in homes and incidentally in hospitals. If one disaggregates the process of general medical care into specialized components, the logical possibilities are numerous—medical specialists, physician extenders, hospital nurses, public health nurses, practical nurses, home health aides, home helpers, and so on. Similarly, if one observes a family caring for an impaired older member, this holistic process can be disaggregated into a large number of basic components, each of which can be the basis for a specialized activity for one or another category of professional or quasi-professional persons.

Let us assume that a society concludes (1) that a number of impaired older persons need supportive health and welfare services; (2) that these services can be and should be offered outside institutions (i.e., in the community or at home); and (3) that there should be some public support for these services when individuals do not have the informal social support ordinarily provided by kin and friends. What one would expect to develop is what one currently observes—a specialized service system which reflects the disaggregation of the holistic process into components and the development of specialized programs to deal with these components. Specialized systems of public community and home care are emerging for each element of service ordinarily provided by kin and friend networks e.g., adult family homes, day care, day health, personal care, continuing supervision, congregate care, meals/nutrition, household maintenance, home health, social interaction/recreation, physical therapy, education, housing, transportation, information and referral, special income maintenance, programs and protective services.[19,23] The process of disaggregation could logically go on and on. The availability and use of such services is relatively limited currently; less than 1% of Medicare expenditures are, for example, directed to community and home care.[31] Nevertheless, many components of a noninstitutional care system are already present.

One or more of these types of specialized noninstitutional services currently exists in most communities in the United States, complex combinations of services exist in many communities, and, in a few communities, a comprehensive range of services is found. There is no question that a case can be made for the feasibility and desirability of each type of service, although how much and for whom are very much in doubt. In the typical instance, each discrete service has developed its own justification, manpower estimates, training procedures, and clienteles. In the typical community, moreover, adequate provision is made neither for coordinating the discrete programs administratively and financially nor for articulating them with the dominant health care delivery system. The principal issue regarding community and home services is, therefore, not their feasibility and desirability. The issues are efficiency, effectiveness, financing, and coordination with other elements of the care system.

THE COST-EFFECTIVENESS OF ALTERNATIVES

Public discussions of alternative care programs have concentrated increasingly on the key issues of cost-effectiveness and integration into the existing care system. Conclusions regarding costs have continued to be inconclusive not only because the definitive evidence is lacking but also because the questions being asked are typically the wrong questions. The question typically asked is, "Are community and home alternatives cheaper than institutionalization?" The intuitive answer would certainly be in the affirmative. This answer is misleading, however, because it avoids the issue of the cost implications of particular services for the total system of care. It is intuitively obvious, for example, that individuals with moderate functional impairments requiring limited support services could be maintained in a community or home setting more cheaply than in an institutional setting. This is true, to a considerable degree, because noninstitutional care costs are shifted from the public sector to the private sector, specifically to family and friends.[21,24] It is also intuitively obvious that a minimally impaired person who is for some reason in an institution which provides more than the required care could be managed more economically as well as more appropriately elsewhere. Enthoven,[25] Luft,[32] and Ingelfinger[6] all note the operation of "the technological imperative" in health care institutions; the specialized health care professionals in high technology settings have professional, ethical, and legal reasons for trying one more test or procedure. These observers are convinced that, in high technology settings, the marginal utility of medical treatment, in both a medical and an economic sense of benefits in relation to investment, is frequently reached and often exceeded. Insofar as community and home care removes an individual from the technology typically found in institutional settings, reduction in the cost of care should follow. Health maintenance organizations apparently reduce the total cost of care through rationing access to hospitals[32] and proponents of the hospice movement are explicit in emphasizing care of dying patients which minimizes the use of costly medical technology and maximizes the use of relatively more economical psychosocial supportive therapy.[33] The appropriateness and defensibility of such a removal, however, is clearly a debatable quality-of-care issue which would require far more evidence than is currently available.[34,35,36,37]

The more severe the functional impairment of the individual, the less intuitively obvious the cost-effectiveness of community and home care becomes. A critical issue in assessing the cost effectiveness of alternative forms of health and social services is, therefore, a determination of degree of functional impairment and the minimal number and quality of service that would meet acceptable standards of care for persons with a known degree and kind of impairment in ability to perform normal social roles. In exploring such an issue, one can imagine an experimental or quasi-experimental design in which at least four categories of older persons emerge: (1) those whose impairments are so severe that by professional and public consensus, they would need to be in an institutional setting; (2) those whose impairments are moderate and for whom the consensus of professionals is that they might be appropriately managed in either institutional or noninstitutional settings; (3) those whose impairments require supportive services, but clearly in noninstitutional settings; and (4) those whose degree of well-being requires no special services. The second category is the critical one for testing hypotheses about comparative costs of alternative types of care.[38] The first and third categories raise different questions. For example, if a person in the first category were found in the community or a person in the third category were found in a long-stay institution, we would be interested primarily in explaining an inappropriate placement. The issue of the different cost of maintaining third category persons in the community or in an institution is uninteresting because it has a predetermined answer; such persons are almost certainly misplaced in institutions. A person in the first category living in the community or a person in the fourth category residing in an institution is certainly misplaced. With degree of functional impairment specified and reasonable consensus achieved regarding the type and amount of required services specified, one can imagine relatively definitive comparative research which might address the issue of cost-effectiveness of alternative care programs for impaired older persons. A few research studies reflect an understanding of and a response to these necessary conditions for drawing conclusions regarding the relative cost of alternative systems of care.

The General Accounting Office in Cleveland, Ohio, designed a study to assess the impact of defined services on the well-being of a random sample of persons 65 years of age and older in that city.[20,21] The design incorporated a methodology developed at the Duke University Center for the Study of Aging and Human Development.[14,18] The Duke Methodology has three elements: (1) a reliable, valid multidimensional assessment of functional status; (2) a procedure for identifying the number, quantity, and cost of basic components of commonly used services; and (3) a matrix which relates the services actually received by persons of known functional status initially to their functional status at some subsequent time. The Cleveland study found that 60% of the older individuals surveyed had minimal impairments which required no special intervention or, at most, services like transportation, help with housing, social and recreational opportunities, and occasionally home help. At the other extreme, 10% of the sample were severely impaired and required and were receiving an extensive range of supportive services. Of the 60% relatively unimpaired, the average individual received the equivalent of $349 in services each month, with 60% of this amount being provided by family and friends. Of the 10% who were extremely impaired, the average cost per month for services received was estimated to be $845, of which 80% was provided by family and friends. This $845 is considerably above the $597 which was the average monthly cost of nursing home care in Ohio at that time. These data suggest several conclusions:

1. A large number of extremely impaired older persons are maintained in the community;
2. The extremely impaired are maintained at a cost well above the cost of nursing home care;
3. The high cost of noninstitutional care is borne primarily by kin and friends rather than public agencies.

For the extremely impaired older persons in the Cleveland study living in the community, total cost of care in a noninstitutional setting was not less than institutional care, but it was less costly to the public treasury, which assumed responsibility for only 20% of the bill. What about the estimated cost of care for the 30% of older persons lying between the classifications *unimpaired* and *extremely impaired*? Such persons in Cleveland were receiving services valued at an average of $323 per month, 70% of which was provided by kin and friends. The total cost of services for this category was about half the cost of nursing home care, even if it had been paid entirely from public resources. Since some persons in nursing homes—possibly 12–14%[15,19]—have an intermediate degree of functional impairment, this category is clearly critical in assessing the potential cost savings that would come from insuring that needed care is provided outside institutions.

The estimate of 12–14% of older persons in nursing homes whose functional impairments might be managed in noninstitutional settings is a plausible and conservative estimate based on admittedly/limited data. Estimation of persons inappropriately institutionalized or receiving more than re-quired care in institutions has varied considerably from study to study, depending on the procedures used to assess impairment and to determine appropriateness of care in relation to the degree of impairment assessed. Some estimates of inappropriate care in institutions have ranged as high as 40%.[19] Current evidence does not permit a resolution of the reported variance in estimates. The consensus is only that the rates of unnecessary institutionalization and of inappropriately high levels of care are significant. Further research is clearly needed. Several existing studies do, however, provide relevant illustrations of the problems of producing definitive information and present some suggestive findings.

Hurtado and his colleagues[16] at the Kaiser facility in Portland, Oregon, have reported the economic effects of introducing an extended care facility and a home care service into a comprehensive prepayment health plan with a history of low hospitalization utilization among subscribers. The effect on Medicare subscribers was of particular interest. The authors demonstrated that, with these new services administratively and spatially an integral part of the comprehensive care organization, hospital utilization of Medicare patients was reduced by 27%. Most of the observed reduction was attributable to the use of the extended care facility rather than the home care service. Moreover, the total cost of the services to Medicare patients outside the hospital service was greater than the savings from the reduced hospitalization; that is, while hospital days were reduced, less expensive extended care and home services were used for longer periods of time, these tending to equalize the cost of illness episodes managed primarily inside or outside the hospital service.

Similarly, Weiler and Rathbone-Mc-Cuan,[23] who are advocates of community-based care for older persons, summarize research on the cost of ten day care facilities that variously emphasized rehabilitation or social support services. The observed range of average daily cost was from $11 to $61 and an average for the 10 facilities was about $25. This average cost for adult day care was above the national average cost of about $19 per day for nursing home care at the time of the comparison. It is important to note that the day care program cost reported did not include an estimate of the out-of-pocket cost of living expenses of program participants. Alan Sager[24] has provided an imaginative pilot study of the cost of alternative forms of care for impaired older persons which illustrates the problems of cost estimation. Working with a sample of individuals at the point of discharge from a hospital, he had nine professionals experienced in discharge planning estimate whether home or nursing care would be the more appropriate assignment. Home care was estimated to be more appropriate for 12%. The assessors then proposed detailed care plans. Reasonable consensus was achieved among planners for each individual and the the estimated cost of implementing the recommended care plans was determined. The average daily cost of the estimated home care plans, with maintenance cost of board and lodging factored in, was about $52. Assessors were also asked to prescribe an alternative care plan for each individual if the person were institutionalized. The estimated cost of the services proposed for delivery in a nursing home proved to be almost exactly the same as for home care. By happenstance, nine subjects for whom home care and nursing home care plans had been developed were in fact institutionalized; the actual average cost per day was about $60. The conceptualization of this study warrants special comment. First, careful attention was given to establishing professional consensus on appropriate service requirements regardless of the service site chosen. Second, total cost of services, whether public or private, was estimated. Third, experienced professional service planners proposed alternative care plans in both nursing home and home settings which proved to have the same total cost, although the actual cost of nursing home care proved to be above the estimated

cost. And, fourth, at the point of discharge from the hospital, a large majority (almost 90%) of older patients considered for inclusion in the study were judged to be inappropriate for home care.

Medicus Systems Corporation,[22] under a federal contract, attempted to implement an ambitious controlled trial of the outcome of assigning appropriately selected individuals being discharged from hospitals to day care or home care programs, to a combination of both, or to a "no special care" control condition. The cost of additional services for the experimental subjects assigned to day care or home service was provided by special federal financial arrangements. For various reasons the research study did not meet the stringent conditions of a controlled clinical trial. True random alternative assignment of subjects proved to be difficult, services received by controls could not be monitored carefully, and cost determination was inadequate. However, within the constraints of the data noted, considerable variation in cost of services between presumably similar programs was observed. The general conclusion reached was that extended benefits available to participants in noninstitutional programs did appear to lower the utilization of traditional health services appreciably. There was some indication that total cost of care increased on the average. These conclusions are similar to those reached by Hurtado and his colleagues.

The most adequate information on the cost of community and home programs designed as alternatives to institutionalization, while clearly not definitive, does not confirm the hopes of the advocates of alternative forms of care. The assertion that community and home care lowers average daily cost or total system cost is not confirmed when there is some control for the level of functional impairment of the older individual involved and for the cost accounting procedures used. It is also evident that community and home care appears most favorably in comparison with institutional care where only public cost is considered and basic maintenance cost and other non-public contributions are not factored in. Further, and this is a critical issue, such evidence as there is does not indicate that total system cost is reduced by community-based care programs. On the contrary, total cost appears to be the same or perhaps slightly higher.

The current evidence on cost-effectiveness of community care does not provide a decisive argument against such care. Economic cost is not necessarily the only or the most important consideration. It is quite possible, for instance that cost being equal, community and home care provide good value for money invested because the care provided is more appropriate than institutional care, is of better quality, or is more effective in the long run. Or the long-run implications may be more favorable for noninstitutional care than short-term studies have indicated. Or public policy might favor noninstitutional care, not because its total cost is less than institutional care, but because noninstitutional care transfers a significant part of the cost to the private sector. Or, by removing impaired individuals from high-technology environments, public policy which emphasizes noninstitutional care may reduce long-run system cost through reducing the use of high-cost interventions of questionable value. Each and all these explanations is plausible and future research must sort out the facts. Concentration on cost may, however, divert attention from what many observers believe to be the more salient problem—the organization of care.

THE ORGANIZATIONAL CONTEXT OF HEALTH CARE

We have argued above that community and home care for impaired older persons is needed and feasible and that such care is not demonstrably more economical than institutional forms of care when degree of functional impairment is controlled and total cost is determined. However, the cost-effectiveness of noninstitutional care is probable, we have argued, for perhaps 30%

of older persons who are moderately but not severely impaired. Essential evidence does not exist that cost-effective noninstitutional care of appropriate quality can be provided for this significant cateory of impaired elderly within the care system as presently organized This is so primarily for two reasons. First, currently the care system and its financing have a decidedly medical and institutional emphasis. That is, the care system is most easily accessed by individuals with a medically certifiable impairment, and access to some community services is contingent on the individual's having been institutionalized. Community and home services, while recognized in Medicare legislation, continue to be a negligible fraction of the services financed. The concept of preventive care and social support services are essentially foreign to Medicare; mental health services are limited.[39,40,41,43]

Contemporary discussions of health usually stress the desirability of taking a broad view of health in terms of functional capacity and the total well-being of individuals. That is, a philosophic interest in the social components of health and well-being is frequently expressed, and strong cases have been made for preferring social models of care to medical models.[37,12,7] Philosophic preferences aside, the dominant care system available to older persons has a decidedly medical focus. Second, the dominant care system is highly specialized, fragmented, uncoordinated, and without a single point of entry to provide systematic, comprehensive assessment of impairment and assignment to appropriate services. One result is that each segment of the care system competes for public resources which are known to be limited but are treated as unlimited. Hence, each program tends to add to total system cost rather than to substitute for the cost of some other service. A striking characteristic of the care system of the United States is that its implied total annual budget is unlimited, is determined by the cumulative cost of all care programs, and is known only after the costs have been incurred. This is in contrast to nationalized systems and, in fact, to prepaid comprehensive programs in this country, which assume a fixed annual budget which must be allocated among the alternative components of the system.

At the beginning of this decade, the Department of Health, Education and Welfare[42] distributed an analysis of what was described as "the crisis of health care." This document asked whether the perceived crisis was produced by (1) inferior health care as reflected in the assessed well-being of citizens; (2) the absence of essential resources; or (3) both of these. The answer in each case was negative. While mortality, morbidity statistics and life expectancy in this country are below most Western European countries, they are tolerable by most standards and are most distinctively different from these countries in regard to variations by race, socioeconomic status, and geography. Health indicators of white, middle-class, urban populations in this country generally compare quite favorably with European populations; nor does this country lack resources. Our health personnel/population ratios are favorable, our hospital bed/population ratios are favorable, and our commitment of percentage of GNP to health (over 8%) is among the highest in the world. Again the most evident problem is in maldistribution of resources, particularly primary care resources, rather than absence of resources. There are, for example, 82 active physicians per 100,000 population in Mississippi and 228/100,000 in New York. Large metropolitan areas average 2½ times more physicians per unit population than rural areas. In recent decades the proportion of primary care physicians has declined to the point that, at the beginning of this decade, more than 6 in 10 active physicians were in specialty practice. The report concluded that the crisis is best described as organizational. The nation suffers, according to this analysis, from excessive fragmentation and poor coordination of existing resources. Significantly, the report did not comment directly on what Wildavsky calls the Great Equation (Medical Care Equals Health), although this idea is implicit. For instance, the report does stress the importance of environmental factors that affect health, preventive care, and health education. The central illustration of a possible solution to the organizational problem identified was Health Maintenance Organizations (HMOs). This preference was justified in the report by evidence then available that HMOs are cost effective, a conclusion supported also by current evidence.[31]

Following the HEW report, legislation intended to foster HMOs emerged. The concept has been politically controversial, has had limited public acceptance, and has generated a considerable amount of rhetoric *for* and *against*.[10] Recent articles by Enthoven[25] and Luft[32] summarize the issues and the evidence. Enthoven correctly notes the absence of controlled trials in comparing alternative care systems and the consequent inability to draw definitive conclusions regarding the cost-effectiveness and quality of care provided by competing alternatives. He reviews the incentive structures of alternative care systems and concludes that fragmented, uncoordinated systems lack any obvious incentive for control of cost. Further, if a fragmented, uncoordinated collection of health care programs is dominated by high technology institutions, the probability is high that a "technological imperative" will operate. That is, the availability of technology encourages high rates of use even in the face of evidence that its use has low marginal utility. This conclusion leads Enthoven to argue that, within a total system of care, there should be alternative care sites, some of which remove individuals from the high technology care centers. Such removal reduces the opportunity, and the inclination, to introduce types of care whose return in terms of increased functioning is demonstrably low. By implication, then, Enthoven argues that community and home care might achieve economies precisely because individuals in such settings are not, and presumably are appropriately not, at risk for high technology therapeutic intervention. Enthoven does, however, introduce the caution that his general argument for alternative forms of care is not an endorsement of any specific form of care in the absence of controlled trials which take into consideration quality as well as cost. It is worth noting in this context that some proponents of the hospice movement appear to reach a similar conclusion.[33] In high technology settings, there are a variety of incentives—professional, ethical, and legal—to make extraordinary efforts to extend life by any available means and at any cost. Proponents of hospices commonly argue that such efforts are not only patently artificial but also, in the final analysis, inhumane. This conclusion leads to the deliberate exclusion of advanced technology from the hospice to a specific emphasis on the social and behavioral rather than medical components of care. Medical technology is emphasized in the hospice movement, if at all, in connection with the reduction of pain rather than with the extension of life.

An article by Luft[32] reviews the rhetoric and the evidence regarding the reputed savings attributed to HMOs and concludes that the claimed economies are probably real and substantial. These reported savings in the total cost of care apparently are attributable primarily to the lower rates of hospitalization in HMOs and not to differences in the utilization of ambulatory care services or length of stay in hospitals. The studies Luft reviews are relatively compelling because they are methodologically adequate, taking into consideration standardized age and sex rates and case mixes; he is not altogether certain why the apparent cost-effectiveness is observed. Possibly, he argues, the HMO client is less sick or differently disposed to utilize available care, although most evidence suggests that this is not the case; on the contrary, some evidence suggests that prepaid plans tend to attract a disproportionate number of chronically ill persons. Or perhaps HMOs undertreat their patients, although evidence that this is so is lacking. It should be recalled here that the research of Hurtado et al.[16] did not find cost savings in

an experiment with alternative forms of service within a particular comprehensive prepaid medical plan. One might conclude that the Hurtado study suggests the possibilities of different, possibly more appropriate, forms of service within an existing cost. This study however, assessed only the cost, not the quality, of alternative forms of care.

HMOs do appear to provide some of the best evidence available of the cost and quality of care implications of a comprehensive system of care. Such a conclusion would not, however, challenge Wildavsky's Great Equation, because HMOs illustrate a predominantly medical model of care. Federal financing of care for older persons continues to concentrate on Medicare and Medicaid and reinforces the dominant fee-for-service principle which undergrids medical care in this country. As will be noted in the next section, however, an HMO strategy may lend itself reasonably well to the development of a model of care which melds social and medical components of care.

CONSTRUCTING THE FUTURE

As noted earlier in the discussion of Perrow's analysis of the three factors which affect service delivery organizations, cultural and ideological factors dominate when the technology for achieving preferred social goals is unavailable and when existing organizational structure affect adversely the application of such technology as exists. Many people, including many expert observers, believe that community and home care are forms of noninstitutional service delivery which are both desirable and feasible; this belief is bolstered by a number of factors, including evidence from this country and abroad (1) that programs of care for older persons outside institutional settings can be efficient and effective; (2) that care in institutional settings not only is very expensive but also that such care provides too much service for some older people and not enough for others who could benefit from minimal supportive care; and (3) that appropriate technology and model organizational forms of community-based care exist which provide the basis for future development of an adequate comprehensive care system.

Beliefs, Technology, Organization

In spite of the attractiveness of these beliefs, community and home care have been developed slowly and with considerable cautiousness in the United States. The explanation is suggested by Perrow's analysis. At the cultural level, the attractiveness of low technology community and home care is matched by the appeal of high technology medical care. In the abstract, both health care providers and consumers would surely respond favorably to the prospect of more noninstitutional forms of care of high quality and at low cost. In the concrete, it is not at all clear that either would respond affirmatively to more non-institutional care if this meant fewer hospital beds, rationed access to hospitals and physicians, or reduction in the specialized tests and therapeutic procedures that are in the heart of contemporary diagnosis.[4] That is, if given the choice of a fixed amount of money to be allocated to health and welfare with more community care resulting in less institutional care, it remains to be seen where public beliefs lie.

The critical question is *not* whether reallocation of resources to alternative forms of care is possible. Most countries in Western Europe provide illustration of successful community care programs as integral components of their systems of care. And the question is *not* whether the health of populations suffers impossibly from extensive use of noninstitutional services. It does not. Every country in Western Europe has gross indicators of mortality and morbidity which compare favorably with our own.[42] The question *is* whether health care personnel and the people of the United States they serve can live with the implications of a changed health care system in which access to medical and hospital care would be rationed and the autonomy, perceived or real, of both professionals and their patients/

clients would be reduced.[44] The evidence and the speculation are variable and suggest that American values and attitudes regarding health care are essentially contradictory. Some social survey evidence suggests that a majority of adult Americans perceive a crisis in health care delivery and identify the inaccessibility of primary care and the cost of health care as their primary concerns.[10] Fox[4] argues that, while Ivan Illich's radical critique of "medicalization" of society and his plea for "demedicalization" have some merit, health remains a central preoccupation of this society. Saward and Sorensen[7] document the continuing societal preoccupation with curative rather than preventive medicine. Individuals continue to resist modifying behavior and lifestyles which increase the risk of morbidity and mortality—cigarette smoking, overeating, physical inactivity, nonuse of auto seat belts, for example. Of special interest are indications that social controls intended to modify risky behavior or noxious environmental factors are widely interpreted as infringements on personal freedom. It is as though, these authors conclude, freedom from regulations is more dear than life itself. Wildavsky's caustic, pessimistic essay "Doing Better, Feeling Worse"[3] is preoccupied with the contradictory, the ironic, indeed what he believes to be the pathological aspects of health care in this country. In addition to persistent belief in the wrongheaded "Great Equation," he notes the "Paradox of Time: Past Success Leads to Future Failure." For example, increased longevity is a human triumph which precipitates the crisis of an aging society. To save our shaky belief that investment in medicine insures health, we displace our goals; interest in curing is displaced by interest in caring, and caring becomes equated with demonstrating we have access to ineffective services. Every move to increase equality in one dimension of health care increases inequality in another dimension. No society is willing and no care system is able, Wildavsky argues, to provide as much care as a population is willing to consume. We are driven by a technological imperative; there is always one more procedure to try. Cost of health care inevitably rises to a total which is provided by private insurance and federal subsidy. One is hardly surprised by the bottom line of Wildavsky's diagnosis: The politics of health care in the United States can only be described as conflicted, ambivalent, pathological. The prognosis is not encouraging. No definitive treatment is available.

Perrow's analysis suggests that the persistent ideological quality of contemporary discussion about health care constitutes evidence of the inadequacy of available technology and organizational arrangements for insuring either curing or caring at a tolerable social cost. Our love affair with medical technology apparently is not over, but it is pursued with less enthusiasm than formerly. The evidence of decreasing marginal utility of costly applications of medical technology is simply too great to be ignored.[6,7,35,36] Yet there are few signs that continued discussion of "the crisis of health care" portends a radical reorganization and reallocation of health resources. After all, there is not yet even consensus about legislation on one or another form of national health insurance.[16]

For the foreseeable future, for better or worse, the United States seems destined to tinkering incrementally with its fragmented, uncoordinated nonsystem of care. Incrementalism—a euphemism for only minor modifications of existing programs which the British call "muddling through"—has some merit in stable, democratically controlled societies.[45] Several incremental changes at selected points in the current system of care affecting older persons do warrant at least some basis for guarded optimism about the future.

Adaptive Responses

Public acceptance of unconditional professional autonomy and a medical monopoly of health care resources have been increasingly challenged. The origins of this challenge lie in the distant past as Chapman[44] has documented. The legal basis of laws regarding professional malpractice can be traced to the fourteenth century. In the intervening centuries public challenge of uncontrolled professional autonomy and monopoly has been expressed through laws dealing with due process, licensure, restraint of trade and quality control. Willingness of legislatures to limit the autonomy of medical professionals has been clearly demonstrated. Physicians, hospitals, and long-term care institutions will continue to play a vital role in the continuum of care which older persons require and in decisions about the allocation of resources to various components of the care system. The issue therefore is not the involvement of physicians and medical institutions in designing health care for the future but the increasing involvement of nonmedical professions and nonmedical, community-based facilities in designing that future. Legislators have been reluctant to control access to high technology medicine; 'to limit the proliferation and geographic concentration of highly specialized health personnel; to develop a plan for national health insurance; to involve government as a prudent buyer and not just an insurer of desired health and social services with emphasis on preventive and primary care; to undertake large-scale experimentation in comprehensive, prepayment care systems which integrate health and social services; and orient consumers to alternative expectations regarding care delivery. Belief in the desirability and feasibility of more community-based services is increasing but nothing approximating a national consensus regarding the reorganization and financing of a comprehensive health care system designed to serve older persons is evident.

Organizational Development

Pragmatic, incremental experience with the organization of care in the United States has produced an outcome which, while not altogether satisfactory, is satisfactory enough to militate against radical reorganization of care delivery in the immediate future. This same pragmatic, incremental orientation does, however, permit experimentation and model building which can provide public standards for assessing effectiveness and efficiency. In this country elaboration of the Health Maintenance Organization concept appears to have particular merit for responding to needs of older persons for comprehensive care.

The cost-effectiveness of HMOs has been reasonably established and this effectiveness is usually attributed, not to restriction of access to care generally but to reduction of institutionalization.[32] The HMO concept also emphasizes comprehensiveness of care within a fixed budget. Consider, for example, Fig. 23-1.[27] In this figure *health* is defined broadly as *well-being,* and attention is given to social as well as medical aspects of care and to preventive maintenance as well as sick care. An integral and important aspect of this care system is the availability of initial screening for purposes of triage, although there is provision for bypass of screening when alternative assignment to health care, preventive maintenance, and sick care are clearly indicated. Another striking feature of this conceptualization of a care system is that, while traditional

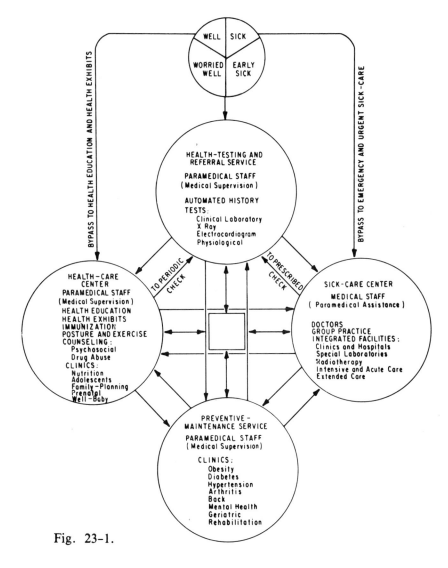

Fig. 23-1.

medical services are considered basic, social and psychological dimensions of care are equally basic and integral to the system. Given the origins of HMOs within the dominant medical model of care, one is hardly surprised that reference is made to *paramedical* staff and services with *medical* supervision. No violence is done to the concept by the substitution of such concepts as *paraprofessional* staff with *professional* supervision in order to transform this conventional medical model into a professional model which can include experts in social and psychological dimensions of care. Special attention is called in Fig. 23–1 to programs of health education, exercise, and psychological counseling in the health care center component of the model; to provision of extended care, which could include community and home care for the impaired elderly, in the sick care component; and to geriatric clinics in the preventive maintenance component.

The HMO model of a comprehensive health maintenance organization is similar to, and is in fact, more comprehensive than the system of geriatric care currently operating in Glasgow, Scotland, as described by Sir Ferguson Anderson and his colleagues.[46,12] The Scottish model has as its focal point a primary care health center manned by general practitioners, visiting nurses, and social workers who have been trained to work as a team. The health center personnel in this setting have access to an impressive continuum of alternative care settings, including in-home services, day care, day hospitals, sheltered housing, and inpatient hospital services with both general and specialized hospital wards, including geriatric psychiatry. Moreover, in Glasgow, community programs supplement the health services by providing special health education and a health examination coincident with retirement and a variety of community support programs. The Scottish Home and Health Service, as a part of the British National Health Service, has a long tradition of integrating medical and social services and is, by definition, a comprehensive, prepaid care system. In Glasgow, professionals appear to use alternative placement of older persons judiciously and to place the impaired elderly at sites where the most appropriate care is available. Although detailed information about the cost of a comprehensive service such as that in Glasgow is not available, in general the British investment in the delivery of care runs about 2% of Gross National Product less than in the United States.

A systematic investment of governmental resources in the development of model HMOs to include assessment, health care, sick care, and preventive maintenance care for older persons appears to be indicated and is to be recommended. Such a decision would not preclude alternative investments in other forms of care. Yet the existence of a comprehensive system of care could provide a specific context for comparing the efficiency and effectiveness of alternative programs.

Technological Development

Our national fascination with technology and its implementation could appropriately be directed increasingly to problems of special relevance to caring for older persons. In the interest of serving older persons more effectively, primary attention might be given to the implementation and specific applications of two existing types of technology. Badly needed are (1) a reliable, valid, economical procedure for identifying the existence and pattern of functional impairment among older persons;[47] and (2) the development of information systems which will facilitate the monitoring and evaluation of the efficiency and effectiveness of alternative systems of care.[34,35,37,18,48] Assessment of the effectiveness and efficiency of care in alternative settings is contingent on the appropriateness of matching level and type of functional impairment with resources intended to maintain or restore function. Adequate procedures for systematic, comprehensive assessment of functioning exist but the available procedures are not widely available or consistently applied. As one might expect in the fragmented, uncoordinated array of services which characterize the situation in the United States, there is no tradition of single points of entry into the care system which could provide assessment, triage, and monitoring of the outcomes of services. Experiments which provide systematic assessment, triage, and monitoring are clearly feasible and warranted.

While explicit experiments in new forms of comprehensive care delivery for older persons are feasible and warranted, the opportunity to benefit from existing care programs should not be underestimated. Legislated governmental programs of care constitute social experiments from which important information can be derived[18,36,49] if several conditions can be met. The efficiency and effectiveness of any service program can be assessed if (1) the functional status of participants can be measured at several points in time, and (2) the components of service to which participants are exposed can be specified. There is no longer any question that these conditions can be met in reasonably economic ways and in ways which are based on the types of information care programs routinely gather or could gather.

As a sense of crisis about the cost and effectiveness of care for older persons escalates in the years ahead, experimentation with alternative systems of care will increase. The nation has the resources and the technology to develop an effective and efficient system of care for older persons at a bearable cost. Our capacity to develop an adequate system will hinge on our ability to reorganize the resources already at our disposal.

REFERENCES

1. U. S. Senate, Special Committee on Aging. 1977. *Older Americans: The 'Alternatives' Issue, I & II.* Washington, D.C.: Government Printing Office.
2. Perrow, C. 1965. Hospitals: Technology, structure, goals. In J. G. March (ed.) *Handbook of Organizations.* Chicago: Rand McNally and Company.
3. Wildavsky, A. 1977. Doing better and feeling worse: The political pathology of health policy. In John H. Knowles (ed.) *Doing Better and Feeling Worse: Health in the United States,* pp. 105–124, New York: W. W. Norton.
4. Fox, Renée C. 1977. The medicalization and demedicalization of American society. In John H. Knowles (ed.) *Doing Better and Feeling Worse: Health in the United States,* pp. 9–22, New York: W. W. Norton.
5. Maddox, G. L. 1977. Community and home care: The unrealized potential of an old idea. In A. N. Exton-Smith and J. G. Evans (eds.) *Care of the Elderly: Meeting the Challenge of Dependency.* New York: Grune and Stratton.
6. Ingelfinger, F. J. 1978. Medicine: Meritorious or Meritricious? *Science, 200,* pp. 942–945.
7. Saward, E., and Sorensen, A. 1978. The current emphasis on preventive care. *Science, 200,* pp. 889–894.
8. Culliton, B. J. 1978. Health care economics: the high cost of getting well. *Science, 200,* pp. 883–885.
9. Walsh, J. 1978. Federal health care spending passes the $50–billion mark. *Science, 200,* pp. 886–888.
10. Lewis, C. E., Fein, R. and Mechanic, D. 1976. *A Right to Health: The Problem of Access to Primary Medical Care.* John Wiley and Sons.
11. Knowles, J. H. (ed.) *Doing Better and Feeling Worse.* New York: W. W. Norton.
12. Kane, R. L., and Kane, R. A. 1978. Care of the aged: Old problems in need of new solutions. *Science, 200,* pp. 913–918.
13. Maddox, G. L. 1975. Families as context and resource in chronic illness. In Sylvia Sherwood (ed.) *Long-Term Care: A Handbook for Researchers, Planners, and Providers.* New York: Spectrum Publications, pp. 317–348.
14. Maddox, G. L. 1972. Interventions and outcomes: Notes on designing and implementing an experiment in health care. *International J. of Epidemiology,* 1: 4:339–345.
15. Laurie, W. F. 1978. Employing the Duke OARS Methodology in Cost Comparisons; Home Services and Institutionalization. In *Duke University Center Reports on Advances in Research,* Vol. 2: 2 (whole issue).
16. Hurtado, A., Greenlick, A., and Saward, E. 1971. Home and extended care in a comprehensive prepayment plan. Chicago: Hospital and Research Educational Trust.
17. Maddox, G. L. and Karasik, R. 1975. *Planning Services for Older People.* Durham, N.C.: Duke University Center for the Study of Aging and Human Development.
18. Maddox, G. L. and Dellinger, D. C. 1978. Assessment of functional status in a program evaluation and resources allocation model. *Annals of the American Academy of Political and Social Sciences,* 438: 59–70.
19. Health Policy Analysis Program, 1978. *Long Term*

Care for the Elderly in Washington. Seattle: Department of Health Services, University of Washington.

20. Comptroller General of the United States. 1977a. *The Well-being of Older People in Cleveland, Ohio.* A Report to the Congress, April 19, 1977. Washington, D.C.: U.S. General Accounting Office.

21. Comptroller General of the United States, 1977b. *Home Health—The Need for a National Policy to Better Provide for the Elderly.* A Report to the Congress, December 30, 1977. Washington, D.C.: U.S. General Accounting Office.

22. Medicus Systems Corporation. 1977. *Evaluation of Day Care and Homemaker Demonstrations: Executive Summary: Report No. 36.* Chicago: Medicus Systems Corporation.

23. Weiler, P. G., and Rathbone-McCuan, E. 1978. *Adult Day Care: Community Work with the Elderly.* New York: Springer Publishing Company.

24. Sager, A. 1977. Estimating the cost of diverting patients from nursing homes to home care. Waltham, Mass.: Levinson Policy Inst., Brandeis Univ.

25. Enthoven, A. C. 1978. Cutting cost without cutting the quality of care. *New England J. of Medicine,* **298:** 22:1229–1238.

26. Ball, R. M. 1978. National health insurance: Comments on selected issues. *Science,* **200,** pp. 864–870.

27. Garfield, S. R. 1970. The delivery of medical care. *Scientific American,* **222:** 4, pp. 15–23.

28. DHEW. 1977a. Current estimates from the health information survey, United States, 1975. *Vital and Health Statistics.* Series **10:** 115.

29. Shanas, E., and Maddox, G. L. 1977. Aging, Health and the Organization of Health Resources. In R. Binstock and E. Shanas (eds.) *Handbook of Aging and the Social Sciences.* New York: Van Nostrand Reinhold.

30. Maddox, G. L. and Wiley, J. 1977. The Scope, Concepts, and Methods in the Study of Aging. In R. Binstock and E. Shanas (eds.) *Handbook of Aging and the Social Sciences.* New York: Van Nostrand Reinhold.

31. DHEW, 1977b. Medicare: utilization of home services, 1974. *Health Insurance Statistics,* November 2, 1977.

32. Luft, H. S. 1978. How do Health Maintenance Organizations Achieve Their 'Savings'? *New England J. of Medicine,* **298:** 1336–1343.

33. Berdes, C. 1978. *Social Services for the Aged Dying and Bereaved in International Perspective.* Washington: International Federation on Aging.

34. Donabedian, A. 1978. The quality of medical care. *Science,* **200,** pp. 856–863.

35. Frazier, H. S. and Hiat, H. H. 1978. Evaluation of medical practices. *Science,* **200,** pp. 875–879.

36. Tancredi, L. R. and Barondess, J. A. 1978. The problem of defensive medicine. *Science,* **200,** pp. 879–883.

37. Breslow, L. 1978. Risk factor intervention for health maintenance. Science, **200,** pp. 908–912.

38. Smyer, M. A. 1977. Differential usage and differential effects of services for impaired elderly. *Duke University Center Reports on Advances in Research.* **1:** 4 (whole issue).

39. Blazer, D. and Maddox, G. 1977. *Developing Geriatric Services in a Community Mental Health Center: A Case History of a University-Based Affiliate Clinic.* Durham, N.C.: Duke University Center for the Study of Aging and Human Development.

40. Glasscote, R. 1976. *Old Folks at Home: A Field Study of Nursing and Board and Care Homes.* Washington: Joint Information Service of the American Psychiatric Association and the National Association of Mental Health.

41. Glasscote, R., Gudeman, J. E. and Miles, D. 1977. *Creative Mental Health Services for the Elderly.* Washington: Joint Information Service of the American Psychiatric Association and the Mental Health Association.

42. DHEW. 1971. *Towards a Comprehensive Health Policy for the 1970s.* Washington, D.C.: US DHEW.

43. Berger, P. A. 1978. Medical treatment of mental illness. *Science,* **200,** pp. 974–981.

44. Chapman, C. B. 1978. Doctors and their autonomy. *Science,* **200,** pp. 851–855.

45. Maddox, G. L. 1971. Muddling through: Planning for health care in England. *Medical Care,* **9:** 5, pp. 439–448.

46. McLachlan, G. 1971. *Problems and Progress in Medical Care.* Oxford: Oxford University Press.

47. Institute of Medicine. 1977. *The Elderly and Functional Dependency.* Washington, D. C., National Academy of Science.

48. Maddox, G. L. 1978. Aging, social change and social policy. In M. Yinger, H. Mausch, and S. Cutler (eds.) *Major Social Issues: A Multidisciplinary View.* New York: The Free Press.

49. Schoolman, H. M., and Bernstein, L. M. 1978. Computer use in diagnosis, prognosis, and therapy. *Science,* **200,** pp. 926–930.

Chapter 24
The Future of Geriatric Psychiatry

Ewald W. Busse, M.D.
Duke University Medical Center

Dan Blazer, M.D.
Duke University Medical Center

INTRODUCTION

Geriatrics in general and geriatric psychiatry in particular have clearly become established as special areas of medical attention, knowledge and medical practice. This development is a response to an increase in our older population, their health and psychiatric problems, and society's efforts to meet their human needs. Geriatric psychiatry will continue to grow as the percentage of older people in this country (10% at present) gradually grows, and the absolute number of older people increases remarkably.[1] Since the turn of the century, this growth in the number of older people has been influenced by dramatic advances in infant survival, the decline in birth rate in recent years, and to a lesser extent upon in-

Preparation of this chapter was supported in part by Research Career Development Award #1 K01 MH 00115–01A1 (Dr. Blazer).

Preparation of this chapter was supported in part by Grant #5 P01 AG00364 from the National Institute on Aging (Dr. Busse).

creased longevity. Regardless of the causes of these changing demographics, it is certain that physicians will encounter many more older people who are afflicted with chronic as well as acute illnesses. The incidence of organic mental syndromes increases with advancing age, and as the number of "old-old"[1] continues to grow, physicians will encounter more such patients.

Aging also has "come of age."[2] The concepts of aging in this society are changing slowly but surely and the problems of aging are no longer something to be ignored or avoided. Sociologists, economists, political scientists and educators, in addition to physicians, have been forced, or have chosen to address issues associated with the increased numbers of older people and the importance of adequately describing and planning for these older persons in our society. Issues being addressed include compulsory versus voluntary retirement, the dependency ratio (Chapter 1), changes in life styles and living arrangements among the elderly, the emerging role of the elderly as a political force, and economic well-being of the elderly, especially as it relates to the ability and desire of older persons to purchase services (Chapter 10). Social and behavioral scientists are increasingly recognizing the continued importance of relationships of the elderly with family members and the changing patterns of these relationships.[3] (Chapter 9) Physicians and others included in health care must address two important questions. First, Should geriatrics (and geriatric psychiatry) become distinct medical specialties? Second, what issues in research, training, practice, and planning are pertinent to the future physician who seriously undertakes the management of the physically and mentally impaired elderly?

GERIATRIC MEDICINE AND GERIATRIC PSYCHIATRY AS SPECIALTIES

A discussion of the future of geriatric psychiatry would not be complete without some discussion of the future of general health care. One of the most important trends in modern health care in America that relates specifically to the elderly is the increased emphasis placed on "primary health care." Dr. Harvey Estes gives the following definition: "Primary health care is accessible, comprehensive, coordinated and continual care delivered by accountable providers of personal health services. It is usually associated with the care of the 'whole person' rather than a particular illness. It is distinguished from others levels of health care by the nature of the services provided, not by the particular specialty training of the provider."[4] According to Dr. Estes, primary health care providers not only include physicians but also physician's associates and nurse practitioners.[5] Special knowledge of epidemiology and the behavioral and social aspects of patient care are most important to the primary health care provider. In many ways the definition of primary health care closely resembles the basic characteristics of a good geriatrician and geriatric psychiatrist. A good geriatrician should also be aware of those aging changes that affect the human organism and

alter its capacity to respond to stress, disease, and trauma and that eventually may result in death. In other words, the geriatrician and geriatric psychiatrist often function within the framework of primary health care with special attention to the age change of the organism as it encounters its environment. In many ways geriatric psychiatry has a similar orientation, if not the specific procedures of therapy, as the other developmentally oriented subspecialty, child psychiatry.

Geriatrics is rapidly moving to the status of a subspecialty, particularly in the established fields of internal medicine and family practice. Although psychiatry has provided leadership in geriatric research, service and training have lagged. The recent increase in the number of training grants for the specific purpose of training psychiatric residents and fellows in geriatric psychiatry should increase the number of psychiatrists with competency in the field. These developments are a rational and orderly response to the history of an accumulation of knowledge, theory, and practice in aging and, at this stage, will best meet the realistic needs of the older population. However, the overall care of the elderly should not be removed from the purview of the primary care physician, and if geriatric medicine were to be made a distinct specialty at this time, it would suffer the isolating effects of specialization. The strength of geriatric medicine and geriatric psychiatry has been the application of knowledge gained through scientific endeavors in the mainstream of medical science and practice. Isolation would seriously jeopardize this process.

Those who advocate the development of a specialty in geriatrics frequently point to developments in Great Britain where a more or less distinct discipline of geriatrics has emerged.[6] The emergence of the British geriatrician, a hospital-based rather than a primary care physician, has spanned a period of 20 years and is tied to a system of health insurance and social assistance that may or may not be acceptable in the United States. If geriatric medicine is considered a distinct discipline in medicine, then one must ask, "Is a geriatrician a primary care physician or does he or she represent a specialty such as cardiology, dermatology, neurosurgery, psychiatry, etc.?" All of these, incidentally, were subspecialties of internal medicine and surgery at some point in their history. In other words, geriatric medicine may be more appropriately considered a subspecialty and not a specialty standing in its own right.

Those who advocate geriatric medicine as a distinct specialty are probably attempting to develop an answer to the obvious need to deliver better health care to older persons. One must applaud this motivation, but it carries with it considerable risks. It is quite possible that geriatric medicine and psychiatry do not, at this time, have the breadth of scientific knowledge, the distinct service component, and the theoretical base which characterize specialties in medicine. Geriatric medicine would therefore, more appropriately, be a subspecialty of internal medicine and/or family practice, and geriatric psychiatry would appropriately be a subspecialty of psychiatry.

Reimbursement for health care in the later years begins around the age of 65.[7] This has introduced an arbitrary distinction between individuals older than 65 and those who are younger than 65. It is well known, however, that the health of those between 65 and 75 closely resembles that of individuals between 55 and 65.[8] It is only after the age of 75 that there is a distinct change in the health and well-being of most individuals. The incidence of disability increases dramatically. Therefore, those practicing geriatric medicine and psychiatry in part take care of a segment of the population which more closely resembles middle age, at least in health characteristics, than those who are defined as "the elderly." Even after the age of 45 a number of biological changes, which are gradually moving to a point where they interfere with the individual's ability to function, begin to appear. However, these changes are not likely to become significant in the majority of individuals until after the age of 70. Yet they have significance to practicing physicians, for they influence drug metabolism, nutritional and sleep requirements, etc. Defining a specific age group as the unique purview of the "geriatrician" becomes quite difficult. Pediatrics is a viable specialty, so geriatrics, which focuses on the opposite end of the life cycle, might survive as a viable specialty. Though this is a strong argument for the emergence of geriatrics as a specialty, at least two concerns arise. Would it be acceptable to the insurer and consumer to have an additional medical specialty when specialists are believed to contribute to the high cost of medical care? Does geriatrics have the basic knowledge that makes it a distinct discipline? In addition, the older person may prefer to remain with the internist or family practitioner with whom he or she has related for many years of adult life. If we achieve the goal of placing primary care physicians throughout our population, then it is quite likely that a strong relationship will develop between patient and physician which will transcend the later years. If this is true, then the geriatrician will not be a primary care physician, (as the care will remain in the hands of the family practitioner or the internist), but will become a type of a consultant as in England and Scotland confined to facilities limited to the health care of the elderly. This, in all probability, would be undesirable from the physician's viewpoint, for a physician who becomes isolated in such restricted medical environments usually loses contact with the mainstream of medicine. There are very few physicians who are comfortable with the idea of serving a very limited type of population such as the very old or those who are being taken care of by a hospice.

These comments about geriatric medicine also apply to geriatric psychiatry. Geriatric psychiatry will undoubtedly follow the future of geriatric medicine as a subspecialty within the health care system. Yet the geriatric psychiatrist must remain a consultant specialist, who participates in the treatment team but who is not considered the primary care physician. The geriatric psychiatrist could literally be in double jeopardy for the isolating effects described above. Not only may he or she be isolated from the primary provision of health care to the older person (available to the primary care physician and/or geriatrician) but could also become isolated from the field of psychiatry itself. Geriatric psychiatrists may always find themselves in the position of liaison between the specialty and primary care. As is true of the liaison psychiatrist, a special set of skills is required to accomplish the translation of psychiatric and gerontological knowledge into effective patient management and treatment procedures for the elderly.[9] In addition, there is a necessity to translate this knowledge and approach into a language understandable by the entire health care team, as the treatment of the mental disorders of late life requires the intervention of individuals from numerous backgrounds (from physician to nurse's aid). This can best be accomplished when the geriatric psychiatrist becomes an integral member of the health care team (as the liaison psychiatrist becomes a member of the primary care team). As has been recognized by liaison psychiatrists, the development of a specialty of "liaison psychiatry" is actually an antipathy to the development of an effective role on the health care team.[8]

THE ROLE OF GERIATRIC PSYCHIATRY IN FUTURE HEALTH CARE

Psychiatry in general and geriatric psychiatry in particular seem to be caught in a persistent crisis of identity. This crisis directly relates to the changing role of psychiatry as it interfaces with medicine and the behavioral and social sciences. The geriatric psychiatrist must consider social and economic factors in his or her patients as well as mental health and physical health factors. If we might avoid debate about what is the medical model and its applicability to psychiatry, the description of three major medical models by Siegler and Osman[10] (scientific, clinical, and public health) provides a useful framework for considering the future roles of the geriatric psychiatrist. By adding a fourth role, namely that of educator, the framework is even more complete.

The Geriatric Psychiatrist as a Scientist

Though many areas of inquiry are of importance to geriatric psychiatry, some consideration must be given to the methodology of research design. In particular, aging is a process and never remains static. Researchers at Duke University Center for the Study of Aging have concluded that a longitudinal approach to the study of the elderly (both normal and abnormal) is essential to gaining knowledge of the aging process.[11] Some of the values of longitudinal research are as follows:[11]

1. Comparisons can be made between the decline in functioning of the whole person and the variations found in rates of decline of organs and systems which comprise the whole person.

2. Early signs and symptoms can be recognized which are contributing and/or causative factors that precede the appearance of disability, disease, or death (i.e., identification of the effects of antecedent events).

3. Observations over time reduce the possibility of retrospective falsification, as encountered in the collection of medical and social histories in cross-sectional studies. This may be especially a problem with elderly individuals whose memories are attenuated secondary to chronic organic mental syndromes.

4. The aging of the individual as a different, distinct, and perhaps unique organism is observed. Hence, the individual serves to some extent as his or her own control and baseline, yet the differences in regard to others in the group can also be studied.

5. Longitudinal studies permit validation by prediction. It is very important to the researcher to have some measure of the success of prediction of outcomes

related to antecedent variables. The clinician is constantly being called upon to predict outcomes given certain physical and mental symptoms and certain types of intervention.

6. Longitudinal studies provide an opportunity to attempt to distinguish senescence (primary aging) from senility (secondary aging), i.e., which declines in function are inherent and appropriate with the passage of time, and which are directly related to disease and trauma.

7. Age differences, the cohort effect, can be distinguished from age changes.

The researcher in aging also must pay attention to the relative importance of genetic versus environmental variables that relate to either normal processes in aging or disease processes.[12,13] Genetic variation is quite likely to contribute to psychiatric disorders and genetic heterogeneity is likely to exist for any single disorder. (Yet genetic factors may play less of a role in the onset of psychiatric illness for the first time in late life as opposed to the onset earlier in life). To achieve a better understanding of late onset genetic determinants, studies are needed that include related individuals, twins, separated relatives, nuclear families, and/or extended pedigrees. This is especially true in Alzheimer's type of dementia, as there is some scattered evidence that genetic factors play a role in its etiology.[14,15] Ultimately such studies should include traits that bridge the gap between the genetic predisposition to a given condition and the diagnostic presentation (i.e., phenotype).

A number of specific issues are being addressed (or can be addressed in the future) that directly relate to geriatric psychiatry. Major research needs that remain unresolved in the biomedical area include:

1. The need for an increased understanding of longevity, with emphasis placed on explaining specific phenomena such as the disproportionate longevity of females. (Chapter 1)

2. The need to understand and have better measures of aging functional assessment criteria rather than chronological age, i.e., cardiac rate and output, muscle mass and strength, perceptual changes, speed of response, etc. (Chapters 6 and 7)

3. The need to obtain a greater understanding of the genetic and biological predisposition to mental illness in later life, especially in depressive illness and organic mental syndromes.[14] (Chapters 1, 2, and 3)

4. The need for research into the pharmacology of late life, i.e., the changes in the responsiveness to various pharmacological agents with normal and abnormal aging, such as the increased response to cholinergical agents in the organically mentally impaired. (Chapter 5)

5. The need of age-adjusted criteria for clinically relevant variables, such as perceptual changes accompanying psychiatric illness and normal aging.[16] (Chapters 8 and 13)

Research into psychosocial aging is also of great importance. The major needs include:

1. The need for a greater understanding of the personality development of the adult male and female, specifically the relationship of personality style in middle and early life to adaptive and maladaptive behavior in late life. (Chapter 8)

2. The need for a greater understanding of the relationship of social support and social stress to adaptation in late life, e.g., the stress of poverty, retirement, etc. as they interrelate with social support networks, in particular the family. (Chapter 9 and 10)

3. The need for age-adjusted criteria for psychological tests commonly used, e.g., the Wechsler Adult Intelligence Scale, Rorschach test, etc. (Chapter 13)

4. The need for an increased knowledge of the epidemiology of mental illness in late life[17] as the prevalence, incidence, and distribution of mental illness among the elderly is not well under-

stood. Operational differentiation of the various psychopathological conditions in late life have not been as successful as might have been hoped for. Therefore much of the epidemiological work that has been done in the past suffers from a lack of the ability to differentiate between the various conditions studied. For example, when we speak of the "depressions" of late life, these conditions must be separated into (1) those individuals who have definite depressive illness; (2) individuals suffering from dysphoric symptoms from environmental stress; and (3) individuals who have dysphoric symptomatology accompanying physical illness.[18] If such differentiation can be made, additional consideration must be given to the prevalence of disorders that are not so severe but where intervention at a given point in time may, in fact, prevent a decline. (Chapter 10)

5. The need for careful studies of life histories to identify events, physical and environmental, which predispose the older patient to such disorders, to recurrent and serious depressions, as well as suicide. This is necessary to devise and test techniques of early intervention and their effectiveness and perhaps at some point, actual prevention. (Chapter 10)

Advances in biomedical science are often propelled by the appearance of technological advances that open new frontiers. It is highly likely that such an important advance is the development of positron emission tomography (PET). Until recently the intact central nervous system, particularly the human brain and nervous system, has not been accessible for precise quantitative study. This new technical ability will allow for careful *in vivo* studies of cerebral perfusion and metabolism. In many respects it offers for research in cerebral metabolism what the CT scanner has provided for study in *in vivo* cerebral anatomy. Short-lived isotopes, for example, O^{15}, C^{11}, F^{18} and N^{13}, can be incorporated into metabolically ac-

tive compounds including glucose, carbon monoxide, and ammonia. A biologically safe method is available for the *in vivo* monitoring of flow, perfusion, and metabolism in the brains of humans and experimental animals. These studies will add immeasurable important knowledge to our understanding of brain changes with aging and to the differences between cerebral vascular disease and senile dementia. Studies of this type are now being funded by the National Institutes of Health. The positron is a subatomic particle and is one of the 33 + fundamental fragments that are believed to compose an atomic nucleii. A positron and an electron are produced when a photon decays. An electron has a negative charge of 1, and the positron has an electrical charge of positive 1; therefore it is also called an antielectron.[19,20]

The Geriatric Psychiatrist as an Educator

Epidemiological data that have been gathered to date on the prevalence of mental illness among the elderly strongly indicate the need for increased numbers of professionals who have training in the treatment of mental illness in later life. Though no truly meaningful quantitative estimates of the number of geriatric psychiatrists needed for the future can be made at this time, it is certain that the field of geriatric psychiatry will not be overpopulated with physicians within the near future.[21] The scarcity of psychiatrists with a specific interest and/or expertise in aging, makes the role of an educator an imperative for the comprehensive psychiatrist who subspecializes in geriatrics. It should be emphasized from the outset that the role of the geriatric psychiatrist as an educator is predicated upon the fact that a useful knowledge base does exist at the present time in gerontology and geriatric psychiatry.

Education in geriatrics and in geriatric psychiatry should begin in the early years of medical school. Special courses are undesirable; rather information regarding the aging processes should be included in physiology, pharmacology, and human behavior—the basic science curriculum of medical students.[22] Aging is a dynamic variable, and must be considered by the clinician as it influences many decisions for treatment. Specific clinical experiences such as a nursing home rotation can be offered within clinical rotations, and both age-related basic science and clinical electives should be available to the medical student. The curriculum that offers only electives and neglects the need to integrate information about the aging into the mainstream of medicine will lose a most important component of medical education.

Once the medical student has reached the clinical years, there is a need for a greater emphasis on rehabilitative and supportive medicine within multidisciplinary settings. The truly broad-based clinical curriculum will place emphasis on the concept of supportive care in addition to the cure of individuals through high technology medicine. For example, nutrition, exercise, and physiotherapy as well as integration of the older person into a supportive social network are just as much a part of the treatment plan of an elderly individual with psychiatric and/or physical illness as the use of medications or a surgical procedure.

Postgraduate specialty training in the primary care specialties of family practice and internal medicine particularly requires emphasis upon the integration of biological age changes, disease processes, and the social, psychological, and behavioral aspects of aging. Though psychiatry is not usually considered a primary care specialty, we might expect that the general psychiatrist will have a high probability of being consulted frequently about the management of the older person with common psychiatric problems. Medical students and postgraduate trainees also need instructions in specific conditions that frequently affect the elderly. These include spontaneous hypothermia, incontinence, normal pressure hydrocephalis, constipation, sleep disorders, and organic mental syndromes. In spite of the high frequency of these symptoms and illnesses, it is surprising how little attention is paid to their diagnosis and management in typical training programs.

Yet the best laid plans of any curriculum committee in a medical school or postgraduate program will prove unfruitful if well-trained and respected role models are not available for the clinical training of students and trainees.[23] One of the greatest deficits in American geriatric medicine and geriatric psychiatry is the lack of individuals who are proven sound clinicians within a given specialty and who have expressed a definite interest in the treatment of the elderly. Role models are the key factor in the education of the physician and will continue to be. Unfortunately, no program can assure the development of these role models though certain approaches may be of help. Well established clinicians with research and/or clinical interest in aging and the care of the elderly should be encouraged, as they are effective instructors in geriatric medicine and geriatric psychiatry. Dr. Robert Butler, Director of the National Institute on Aging, says that "Perhaps less than 15 of an estimated 25,000 faculty members of American medical schools have a genuine expertise in geriatrics."[23] Though the number has undoubtedly increased in the last 2 or 3 years, the deficit still is a great one.

The Geriatric Psychiatrist as a Clinician

Future geriatric psychiatrists must have a multidimensional orientation. Diagnostic criteria for illnesses should be age adjusted for elderly patients, and the chronic and multifactoral etiology of illness in late life should remain paramount in the clinician's mind. This multidimensional approach should enable the geriatric psychiatrist to work effectively with the treatment team (primary care physician, nurse, social worker, physician's associate, etc.). In fact, the geriatric psychiatrist may be a key figure in developing and maintaining the team approach to the care of the older patient.

The geriatric psychiatrist must be skilled in the use of pharmacological agents with the elderly. If there is any unique skill that a psychiatrist contributes to the overall care of older patients it is the proper use of psychotropic medications. As new agents are coming on the market for the treatment of organic mental syndromes, the geriatric psychiatrist should be in a position to treat and monitor the treatment of an illness that has, to date, proven quite frustrating to the medical profession. In addition, the emergence of antidepressant agents with fewer side effects will enable the geriatric psychiatrist to more effectively treat depressive illness in the medically ill as well as in healthy older persons.

The clinical geriatric psychiatrist must broaden his or her scope of psychiatric therapy in the elderly. The traditional one-on-one interaction within a psychiatrist's office must be complemented by programs that include nutrition, exercise, social involvement, and even financial management (not to mention physical health care). Clinicians must therefore maintain a flexible approach to the therapy of the older person, not being bound to preconceived notions of the proper intervention of a psychiatrist. It is especially important to note that the geriatric psychiatrist of the future will include the family in therapeutic planning and implementation. Family therapy has begun to take an increasingly important role in the total training and intervention of psychiatrists, especially those psychiatrists who find themselves closely associated with primary care environments. Skill in family therapy and family support is of great benefit to the geriatric psychiatrist. (Chapter 19)

There is also a need for new models of psychotherapy in working with the elderly patient. Recent emphasis on the understanding of adult personality development coupled with a long-standing knowledge of psychological issues in late life will make psychotherapy with the elderly an intriguing and interesting area of practice in the future. Psychotherapy with an older person can be a rewarding and useful experience for both patient and physician. (Chapter 19)

The advent of behavior techniques in working with psychiatric patients should be of particular use with the elderly. Techniques of controlled environmental input on an inpatient ward coupled with improvement in reality orientation practice should, in the future, prove to be a most helpful approach to working with geriatric patients with mental illness. Though such techniques may be especially valuable in working with patients with organic mental syndromes, they certainly are not exclusively limited to this syndrome. For example, behavioral techniques that encourage activities and interaction in the ward milieu by individuals who are depressed, are being shown to be very helpful in treating the depressed elderly. (Chapter 20)

The foundations for successful clinical geriatric psychiatry may be predicated on the changed orientation of the clinician (as emphasized repeatedly throughout this book). The concept of ill versus well needs to be replaced with concepts such as impaired versus unimpaired. Most older individuals have at least one "chronic illness" and all have developed biological and psychological changes that may be considered to be "ill" in relation to early life. Chronic illnesses and their accompanying impairments are often not disabling to the point of interfering with successful social adaptations and a rewarding and satisfying life. Though older individuals certainly develop conditions that require acute medical intervention and where a complete cure is highly probable, the geriatric psychiatrist is much more likely to encounter conditions where "cure" is not possible. A major goal of the geriatric psychiatrist is to permit a greater degree of functional independence, as opposed to cure. For example, the chronically depressed older patient with intermittent depressive illness may never overcome depressive symptomatology. Yet such individuals have been shown to have decreased activities of daily living in spite of adequate physical health. A therapeutic approach that emphasizes increased independence in activities of daily living may prove to be the most effective intervention for such individuals.

The Geriatric Psychiatrist and Public Health

Given the large numbers of older persons in our society and the limited resources available, the geriatric psychiatrist of the future, of necessity, must have an interest in and understanding of the prevalence and distribution of mental disability in the population and the delivery of mental health services. If a representative elderly person is considered to have a certain potential for developing mental illness in late life and, on the average, declines in function secondary to that mental illness over time, then the intervention of mental health care personnel may take place at one of three points in the natural course of the disability. These points correspond to the three types of prevention outlined by public health specialists, i.e., primary, secondary, and tertiary prevention.[24] The geriatric psychiatrist can engage in primary prevention by identifying hostile events and elements present in the social and physical environment that occur in the community, hospitals, and long-term care facilities. The geriatric psychiatrist then can encourage the elimination of these negative features. Further, the education of medical colleagues in the proper use of psychotropic medications to avoid the occurrence of acute organic brain disease and the encouragement of early and effective support to the bereaved are examples of primary prevention. If the geriatric psychiatrist intervenes in order to prevent the development of an illness once it has occurred (secondary prevention), he might facilitate the early diagnosis and treatment of disorders such as depressive illness, organic mental syndromes, and paranoid disorders. It is at this level that the geriatric psychiatrist may have the greatest impact, given limited resources. The third point of intervention would be activities directed toward preventing the sequelae of mental illnesses (tertiary prevention). Rehabilitation techniques are espe-cially important in long-term care facilities (e.g., reality orientation and physical therapy). Such activities may not be the direct responsibility of the geriatric psychiatrist, but he or she should aid in the planning of these services. If all of the possible types of intervention are considered at each of these points, it becomes obvious that the geriatric psychiatrist cannot work alone. A "team approach" is necessary for effective intervention and prevention techniques. The team should consist of professionals (e.g., nurses, social workers, psychologists, etc.), paraprofessionals, (e.g., nurse's aids, physician's associates) and lay personnel in the community e.g. lay counseling groups, pastoral counselors. The geriatric psychiatrist may intervene more directly at certain points and indirectly at others, but the treatment and prevention aspects of intervention must be considered as a whole.

In addition to conceptualizing intervention at various points in the natural history of mental illness in late life, the geriatric psychiatrist must consider the delivery of mental health care in a variety of settings. A practice made up of elderly persons should not be limited to the office. The inpatient unit is a critical site where expertise is required to maximize treatment capabilities. The geriatric psychiatrist will also be asked to consult frequently in long-term care facilities. Such consultations could easily become stagnant through an overburden of individual patient contacts. The development of staff conferences to discuss the key management issues of the mental health problems among the elderly and group therapy should make long-term care consultations more interesting and effective. There is a need for the geriatric psychiatrist to extend his or her services into the community. Consultation services may be set up in retirement communities, multipurpose senior centers, the office of primary care physicians, and the outpatient clinics of medical centers. Special clinics for the elderly (such as the OARS Geriatric Evaluation and Treatment Clinic at Duke University Medical Center) may be developed with specific emphasis placed on the assessment and treatment of the elderly. Yet the geriatric psychiatrist will ultimately be forced to meet patients where they are most likely to present themselves within the health care system.

As has been emphasized throughout this book, there is a need to coordinate the delivery of psychiatric service with other medical specialists and nonmedical human services personnel. Specific relationships that may prove to be of great importance include homemaker/home health aid service, visiting nurse associations, the Department of Social Services, senior citizen programs, programs involved in Meals-on-Wheels, primary care physicians, and the administrators of long-term care facilities. Within this context, the geriatric psychiatrist can contribute to the planning of mental health services. Epidemiological data can be of great value in such a planning activity.[25]

The geriatric psychiatrist must be aware that lack of funding may be the primary barrier to the development of effective geriatric psychiatry services. Because of the high risk of developing disabilities in late life, catastrophic comprehensive health insurance coverage is often not available. The most visible funding for medical and psychiatric services in late life are the Medicare and Medicaid programs. The hospital insurance portion of Medicare provides coverage for psychiatric hospitalization. This coverage, however, favors treatment within the general hospital as opposed to the psychiatric hospital.[7] In fact, there is a 190-day lifetime limit applied to psychiatric hospitals. In addition, Medicare provides only a portion (45%) of the total payment of health care for the elderly. The amount paid for psychiatric services is quite low. In theory, Medicaid would "take up the slack" of Medicare payments for psychiatric services to the poor. Yet the Medicaid rates are so low and reimbursement is so delayed that many psychiatrists believe the system is not cost-effective and do not treat those covered by Medicare and Medicaid only. In addition, it has been the experience of the OARS Clinic at Duke that indigent individuals utilize services when mental health services are provided free of charge but, for various reasons, do not utilize services when Medicare and Medicaid payments are required. Needless to say, these federally sponsored programs do not insure the adequate utilization of mental health services.

Other federal monies are potentially available for delivering mental health services. One source of funding is Title XX monies. The OARS Clinic at Duke University Medical Center, as an affiliate clinic of the Community Mental Health Center in Durham County, utilized Title XX funds from the Department of Human Resources in the State of North Carolina to fund mental health services. Though these funds were not dependable in the long run, they were potentially available when a coordinated effort was made by all human resource personnel. The comprehensive goals of the clinic, which included the coordination of the delivery of human services not typically considered as "mental health services," allowed a flexibility of funding not previously available.[25] Third-party payments certainly provide coverage for certain older persons, but these individuals suffer from the same problems of individuals at other points in the life cycle in obtaining psychiatric coverage through third-party payers.

A special problem for the geriatric psychiatrist is the difficulty in being reimbursed for consultation in nursing homes and any additional activities that remove mental health care from the clinic or hospital. Those activities which indirectly lead to better mental health care are rarely reimbursed, except on a contract basis. Though one staff conference at a nursing home may prove more effective than seeing 10 patients, there is no usual mechanism to finance this one conference through Medicare, Medicaid, or third-party payments.

Most health insurance programs have placed emphasis on services that are readily identified as being of direct medical benefit. The general services offered by mental health professionals to elder persons have a somewhat broader orientation, especially to those who see services such as service coordination, education, etc. as necessary to meet the mental health needs of the elderly. These services have not been funded through usual mechanisms. In the future, greater emphasis should be placed on providing services that can enable an individual to remain in the home setting and that will maximize the probability that health care professionals will coordinate their activities in developing a comprehensive health care program (including mental health).

The geriatric psychiatrist will, naturally, not directly deliver many of these broad-based services. Yet he or she, of necessity, will be the key member of the mental health team and a key member of the overall treatment team. One approach to the above difficulties is the development of geriatric assessment clinics. Such clinics would not overlap existing medical and mental health services and would provide a setting where various care givers, especially the primary care physician, the geriatric psychiatrist, the gerontological nurse, and the social worker could begin to interact as a team in the assessment of the older adult and the development of a treatment plan. The team could be located in each county (as in the State of Maryland) and could be made up of practicing clinicians within the community. Funding might be achieved through third-party payments and state or federal funds. The establishment of special clinic settings to assess and recommend treatment for multifactoral impairments is one of the major thrusts in health care in recent years such as pain clinics, clinics for "hypochondriacs," and cancer clinics.

Geriatric psychiatry is an expanding area of medical responsibility and knowledge. Medicine and psychiatry should foster its rapid development as it is necessary to insure that skillful clinicians can provide the medical care that our older population needs and deserves.

REFERENCES

1. Harris, C. S. *Fact Book on Aging.* Washington, D.C.: National Council on Aging, 1978.

2. de Beauvoir, S. *The Coming of Age.* New York: Putnam, 1972.

3. Sussman, M. B. The family life of old people, In R. H. Binstock, and E. Shanas, (eds.), *Handbook of Aging and the Social Sciences.* New York: Van Nostrand, pp. 218–243, 1976.

4. Estes, E. Harvey. A manpower policy of primary care. *Tar Heel Practitioner,* Summer, 1978. pp. 13–15.

5. Estes, E. Harvey. Primary care in medicine. National Academy of Sciences, Institute of Medicine, Washington, D.C., June, 1977. E. Harvey Estes, Chairman.

6. Anderson, W. F. and Judge, T. G. *Geriatric Medicine.* New York: Academic Press, 1974.

7. Gipson, R. W. Insurance coverage for treatment of mental illness in later life, In E. W. Busse, and E. Pfeiffer, (eds.) *Mental Illness in Later Life.* Washington, D.C.: American Psychiatric Association, pp. 179–198, 1973.

8. Busse, E. W. and Pfeiffer, E. *Behavior and Adaptation in Late Life* (Second Edition). Boston: Little, Brown and Company, 1977.

9. Greenhill, M. H. The development of liaison programs, in G. Usden, (ed.), *Psychiatric Medicine.* New York: Brunner/Mazel, 1977.

10. Siegler, M. and Osmund, H. *Models of Madness, Models of Medicine.* New York: Macmillan, 1974.

11. Busse, E. W. The Duke study: the electroencephalogram in senescence and senility. Paper presented at the Symposium on Longitudinal Studies, XIth International Congress of Gerontology, Tokyo, Japan. August, 1978.

12. Kidd, K. K. and Matthysee, S. Research designs for the study of gene environment interactions in psychiatric disorders. *Arch. Gen. Psychiatry,* **35:** 925 (1978).

13. Schneider, E. L. *The Genetics of Aging.* New York: Plenum Press, 1977.

14. Katzman, R., Terry, R. D. and Bick, K. *Alzheimer's Disease—Senile Dementia and Related Disorders.* New York: Raven Press, 1978.

15. Larsson, T., Sjogren, T. and Jacobson, G. Senile dementia. *Acta. Psychiatri. Scand.,* **39** (Suppl. 167): 3 (1963).

16. Rowe, J. W. Clincial research on aging: strategies and directions. *New England J. Med.,* **297:** 1332 (1977).

17. Blumenthal, M. D. Research problems in mental health and illness of the elderly. *Research Task Force President's Commission on Mental Health,* 1978.

18. Blazer, D. Epidemiology of late life dysphoria and depression. (Unpublished manuscript), 1978.

19. Life Science Library. Matter, New York: Time Life Books, 1968.

20. Schwitters, Roy F. Fundamental particles with charm, Scientific American, **237:** 56–59 (1977).

21. Verwoerdt, A. Training in geropsychiatry, In E. W. Busse and E. Pfeiffer, (eds.) *Behavior and*

Adaptation in Late Life (Second Edition). Boston: Little, Brown and Company, 1977.

22. *Our Future Selves: A Research Plan Toward Understanding Aging.* DHEW Publication No. (NIH) 78-1446, 1978.

23. Butler, R. N. *Why Survive: Being Old in America.* New York: Harper and Row, 1975.

24. Zussman, J. Primary prevention, in A. M. Freedman, H. I. Kaplan and B. J. Sadock (eds.) *Comprehensive Textbook of Psychiatry/II.* Baltimore: Williams and Wilkins, 1975.

25. Blazer, D. and Maddox, G. *Developing Geriatric Services in a Community Mental Health Center: A Case History of a University-Based Affiliate Clinic.* Durham, North Carolina: Center for the Study of Aging and Human Development, 1977.

Index

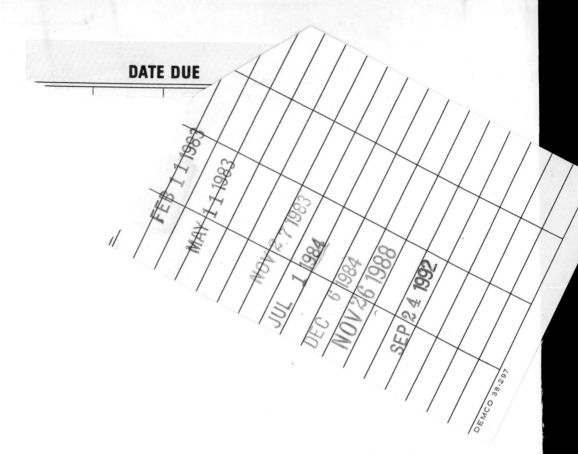